Scrub Nurse in Minimally Invasive and Robotic General Surgery

Marco Milone • Ferdinando Agresta
Mario Guerrieri • Wanda Petz
Alberto Arezzo • Salvatore Casarano
Editors

Scrub Nurse in Minimally Invasive and Robotic General Surgery

Endorsed by the Italian Society of Endoscopic and Laparoscopic Surgery & New technologies and by the Italian Association of Scrub Nurses

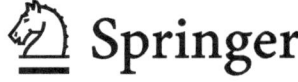 Springer

Editors
Marco Milone
Clinical Medicine and Surgery
University Federico II
Naples, Napoli, Italy

Mario Guerrieri
Dpt Experimental and Clinical Medicine
Marche Polytechnic University
Torrette di Ancona, Italy

Alberto Arezzo
Dipartimento di Scienze Chirurgiche
Università Degli Studi Di Torino
Torino, Italy

Ferdinando Agresta
Department of General Surgery
AULSS2 Trevigiana del Veneto
Vittorio Veneto (TV), Italy

Wanda Petz
Gastrointestinal Surgery Division
European Institute of Oncology IRCCS
Milan, Italy

Salvatore Casarano
scientific coordinator of AICO
University of Bari
Lecce, Italy

ISBN 978-3-031-42256-0   ISBN 978-3-031-42257-7   (eBook)
https://doi.org/10.1007/978-3-031-42257-7

This Springer imprint is published by the registered company Springer Nature Switzerland AG
The registered company address is: Gewerbestrasse 11, 6330 Cham, Switzerland

Paper in this product is recyclable.

Preface

It has already been said that laparoscopy is the evolution of surgery! Continuous evolution, evolution that doesn't stop, so much evolution as to become Robotic surgery. Because robotic surgery is laparoscopic surgery itself, done, indeed, mediated, by a Robot.

Evolution! But not only. Revolution, more than Copernican!

Because the "Earth planet" Surgeon has become a (integral) part of that system which is the surgical team (e.g. nurses, anaesthesiologists, young surgeons in training), which has a truly unique "Sun" at its centre: (our) patient.

Evolution/Revolution also in the way of teaching and transmitting the Art: no longer perched and distant, but everyone, really everyone, watching the same Monitor, really following every single moment of the surgical act "step by step".

But even revolution/evolution must have its written rules. We are not referring to those of EBM and that is not the task of this book.

The first rule is precisely the "before": every single intervention is a journey that must be known and planned in detail beforehand, always ready for any "variations" of the route. The second rule, so current today given the power of the media, is sharing. The third: continuous testing and re-discussing!

Hence the idea of this book: a technique experienced by those who have already undertaken this journey for a long time and continue to do so every day; to be shared with those who since always travel with us, our fellow nurses, and with those who, only by age, has recently joined the adventure (the young colleagues).

This book on laparoscopic technique and its natural Robotic evolution, endorsed by the Italian Society for Endoscopic and Laparoscopic Surgery and New technologies (SICE) and the Italian Association of Scrub Nurses (AICO), has been written precisely by "four hands", surgeons and operating theatre nurses.

It is geared to scrub nurses, junior surgeons, and anyone who wants to re-discuss their professional journey.

So: Happy Reading…or better: Happy Travelling!

Naples, Napoli, Italy	Marco Milone
Vittorio Veneto (TV), Italy	Ferdinando Agresta
Torrette di Ancona, Italy	Mario Guerrieri
Milan, Italy	Wanda Petz
Torino, Italy	Alberto Arezzo
Lecce, Italy	Salavatore Casarano

Contents

Part I

Scrub Nurse in Minimally Invasive and Robotic General Surgery

The Evolution of the Scrub Nurse in Laparoscopic and Robotic Surgery

1

Rosanna Zeccardo and Fabio Ferraiuolo

1.1 The Laws About Nurses, Professional Autonomy and Professional Profile

Rosanna Zeccardo and Fabio Ferraiuolo

The nursing profession over the years has undergone a series of changes that have resulted in a modernization of the nursing figure in Italy and in the world. The modern nurse is a professional with university education, professional autonomy and professional responsibility [1].

Abolished since 1999 with law 42, the job description assigned to nurses the nomenclature of 'auxiliary health profession', giving them a list of tasks limiting autonomy [2].

Its abolition has allowed the nurse to move in a legislative view with specific references that recognize its centrality in the health landscape. The foundation of modern nursing is the 'code of ethics', which represents the document that dictates the rules of conduct and ethics of the nurse in his professional activity [1]. It constitutes a point of reference for the individual and for the community because it defines the behavioural models of nurses. The code identifies the health professional as the sole responsible for nursing care. The field of action of nursing care is outlined (preventive, curative, palliative, rehabilitation and of a technical nature, relational, educational; know, knowing how to do, knowing how to be), the functions (prevention of disease, care of the sick and disabled people of all ages and health education) and the consequent responsibilities, also linked to the planning, design, implementation and valuation of the activities related to the functions [1, 3].

Another important principle of nursing is the Ministerial Decree No. 739 of 1994 in which the nurse is responsible for general nursing care and a fundamental concept of autonomy is introduced. It is at this moment that the nurse sees the auxiliary character disappear to fully evolve as a 'health professional' [3].

1.2 Modern Nursing, Roles, Responsibilities

Today the nurse is the health professional who, with his own field of activity, assists, treats and takes care of the patient in a global way. He is a graduate professional who, enrolled in the professional order, carries out prevention functions, assistance, therapeutic education, management, training and research [1]. Today the nurse is an independent professional, trained and responsible [1, 4]. Over the past 20 years nurses have worked in a rapidly evolving legislative scenario

R. Zeccardo
Sassuolo Hospital, Sassuolo, MO, Italy

F. Ferraiuolo (✉)
Madonna del Soccorso Hospital,
San Benedetto del Tronto, Italy

© The Author(s), under exclusive license to Springer Nature Switzerland AG 2024
M. Milone et al. (eds.), *Scrub Nurse in Minimally Invasive and Robotic General Surgery*,
https://doi.org/10.1007/978-3-031-42257-7_1

that has also seen the side of professional responsibility evolve. Each nurse assumes the responsibility of their profession according to the level of competence reached, which cannot be considered static but dynamic, in continuous construction through training and research. A modern nurse must apply the scientific method and must have a logical and critical reasoning to be able to be autonomous not only at the legislative level but in the concrete of every day [4]. The modern role of the active team nurse is to be considered a change achieved gradually and deservedly. Finally, the legislative and professional evolution has led to the transformation of the colleges into orders and the equalization of responsibilities for all health roles [5]. The Law 24 of 2017, known as the 'Gelli law', reforms the responsibility penal and civil for health professionals by modifying the burden of proof and attributing an important role to the guidelines and good clinical-care practices where compliance with which it becomes fundamental in the giving of responsibility of the health personnel also of a penal nature [6].

1.3 Ethics and Legal Aspects in Scrub Nursing

Ethics, but more properly the discipline of bioethics, understood as 'the systematic study of human behaviour in the sciences and life and health care examined in the light of values and moral principles', is a method for finding answers to the new problems arising from the operator-patient relationship. The daily practice of health care and assistance to the sick is full of perplexity and forces nurses to make choices and decisions with important moral values [7]. Another criticality is represented by the times within which these decisions must be made: there is often no time to consult the experienced colleague or the company ethics committee. The instrumental nurse is responsible for maintaining the sterility of himself and the operating field and dressing the surgeon [8].

The instrumental nurse is the health professional responsible for the preparation and of the correct intraoperative management of all devices and useful materials for operation.

He is the guarantor and supervisor of the sterility of the operating field and surgical aids and has a fundamental role in coordinating the intraoperative phase towards all members of the surgical team [8]. The instrumental nurse participates actively in the surgical operation, collaborates with surgeons and manages, promptly and safely, the materials and instruments required, in observance of the guidelines, operating instructions and company [8].

The professional role imposes relational and communicative competences, producing a climate of collaboration between the various professionals which are indispensable for preventing operator accidents and the success of the intervention [8].

In a teamwork such as that of the operating room, each professional should trust and rely on the other, and in fact according to the relevant jurisprudence, the only general criterion for the division of competences and responsibilities within the teamwork, it is the principle of trust.

This principle dictates that each member of a group engaged in a surgery operation should be able to rely on the ability of the collaborators to fulfil their role with the necessary competence and diligence, without prejudice to the power of control of those who, at a given moment, take up the qualification as group leader or team leader.

Each health professional must constitute a guarantee for the conduct of the other components and remedy any errors of others, as long as they are evident for an average professional and non-sectoral of a specific discipline unrelated to his knowledge.

References

1. FNOPI. Deontological Code of Nursing Professions 2019 [05/05/2022]. Available from: https://www.fnopi.it/norme-e-codici/deontologia/#1695646156049-90af3813-bfc5.
2. LAW 42 OF 26 February 1999 "Provisions Concerning Health Professionals".

3. Health Mo. Decree 14 settembre 1994, n. 739. Regulations concerning the identificati on of the figure and the relative professionale pirofile of the nurse Official Gazette General Series. (6).
4. Law 10 August 2000, n 251. Discipline of the nursing, technical, rehabilitation, prevention and obstetric professions.
5. Healt Mo. Decree, 11 jenuary 2018 (Lorenzin Law).
6. Provisions on the safety of care and the assisted person, as well as on the professional responsibility of the health professions. sanitary. Law 24 april 2017 (Gelli Law).
7. Jonas H. Technique, medicine and ethics: Giulio Einaudi Editore; 2016.
8. A.I.C.O. Italian Operating Room Nurses Association. Available from: https://www.aicoitalia.it/

Part II

Instruments and Technologies: The Nurses' Point of View

The Management of Instruments and Technologies

2

Fabio Ferraiuolo (ORCID)

2.1 Sterilization

With the promulgation of Legislative Decree No. 46 of 24-2-97 concerning medical devices and with the CEE directive 93/42, the manufacturer is also responsible for all the phases of the sterilization process [1].

This decree leaves or refers to the responsibility for the production cycle of sterile material to hospitals that carry out their own sterilization activities.

Sterilization is the final result of a process that must guarantee the condition in which the survival of microorganisms is highly unlikely: a surgical instrument is defined sterile if the safety level of sterility (SAL) is less than 10^{-6}, that is, when the probability of finding a microorganism is less than one in a million and is established in the technical standard UNI EN 556–1 [2].

Sterilization procedures represent one of the main and fundamental moments in the prevention and control of infections.

Sterilization is the denaturation of proteins and nucleic acids and the degradation of membrane components and cell wall, causing the lethal alteration of some of their essential components.

Till today in the health sector, for sterilization, reference has mostly been made to Legislative Decree 46/97, transposition of European legislation 43/98/CEE [3].

Structurally, a sterilization station has three distinct macro zones:

- Septic area.
- Aseptic area.
- Sterile area.

Septic Area: it is the area where all the instruments and/or other contaminated devices coming from the operating room are collected, for example, used during an operation, and/or by the various departments and/or wards of hospitalization inside containers or baskets.

The rooms pre-sterilization and post-sterilization must be at least in class ISO 8.

The controlled room must have an entrance door for staff and an entrance door for raw materials with a double door. The exit of sterilized materials must be with a door and double door and must be dedicated exclusively to the materials and to those who access in a clean place. The controlled room must not have inaccessible surfaces parallel to the floor (e.g., suspended neon that could accumulate dust, corners on the floor, etc.).

The controlled room must have walls adequately coated without continuous solutions in order to proceed with cleaning operations with-

F. Ferraiuolo (✉)
Madonna del Soccorso Hospital,
San Benedetto del Tronto AP, Italy

out depositing dust and must not have exposed walls.

The edges must be rounded to facilitate cleaning.

A correct preliminary identification of the nature of the instrument and its intended use is necessary to identify the techniques of most suitable treatment for the sterilization processes.

According to current regulations, sanitary devices and surgical instruments are divided into two categories: 'critical articles' and 'semi-critical articles.'

The first category includes those health devices or surgical instruments which, introduced into the bloodstream and/or in areas of the body that are normally sterile and/or which come into contact with skin and mucous membranes that are not intact, require the requirement of sterility (e.g., surgical instruments, drainage tubes, surgical gloves, catheter for angiography).

The second category includes all those health devices or surgical instruments in which, coming into contact with intact mucous membranes, the requirement is desirable sterility, but in most cases a high-level disinfection guarantees that the article is free of pathogenic microorganisms [4].

Before the real sterilization it is necessary to follow a series of preventive procedures and these have the purpose of decreasing the microbial load and making the sterilizing action more effective.

In 1990 the Joint Commission for Accreditation of Hospitals (JCAH) developed some standards that can be considered a reference point for the correct management of the sterilization process [5]. In particular, these phases are described as follows:

1. Decontamination/disinfection

Article 2 of the Decree of the Ministry of Health from 28/09/1990 rule (DM 28/9/1990—Protection rules for health workers from occupational exposure to bloodborne pathogens, subsequent cleaning and careful drying) states the correct phase of decontamination/preventive disinfection in order to reduce the microbial load present on the instruments, making manipulation by operators less risky [6].

Before this there is the collection of the material used, instruments, and contaminated devices that must undergo a disinfection cycle before there are coagulation and encrustation of blood or serum on them. Decontamination allows the removal of organic residues present on the instruments [6].

2. Cleaning/washing

The correct washing of the material is the basis of any sterilization process, because the simple mechanical removal of dirt reduces the initial microbial load by at least 90%.

According to the probabilistic definition given, the more the number of microorganisms present on an object is reduced, the more effective the selected sterilization procedures will be.

Once the decontamination process has been undergone, the instruments must be washed with special detergents that eliminate dirt residues and the organic substances present [9].

This process can be done manually if it is not possible to use appropriate machines using detergents and brushes and pipe cleaners under a jet of water at 45 °C up to 95 °C to avoid the coagulation of residues of protein material.

With ultrasound machines, combining the disinfection phase and cleaning, it allows to minimize the manual intervention by the operator.

The process allows, through cavitation, to clean areas that are difficult to access such as interstices or hollow bodies and the action of the disinfectant solution is also enhanced by the possibility of raising the temperature of the water [7].

The water used in the operations of decontamination/washing must have particular qualitative characteristics that must meet the requirements of the rule UNI EN 285 [8].

Ultrasounds at 40–45 °C allow disinfection in just 15 min, reducing the time required by 80%, and finally, with a thermodisinfector that allows to gather the disinfection phase, cleaning, and washing. Normally, a 10-minute cycle is performed at 93 °C with washing of detergent solutions and disinfectant and rinsing and drying are also often included in the cycle [8].

3. Rinsing

After cleansing, rinsing is a simple phase but fundamental; the instruments must be washed under running water to remove the last residues of organic material and disinfectant.

4. Drying

Drying must be carried out accurately to eliminate all moisture with paper clothes or canvas clothes that do not release fibers or with the use of compressed air guns (especially for cannulated instruments).

During the drying phase both macroscopic control and maintenance of the instruments must be carried out.

The last three phases described, in modern sterilization centers, are performed inside an instrument washer whose programs allow an extremely satisfactory and functional result.

Aseptic Area: After cleaning and automated disinfection, containers and surgical instruments are not sterile, but are safe to handle and ready to be sorted, inspected, and packaged.

5. Packaging

Before packaging, maintenance of the instruments is carried out if required.

The instruments and the treated devices are placed inside sterile barrier systems (container, envelope, or medical paper) suitable for the sterilization process and for maintaining the sterility of the contents until the moment of its use.

Generally, the packages must be of such size as to allow a single use.

The baskets must not exceed the dimensions $30 \times 30 \times 60$ cm and the weight of 5 kg for the drapery and 10 kg for the instruments, and their packaging inside bags or containers allows to maintain the sterility of the material usually 30 days obviously if stored in a dry environment and without sudden changes in temperature [9, 10].

The packages and containers must contain an external indicator, such as tape and/or label, to distinguish the material already subjected to sterilization from that not yet started and an internal one of class 5 or class 6 for the verification, at the moment of use, of the penetration of the sterilizing agent [9, 11].

Therefore, each bag or container is equipped with both process indicators and an adhesive label on which are reported: packaging date and sterilization, code of the operator who performed the sterilization, and progressive number of the cycle, number of the sterilizing machine, description of the article, operating unit of origin, and expiry date.

2.1.1 Sterilization Methods

The sterilization of medical devices represents one of the main moments in the prevention process and infection control.

There are several sterilization methods: saturated steam, ethylene oxide, hydrogen peroxide, and peracetic acid.

The phase of loading of the equipment into the autoclave must respect precise instructions to allow the sterilizing agent to circulate freely and penetrate indistinctly from the type of package/container.

The load categories are classified according to the difficulty of exposure to saturated steam and are as follows:

(a) Solid, without hollow spaces.
(b) Hollow type A, with deep hollow spaces and narrow (whose ratio diameter/depth varies from 1/5 to 1/750) [12].
(c) Hollow type B, with hollow spaces shallow and wide.
(d) Porous or complex loads that retain air before the cycle and humidity after.

Autoclaves of class B are able to sterilize any type of load and autoclaves class N only solid unwrapped load; autoclaves class S fill the gap between B and N and their capacity must be specified by the manufacturer [8].

Each load must be identifiable with respect to the date of sterilization, to the machine used, and to the operator who conducted the cycle in order to be able to easily trace the material in the event of cycles of dubious effectiveness. Below are the two sterilization methods that are mostly used in Italy.

2.1.2 Moist Heat

Saturated steam under pressure in autoclaves is the most used, least expensive, and most effective for sterilization of most surgical instruments in the health sector.

It is the method of choice for the sterilization of health articles critical and semi-critical. The sterilization cycles normally used are as follows:

- Cycle to 121 °C suitable for rubber materials, low-melting plastics (e.g., pure polyethylene), and all materials that would be damaged by higher temperatures.
- Cycle to 134 °C for all materials resistant to heat such as surgical instruments, drapes, and dressings [8].

2.1.3 Gas Plasma

Plasma gas to low temperature consists of a reactive cloud of ions, electrons, and neutral atomic particles that can be produced through the action of a strong electric or magnetic field.

The sterilization system uses the synergistic action of hydrogen peroxide and low-temperature plasma gas to rapidly destroy microorganisms.

At the end of the sterilization process, no toxic residues remain in the treated materials.

The method is particularly suitable for the sterilization of instruments sensitive to heat and to humidity since the process temperature does not exceed 50 °C and the sterilization is done in a practically dry place in just over 1 h.

Sterile Area: After the sterilization treatment, the instruments released in the sterile area are available for immediate transport towards their subsequent reuse or are stored awaiting collection.

2.2   Storage 2.3 Activation and Functioning

Appropriate documented company procedures describe the storage phase of the products (intermediate and final) during the entire manufacturing process:

The document drawn up must specify the correct procedure for checking products with a limited life or requiring special storage conditions.

Product storage must include:

(a) Identification.
(b) Handling.
(c) Packaging.
(d) Storage.
(e) Protection.

Everything must necessarily also be applied to the component parts of a product. These conditions must be checked, documented, and registered. The records that the organization must keep are at least those relating to the validation of washing, decontamination, sterilization, packaging, and records relating to the checks carried out on each washing cycle, decontamination, sterilization, and packaging. The organization must ensure that the documents certifying how the medical device has been produced and tested are available at least for the life of the product, but not less than the storage period established by the mandatory legislation. It is necessary to identify and maintain a warehouse (suitable rooms for the storage of equipment) for the collection of the finished product; a rotation of this warehouse must be carried out, with a periodic frequency indicated in the procedure, to avoid reaching the expiry date of the stored products.

The sterilized surgical instruments must be stored in closed cabinets that protect them from dust and humidity and the storage rooms must have a controlled temperature (18°/20 °C), humidity of 35/50%, and limited access.

The cabinets containing the sterile material must be raised from the ground by at least 20 cm, separated from the ceiling by 50 cm and from the wall by 10 cm to facilitate sanitization maneuvers.

Table 2.1 Steam sterilization

Steam sterilization	Duration
Container	30 days
Single envelope medical grade	30 days
Double envelope medical grade	60 days
Gas plasma	
Single envelope Tyvek	6 months
Double envelope Tyvek	1 year

Packages that are damaged, fallen to the floor, come into contact with wet surfaces, and expired are to be considered non-sterile; therefore, they must be repackaged and processed again [13].

It should be remembered that maintaining the sterility of a packaging system is in fact linked more to events than to time Table 2.1 [9].

To date, saturated steam sterilization is the safest method because this steam, condensing on the surface of the object to be sterilized, effectively releases energy and causes nonreversible damage to microorganisms. There are four phases that compose a sterilization cycle in autoclave:

Vacuum generation: which includes the initial vacuum phase or high vacuum or fractional vacuum. In the vacuum phase, a series of fractionated vacuums are performed which have the aim of totally removing the air from inside the sealed chamber of the autoclave to ensure the effectiveness of the sterilization process.

Heating: thanks to saturated steam, every tiny component of the instruments that need to be sterilized reaches the necessary temperature.

Sterilization: the injection of steam into the sealed chamber of the autoclave leads to an internal temperature of 134 °C and a pressure of 3 bar.

The exposure times and temperatures are indicated in the standards EN285:98 and EN13060:05. The EN 285 standard (like EN13060) [8] also states that the holding times must not be less than:

(a) 15 min for 121 °C
(b) 10 min for 126 °C
(c) 3 min for 134 °C.

Cooling: which includes the cooling phase and baric balancing.

It is the last phase of the sterilization process and corresponds to a vacuum phase that eliminates the steam and starts drying of the load with the removal of most of the condensed steam.

This phase is fundamental for a correct sterilization because a humid and wet load undergoes microbial contamination.

The baric balance guarantees the return to atmospheric pressure.

The advantages of this method are that surgical instruments, metal instruments, textile material, and non-thermolabile rubber material can be treated.

The disadvantages of this method are that it is not possible to treat endoscopic equipment, non-water-soluble substances, and thermolabile material.

When loading the autoclave, some general precautions must be followed:

– Never obstruct the drain of equipment.
– Never cover areas of the valves of baskets and those of the filters.
– Never overlap the instruments to be sterilized.
– Avoid that the instrument bags can touch the internal walls of the autoclave.

The bags used for sterilization must be arranged "cut," in a position parallel to the flow of steam.

These envelopes must also be placed close together without pressing them.

Finally, the porous part must be turned upwards, using the perforated trays suitable for containment.

The non-overloading of the autoclave is of absolute importance.

Once the phases described have been completed, the biological and/or chemical control tests must be inserted into the autoclave before the door is closed, and then start the appropriate sterilization cycle.

The other most widespread method in Italy is gas plasma sterilization which is one of the most recent methods of cold sterilization of health centers.

Plasma gas is a gas with large internal energy with a neutral power band that emits free radicals when external electrons are hit by electromagnetic discharges, radio frequencies, or microwaves.

This ensures fast sterilization and effective on many health devices, leaving no toxic residue.

As for saturated steam under pressure, also for plasma gas the sterilization cycle is divided into the following phases:

Vacuum generation: when the material is correctly positioned inside the sealed chamber of the autoclave, the system first of all proceeds to create a vacuum state.

In this first phase the pressure of the treatment chamber is reduced up to 300 millitorr.

The operation of creating the vacuum state is performed in a variable time from 5 to 20 min depending on the humidity present.

Injection: a water solution of hydrogen peroxide is injected and vaporized inside the treatment chamber which spreads rapidly.

Diffusion: the phase of diffusion of gas inside the treatment chamber allows the uniform diffusion of hydrogen peroxide around the devices to be sterilized.

Plasma: the gas, hit by electromagnetic waves, in the presence of water, decomposes into many active free radicals and spreads on the surfaces and in the internal parts.

The active gaseous molecules (essentially free electrons and ions) kill the bacteria and microorganisms present.

Ventilation: at the end of the sterilization process, the pressure inside the chamber returns to the atmospheric one, and the particles recombine in water and oxygen, even with the aid of disintegrating UV rays, without any residue for the surrounding environment.

The advantages of this method are that it is possible to treat plastic materials, metals, optical fibers, electronic components, and very delicate instruments (microsurgery). Furthermore, sterility is preserved for up to 12 months.

The disadvantages are that materials capable of absorbing peroxide such as cellulose (paper and cloth), liquids, and powders [8] cannot be used.

References

1. Legislative Decree No. 46 of 24–2-97. Implementation of Directive 93/42/EEC concerning medical devices 1997 [46]. Available from: https://www.gazzettaufficiale.it/atto/serie_generale/caricaDettaglioAtto/originario?atto.dataPubblicazioneGazzetta=1997-03-06&atto.codiceRedazionale=097G0076
2. UNI EN 556–1. Sterilization of medical devices—Requirements for medical devices marked "STERILE"—Requirements for terminally sterilized medical devices; 2021.
3. Legislative Decree 46/97. Implementation of Directive 93/42/EEC concerning medical devices; 1997. Available from: https://www.gazzettaufficiale.it/atto/serie_generale/caricaDettaglioAtto/originario?atto.dataPubblicazioneGazzetta=1997-03-06&atto.codiceRedazionale=097G0076.
4. Seavey R. High-level disinfection, sterilization, and antisepsis: current issues in reprocessing medical and surgical instruments. Am J Infect Control. 2013;41(5):S111–S7.
5. The Joint Commission. Available from: https://www.jointcommission.org.
6. Health Mo. Decree of the Ministry of Health of 28-09-1990. Rules of protection from professional HIV infection in public and private health and assistance structures; 1990. Available from: https://www.gazzettaufficiale.it/eli/id/1990/10/08/090A4288/sg.
7. UNI EN ISO 15883. Washing and disinfecting equipment—Part 5: Performance requirements and test method criteria to demonstrate cleaning effectiveness; 2021.
8. UNI EN 285. Sterilization—steam sterilizers—large sterilizers;.2021.
9. UNI EN ISO 11607-1. Packaging for terminally sterilized medical devices—Part 1: Requirements for materials, sterile barrier systems and packaging systems; 2020.
10. UNI EN 868–2. Packaging for terminally sterilized medical devices—Part 2: Sterilization wrap—Requirements and test methods; 2017.
11. AopR N. Recommended practices for selection and use of packaging systems for sterilization. AORN J. 2007;85(4):801–12.
12. UNI EN 13060. Small steam sterilizers; 2019.
13. DIN 58953. Sterilization—sterile supply—Part 6: Microbial barrier testing of packaging materials for medical devices which are to be sterilized; 2016.

Part III

Access Techniques in Minimally Invasive Surgery

Open and Close Laparoscopic Access

3

Wanda Petz and Ferdinando Agresta

3.1 Introduction

The term laparoscopy derives from the ancient Greek words *laparo* (abdomen) and *scopein* (to examine); it initially indicated the technique of examining the abdominal cavity and its contents, but rapidly evolved from a diagnostic procedure to a surgical approach employed by numerous disciplines to perform various surgical interventions.

Laparoscopy requires the insertion of a cannula through the abdominal wall, the distention of the abdominal cavity with gas or air (pneumoperitoneum), and the visualization of the abdomen's contents with an illuminated telescope.

Access to the abdominal cavity is one of the challenges of laparoscopy, as it involves the insertion of surgical instruments through small incisions; many complications may occur during this very first phase of the procedure, in particular injuries to the gastrointestinal tract, to other organs (liver, spleen), or to major vessels [1–4].

These complications may jeopardize the achievement of a minimally invasive procedure; therefore, a safe technique of trocar insertion must be very well known by the surgical staff.

Different techniques of access to the abdominal cavity for laparoscopic and robotic surgery have been described, the main difference being the insertion of the first cannula (trocar) under direct vision (open technique) or without direct vision (closed technique).

In this chapter these two techniques and some variants will be described in detail, focusing in particular on the aspects that could more be interesting for the scrub nurses.

Moreover, a summary of consequences of pneumoperitoneum on the patient and a brief analysis of the different available trocars for laparoscopy will be addressed.

3.2 Closed Laparoscopic Access

The closed laparoscopic access requires cutting of the abdominal skin with a scalpel, insufflation of air or gas into the abdomen to establish pneumoperitoneum, and the insertion of a sharp trocar into the abdomen.

Insufflation of gas in the peritoneal cavity can be done by blindly inserting the first trocar in the abdomen or by means of the Veress needle.

W. Petz (✉)
Department of Digestive Surgery, European Institute of Oncology IRCCS, Milan, Italy
e-mail: wanda.petz@ieo.it

F. Agresta
Department of General Surgery, AULSS2 Trevigiana del Veneto, Ospedale di Vittorio Veneto, Vittorio Veneto, Italy

3.2.1 The Veress Needle

The Veress needle is a sterile disposable cannula made of surgical stainless steel and has an atraumatic protective cap, an ergonomically shaped handle, and a particularly flexible spring. The atraumatic protective cup is pushed back when the surgeon first presses the needle onto the abdominal wall; then the sharp hollow needle is exposed. If the peritoneum is penetrated, the cap automatically jumps forward again and covers the needle tip. In this way, organ injuries should be avoided. The Veress needle is available in different sizes: 118 and 150 mm.

The first description of the utilization of a Veress needle to induce pneumoperitoneum was made by the French surgeon Raoul Palmer in 1947 [5]: he suggested the site of needle insertion to be situated 3 cm below the left subcostal border in the midclavicular line (the nowadays so-called Palmer point), with the necessary precaution of the emptying of the stomach by nasogastric suction and of inserting the needle perpendicularly to the skin.

The Palmer insertion point is particularly useful in case of patients with previous laparotomies, but caution must be taken in using this access in patients with previous splenic or gastric surgery, significant hepatosplenomegaly, portal hypertension, or gastropancreatic masses.

The most commonly used alternative site of insertion of Veress needle is the umbilical area, in the midsagittal plane; however, this could be dangerous in very thin patients and in obese women: in very thin patients, especially those with a prominent sacral promontory and android pelvis, the great vessels lie 1–2 cm underneath the umbilicus, and in obese women, the umbilicus is shifted caudally to the aortic bifurcation.

Therefore, in these two categories of patients a Veress needle insertion through the umbilicus should be avoided.

Different techniques may be used to check the correct placement of the Veress needle in the abdominal cavity. These include:

– **The double-click sound test:** A double click is heard when the needle passes through the anterior and the posterior fascia if it is inserted in the Palmer point.
– **The aspiration test** [6]: By connecting a syringe to the needle, before induction of pneumoperitoneum the pressure of the peritoneal cavity is inferior to the atmosphere pressure: this difference may be appreciated with the aspiration test. On the contrary, the eventual aspiration of blood or intestinal liquid means the wrong position of the needle.
– **the hanging drop of saline test** [7]: The normal outflow of saline solution through the Veress needle indicates its correct positioning.
– **The "hiss" sound test** [8]: When the needle is inserted and the pneumoperitoneum is induced, by opening the valve a hissing sound can be heard, confirming the proper insertion of the needle.

Besides these tests, it is of extreme importance that the surgeon carefully observe the increase of intra-abdominal pressure, depicted on the insufflator: pressure must raise progressively to reach the desired value (usually not higher than 12 mmHg). If immediately after the starting of insufflation the intra-abdominal pressure is too high, this means that the Veress needle is not in the peritoneal cavity but more probably in the abdominal wall in the preperitoneal space.

After establishment of the pneumoperitoneum, the camera trocar is introduced either blindly with a nontransparent cannula or with a transparent cannula containing the laparoscope that can show to the surgeon a cascade of color sequences that represent different abdominal wall layers: subcutaneous fat appears yellow, fascia white, anterior rectus muscle red, and peritoneum translucent or shiny bright.

The other trocars are then inserted under direct vision.

Surgical instruments needed for a closed laparoscopic access with Veress needle are the following:

– One scalpel (blade 11)
– One Veress needle (118 mm or eventually 150 mm in obese patients)
– One 5-mL syringe for saline drop test or aspiration test

3.2.2 Variants of Veress Needle

Some modifications of the Veress needle have been described, like, for example, a pressure-sensor-equipped needle that provides the surgeon immediate feedback the moment the tip enters the peritoneal cavity [9] or the optical needle, which has a diameter of 2.1 mm that allows insertion of a thin (1.2-mm-diameter), zero-degree, semirigid fiberoptic minilaparoscope [10].

3.2.3 Direct Trocar Entry Technique

With the aim of avoiding complications related to the use of the Veress needle, as failed pneumoperitoneum, preperitoneal insufflation, intestinal insufflation, or the more serious CO_2 embolism, the **direct trocar entry technique without prior pneumoperitoneum** has been proposed [11].

The technique begins with an infraumbilical skin incision wide enough to accommodate the diameter of a sharp trocar. The anterior abdominal wall must be adequately elevated by hand, and the trocar is inserted directly into the cavity, aiming towards the pelvic hollow. Alternatively, the abdominal wall is elevated by pulling on two towel clips placed 3 cm on either side of the umbilicus, and the trocar is inserted at a 90° angle. On removal of the sharp trocar, the laparoscope is inserted and the correct position of the trocar is confirmed.

Potential benefits of direct trocar entry include shorter operating times, immediate recognition of bowel or vascular injuries, and immediate recognition of failed entry.

Among closed access techniques, trocars for direct vision to visualize passage of the trocar through the abdominal wall layers have been conceived to reduce complication rates, as trocars are not inserted blindly [12].

3.3 Open Laparoscopic Access

The first description of an open access for laparoscopy was made by Hasson in 1971 [13].

With this technique, through a small transverse or longitudinal periumbilical incision tissues are dissected and the fascia and the peritoneum are incised.

The first blunt trocar is therefore inserted in the peritoneal cavity under direct vision.

The trocar can be secured to the fascia by means of two stitches or by a purse-string suture.

After insertion of the first trocar, pneumoperitoneum is induced, the laparoscope is inserted, and the remaining trocars are inserted under laparoscopic vision.

At the end of the surgical procedure, the fascial defect is closed and the cut is re-approximated.

This technique has been proposed with the aim of reducing inadvertent visceral or vascular injuries that may be a consequence of a closed laparoscopic access (Veress needle to induce pneumoperitoneum and then blind insertion of the first trocar, or direct trocar entry).

Surgical instruments needed for a closed laparoscopic access are the following:

- One scalpel with stainless steel blade (usually size 11)
- One monopolar electric scalpel
- Two Farabeuf retractors
- Two Kocher clamps
- Two Klemmer clamps
- One Mayo curved scissors
- Two toothed forceps
- Two anatomical tissue forceps
- One needle holder
- Two Vicryl 0 sutures
- Two mosquito curved forceps

3.3.1 The Fingertip Technique

This is a particular type of open access first described by Sahan in 2020 [14].

With this approach, the skin is marked with a 10-mm empty disposable trocar tip to prevent excessive incision. The skin is vertically incised at the boundaries of the marked area until the subcutaneous adipose tissue can be seen. Then, blunt dissection is done with the index finger down until the upper sheet of the abdominal fascia is felt. A 15-mm scalpel is placed on the inside of the index finger and held with the proximal part of the thumb.

The tip of the scalpel should not exceed the tip of the finger. After that, the finger and the scalpel are held perpendicular to the fascia while applying mild pressure on the fascia.

The finger and scalpel are bent 30° medially, without moving the tip of the finger or the scalpel. Due to the softness of the fingertip, the scalpel passes the fingertip by only a few millimeters and incises the fascia. Only mild pressure on the layer during the maneuver is needed to achieve a 3- to 4-mm incision. Then, the abdominal muscle is dissected bluntly with the index finger.

Finally, the peritoneal layer is incised again using the fingertip technique and enlarged bluntly with the index finger to enter the abdomen. Then, the abdominal wall is elevated bilaterally next to the incision, and a 10-mm trocar is inserted bluntly through the incision.

Since the port size is at least 10 mm at the entry site of the fingertip technique, the port defect is closed at the end of the operation either by traditional methods or by a trocar closure device.

3.4 Literature Evidences About Different Techniques of Laparoscopic Access

There is no uniform consensus regarding the better technique of laparoscopic entry and many studies have been published in recent years.

The most definitive evidence derives from a recent Cochrane review of 57 randomized clinical trials [15] including a total of 9865 patients.

The main comparisons made in this review were the following:

- Open-entry technique versus closed-entry technique
  - Open-entry versus direct trocar entry
  - Open-entry versus Veress needle entry
- Direct trocar entry versus Veress needle entry
- Direct vision entry versus Veress needle entry
- Direct vision entry versus open-entry technique

Outcomes analyzed were major (mortality; vascular, visceral, or solid organ lesions; gas embolism; and failed entrance in the abdomen) and minor (extraperitoneal insufflation, trocar site bleeding or infection, incisional hernia, omentum injury, uterine bleeding) complications.

Overall, evidence was insufficient to support the use of one laparoscopic entry technique over another: incidence of complications did not differ significantly between the techniques analyzed, as it was expected given the very low rate of reported complications and the consequent too big sample sizes that would have been needed to identify plausible differences in rare but serious adverse events.

Results only showed an advantage of direct trocar entry over Veress needle entry in terms of lesser incidence of failed entry.

3.5 Pneumoperitoneum

To create the surgical space needed to perform a laparoscopic surgical procedure or even a simple exploration of the abdominal cavity, the abdominal wall has to be separated from the intra-abdominal organs.

This is done by the insufflation of gas in the abdominal cavity, i.e., the creation of pneumoperitoneum.

Although necessary for the intervention, the insertion of carbon dioxide into the intraperitoneal space during surgery may lead to relatively not serious complications as pneumothorax, hypoxemia, hypercarbia, respiratory acidosis, and subcutaneous emphysema, or to more serious adverse events due to the increase in intraperitoneal pressure [16]. This causes the diaphragm to move cephalad, leading to increased intrathoracic pressure and mean airway pressure as a result. The intra-atrial pressure increases as intrathoracic pressure increases, and the resulting decrease in venous return reduces cardiac output. Moreover, as carbon dioxide is absorbed in the blood, minute ventilation increases and mean airway pressure increases even more as a result.

In this situation, a position change to head down or to the Trendelenburg during certain laparoscopic procedures (colectomy, rectal resection, prostatectomy) can further significantly reduce the lung volume.

Compression atelectasis may therefore occur during laparoscopy, so that a special caution should be taken in obese patients or patients suffering from chronic obstructive pulmonary disease.

A general precaution is that of inserting carbon dioxide to an appropriate pressure after checking respiratory changes at the beginning of surgery rather than injecting the same pressure en bloc, for safe and appropriate respiratory management.

An increase in cerebral blood flow, intracranial pressure, and intraocular pressure is also observed during laparoscopy, especially in procedures requiring a steep Trendelenburg position [17].

Therefore, patients with a complicated glaucoma may not be ideal candidates to these procedures.

In case of intraoperative difficulties in assuring an adequate lung expansion and ventilation, surgeons should temporarily decrease the intra-abdominal pressure or change patient position.

Different gases have been proposed to obtain pneumoperitoneum: nitrous oxide, helium, room air gas, and carbon dioxide, which is at the moment the most frequently used.

An ideal gas for insufflation of the abdominal cavity should be cheap, colorless, not flammable, inexplosive, easily removed by the body, and completely nontoxic to participants.

A recent Cochrane review of trials comparing carbon dioxide to the less frequently used nitrous oxide, helium, and room air failed to clarify if those gases are superior, equivalent, or inferior to carbon dioxide with regard to the incidence of heart or lung complications, surgical complications, or serious unwanted events [18].

3.6 Types of Trocars for Laparoscopy

There are many variants of cannulas (trocars) used to introduce the laparoscope and the other surgical instruments in the abdomen; some of them are the following:

3.6.1 Disposable Shielded Trocars

Disposable shielded "safety" trocars are designed with a shield that partially retracts and exposes the sharp tip as it encounters resistance through the abdominal wall. As the shield enters the abdominal cavity, it springs forward and covers the sharp tip of the trocar.

These trocars are intended to prevent the sharp tip from injuring intra-abdominal contents. However, it must be pointed out that even when a shielded trocar functions properly and is used according to the specifications, there is a brief moment when the sharp trocar tip is exposed and unprotected as it enters the abdominal cavity.

In the presence of pneumoperitoneum, disposable shielded trocars have been shown to require half the force needed for a reusable trocar. Increased entry force frequently results in loss of operator control and overthrusting of the trocar, which is a potential cause of serious vascular and visceral injuries.

3.6.2 Radially Expanding System

The radially expanding access system (Step, InnerDyne, Sunnyvale, CA) consists of a 1.9-mm Veress surrounded by an expanding polymeric sleeve. The abdomen may first be insufflated using the Veress needle. The needle is removed, and the sleeve acts as a tract through the abdominal wall that can be dilated up to 12 mm by inserting a blunt obturator with a twisting motion. The force required to push this trocar through the abdomen in pigs is 14.2 kg compared with forces of 4–6 kg needed for disposable trocars.

Advantages of this system include elimination of sharp trocars, application of radial force, stabilization of the cannula's position (cannula does not slide in and out), avoidance of injury to abdominal wall vessels, and elimination of the need for suturing of fascial defects.

3.6.3 Disposable Optical Trocars (Visual Entry Systems)

These single-use visual trocars trade blind sharp trocars for a hollow trocar, in which the laparoscope is loaded for the distal crystal tip to transmit real-time monitor images while transecting abdominal wall tissue layers. Their application recruits significant axial thrust through the surgeon's dominant upper body muscles to transect abdominal myofascial layers.

3.6.4 Endopath Optiview Optical Trocar (Ethicon Endo-Surgery, Inc., Cincinnati, OH)

The Endopath Optiview optical trocar comprises a hollowed trocar and a cannula. When insufflation is complete, the Veress needle is withdrawn, and the subcutaneous fatty tissue is dissected off, using peanut sponges, to expose the white anterior rectus fascia. A 5-mm incision is then made with a scalpel to accommodate the visual trocar's pointed tip.

When the Endopath optical trocar is used directly, without pre-insufflation, two anterior rectus fascia stay sutures are placed at 3 and 9 o'clock and held with snaps. The fascia is then divided between the stay sutures over a length of approximately 5 mm. During insertion, the stay sutures are pulled to lift the abdominal wall against the advancing trajectory and facilitate proper port site closure at the end of the operation. Alternatively, the assistant may grasp the abdominal wall with towel clips, while the surgeon negotiates the visual trocar.

Twisting the handle advances the hydrophobic and winged trocar tip to dissect successive tissue layers on its way towards the abdomen. The cascade of generated entry images displayed on the monitor demonstrates the level of penetration.

Some surgeons advocate the use of visual trocars during gasless laparoscopy, in which abdominal wall lifting devices are used to tent the abdominal wall before the primary visual trocar is inserted under visual control. Experience with such methods is limited, and large-scale studies are lacking.

The retention of the push-through trocar design necessitates considerable axial force to propel the trajectory, with no mechanism to offset overshoot. Given the winged trocar tip, the generated axial force dents tissue layers, and compression renders layer recognition more difficult.

3.6.5 Visiport Optical Trocars (Tyco-United States Surgical, Norwalk, CT)

The Visiport optical trocar is a disposable visual entry instrument that comprises a hollow trocar and a cannula. Every trigger squeeze advances the sharp cutting knife 1 mm to transect tissue in contact with the crystal tip and swiftly retracts back into the crystal hemisphere. It is advised that, as with other visual trocars, the Visiport optical trocar is to be applied only after CO_2 insufflation.

When insufflation is complete, the Veress needle is withdrawn, and subcutaneous fatty tissue is dissected off the white anterior rectus fascia using peanut sponges. The Visiport optical trocar is palmed by the surgeon's dominant hand and held perpendicular to the supine patient's CO_2 distended abdomen. Once the exact anatomical position of the trocar tip is verified on the monitor, downward axial pressure is applied while activating the trigger. Then downward pressure is relieved, the trigger released, and the trocar tip position verified on the monitor again. This entry sequence is repeated until the peritoneal cavity is entered. The trigger is not fired until the exact anatomical position of the trocar tip is known.

The push-through entry design requires significant perpendicular force to drive a trajectory across tissue planes with no means of avoiding trocar overshoot. Sometimes, the anterior abdominal wall may be grasped with the nondominant hand of the surgeon and lifted to offer counterpressure against the advancing trocar. The Visiport optical trocar comes in only one diameter and accommodates only a 10-mm laparoscope.

3.6.6 EndoTIP Visual Cannula

The endoscopic threaded imaging port, EndoTIP (Karl STORZ Endoscopy, Tuttlingen, Germany), is a reusable visual cannula system that allows real-time interactive port creation, when port dynamics are archived, for recall and analysis. The principal differentiating aspects of EndoTIP include reduction of push-force, visually controlled entry, elimination of overshoot, and lack of sharp trocar.

Conventional primary trocar insertion requires application of considerable axial push-force (2–14 kg) to the trocar and cannula where the anterior abdominal wall dents towards the viscera; entry is blind. The EndoTIP consists of a stainless steel cannula with a proximal valve segment and distal hollow threaded cannula section. The conventional valve sector houses a standard CO_2 stopcock, and the cannula's outer surface is wrapped with a single thread, winding diagonally to end in a distal blunt notched tip. The cannula is available in different lengths and diameters for different surgical applications. A retaining ring keeps the mounted laparoscope from sliding out of focus during insertion.

The EndoTIP visual cannula system requires no trocar and has no crystal tip compressing and distorting monitor images at the tissue–cannula interface. Interpretations of observed monitor images are identified, layered entry, and real-time interactive.

A generous umbilical skin incision is made using a surgical blade to avoid skin dystonia. Ribbon retractors and peanut sponges are used to expose the white anterior rectus fascia. As when using the optical trocar, insertion starts at the fascial level. A 7-mm rectus fascial incision is then made under direct vision, and the Veress needle is inserted through the fascial incision with the CO_2 stopcock in the open position.

When insufflation is complete, the surgeon holds the laparoscope with the mounted cannula perpendicular to patient's supine abdomen, using the nondominant hand. The unit (laparoscope and mounted cannula) with the CO_2 stopcock in the closed position is then lowered into the umbilical wound. The surgeon uses the muscles of the dominant wrist to rotate the cannula clockwise while keeping the forearm horizontal to the patient's abdomen. Downward axial pressure during rotation is kept to a minimum.

The blunt cannula's notched tip engages the anterior rectus fascial window and stretches it radially. Rotation applies Archimedes' principle to lift the anterior abdominal wall and transpose successive tissue layers onto the cannula's outer thread. The white anterior rectus fascia, red rectus muscle, pearly white posterior rectus fascia, yellowish preperitoneal space, and transparent greyish peritoneal membrane are all observed sequentially on the monitor.

As the cannula has no cutting or sharp end, tissue layers are not transected; instead, they are taken up along the outer pitch. The parted tissue layers preserve port competence and result in a smaller fascial entry wound area with less muscle damage than with pyramidal trocar wounds.

Further clockwise rotation parts the peritoneal membrane radially to advance the cannula incrementally into the peritoneal cavity under direct visual control while avoiding cannula overshoot.

In 2015 a Cochrane review [19] analyzed major and minor complications related to the use of five different trocar types: radially expanding, cutting, conical blunt-tipped, single-bladed, and pyramidal-bladed trocars.

No advantage was observed with the use of a specific trocar design to minimize major trocar-related complications like vascular and visceral injuries, mortality, conversion to laparotomy, intensive care admission, or any reintervention.

Concerning minor trocar-related complications, very-low-quality evidence demonstrated a lower risk of trocar site bleeding with the use of radially expanding trocars in comparison to cutting trocars and very-low-quality evidence suggested less postoperative pain after the use of radially expanding trocars compared to cutting trocars.

For the remaining minor trocar-related complications analyzed, as trocar site herniation, trocar site infection, extraperitoneal insufflation, and other injuries that did not require IC or ICU management or a subsequent surgical, endoscopic, or radiological intervention under general anesthesia, no difference was demonstrated between different trocar designs.

References

1. Alkatout I. Complications of laparoscopy in connection with entry techniques. J Gynecol Surg. 2017;33:81–91.
2. Jansen FW, Kapiteyn K, Trimbos-Kemper T, Hermans J, Trimbos JB. Complications of laparoscopy: a prospective multicentre observational study. Br J Obstet Gynaecol. 1997;104(5):595–600.
3. Jansen FW, Kolkman W, Bakkum EA, de Kroon CD, Trimbos- Kemper TC, Trimbos JB. Complications of laparoscopy: an enquiry about closed versus open entry technique. Am J Obstet Gynecol. 2004;190(3):634–8.
4. Bhoyrul S, Vierra MA, Nezhat CR, Krummel TM, Way LW. Trocar injuries in laparoscopic surgery. J Am Coll Surg. 2001;192:677–83.
5. Palmer R. Instrumentation and technique of gynecological laparoscopy. Gynecol Obstet (Paris). 1947;46(4):420–31.
6. Semm K, Semm I. Safe insertion of trocars and Veress needle using standard equipment and the 11 security steps. Gynaecol Endosc. 1999;8:339–47.
7. Fear RE. Laparoscopy: a valuable aid in gynecologic diagnosis. Obstet Gynecol. 1968;31:297–309.
8. Lacey CG. Laparoscopy: a clinical sign for intraperitoneal needle placement. Obstet Gynecol. 1976;47:625–7.
9. Anicki TI. The new sensor-equipped Veress needle. J Am Assoc Gynecol Laparosc. 1994;1(2):154–6.
10. Riek S, Bachmann KH, Gaiselmann T, Hoernstein F, Marzusch K. A new insufflation needle with a special optical system for use in laparoscopic procedures. Obstet Gynecol. 1994;84:476–8.
11. Dingfelder JR. Direct laparoscopic trocar insertion without prior pneumoperitoneum. J Reprod Med. 1978;21:45–7.
12. Mettler L, Ibrahim M, Vinh VQ, Jonat W. Clinical experience with an optical access trocar in gynecological laparoscopy-pelviscopy. JSLS. 1997;1(4):315–8.
13. Hasson HM. A modified instrument and method for laparoscopy. Am J Obstet Gynecol. 1971;110:886–7.
14. Sahan A, Orkunt O, Alkan C, Mete K, Oktay A. A novel open abdominal entry method: fingertip technique. Videourology. 2020;34(4).
15. Ahmad G, Baker J, Finnerty J, Phillips K, Watson A. Laparoscopic entry techniques. Cochrane Database Syst Rev. 2019;1(1):CD006583.
16. Park JS, Ahn EJ, Ko DD, Kang H, Shin HY, Baek CH, Jung YH, Woo YC, Kim JY, Koo GH. Korean effects of pneumoperitoneal pressure and position changes on respiratory mechanics during laparoscopic colectomy. J Anesthesiol. 2012;63(5):419–24.
17. Sahay N, Sharma S, Bhadani UK, Singh A, Sinha C, Sahay A, Ranjan A, Agarwal MJ. Effect of pneumoperitoneum and patient positioning on intracranial pressures during laparoscopy: a prospective comparative study. Minim Invasive Gynecol. 2018;25(1):147–52.
18. Yang X, Cheng Y, Cheng N, Gong J, Bai L, Zhao L, Deng Y. Gases for establishing pneumoperitoneum during laparoscopic abdominal surgery. Cochrane Database Syst Rev. 2022;3(3):CD009569.
19. la Chapelle CF, Swank HA, Wessels ME, Mol BWJ, Rubinstein SM, Jansen FW. Trocar types in laparoscopy. Cochrane Database Syst Rev. 2015;(12):CD009814.

Part IV

Instruments and New Technologies

High-Energy Devices

4

E. Botteri and N. Vettoretto

4.1 Introduction

Surgical activities rely on a safe section and dissection of the human tissues. A good hemostasis is crucial to maintain the homeostasis of the patient during the procedures, but also it enables better visualization of the surgical field. From the simple "tie and knot" to the use of complex devices in which different energies are involved, there are several possibilities for a surgeon to reach a safe and rapid hemostasis. In 1928, William Bovie, a physicist, and Harvey Cushing, a neurosurgeon, developed an electrosurgical unit (ESU) capable of cutting and coagulating. Even if the original Bovie unit is nowadays abandoned, it could be conferred as the precursors of modern energy devices. At present electrosurgery is the most commonly used form of surgical energy both in minimally invasive and open surgery. With the term of high-energy devices (HEDs), we refer to a group of surgical tools that exploit the interactions between tissue and applied energy to allow different biological effects such as coagulation, vessel sealing, and section. Less blood loss and the reduction of operative time probably represent the strongest advantages [1–4]. Next to these benefits we could argued about the costs, the smoke production, the risks of col-

lateral injuries, and the global sustainability of the use of HED. This chapter presents the most important HEDs analyzing the energy involved, its biological effects, and the clinical employment.

4.2 Electrosurgery

The interaction between tissues and electricity is well described by the Joule effect where the energy of an electric current is converted into heat as it flows through a resistance. In particular, when the electric current flows through a solid or a liquid with finite conductivity, electric energy is converted to mechanical energy because of the back and forth movements of the high-frequency alternating current making the cellular ions oscillate creating frictional heat.

The physics of electrosurgery is regulated by three parameters: current, voltage, and resistance. The *current (I),* measured in amp (ampere), is defined as the flow of electrical charges. Without current flow, no electrosurgical action would happen. To move the charges it is necessary to create a difference in the potential between the starting point and the arrival. It is expressed in volt and the *voltage (V)* is the amount of work an electrosurgical generator must perform to force the current through the resistance of the tissue. Impedance to the conduction of electrical current through a given medium is referred to as *resis-*

E. Botteri · N. Vettoretto (✉)
Montichiari Surgery, ASST Spedali Civili Brescia, Brescia, Italy

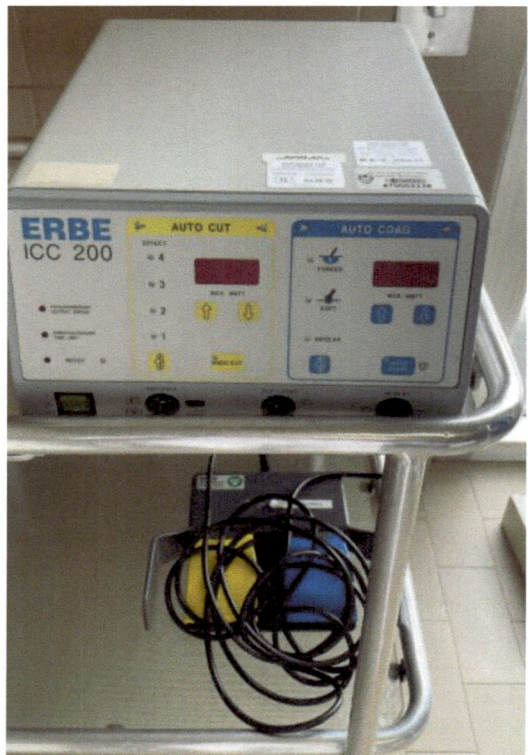

Fig. 4.1 Example of electrosurgical unit

tance (R) and is expressed in ohms. The relationship of current, potential, and resistance is expressed as Ohm's law: $V = IR$.

The household electricity has a low frequency (50–60 Hz) and it is converted by electrosurgical units (Fig. 4.1) to higher frequencies (5,000,000–3,000,000 Hz). At this level of frequencies the Faradic effect of neuromuscular stimulation is inhibited leading to a more controllable and predictable tissual effect. Generators are able to produce three fundamental waveforms: cut, coagulation, and blend. In addition they control wattage, voltage, and duty cycle. A precise adjustment of these parameters is crucial for a safe use of electrosurgery.

4.3 Monopolar Services

Using a pencil instrument, monopolar electrosurgery can be used for several working modalities including cut, blend, desiccation, and fulgura-

tion. The current in a monopolar scalpel runs from the probe electrode to the return pad attached to the patient passing through the body. The target tissue is touched by the pencil producing the biological effect. Every monopolar scalpel can be associated to different tips (needle, plane, or ball) depending on the required use (Figs. 4.2 and 4.3).

Monopolar devices are most commonly used because of its versatility, affordability, and effectiveness. The main drawback connected to the use of monopolar devices is its incompatibility with implanted pacemaker or ICD. The increased risk of injuries caused by lateral thermal spread, direct coupling, inadvertent activation, or dispersive electrode burns suggests constant caution during the use of monopolar devices.

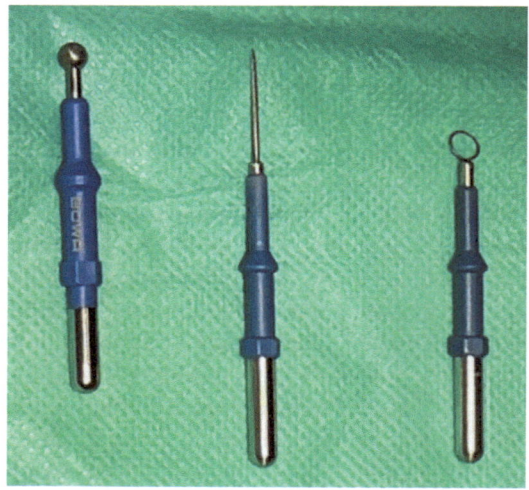

Fig. 4.2 Example of tip a monopolar device can mount

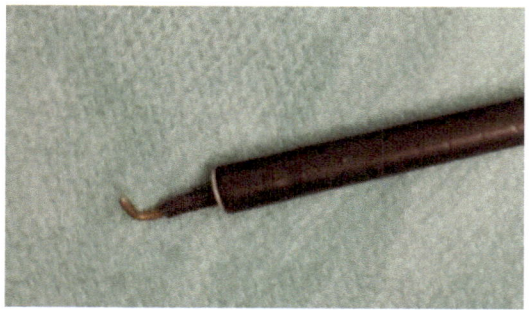

Fig. 4.3 Monopolar hook for laparoscopic surgery

4.4 Bipolar Devices

In bipolar instruments, the electrodes between the current flows are located on the same devices (usually a forceps, a scissor, or a tweezer) (Fig. 4.4). There is no need of a pad attached to the patients because the electrical circuit is close when the surgeon holds an amount of tissue between the electrodes and the current only passes through this thickness. Bipolar electrosurgery uses lower voltages, so less energy is required.

The current flow in bipolar electrosurgery is restricted to just the tissue between the arms of the forceps electrode. This gives a better control over the target area preventing injuries to the nearby spaces.

Because the path of the electrical current is confined to the tissue between the two electrodes, it can be used in patients with cardiac stimulating implanted devices to prevent electrical current passing through the device causing a short circuit or misfire.

It has limited ability to treat large bleeding areas, so it is helpful in those situations where target tissue can be easily grabbed by the forceps.

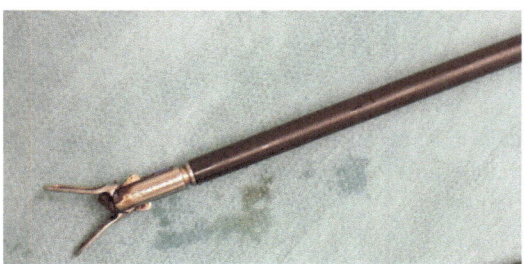

Fig. 4.4 Bipolar device for laparoscopic surgery

4.5 Radiofrequency Devices

Radiofrequency (RF) devices share the same physical basis of bipolar ones (Fig. 4.5). In fact, an RF instrument combines bipolar high electric current (4 A) at a low voltage (<200 V) with the pressure of the tissue between the jaw. Energy denatures the collagen and elastin within the blood vessel wall, but during the cool-down phase, cross link reoccurs creating a new solid wall of collagen and elastin tissue. In this way an RF instrument can seal vessels with a diameter of up to 7 mm [5, 6]. It works with an average cycle of 2–4 s and the vessel sealed has a burst pressure greater than three times the normal systolic blood pressure. The generator is projected to adjust the energy delivered and optimal time of use to achieve a safe and consistent vessel closure.

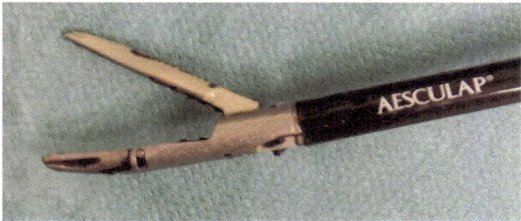

Fig. 4.5 Example of a radiofrequency device

4.6   Ultrasound Devices

With the term of piezoelectric effect we refer to the physical phenomenon in which a crystal, if mechanically deformed, can produce a voltage. A harmonic scalpel (HS) is based on a reverse piezoelectric effect.

Electric energy provided by the generator produces the vibration of a blade (about 55,000 Hz) so the vibrating blades allow the denaturation of hydrogen bonds in tissue and blood vessel proteins with the result that the coagulum seals the lumen of vessels up to 5 mm in diameter while the pressure of the blade cuts the tissue. The temperature developed during the use of an HS is less compared to RF instruments (50–90 °C versus up to 400 °C). This reduces the risk of lateral spreading of thermal injuries. Another potential effect of the use of HS is the total absence of electrical energy in the patients resetting the possibility of interferences with cardiac stimulating devices [7].

4.7   Hybrid Devices

Nowadays, a device that integrates both US and advanced bipolar energy in a unique instrument (H-US/RF) is available: it allows to cut tissue with US energy, on the one hand, and seals vessels with bipolar energy, on the other hand.

4.8   Risk Related to the Use of HED

The HEDs are nowadays widely spread in clinical practice [4] and doubtless they represent an evolution in surgical activities determining less operative time, less blood loss, and in some cases less complications [8]. Nevertheless, during the use of an HED both surgeon and scrub nurse have to pay attention to some potential risks related to the use of HEDs. These risks are addressed to the patients but also to the operating room staff.

4.8.1   Lateral Thermal Spread

It is due to the spreading of high temperature next to the working area of an HED. Lateral thermal spread is the most common cause of electrosurgical unintended burns. Monopolar devices generate more lateral thermal spread during coagulation compared to the bipolar and ultrasonic ones [9].

4.8.2   Residual Heat

The blades or the jaws of an HED retain heat after deactivation for a variable length. Ultrasonic devices have the highest residual heat [9].

4.8.3   Inadvertent Activation

Inadvertent activation of electrosurgical devices may result in unintended burns for patients or operating room staff. During minimal invasive surgery, it can produce injuries to organs or vessel especially when they are out of the field of view [9].

4.8.4   Direct Thermal Extension (Pedicle Effect, Funnelling)

It occurs when the active electrode touches a structure with a narrow pedicle or a narrow band of adhesion. The increased current density at that remote narrow area causes an unintended burn [9].

4.8.5   Dispersive Electrode Burns

High current density results in skin burn. To dissipate the current safely, the dispersive electrode is provided with a wide surface area to create low current density. Usually it is applied to an area with low impedance away from metal prothesis. It should be close to the operation site but away from any metal prosthesis or irregular body contour, bony prominences, fat, scar tissue, and hairy skin. Dispersive electrode burns occur when there is inadequate electrode contact with the patient due to either partial detachment of the dispersive electrode or high impedance at the skin application area [9].

4.8.6 Insulation Failure

A defect in the insulation layer of an active electrode is like having an extra active tip that can transmit the wattage to nearby tissues. Insulation defect can occur during the surgery when high voltage is used. The majority of these defects are too small to be detected by inspection and lead to high current density and severe burns. The critical area is the distal third [9].

4.8.7 Direct Coupling

It occurs when the activated electrode touches another metal instrument that may be in contact with some tissue as bowel [9].

4.8.8 Capacitive Coupling

A capacitor is formed when the active electrode induces current through its intact insulation in a nearby conductor. The magnitude of such induced current increases with the proximity of the two conductors, thinner insulation, increased voltage, and longer activation time [9].

4.8.9 Antenna Coupling

This phenomenon is caused by the emission of electromagnetic energy from the active electrode cord (emitting antenna) captured by a nearby inactive cord (receiving antenna). It is similar to capacitive coupling and can lead to patient burns [9].

4.8.10 Electrical Shock and Glove Burns

Even if surgical gloves are used primarily to protect patients and the surgical team from biological hazards, preexisting holes in surgical gloves are responsible for the occasional shocks and burns that surgeons and assistants may receive during electrosurgery [9].

4.8.11 Surgical Smoke

Smoke with high levels of small particles reduces laparoscopic visibility which can lead to unintended complications. Bipolar and ultrasonic devices produce less smoke with less affected visibility compared to the monopolar ones [9].

4.8.12 Surgical Fires and Explosions

Although operating room fires and explosions are rare events, they still occur and can potentially cause devastating outcomes. The high concentration of supplemental oxygen is the most important risk factor [9].

References

1. Kennedy J, Buysse S, Lawes K, et al. Recent innovations in bipolar electrosurgery. Minim Invasive Ther Allied Technol. 1999;8:95–9.
2. Carroll T, Ladner K, Meyers AD. Alternative surgical dissection techniques. Otolaryngol Clin North Am. 2005;38:397–411.
3. Devassy R, Gopalakrishnan S, De Wilde RL. Surgical efficacy among laparoscopic ultrasonic dissectors: are we advancing safely? A review of literature. J Obstet Gynaecol India. 2015;65:293–300.
4. Botteri E, Podda M, Arezzo A. Current status on the adoption of high energy devices in Italy: an Italian Society for Endoscopic Surgery and New Technologies (SICE) national survey. Surg Endosc. 2021;35:6201–11.
5. Harold KL, Pollinger H, Matthews BD, et al. Comparison of ultrasonic energy, bipolar thermal energy, and vascular clips for the hemostasis of small-, medium-, and large-sized arteries. Surg Endosc. 2003;17:1228–30.

6. Campbell PA, Cresswell AB, Frank TG, et al. Real time thermography during energized vessel sealing and dissection. Surg Endosc. 2003;17:1640–5.

7. Person B, Vivas DA, Ruiz D, Talcott M, et al. Comparison of four energy-based vascular sealing and cutting instruments: a porcine model. Surg Endosc. 2008;22:534–8.

8. Vettoretto N, Foglia E, Gerardi C, Lettieri E, Nocco U, Botteri E, Bracale U, Caracino V, Carrano FM, Cassinotti E, Giovenzana M, Giuliani B, Iossa A, Milone M, Montori G, Peltrini R, Piatto G, Podda M, Sartori A, Allocati E, Ferrario L, Asperti F, Songia L, Garattini S, Agresta F, HTA-HED Collaborative Group. High-energy devices in different surgical settings: lessons learnt from a full health technology assessment report developed by SICE (Società Italiana di Chirurgia Endoscopica). Surg Endosc. 2023;37(4):2548–65. https://doi.org/10.1007/s00464-022-09734-5. Epub ahead of print. PMID: 36333498; PMCID: PMC9638482.

9. Feldaman L. Fuchshuber P, Jones DB. The SAGES manual on the fundamental use of surgical energy (FUSE). Springer; 2012.

The Robotic Platform

5

Wanda Petz

5.1 The Robotic Platform

The term "robot" derives from the Czeck word *robota*, meaning slavery, and was first introduced in 1920 by the Czech Karel Čapek in the three-act scientific fiction drama R.U.R (Rossum's Universal Robot).

In that drama, robots were replicating androids designed to free humans from the bondage of physical fatigue.

Even if nowadays there are no robotic machines capable of autonomously carrying out complex activities, robotic surgery is carried out thanks to sophisticated technologies that involve the use of computers and a remote manipulation system capable of reproducing, by miniaturizing them, the movements of the human hand.

Robotic surgery was developed with the aim of overcoming the technical limitations of traditional laparoscopy such as:

- Two-dimensional view on the screen
- Paradoxical movements of manually operated instruments through the trocars
- Unnatural positions of the surgeon
- Dissociation between instrument control and vision control (video camera operated by an assistant)

- Difficulty in carrying out high-precision microsutures
- Reduced degrees of freedom of the instruments with respect to the hand and wrist
- Physiological tremor

In the case of robotically assisted minimally invasive surgery, instead of directly moving the instruments, the surgeon uses a computer to control the robotic arms and its end effectors; one of the advantages of this method is that the surgeon does not have to be present, leading to the possibility for remote surgery.

From the early 1980s, different robotic platforms have been developed and employed in various surgical procedures; the most sophisticated and the most widespread is the Da Vinci® surgical system.

The Da Vinci® robotic platform has three components:

- The patient cart
- The vision cart
- The surgeon console

5.2 Patient Cart

The patient cart is the only sterile component during surgery; the cart of the most recent Da Vinci® system (the Xi® robotic platform) is provided with four articulated arms that can har-

W. Petz (✉)
Department of Digestive Surgery, European Institute of Oncology IRCCS, Milan, Italy

bor surgical instruments; the arms are connected with robotic 8-mm trocars so that instruments, included the camera, can be interchangeable between the arms.

The Xi® system has been conceived to be suitable for multiquadrant surgery as its thin arms minimize external conflict and its boom-mounted architecture and multi-position setup joints maximize the surgical workspace internally and externally.

5.3   Vision Cart

The vision cart is the "brain" of the system. Inside, the processor elaborates the surgeon's movements and transmits them to the arms and robotic instruments. The images are processed and continuous security checks on the functioning of the system are carried out.

5.4   Surgeon Console

The surgeon console is the control center of the da Vinci Xi® system. The surgeon seated at the console controls all movements of the instruments and the endoscope using two hand controls and a set of pedals, performing natural movements that are reproduced in real time by the instruments on the patient cart. The surgeon views the endoscopic image on a three-dimensional (3D) viewer, which provides a view of the patient's anatomy and instrumentation as well as icons and other user interface elements.

5.5   The Da Vinci Xi Platform Setup

A proper setup is key to a successful robotic procedure. The five fundamentals of robotic setup are the following:

1. Port placement
2. Deploy for docking
3. Drive laser lines to endoscope port
4. Perform targeting

5. Perform manual arms adjustments

Following the five setup fundamentals provides important advantages, because instrument tips are enabled to reach where needed to complete the procedure, the da Vinci is adjusted to an appropriate starting position, the setup is reproducible, external arm-to-arm interferences are minimized, and intraoperative range-of-motion limits are maximized.

5.5.1   Port Placement

First, the surgeon must identify the surgical workspace, or where the instrument tips must reach, in order to complete the procedure. If the surgical workspace of any procedure requires access to more than two quadrants, a dual docking should be considered.

Then the target anatomy has to be determined: the target anatomy is not the pathology but it is the area where the midline of the surgical workspace intersects the far edge of the surgical workspace boundary.

The initial endoscope port must be placed 10–20 cm back from the target anatomy, on the opposite edge of the surgical workspace boundary.

The surgeon can decide whether to control two instruments with the left hand or with the right hand, as this determines port placement. Two *da Vinci* instrument ports will go to one side of the initial endoscope port, and one *da Vinci* instrument port will go to the other.

The remaining ports are placed 8 cm apart, along a line perpendicular to the target anatomy; port distance should range between 6 and 10 cm and can be adapted according to patient body habitus. Ports should be placed at least 2 cm away from bony structures and no port should be placed between other ports and the target anatomy.

The assistant port can be placed as needed, as far away as possible from robotic ports (at least 7 cm) and usually lateral to the robotic ports or triangulated between the robotic ports.

The location of assistant port should enable the surgeon to reach the desired anatomy, and the assistant must have physical access to it.

5.5.2 Deploy for Docking

After port placement, the anatomic region of the desired surgical workspace and the cart location, or how the patient cart will approach the patient (from patient right, patient left, or patient legs), must be selected on the patient cart helm.

Then, pressing and holding the "deploy for docking" button, the robotic arms and boom will move automatically and they will adjust to an appropriate starting position: the cart is so ready to be driven to the patient.

5.5.3 Drive Laser Lines to the Endoscope Port

A staff nurse grasps the handlebars and slowly drives the patient cart to the operating table, monitoring patient clearance. The angle of the patient cart base relative to the operating table is not critical but it is important to avoid setting up the system with the boom rotated 180° opposite the base. For example, it has to be avoided to position the cart on the patient's left side for right-sided procedures or vice versa, as in this configuration, access to the patient is limited and assistants have their backs close to the sterile draped column.

The laser line must be driven within 5 cm of the initial endoscope port. This positions the center of the *da Vinci* boom over the initial endoscope port.

5.5.4 Perform Targeting

The initial endoscope arm is docked to the initial endoscope port and the endoscope is inserted; the endoscope must be rotated to a "neutral" horizon position before performing targeting.

The cannula is held with one hand to support it during motion; by pressing and holding the targeting button on the endoscope, the boom will automatically rotate and orient itself toward the target anatomy. The targeting button must be held until the audible countdown completes and motion stops.

Performing targeting simultaneously adjusts column height, boom extension, and boom rotation and achieves the following:

- Centers boom over the initial endoscope port
- Rotates boom to point toward the target anatomy
- Adjusts column height to maximize sterility and ensure arms reach to all ports for docking

Targeting does not move the flex joints.

To enable successful targeting, the operating table height must be lowered prior to docking and the laser lines must be driven within 5 cm of the initial endoscope port without manually adjusting the boom.

5.5.5 Perform Manual Arm Adjustments

The remaining arms are docked to the robotic ports, and manual adjustments are done to maintain at least the space of one fist between arms and between the arms and patient body.

5.6 Robotic Instruments

EndoWrist instruments offer a wider range of motion than natural hands, allowing for greater precision during surgery.

Different EndoWrist instruments are available for general surgery:

- Monopolar hook
- Monopolar curved scissors
- Bipolar forceps
- Needle holders
- Clip appliers
- Normal (Cadière) and long (tip-up) graspers
- Staplers
- Vessel sealer
- Harmonic scalpel

Moreover, the robotic platform has an integrated fluorescence imaging system (Firefly) that allows to switch the vision from normal light to fluorescent images using indocyanine green.

Of interest is the functioning of the **robotic staplers**, which have the so-called smart firing technology that measures tissue compression before and during firing; it uses more than one thousand measurements per second to make automatic adjustments to the firing process, as staples are being formed and as the transection is being made.

Once the firing has started, there are different messages that may appear on the screen:

– The "*pausing for compression*" message: it appears if the system determines that an additional compression is needed for optimal staple formation. In this case, the firing pauses, the surgeon receives an audio feedback, and the jaws of the staple will apply extra compression to the target tissue. Then firing will resume once the appropriate compression is gained on the target tissue.

– The "*tissue too thick to continue*" message: it appears if the tissue cannot be compressed adequately for optimal staple formation, based on the reload selected: in this case, the firing pauses and a progress bar will display how far the firing cycle progressed before being unable to proceed. The surgeon has to unclamp, ensure that there are no obstructions to the target tissue, and eventually consider to change the reload color before continuing.

ICG 4.4, Optical Devices

6

Ludovica Baldari, Luigi Boni,
Massimiliano Della Porta, and Elisa Cassinotti

6.1 Fluorescence-Guided Surgery

During the last years, several technologies have been introduced in surgery, in order to elevate the level of precision and efficiency of clinical practice. New surgical devices have been integrated into the operating theatre, changing its classical setting. One of the most innovative technologies is fluorescence-guided surgery.

The term fluorescence-guided surgery (FGS) describes a medical technology based on real-time imaging intended to help and guide the surgeon during his operating practice, identifying areas invisible by the naked eyes, using a fluorophore (Fig. 6.1). This emerging field promises to be a powerful enhancement to traditional low-contrast white-light visualization, offering real-time highlighted delineation of complex anatomic structures. Basically, enhancing the visual differences between tissues, by using fluorescent probes based on structure or disease, could be

equated to color-coding the surgical field. Improved visualization will lead to more complete removal of disease, decreased inadvertent injuries to vital structures, and improved identification for repair of damaged tissues. This is the reason why FGS could represent a major contribution to intraoperative decision-making during surgical procedures [1, 2].

6.1.1 Fluorophores

Fluorophores are molecules that can emit fluorescence when stimulated by different-wavelength light source. If this specific molecule allows to study and gives information about the structure and/or a system, it is named "fluorescent probe" [3, 4].

Fluorescent probes are basically contrast agents able to enhance a specific structure of tissue from the surrounding ones. Based on their fluorescence emission spectra, clinically evaluated dyes can be separated into three groups. The first group includes probes emitting fluorescence in the visible part of the light spectrum (400–650 nm) (Fig. 6.2). The second group consists of dyes emitting in the far-red region of the light spectrum (650–750 nm). The last group consists of near-infrared (NIR)-emitting cyanine dyes (750–1000 nm), such as indocyanine green (ICG) that is the most used fluorescent dye in clinical practice [3, 5].

L. Baldari (✉) · M. D. Porta
Department of General and Minimally Invasive Surgery, Fondazione IRCCS Ca' Granda Ospedale Maggiore Policlinico, Milan, Italy

L. Boni · E. Cassinotti
Department of Surgery, Fondazione IRCCS Ca' Granda Ospedale Maggiore Policlinico, Milan, Italy

Department of Scienze Cliniche e delle Comunità, University of Milan, Milan, Italy

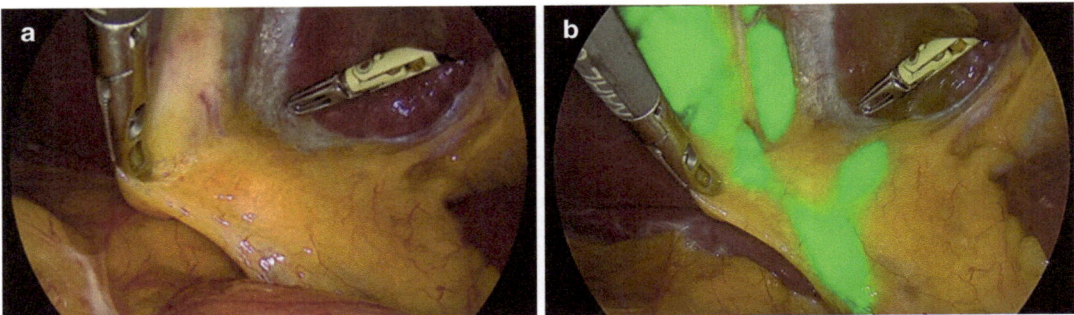

Fig. 6.1 Endoscopic visualization of the gallbladder with standard white light (**a**) and with near-infrared fluorescence (**b**)

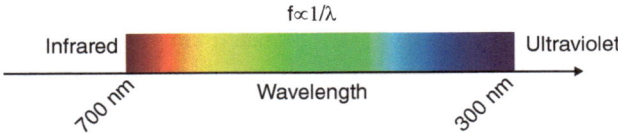

Fig. 6.2 Electromagnetic spectrum and its relation to visible, ultraviolet, and infrared light: wavelength (λ) and frequency (f) (*nm* nanometer)

6.1.1.1 Indocyanine Green

It is a water-soluble tricarbocynanine dye that has been used clinically for over 50 years for hepatic clearance, cardiovascular function testing, and retinal angiography on the basis of its dark green color [6]. Indocyanine green is a negatively charged ion that belongs to the large family of cyanine dyes. Dry ICG is stable at room temperature. In aqueous solutions, ICG molecules tend to aggregate, which influences their optical properties. The aggregation depends on the concentration and time. Spectral stabilization is fastest when ICG is dissolved in distilled water, and thus, some authors do not recommend adding isotonic saline and/or albumin to the injectate, when fast spectral stability is essential, for example, when using ICG for quantitative purposes. IGC is hydrophobic and, thus, it frequently bounds to proteins in plasma (especially albumin), which confines ICG to the intravascular space and makes it especially suited for angiographic applications [7, 8].

The binding to plasma proteins does not seem to alter protein structures, which is one sign of nontoxicity. ICG does not have any known metabolites, and it is quickly extracted by the liver into bile juice [6–8]. A peculiar feature is the low toxicity (LD50 after a single IV dose of 50–80 mg/kg for animals). No significant toxic effects have been observed in humans with the high dose of 5 mg/kg of body weight. ICG for injection contains sodium iodide and should be used with caution in patients who have a history of allergy to iodides because of the risk of anaphylaxis.

The commercially available instrumentation used for ICG detection is adjusted for the characteristics that ICG displays in plasma (peak excitation wavelength of 807 nm and peak emission wavelength of 822 nm) [6, 9].

6.2 Near-Infrared Fluorescence Surgical Systems

Fluorophores with excitation and emission spectra in the nearinfrared wavelength range (700–900 nm) have attracted the most attention owing to their improved depth penetration range compared with fluorophores that emit electromagnetic radiation of shorter wavelengths. Since NIR fluorescent light is essentially invisible to the human eye, special imaging systems are required

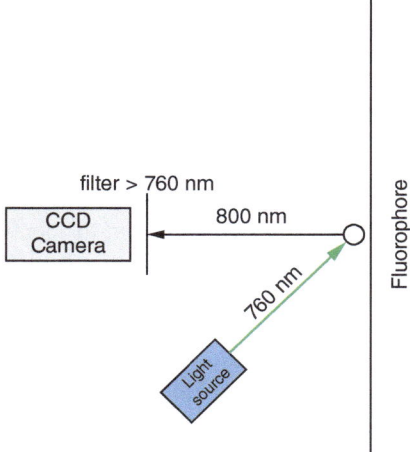

Fig. 6.3 Operating principle of fluorescence-guided surgery (FGS)

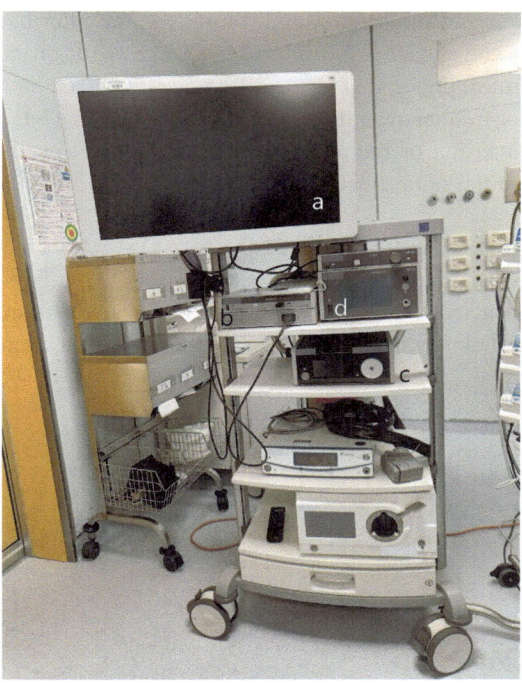

Fig. 6.4 Components of a near-infrared endoscopic fluorescence system: screen (**a**), camera control unit (**b**), light source (**c**), and insufflator (**d**)

to excite the NIR fluorophores within the surgical field and to collect emitted photons. Well-designed NIR fluorophores are needed to highlight the specific structures desired by the surgeon [10].

Indeed, ICG becomes fluorescent once excited with NIR light or with a dedicated laser beam. The fluorescence can be detected using specific scopes and cameras and then transmitted to a standard monitor allowing identification of anatomical structures where the dye is present (i.e., biliary ducts, vessels, lymph nodes, etc.) (Figs. 6.3 and 6.4) [11].

6.2.1 Components of Near-Infrared Fluorescence Surgical Systems

Fluorescence technology used in the surgical system is based on methodology already defined in fluorescence microscopy and spectroscopy [12]. The system is made of an excitation source, a fluorescent probe (described above), filters, and fluorescent detector.

6.2.1.1 Excitation Source
The excitation source to obtain a fluorescent signal is a light that can be generated by xenon lamps, light-emitting diodes (LEDs), and laser diodes. Even if lamps are flexible, allowing a

wide range of wavelength, they are not the ideal source as they produce heat, requiring a warm-up period, and deteriorate with use with a consequent decrease of brightness. LEDs are more diffused. If compared to xenon lamps, LEDs have longer lifetimes, do not need a warm-up period, have lower consumption, and have a narrow bandwidth. Laser diodes have a narrower wavelength and higher intensity compared with the other two sources. Laser source is more expensive than LED ones, so they are less diffused (Fig. 6.5) [13].

6.2.1.2 Fluorescence System Filters
Excitation and emission filters are necessary to select wavelengths and unwanted signal. For example, emission filters can be used to narrow the fluorescence signal collected to the spectrum of interest. Emission filters' features should be clearly defined and balanced, as a large band allows higher intensity of the signal but less specificity resulting in lower contrast between the tar-

get and the background. Moreover, the filter has to be chosen according to the Stokes shift of the fluorophore, that is, the difference (in wavelength or frequency units) between positions of the band maxima of the absorption and emission spectra of the same electronic transition [13].

6.2.1.3 Fluorescence System Detectors

The aim of the detector is to quantify the fluorescence of the single photons according to quantum efficiency, that is, the ability to convert the inci-

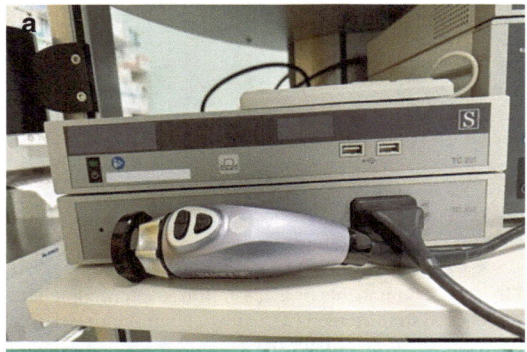
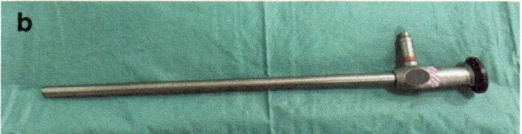

Fig. 6.5 Camera control unit and camera head (**a**) and scope (**b**)

dent light to excited electron, and internal gain, that is, the ability to amplify the signal in a large electrical signal.

To date several systems are currently used to detect photons in the surgical field:

- Photomultiplier tubes absorb the incident photons and produce electrons to obtain the signal.
- Microchannel plate photomultipliers absorb the incident photons and produce electron with an amplification of the signal and improved time resolution of the detection system.
- Charge-coupled devices are made of pixel array that produce a signal proportional to exposure time of incident light, resulting in high sensitivity.
- Single-photon avalanche photodiode generates current quickly after photon absorption thanks to a multiplexed pixel array. The main advantage is the higher quantum efficiency.

Each of these detectors has advantages and disadvantages, and even if single-photon avalanche photodiode has high potential for fluorescence lifetime use, photomultiplier tubes and charge-coupled devices are still currently used [13]. The complex system of filter and detector are inserted into the camera control unit, the camera head, and the scope (Fig. 6.6).

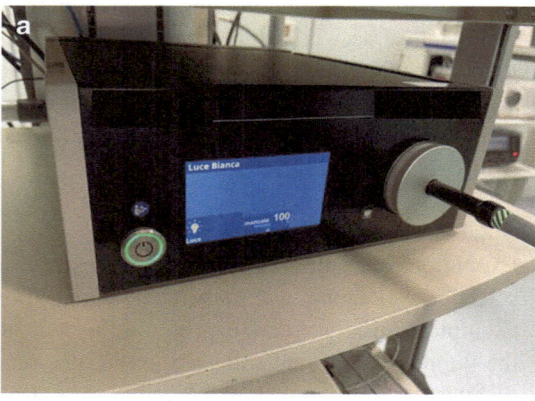
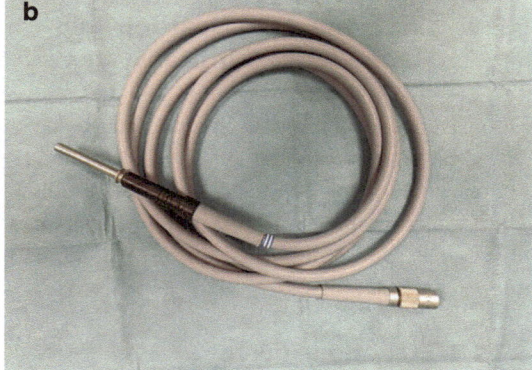

Fig. 6.6 Light source (**a**) and light cable (**b**)

6.3   Currently Available Devices for Fluorescence-Guided Surgery

Nowadays, a growing number of companies are developing new systems for FGS. These systems that are suitable for both near-infrared fluorescence and white-light (WL) imaging, integrating the aforementioned technology, available for both minimally invasive and robotic surgery.

Each system differs from others on some key features:

- The "exciting" light source type (neon light, LED, or laser beam)
- The system of signal detection
- The wavelength emitted and captured
- The optimal distance to visualize fluorescence signal
- The strength of signal to background ratio (SBR)

- The possibility of direct overlay of the NIR images to the WL ones

The different features that characterize each device (field of vision, zoom capability, type of light source, NIR wavelength emitted and captured, etc.) will have an impact on the system performance during surgery. During surgical procedures the alternate exposure to from WL to NIR light (ICG mode) is used to identify anatomical structures, blood perfusion, and other details. The fluorescence imaging systems allow to obtain fluorescent images in a real-time setting. They are quite unexpensive, if compared to some other technological equipment widely adopted in surgery [14]. Table 6.1 reports a selection of the main manufacturers of fluorescence imaging systems used in clinical research for both minimally invasive and robotic surgery.

Table 6.1 Selection of the main manufacturers of fluorescence imaging systems used in clinical research and practise for both minimally invasive and robotic surgery

Imaging system		Image resolution	Use	Visualization mode
Hamamatsu Photonics Co.	Photodynamic eye (PDE) 2	HD Laser-free LED light source	Laparoscopic	– Fluorescence mode – Fluorescence mapping mode – B/W fluorescence mode
University of Texas Health Science Center	FDPM imager	HD Laser diode	Laparoscopic	– Fluorescence mode
Pulsion Medical Systems SE	IC View	HD Laser diode	Laparoscopic	– Fluorescence mode
Stryker	1688 Advanced Imaging Modalities	4K	Laparoscopic	– Green overlay mode – SPY-ENV mode – SPY contrast – IRIS
Karl Storz 1S™	Image 1S™	HD xenon light source	Laparoscopic	– Optical illumination and contrast enhanced modality – No overlay mode
	Image 1S™ Rubina™	4K and 3D Laser-free LED light source	Laparoscopic	– Overlay mode – Intensity map – Monochromatic
Olympus Corp.	EVIS LUCERA Spectrum	HD xenon light source	Laparoscopic	– Fluorescence mode
Olympus Corp.	VISERA ELITE III	4K and 3D Laser free LED light source	Laparoscopic	– Overlay mode – Monochromatic
Arthrex	Synergy *ID* System	4K	Laparoscopic	– Overlay mode – Grayscale – Monochromatic
Da Vinci Surgical System (Intuitive)	Firefly camera system integrated into Da Vinci Si and Xi	3D LED light	Robotic	– Normal imaging and fluorescent modes

6.4 Clinical Application of Fluorescence-Guided Surgery

Near-infrared imaging has been introduced in clinical practice for several intraoperative indications. The most popular current clinical applications in surgery worldwide include fluorescence cholangiography, lymph node identification, real-time cancerous tumor detection [10], and bowel anastomotic perfusion assessment [15–18]. Depending on the clinical application and the target organ, the dye can be administered through several routes such as intravascular injection, the most common, topical, intradermal, intraluminal, or through a catheter.

6.4.1 ICG Fluorescent Cholangiography During Laparoscopic Cholecystectomy

The dye is injected intravenously at least 30 min before surgery to allow the agent to accumulate in bile. Following injection, the agent is concentrated in bile, resulting in visual enhancement of the biliary tree anatomy, especially in Calot's triangle (Fig. 6.1). During laparoscopic cholecystectomy, the use of ICG-enhanced fluorescence imaging under NIR light has proven useful in both elective and acute settings. Employed in an acute setting, diluted ICG should be administered as early as possible (at least 30 min prior to surgery). In such cases, concomitant background fluorescence is anticipated to occur in the liver parenchyma. Even though there is variability between individuals, mainly related to liver function, BMI, and inflammation grade, the ICG standard dose for fluorescence-guided cholecystectomy is 0.0119 mg/kg [1, 15, 19].

Based on the standard protocols published in literature, a 25-mg vial of ICG is diluted using 40 mL of sterile water [20].

- **Elective cholecystectomy**: 0.0119 mg/kg of ICG solution administered 1 h prior to the procedure.

- **Acute cholecystitis**: 0.0119 mg/kg of ICG solution administered at least 30 min prior to the procedure [19].

6.4.2 Intraoperative Assessment of Lymphatic Drainage and Sentinel Lymph Node Detection

ICG-enhanced fluorescence imaging may also be used for mapping lymphatic drainage pathways from various organs. The method has been proposed for sentinel lymph node biopsy in breast surgery and melanoma, lymphadenectomy in gastrointestinal cancer, and tumor of the prostate and endometrium. In these cases, it is recommended to dilute 25 mg of ICG with 20 mL of sterile water. The dye is injected in the peritumoral area (a bolus of 0.5–1 mL used on each quadrant of the tumor) or—given a history of primary tumor removal—in the scar region the day before or at the beginning of the procedure. This is to ensure that proper diffusion into the lymphatic vessels occurs (Fig. 6.7) [21, 22].

6.4.3 ICG Fluorescent Angiography

ICG-enhanced fluorescence imaging may also be used to clarify vascular anatomy and to assess perfusion of solid organs or viscera, e.g., in pro-

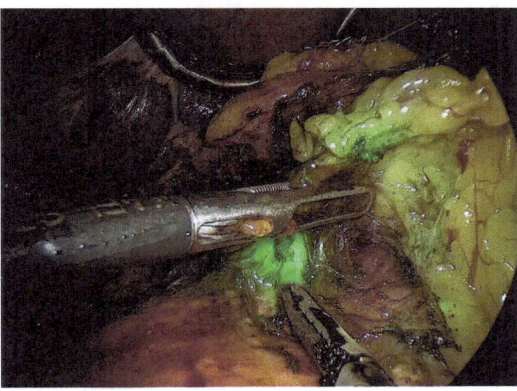

Fig. 6.7 ICG-enhanced fluorescence-guided lymph node mapping during laparoscopic gastrectomy

cedures like laparoscopic gastrointestinal surgery. The angiographic modality is effectively used to facilitate vascular dissection. This has been shown to be helpful under certain conditions when there is reason to suspect anatomical variations, as is the case in nephrectomy, liver resection, splenectomy, or vascular surgery. In such cases, ICG-enhanced fluorescence imaging provides a real-time video image of the individual distributive pattern of vascularity (Fig. 6.8). The technique may also be used for assessment of organ perfusion and ischemia in applications such as liver resection, partial splenectomy, control of perfusion after kidney transplantation, and perfusion assessment of the gastric conduit during esophagectomy, just to mention a few. To perform fluorescent angiography, diluted ICG is injected using multiple boluses of 3 mL, each at a concentration of 0.2 mg/kg (usually a 25-mg vial of ICG diluted with 10 mL of sterile water) [18].

6.4.4 ICG Fluorescence-Guided Resection of Hepatic Metastases

ICG-enhanced fluorescence imaging aids in localizing hepatic metastases, thus enabling a targeted tumor removal in laparoscopic liver resection. An intravenous injection of 0.4 mg/kg ICG solution is given 36 h prior to surgery. After this period, the normal liver parenchyma

has eliminated most of the injected dye, whereas it is retained in adjoining non-diseased cells around the metastatic lesion, which are deficient in normal bile secretion (Fig. 6.9). In this case, ICG-enhanced fluorescence imaging not only helps in localizing metastatic lesions, but also facilitates to determine the resection margins.

6.4.5 ICG Fluorescence Imaging for Visualization of Ureters in Laparoscopic Abdominal Surgery

ICG-enhanced fluorescence imaging can also be used for intraoperative identification of the ure-

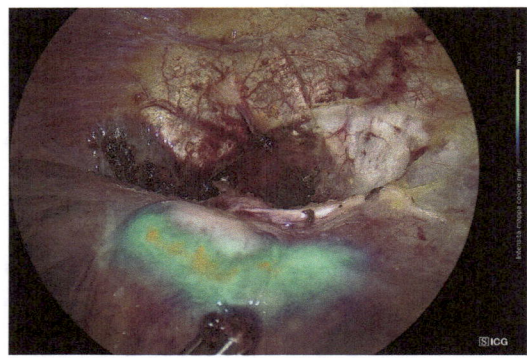

Fig. 6.9 ICG-enhanced fluorescence-guided liver resection for metastatic hepatic lesions

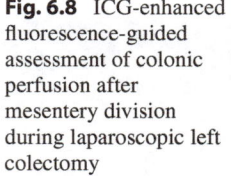

Fig. 6.8 ICG-enhanced fluorescence-guided assessment of colonic perfusion after mesentery division during laparoscopic left colectomy

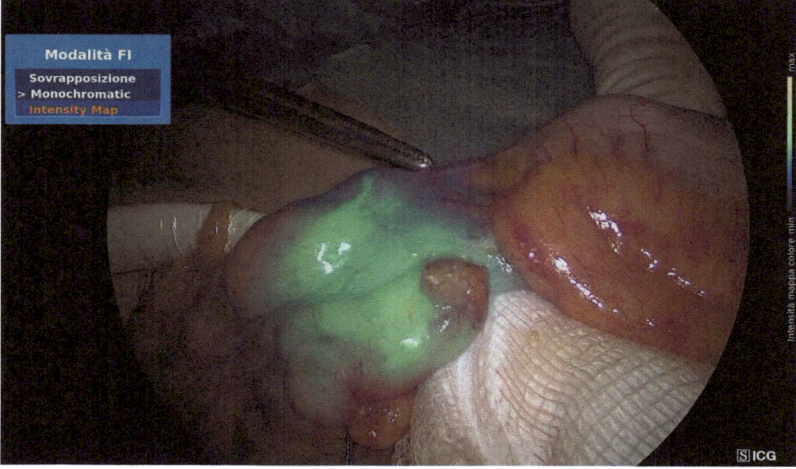

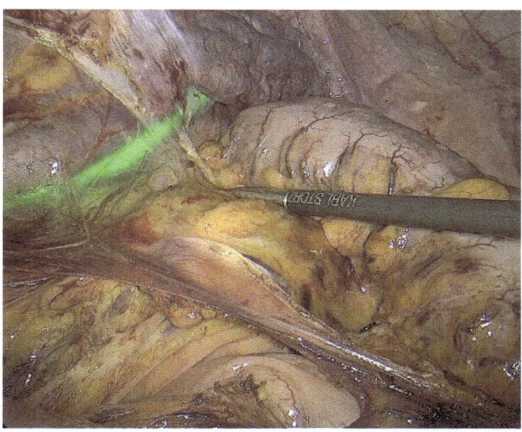

Fig. 6.10 ICG-enhanced fluorescence imaging for visualization of the left ureter during left colectomy

ters. As mentioned above, ICG is excreted in bile; thus, it is not possible to localize the urinary system after intravenous ICG injection. In order to enable identification of the ureters by ICG fluorescence, ureteral catheters (monolateral or bilateral, depending on surgery) are placed with a cystoscope directly before surgery. It is recommended to dilute 25 mg of ICG with 20 mL of sterile water and inject 2–3 mL of the solution into the renal pelvis through the open catheter. Following administration of ICG, the catheter(s) need(s) to be clamped and retracted causing ICG inflow followed by emergence of NIR fluorescence of the ureter(s) (Fig. 6.10). Once the dye is instilled as described, NIR/ICG fluorescence allows to identify the ureters throughout the surgical procedure. The technique has been found to be very useful in complex cases of abdominal and pelvic surgery, like complicated diverticular disease or in the treatment of bulky tumors [23].

References

1. Orosco RK, Tsien RY, Nguyen QT. Fluorescence imaging in surgery. IEEE Rev Biomed Eng. 2013;6:178–87.
2. Nguyen QT, Tsien RY. Fluorescence-guided surgery with live molecular navigation—a new cutting edge. Nat Rev Cancer. 2013;13(9):653–62.
3. Dip FD, Ishizawa T, Kodudo N, Rosenthal RJ. Fluorescence imaging for surgeons concepts and applications. Cham: Springer; 2015. p. 3–23. isbn:978-3-319-35213-8.
4. Valeur B, Berberan-Santos MN. Molecular fluorescence: principles and applications. Weinheim: Wiley-VCH; 2012; isbn:978-3-527-32837-6.
5. Fernandez-Suarez M, Ting AY. Fluorescent probes for super-resolution imaging in living cells. Nat Rev Mol Cell Biol. 2008;9(12):929–43.
6. Alander JT, Kaartinen I, Laakso A, Pätilä T, Spillmann T, Tuchin VV, et al. A review of indocyanine green fluorescent imaging in surgery. Int J Biomed Imaging. 2012;2012:940585.
7. Mordon S, Devoisselle JM, Soulie-Begu S, Desmettre T. Indocyanine green: physicochemical factors affecting its fluorescence in vivo. Microvasc Res. 1998;55:146–52.
8. Desmettre T, Devoisselle JM, Mordon S. Fluorescence properties and metabolic features of indocyanine green (ICG) as related to angiography. Surv Ophthalmol. 2000;45:15–27.
9. Schaafsma BE, Mieog JS, Hutteman M, van der Vorst JR, Kuppen PJ, Lowik CW, et al. The clinical use of indocyanine green as a near-infrared fluorescent contrast agent for image-guided oncologic surgery. J Surg Oncol. 2011;104:323–32.
10. Gioux S, Choi HS, Frangioni JV. Image-guided surgery using invisible near-infrared light: fundamentals of clinical translation. Mol Imaging. 2010;9(5):237–55.
11. Luo S, Zhang E, Su Y, Cheng T, Shi C. A review of NIR dyes in cancer targeting and imaging. Biomaterials. 2011;32:7127–38.
12. Engelborghs Y, Visser AJWG. Fluorescence spectroscopy and microscopy: methods and protocols. In: Methods in Molecular Biology; 2014. https://doi.org/10.1007/978-1-62703-649-8.
13. Stewart HL, Birch DJS. Fluorescence guided surgery. Methods Appl Fluoresc. 2021;9(4).
14. Sevick-Muraca EM, Houston JP, Gurfinkel M. Fluorescence-enhanced, near infrared diagnostic imaging with contrast agents. Curr Opin Chem Biol. 2002;6:642–50.
15. Agnus V, Pesce A, Boni L, Van Den Bos J, Morales-Conde S, Paganini AM, Quaresima S, Balla A, La Greca G, Plaudis H, Moretto G, Castagnola M, Santi C, Casali L, Tartamella L, Saadi A, Picchetto A, Arezzo A, Marescaux J, Diana M. Fluorescence-based cholangiography: preliminary results from the IHU-IRCAD-EAES EURO-FIGS registry. Surg Endosc. 2020;34(9):3888–96.
16. Kusano M, Tajima Y, Yamazaki K, Kato M, Watanabe M, Miwa M. Sentinel node mapping guided by indocyanine green fluorescence imaging: a new method for sentinel node navigation surgery in gastrointestinal cancer. Dig Surg. 2008;25(2):103–8.
17. Zhang RR, Schroeder AB, Grudzinski JJ, Rosenthal EL, Warram JM, Pinchuk AN, et al. Beyond the margins: real-time detection of cancer using targeted fluorophores. Nat Rev Clin Oncol. 2017;14(6):347–64.

18. van den Bos J, Al-Taher M, Schols RM, van Kuijk S, Bouvy ND, Stassen LPS. Near-infrared fluorescence imaging for real-time intraoperative guidance in anastomotic colorectal surgery: a systematic review of literature. J Laparoendosc Adv Surg Tech A. 2018;28(2):157–67.

19. Baldari L, Boni L, Kurihara H, Cassinotti E. Identification of the ideal weight-based indocyanine green dose for fluorescent cholangiography Surg Endosc. 2023;37(10):7616–24. https://doi.org/10.1007/s00464-023-10280-x.

20. van den Bos J, Wieringa FP, Bouvy ND, Stassen LPS. Optimizing the image of fluorescence cholangiography using ICG: a systematic review and ex vivo experiments. Surg Endosc. 2018;32(12):4820–32.

21. Mieog JSD, Troyan SL, Hutteman M, Donohoe KJ, Van Der Vorst JR, Stockdale A, et al. Toward optimization of imaging system and lymphatic tracer for near-infrared fluorescent sentinel lymph node mapping in breast cancer. Ann Surg Oncol. 2011;18(9):2483–91.

22. Miyashiro I, Miyoshi N, Hiratsuka M, Kishi K, Yamada T, Ohue M, et al. Detection of sentinel node in gastric cancer surgery by indocyanine green fluorescence imaging: comparison with infrared imaging. Ann Surg Oncol. 2008;15(6):1640–3.

23. Mandovra P, Kalikar V, Patankar RV. Real-time visualization of ureters using indocyanine green during laparoscopic surgeries: can we make surgery safer? Surg Innov. 2019;26(4):464–8.

Laparoscopic Nissen Fundoplication, Practical Guideline

7

Nicole D. Bouvy and Selwyn van Rijn

7.1 Laparoscopic Nissen Fundoplication

Laparoscopic Nissen fundoplication consists of the following surgical steps:

- Opening lesser omentum towards the left liver lobe; watch out for an aberrant left hepatic artery and vagal nerve branches to the gallbladder.
- Dissection of the peritoneum at the right side of the crus and at the top of the hiatus.
- Dissection of the crus dorsally towards the confluence.
- Then the stomach is moved to the right to dissect the left side of the crus.
- Care should be taken here with traction on the spleen as this may cause capsule tears leading to haemorrhage.
- Dissection of the short gastric vessels with an energy device (vasa brevia) and thereby mobilisation of the gastric fundus.

- The entire hernia sac should be dissected so that the distal part of the oesophagus remains tension-free in the abdominal cavity for at least 2 cm.
- Placement of a small rubber band around the oesophagus for easy manipulation and optimal exposure of the hiatus.
- Hiatal closure with interrupted sutures with a thick (size 0) braded polyester thread or other non-absorbable suture on the dorsal side of the oesophagus in a 4–1 ratio altered with a ventral to the oesophagus closure suture.
- The gastric fundus of the stomach is wrapped 360 degrees around the lower end of the oesophagus and fixed with 3–4 interrupted sutures using a thick (size 0) braded polyester thread or other non-absorbable suture. Care should be taken during this phase that the wrap is not fixed too tight around the oesophagus thereby causing dysphagia.
- During this procedure constant care should be given not to hurt the anterior nor the posterior vagal nerve (Fig. 7.1).

N. D. Bouvy (✉)
Maastricht University, Maastricht, the Netherlands
e-mail: n.bouvy@mumc.nl

S. van Rijn
Rijnstate Hospital, Arnhem, the Netherlands
e-mail: svanrijn@rijnstate.nl

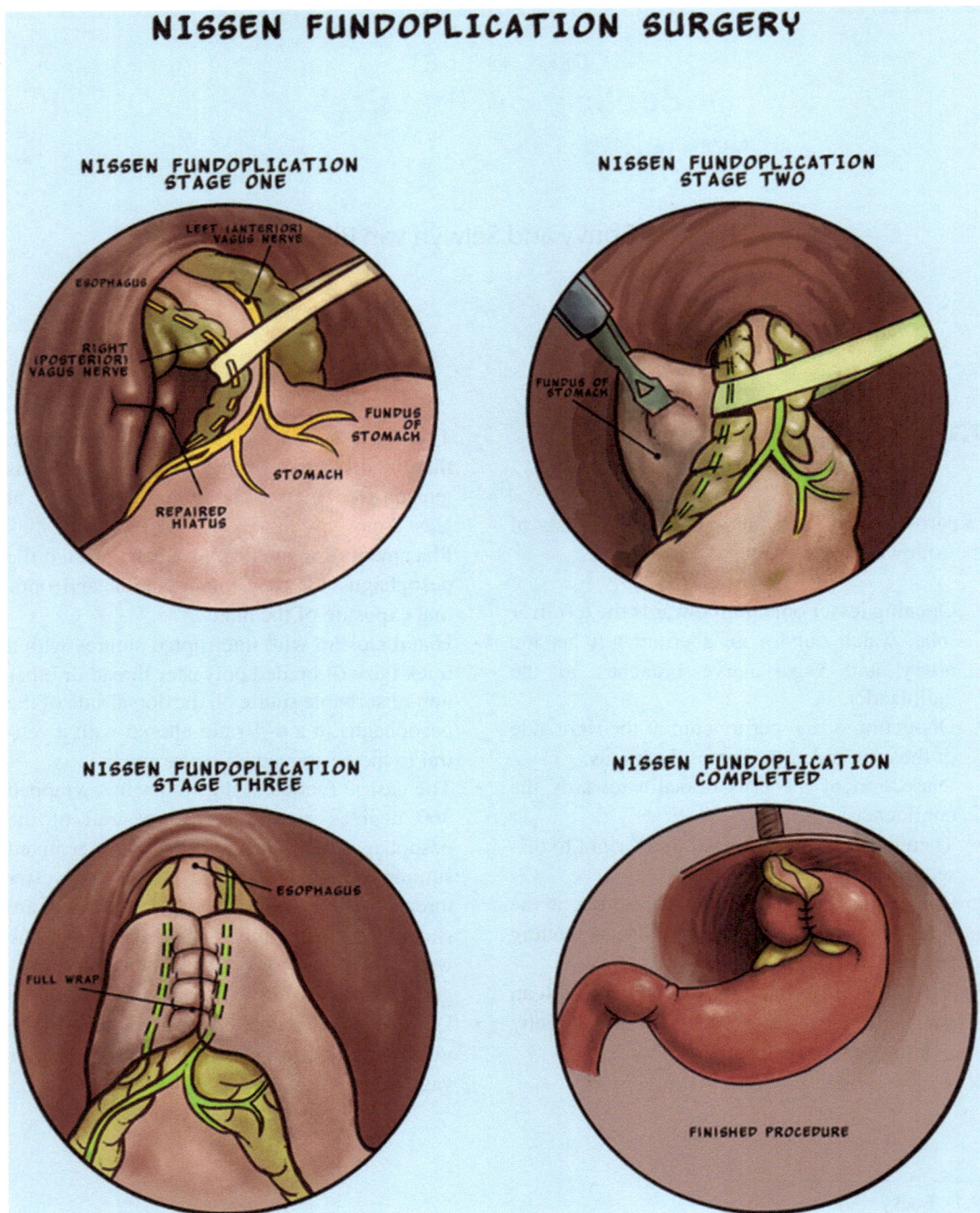

Fig. 7.1 Schematic steps of a laparoscopic Nissen fundoplication

7.2 Patient Positioning and Operating Theatre Setting

The operating theatre setting and patient positioning for a laparoscopic Nissen fundoplication are as follows:

- The patient is positioned in supine position laying on his back (sometimes on a bariatric pillow depending on the patients BMI).
- Both arms can be positioned outward or adducted alongside the patient according to the surgeon's preference.
- Both legs are spread using adjustable leg rests (the patient must be able to be placed in reverse Trendelenburg position up to 20°).
- The two operating screens are placed at the head of the patient.
- The surgeon is positioned between the legs.
- The first assistant, operating the endoscopic camera, is positioned at the right side of the patient.
- The instrument assistant is positioned at the left side of the patient.
- The serving cart is placed at the left side of the instrument nurse.

7.3 Port Placement

Pneumoperitoneum is created either through the Hasson technique (open introduction) or by using the Verres technique (using Verres needle insufflation). The abdomen is inflated until a pressure gradient of 12–14 mmHg is reached.

- Optical 12-mm trocar placement; handbreadth above the umbilicus slightly to the left of the midline.
- 12-mm trocar placed handbreadth to the left of the optical trocar.
- 2 × 5 mm trocar placed handbreadth to the right of the optical trocar with handbreadth distance in between.
- Liver retractor placed subxyphoidal slightly to the left of the midline or in patients with a lower BMI via the 5-mm trocar most laterally

placed underneath the costal margin. Then an extra 5-mm port for retraction of the stomach is placed in the lateral left subcostal margin.

7.4 Surgical Instruments Required

The preparation of the instrument table and the serving cart must be carried out.

Laparoscopic Instruments
- 1× optical trocar (12 mm)
- 1 × 12 mm trocar
- 3 × 5 mm trocar
- Liver retractor (Nathanson), or other 5-mm retractor
- Harmonic ACE curved shears 36 cm or LigaSure Maryland 37 cm
- 3× laparoscopic fenestrated grasping forceps
- 1× endo clinch forceps
- Laparoscopic needle holder
- Laparoscopic dissection/coagulation forceps
- Laparoscopic suction/irrigation system
- Laparoscopic scissors
- Scope warmer

Open Instruments
- 1 scalpel with stainless steel blade (sizes 11–15)
- 1 anatomical tissue forceps
- 2 toothed forceps
- 1 needle holder
- 2 curved Klemmer clamps
- 2 curved Kocher clamps
- 1 Mayo scissors
- 1 Nelson-Metzenbaum dissection scissors
- 2 Langenbeck retractors
- 1 monopolar electric scalpel

7.5 Surgical Steps and Related Instruments

Hasson Technique for Laparoscopic Access
- 1 scalpel (blade 11)
- 2 surgical tissue forceps
- 2 Langenbeck retractors

- 1 Nelson-Metzenbaum dissection scissors
- 2 curved Kocher clamps to grasp fascia and parietal peritoneum

Veress Technique for Laparoscopic Access
- Scalpel (blade 11)
- Veress needle

7.6 Intraoperative Complications

The most frequent intraoperative complications to manage during laparoscopic Nissen fundoplication are basically haemorrhage and injuries of abdominal organs in the operating field (such as the oesophagus, vagal nerve, diaphragm vessels, short gastric vessels, stomach, spleen and liver) [1].

In these circumstances, the instrument nurse must have the following instruments available:

- Laparoscopic suction/irrigation system
- Laparoscopic coagulation forceps/device
- 10 × 10 cm gauze to be passed to the assistant at the request of the surgeon
- Endoscopic clip applier with titanium clips
- Laparoscopic Hem-o-lok applier, with clips already loaded, if the source of bleeding is clearly visible
- Needle holder and monofilament suture with small gauge needle to attempt to stop the bleeding or close the iatrogenic injury
- Laparoscopic vascular clamp
- In case of more severe bleeding, Floseal or instruments to convert to an open procedure

Reference

1. Yadlapati R, Hungness ES, Pandolfino JE. Complications of antireflux surgery. Am J Gastroenterol. 2018;113(8):1137–47.

Robotic Treatment of Functional Esophagogastric Diseases

Antonio Sciuto [ID], Luca Montesarchio [ID], Giuseppina Di Rosa, Felice De Stasio, and Felice Pirozzi [ID]

Functional esophagogastric diseases that are amenable to surgical treatment include primary motility disorders of the esophagus as well as gastroesophageal reflux disease (GERD) and hiatal hernia.

Achalasia is the most common esophageal motility disorder. It is characterized by a functional obstruction at the esophagogastric junction due to the absence of esophageal peristalsis and impaired relaxation of the lower esophageal sphincter (LES) in response to swallowing. Dysphagia, regurgitation, and weight loss are the most frequent symptoms. Surgical treatment of achalasia does not address the issue of decreased motility in the esophageal body but is directed toward relieving the obstruction at the esophagogastric junction. This is achieved by performing a *myotomy*, which was originally described by Ernst Heller in 1913 and involves cutting the muscle fibers of the distal esophagus and proximal stomach, thereby dividing the LES. Since mechanical disruption of the LES can cause symptomatic gastroesophageal reflux, myotomy is usually combined with an anti-reflux procedure called a *fundoplication* which is done by wrapping the fundus of the stomach around the lower esophagus. Typically, a partial (Dor or Toupet) and not a circumferential (Nissen) fundoplication is performed due to poor esophageal motility. The *Dor fundoplication* provides a wrap of approximately 180° anterior to the esophagus, while the *Toupet fundoplication* is a 270° posterior wrap. Without treatment, patients with long-standing achalasia can develop a massive esophageal dilation and atonia (megaesophagus) and finally require esophagectomy [1–6].

GERD is a condition that develops when the reflux of stomach contents into the esophagus causes troublesome symptoms and/or complications. The classic symptoms are heartburn and regurgitation, but patients may also develop respiratory manifestations. From a surgical perspective, GERD is caused by a failure of the anti-reflux barrier at the esophagogastric junction, allowing abnormal backflow of gastric contents and resulting in esophageal injury and/or symptoms. Surgical treatment aims to recreate a barrier that prevents reflux from occurring and involves performing a *hiatoplasty*, which is the surgical repair of the esophageal hiatus of the

A. Sciuto
Department of General Surgery, Santa Maria delle Grazie Hospital, Pozzuoli, Italy

Department of Electrical Engineering and Information Technology, University of Naples Federico II, Naples, Italy
e-mail: antonio.sciuto@aslnapoli2nord.it

L. Montesarchio · G. Di Rosa · F. De Stasio · F. Pirozzi (✉)
Department of General Surgery, Santa Maria delle Grazie Hospital, Pozzuoli, Italy
e-mail: luca.montesarchio@aslnapoli2nord.it;
giuseppina.dirosa@aslnapoli2nord.it;
felice.destasio@aslnapoli2nord.it;
felice.pirozzi@aslnapoli2nord.it

diaphragm, and a fundoplication. The most common type is a *Nissen fundoplication* in which the stomach is wrapped 360° around the lower esophagus, although a Toupet fundoplication may also be performed [1–6].

GERD is often associated with a hiatal hernia. This medical condition refers to a protrusion of any abdominal structure into the thoracic cavity through a widening of the hiatus of the diaphragm. Hiatal hernias are broadly divided into sliding and paraesophageal hernias. Sliding hernias are characterized by the displacement of the gastroesophageal junction above the diaphragm, while paraesophageal hernias entail an upward dislocation of the gastric fundus or any organ other than the stomach (e.g., colon, spleen, pancreas, or small bowel). Patients with sliding hernias may have symptoms of GERD, while paraesophageal hernias usually present with pain, acute or chronic obstructive symptoms, and respiratory symptoms. Sliding hiatal hernias are repaired during surgery for GERD, whereas surgical repair of paraesophageal hernias is usually indicated for symptomatic or complicated hernia. As with sliding hernia, surgery involves performing a hiatoplasty and a fundoplication. Patients with paraesophageal hernias may develop acute gastric volvulus, which is characterized by rotation of the stomach along its long or short axis and may require urgent surgery, with gastrectomy if necrosis or perforation occurs [1–6].

Surgery for the aforementioned diseases is performed through an abdominal approach. Transthoracic procedures for anti-reflux surgery and hiatal hernia repair have been reported but are rarely used in contemporary surgical practice. In this chapter, transabdominal procedures using the da Vinci Xi robotic platform are described.

8.1 Surgical Technique

8.1.1 Cardioesophageal Myotomy for Achalasia

The surgical procedure for the treatment of achalasia can be divided into two phases: myotomy and fundoplication.

8.1.1.1 Heller Myotomy

Myotomy is performed on the anterior wall at the cardia and involves the following surgical steps:

- Division of the phrenoesophageal ligament and dissection along the anterior aspect of the esophagus up to the mediastinum, taking care to identify and preserve the anterior vagus nerve
- Division of the gastrophrenic ligament and short gastric vessels
- Division of the longitudinal muscle fibers 6–7 cm along the distal esophagus and approximately 2 cm onto the proximal gastric wall
- Division of the underlying circular muscle fibers for the same length and exposure of the submucosal plane
- Transoral insertion of a lighted bougie dilator (or endoscope) to check the complete division of muscle fibers and to identify and repair any mucosal perforations.

8.1.1.2 Dor Fundoplication

This is an anterior partial fundoplication and involves the following surgical steps:

- Grasping the gastric fundus and placement alongside the myotomy
- Suturing the medial aspect of the fundus to the left side of the myotomy
- Folding the anterior fundus over the myotomy
- Suturing the fundus to right side of the esophagus and the right crus

8.1.2 Anti-reflux Surgery

The surgical procedure for the management of GERD can be divided into two phases: hiatoplasty and fundoplication.

8.1.2.1 Hiatoplasty

Hiatoplasty involves the following surgical steps:

- Division of the short gastric vessels and dissection of the left crus of the diaphragm

- Division of the gastrohepatic omentum and dissection of the right crus
- Division of the phrenoesophageal ligament and mobilization of the distal portion of the mediastinal esophagus, taking care to identify and preserve the vagus nerves
- Crural closure with sutures and transoral insertion of a bougie dilator to test the adequacy of closure
- Crural reinforcement with mesh when indicated

8.1.2.2 Nissen Fundoplication

This is a complete fundoplication and involves the following surgical steps:

- Grasping and passing the gastric fundus behind the esophagus from left to right to obtain a fold of fundus wall on each side of the esophagus
- Reinserting a bougie dilator to calibrate the fundoplication
- Approximating and suturing the two folds of the fundus wall together anterior to the esophagus
- Securing the fundoplication with additional sutures.

8.1.3   Paraesophageal Hernia Repair

The surgical procedure for paraesophageal hernia repair can be divided into two phases: hiatoplasty and fundoplication.

8.1.3.1 Hiatoplasty

The surgical steps are as follows:

- Dissection of the hernia sac from the mediastinal structures, reduction into the abdominal cavity, and excision
- Division of the short gastric vessels and dissection of the left crus of the diaphragm
- Division of the gastrohepatic omentum and dissection of the right crus
- Mobilization of the distal portion of the mediastinal esophagus

- Crural closure with sutures and transoral insertion of a lighted bougie dilator to test the adequacy of closure
- Crural reinforcement with mesh when indicated

8.1.3.2 Toupet Fundoplication

This is a posterior partial fundoplication and involves the following surgical steps:

- Grasping and passing the gastric fundus behind the esophagus from left to right to obtain a fold of the fundus wall on each side of the esophagus
- Suturing the two folds of the fundus wall to the anterolateral aspect of the esophagus on both sides
- Securing the fundoplication with additional sutures

Two supplementary procedures may be needed during paraesophageal hernia repair:

- A Collis gastroplasty: a procedure used to lengthen the esophagus by removing a portion of the gastric fundus by means of a linear stapler
- An anterior gastropexy: placement of one or more sutures fixing the anterior gastric wall to the inner abdominal wall

8.2   Operating Theatre Setting

The operating theatre for all the above surgeries is set up as follows (Fig. 8.1):

- Operating table in the center of the theatre
- Vision cart to the right of the patient, at the level of the feet
- Supplementary monitor to the left of the patient, at the level of the shoulder (if not available, the vision cart replaces the monitor)
- Patient cart to the right of the patient
- Surgeon at the robotic console
- First assistant at the operating table between the patient's legs

Fig. 8.1 Schematic view of the operating room setup

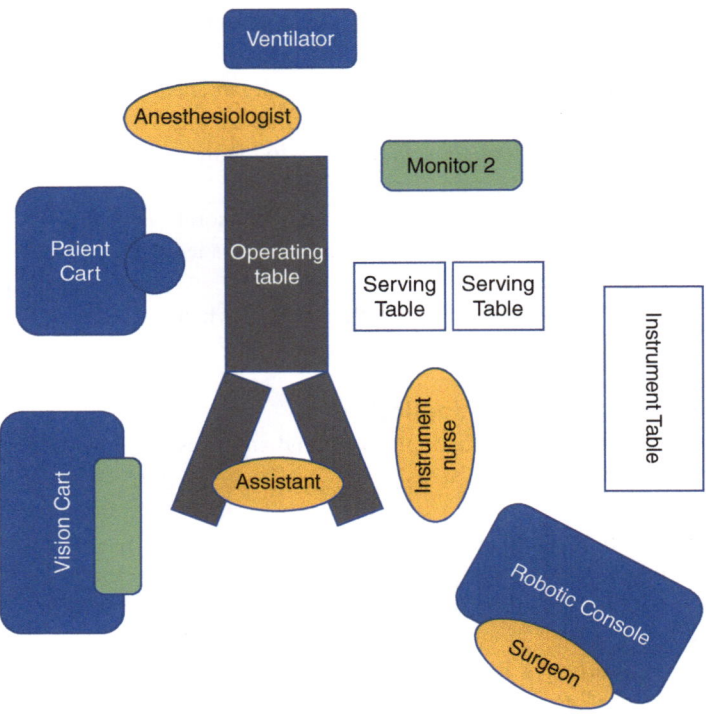

- Instrument nurse to the right of the first assistant
- Serving table to the right of instrument nurse

8.3 Patient Positioning

Surgery is performed under general anesthesia. The patient is positioned as shown in Fig. 8.2:

- Supine with 15–20° reverse Trendelenburg tilt
- Both arms alongside the body
- Legs apart

A viscoelastic mat (CarePad®) is placed on the operating table to prevent the patient sliding throughout surgical procedures and to reduce the risk of pressure injuries.

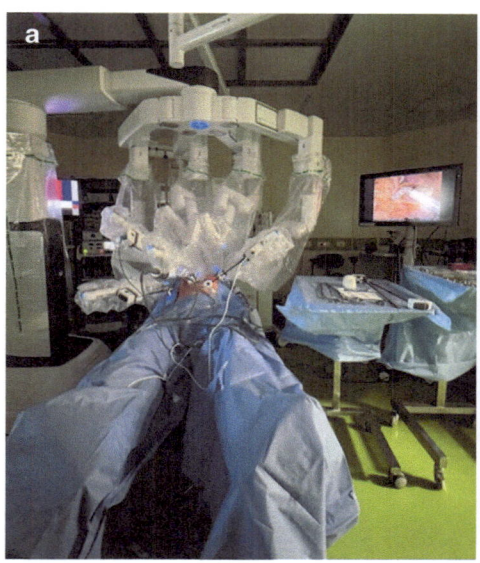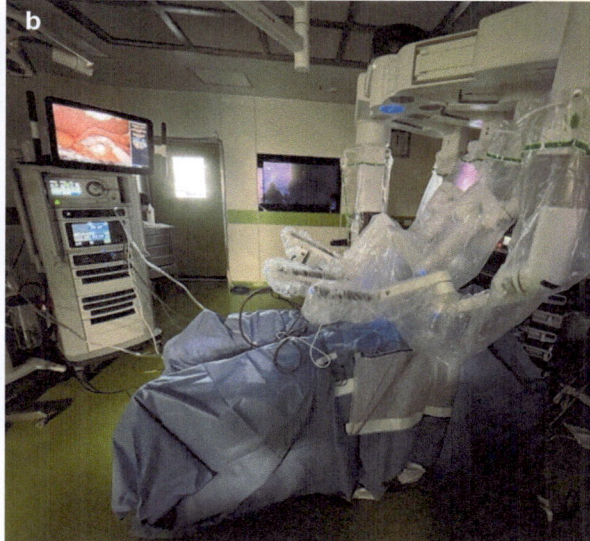

Fig. 8.2 Patient position: frontal view (**a**) and side view (**b**)

8.4   Port Placement and Robotic Docking

A 12-mmHg pneumoperitoneum is achieved by using a Veress needle through a small incision in the left upper quadrant. Subsequently, sterile marker and ruler may be used for drawing bone reliefs and port sites on the patient skin.

Four 8-mm robotic ports and one assistant port (AirSeal® Access Port) are used. Robotic ports are placed at least 8 cm from each other along a transverse line located approximately 4 cm above the transverse umbilical line. The assistant port is placed below the robotic ports, 5–10 cm away, on the left side of the abdomen (Fig. 8.3). However, port location may partially change according to the patient's body habitus and the position of the transverse umbilical line, considering that the distance between the line of the robotic ports and the target anatomy should not exceed 20 cm.

The port for the endoscope is placed first after a saline drop test is performed in the periumbilical area, while the remaining working ports are placed under direct vision. An empty trocar may be used to create an indentation on the patient's skin and subsequently create a skin incision.

A sterile staff member docks the arm used for the endoscope (usually arm no. 3) to the endoscope port and then installs the endoscope onto the port. Next, the endoscope is inserted to point the target anatomy which is the left lobe of the liver. Once targeting—the selection of the target anatomy through the endoscope—is complete, and the endoscope is aligned with the target anatomy, the rest of the arms can be docked and positioned, leaving a fist-width space between the arms and between the patient and the arms. Next, instruments may be inserted.

8.5   Surgical Instruments

The instrument table and the serving cart may be set up as shown in Fig. 8.4. The instruments may vary according to the surgeon's habits and the composition of the surgical containers.

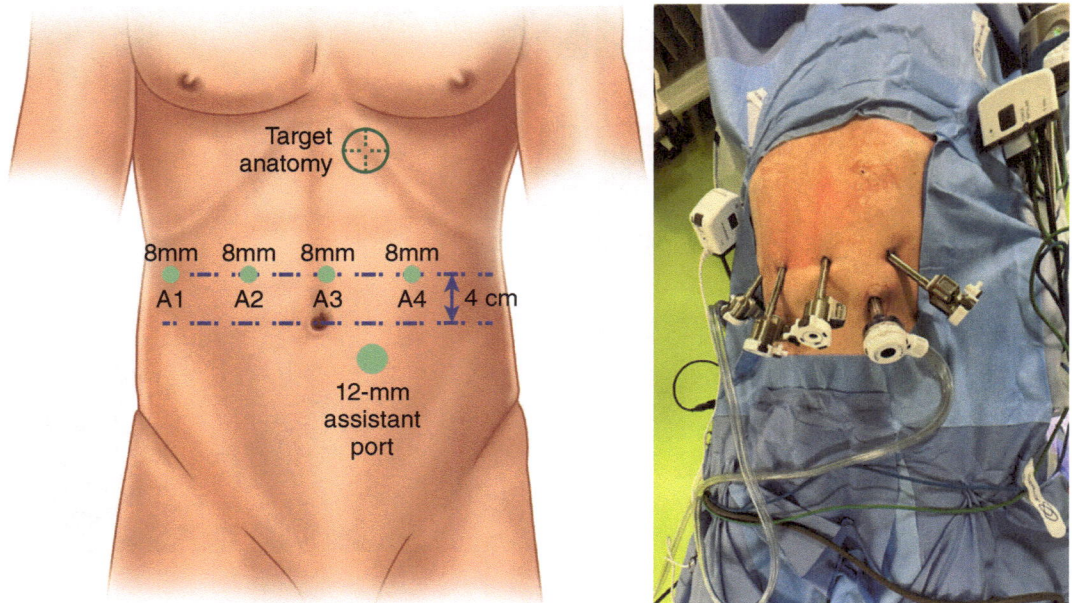

Fig. 8.3 Port placement

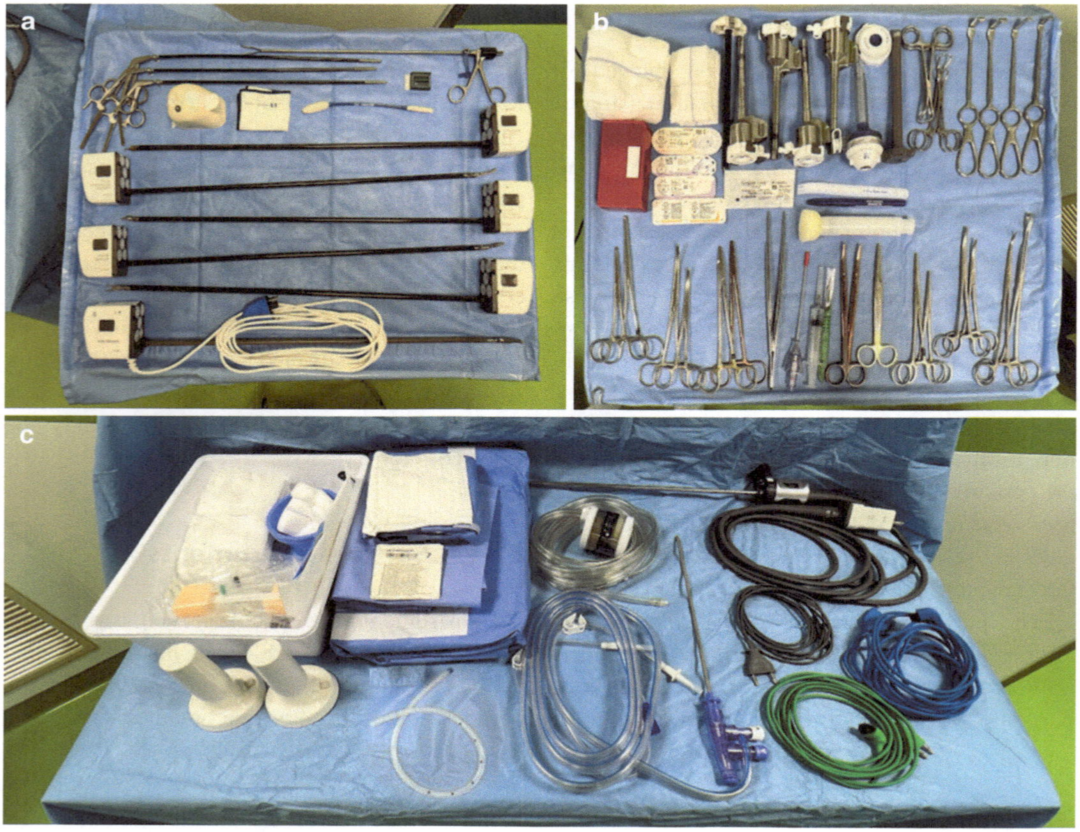

Fig. 8.4 Serving tables (**a**, **b**) and instrument table (**c**)

8.5.1   Robotic instruments

- Four 8-mm ports
- 30° endoscope
- 1 grasping forceps (Tip-Up Fenestrated Grasper®)
- 1 bipolar forceps (Fenestrated Bipolar Forceps®)
- 1 monopolar instrument (Permanent Cautery Hook®)
- 1 sealing instrument (Vessel Sealer® or SynchroSeal®)
- 1 needle holder with suture cutter (Large SutureCut™ Needle Driver®)
- 1 clip applier (Medium-Large Clip Applier® with Hem-o-lok® ligating clips)

One 12-mm port and port reducer and one linear stapler (SureForm™ Stapler® 45 or 60 mm) are needed if a Collis gastroplasty is required.

8.5.2   Laparoscopic Instruments

- One 12-mm assistant port (AirSeal® Access Port) with insufflation tubing
- 2 grasping forceps (Johann forceps)
- 1 suction/irrigation system (Dolphin evo®)
- 1 bipolar forceps

Laparoscopic scissors (or energy devices) are needed if adhesiolysis is performed before robotic docking, while a fibrin glue (Tisseel® or Evicel®) applicator is needed for mesh hiatoplasty.

8.5.3   Open Instruments

- 1 scalpel (no. 11 blade)
- 2 anatomical tissue forceps
- 2 Nelson-Metzenbaum dissection scissors
- 1 Mayo scissors
- 2 needle holders
- 2 curved Klemmer forceps
- 2 straight Klemmer forceps
- 2 curved Kocher forceps
- 2 straight Kocher forceps
- 1 curved Bengolea forceps
- 1 Foerster forceps

- 4 Backhaus clamps
- 2 Langenbeck retractors

8.5.4   Other Devices

- Sterile surgical gloves, gowns, and drapes
- Sterile gauzes (5 × 30 cm and 10 × 20 cm)
- Sterile marker and ruler
- Antiseptic solution (Nex Clorex 2% chlorhexidine/70% alcohol prep applicator)
- 1 Veress needle
- One 10-mL syringe filled with 2 mL of saline
- 1 endoscope cleaning device (Clearify™ Visualization System)
- 1 basin
- 1 surgical loop
- 1 bougie dilator
- 2 or more polyester sutures (2-0 Ethicon Ethibond Excel®)
- Absorbable sutures (0 Coated Vicryl™ *Plus* with 5/8 circle needle; 3-0 Coated Vicryl™ Rapide)
- 1 sharp disposal and needle counter box

If needed:

- Biosynthetic mesh (GORE® BIO-A® Tissue Reinforcement)
- Additional absorbable sutures (3-0 Coated Vicryl™ *Plus*)

8.6   Surgical Steps and Related Instruments

The technique for access to the abdominal cavity as well as port placement and robotic docking is the same for all the surgical procedures described above.

8.6.1   Veress-Assisted Technique for Access to the Abdominal Cavity

- 1 scalpel (no. 11 blade)
- 1 Veress needle
- 1 syringe for saline drop test

8.6.2 Port Placement and Robotic Docking

- 1 sterile marker and ruler to measure the distance between the ports
- 1 scalpel (no. 11 blade)
- Four 8-mm robotic ports
- One 12-mm assistant port (AirSeal® Access Port) with insufflation tubing
- 30° robotic endoscope

The instruments needed to perform myotomy, hiatoplasty, and fundoplication are as follows:

8.6.3 Heller Myotomy

The robotic instruments used by the surgeon at the surgical console are as follows:

- 30° endoscope
- Grasping forceps (Tip-up Fenestrated Grasper®)
- Bipolar forceps (Fenestrated Bipolar Forceps®)
- Monopolar instrument (Permanent Cautery Hook®)
- Sealing instrument (Vessel Sealer® or SynchroSeal®)
- Clip applier (Medium-Large Clip Applier® with Hem-o-lok® ligating clips)

Robotic grasping forceps and energy devices are used for surgical dissection and division of muscle fibers, which is usually performed by using the electrocautery hook or a sealing instrument. The clip applier is used for vessel ligation. The needle holder with suture cutter is required if the esophagus is perforated during the myotomy and the hole is repaired with an absorbable suture.

The laparoscopic instruments used by the first assistant at the operating table are as follows:

- Grasping forceps (Johann forceps)
- Suction/irrigation system (Dolphin evo®)

Grasping forceps are used to assist in exposing surgical structures and for passing and with-drawing gauzes (and sutures if needed). The suction irrigation system is employed to keep the abdominal cavity clear of liquids and blood.

Other devices used during this phase are as follows:

- A gauze soaked in the diluted epinephrine
- A lighted bougie dilator
- Absorbable sutures

The gauze can be placed on small vessels to reduce bleeding during division of muscle fibers, while the bougie is used to check the complete division of muscle fibers and to identify and repair any mucosal perforations.

8.6.4 Hiatoplasty

The robotic instruments used by the surgeon at the surgical console are as follows:

- 30° endoscope
- Grasping forceps (Tip-up Fenestrated Grasper®)
- Bipolar forceps (Fenestrated Bipolar Forceps®)
- Monopolar instrument (Permanent Cautery Hook®)
- Sealing instrument (Vessel Sealer® or SynchroSeal®)
- Needle holder with suture cutter (Large SutureCut™ Needle Driver®)
- Clip applier (Medium-Large Clip Applier® with Hem-o-lok® ligating clips)

Robotic grasping forceps and energy devices are used for surgical dissection, crural closure, and hernia sac excision, while the clip applier is employed for vessel ligation. The needle holder is used for crural closure.

The laparoscopic instruments used by the first assistant at the operating table are as follows:

- Grasping forceps (Johann forceps)
- Suction/irrigation system (Dolphin evo®)
- Fibrin glue (Tisseel® or Evicel®) applicator (for mesh hiatoplasty)

Grasping forceps are used to assist in exposing surgical structures, for passing and withdrawing gauzes and sutures (and mesh if needed), and for removing the excised hernia sac. The fibrin glue applicator is needed to fix the mesh when a mesh hiatoplasty is performed.

Other devices used during this phase are as follows:

- Surgical loop (or Penrose drain);
- Polyester sutures (2-0 Ethicon Ethibond Excel®)
- Bougie dilator
- Biosynthetic mesh (GORE® BIO-A® Tissue Reinforcement)
- Absorbable sutures (3-0 Coated Vicryl™ *Plus*)

A surgical loop (or Penrose drain) is usually placed around the gastroesophageal junction to provide traction by the first assistant. Crural closure is performed by using polyester sutures, and a bougie dilator is used to test the adequacy of closure. A biosynthetic mesh is used for reinforcement of crural closure when needed, and absorbable sutures are employed to fix the mesh in addition to fibrin glue.

8.6.5 Fundoplication

The robotic instruments used by the surgeon at the surgical console are the following:

- 30° endoscope
- Grasping forceps (Tip-up Fenestrated Grasper®)
- Bipolar forceps (Fenestrated Bipolar Forceps®)
- Sealing instrument (Vessel Sealer® or SynchroSeal®)
- Needle holder with suture cutter (Large SutureCut™ Needle Driver®)

Robotic forceps and sealing instruments are used for grasping the stomach, while sutures are placed and cut by employing the needle holder. Energy devices may also be used for hemostasis.

The laparoscopic instruments used by the first assistant at the operating table are the following:

- Grasping forceps (Johann forceps)
- Suction/irrigation system (Dolphin evo®)

Grasping forceps are used to assist in exposing surgical structures and grasping the stomach and for passing and withdrawing gauzes (and sutures if needed). The suction irrigation system is employed to keep the abdominal cavity clear of liquids and blood.

Other devices used during this phase are as follows:

- Surgical loop (or Penrose drain)
- Polyester sutures (2-0 Ethicon Ethibond Excel)
- Bougie dilator.

A surgical loop (or Penrose drain) is used to provide traction on the gastroesophageal junction by the first assistant when circumferential dissection of the esophagus is performed (Nissen or Toupet fundoplication). A bougie dilator is employed for calibration when a complete or Nissen fundoplication is performed.

8.6.5.1 Closure of Abdominal Incision
- Laparoscopic bipolar forceps
- Langenbeck retractors
- Needle holders
- Anatomical forceps
- Curved Klemmer forceps
- Absorbable sutures (0 Coated Vicryl™ *Plus* with 5/8 circle needle; 3-0 Coated Vicryl™ Rapide)

Laparoscopic bipolar forceps are used to control or prevent bleeding from the port sites. Fascial closure is performed at the 12-mm port site by using Langenbeck retractors and 0 absorbable sutures with 5/8 circle needle, while skin incisions are closed with 3-0 absorbable sutures.

8.7 Intraoperative Complications

The most frequent intraoperative complications include bleeding from injury to the upper abdominal vessels or organs (spleen, liver), tear of the esophageal or gastric wall, injury to the vagus nerves, and pneumothorax.

When bleeding occurs, the following instruments should be promptly available:

- Laparoscopic suction/irrigation system
- Bipolar forceps (robotic and/or laparoscopic forceps)
- Gauzes to be passed by the first assistant
- Robotic clip applier with a clip already loaded
- Laparoscopic grasping forceps (or vascular clamps)
- Robotic needle driver with small caliber sutures
- Topical hemostatic agents (e.g., Floseal®, Hemopatch®, etc.)

Life-threatening hemorrhages due to injury to major vessels (inferior vena cava, aorta, left hepatic vein, etc.) or cardiac tamponade are rare and usually require conversion to open surgery or open repair.

Esophageal and gastric tears can be repaired by fine absorbable sutures.

Division of only the anterior or posterior vagus nerve is usually not repaired, as postoperative symptoms (early satiety, bloating, diarrhea, dumping syndrome) rarely occur with a unilateral vagotomy. Otherwise, a pyloroplasty—transverse closure of a longitudinal pyloromyotomy—might be performed.

A pneumothorax can be caused by inadvertent injury to the pleura during mobilization of the distal esophagus. Neither a suture nor a chest tube is required in most patients.

References

1. Ponsky JR, Rosen MJ. Atlas of surgical techniques for the upper gastrointestinal tract and small bowel. Philadelphia: Saunders Elsevier; 2010.
2. Izbicki JR, Broering DC, Yekebas EF, Kutup A, Chernousov AF, Gallinger YI, et al. Surgery of the esophagus. In: Textbook and atlas of surgical practice. Heidelberg: Steinkopff Heidelberg; 2009.
3. Oelschlager BK, Petersen RP. Surgical myotomy for achalasia. In: UpToDate, Post TW, editors. Waltham: UpToDate.
4. Schwaitzberg SD. Surgical management of gastroesophageal reflux in adults. In: UpToDate, Post TW, editor. Waltham: UpToDate.
5. Kohn GP, Price RR, DeMeester SR, Zehetner J, Muensterer OJ, Awad Z, et al. Guidelines for the management of hiatal hernia. Surg Endosc. 2013;27(12):4409–28.
6. Melotti G, Trapani V, Frazzoni M, Varoli M, Piccoli M. Anti-reflux procedures and cardioesophagomyotomy. In: Spinoglio G, editor. Robotic surgery. Updates in surgery. Milano: Springer; 2015. p. 51–8.

Total Minimally Invasive Ivor Lewis Esophagectomy (TMIE)

9

Roberto Quattromani, Francesco Puccetti, Andrea Cossu, Lavinia Barbieri, Lorenzo Cinelli, Umberto Casiraghi, Ugo Elmore, and Riccardo Rosati

9.1 Two-Field Esophagectomy

In 1946, Ivor Lewis introduced the two-field esophageal resection, including the opening of both abdominal and right thoracic spaces [1]. Since then, this procedure progressively evolved up to getting completely performed minimally invasive [2–6].

A comprehensive description of the total minimally invasive Ivor Lewis esophagectomy follows:

9.2 Abdominal Stage (Laparoscopy)

Consecutive sequence of the main stages:

1. *Kocher maneuver,* to obtain a complete duodenal mobilization and a consequent exten-

R. Quattromani · A. Cossu · L. Barbieri · L. Cinelli · U. Casiraghi
Department of Surgery, San Raffaele Hospital, Via Olgettina Milano, Milan, Italy
e-mail: quattromani.roberto@hsr.it; cossu.andrea@hsr.it; barbieri.lavinia@hsr.it; cinelli.lorenzo@hsr.it; casiraghi.umberto@hsr.it

F. Puccetti · U. Elmore (✉) · R. Rosati
Department of Surgery, San Raffaele Hospital, Via Olgettina Milano, Milan, Italy

Vita-Salute San Raffaele University, Milan, Italy
e-mail: puccetti.francesco@hsr.it; elmore.ugo@hsr.it; rosati.riccardo@hsr.it

sion of the proximal stomach up to the upper mediastinum.

2. *Pyloromyotomy and pyloroplasty,* to decrease the pyloric stenosis/resistance to the gastroduodenal passage of bolus after surgery.
3. *The dissection of the lesser omentum,* to allow a complete exposure of the retrogastric and celiac regions.
4. *Extended abdominal lymphadenectomy*, including celiac and lesser curvature stations, such as no. 1, 2, 3, 5, 7, 8a, 9, 11p, 11d, and 12a.
5. *Left gastric vessel ligation with preservation of the right gastric artery,* to create a simultaneous gastric mobilization and adequate pyloric perfusion and patency.
6. *Gastrolysis,* or completion of the stomach mobilization, is achieved by the dissection of the gastrocolic ligament along the greater curvature with preservation of the right gastroepiploic artery (RGA).
7. *Intraoperative fluorescence-mediated angiography* with indocyanine green (ICG) dye to assess the integrity of the gastroepiploic arcade and visceral perfusion of the stomach before fashioning the conduit.
8. *Conduit fashioning,* a four- to five-centimeter-wide gastric conduit is shaped through multiple mechanical linear sutures running parallel to the greater curvature.

9. *Feeding jejunostomy*, this supporting device is routinely placed in all patients presenting with a Nutritional Risk Screening score (Jens Kondrup et al.) higher than two.

10. *Peritoneal colopexy,* the suture between the splenic flexure and the abdominal wall represents a useful way to prevent the diaphragmatic hernia from occurring after esophagectomy. This can be done with Filbloc® 3-0 suture (26 mm 1/2 circle taper point).

11. *The opening of the right pleura and positioning of transdiaphragmatic drainage,* the circumferential dissection/mobilization of the distal esophagus gives access to the right thoracic space and allows the insertion of a suctioning Jackson-Pratt drainage through the hiatal space. During the circumferential dissection of the lower esophagus, a section of the right diaphragmatic pillar can be performed to facilitate the conduit transposition to the chest.

12. *Intraoperative fluorescence-mediated lymphography,* the US-guided ICG injection at the level of inguinal lymph nodes bilateral to achieve a fluorescent lymphography for an accurate thoracic duct identification.

9.3 Abdominal Stage (Laparoscopy), Description

9.3.1 General Anesthesia

The surgical operation requires a general anesthesia and intubation with a double-lumen endotracheal tube (Robertshaw) allowing the possibility of selective pulmonary ventilation.

Further anesthesiological supplies include an artery line (usually at the radial artery) for invasive blood pressure monitoring, a nasogastric double-lumen tube (16- or 18-Fr double-lumen nasogastric tube, Salem type), two peripheric venous lines, a central venous catheter, and a urinary catheter with temperature sensor.

To prevent hypothermia and respective negatives, the patient's temperature is maintained through an active body surface warming system (Bair Hugger) and the fluid administration at 36 °C (hot-line system).

9.3.2 Patient and Operators' Positioning

A lithotomy position (i.e., supine split-leg or French position), as shown in Fig. 9.1, involves patient lying:

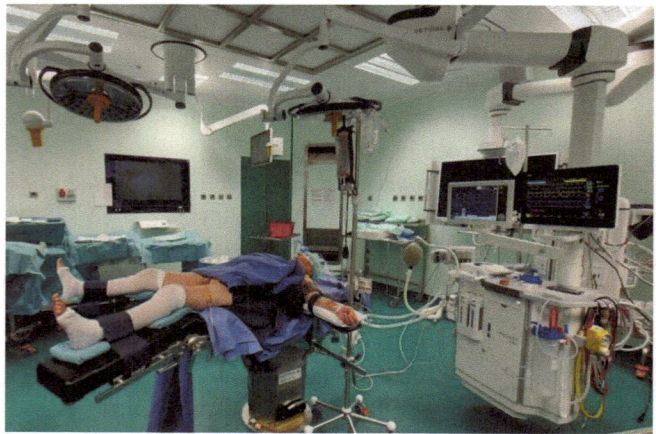
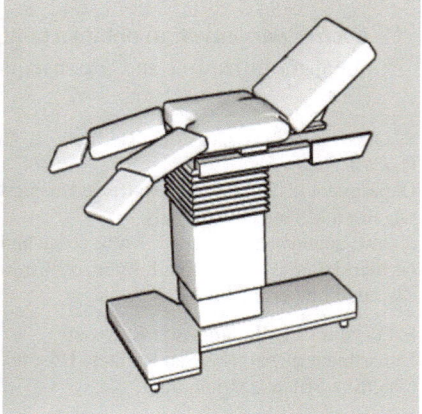

Fig. 9.1 Patient positioning during the abdominal stage

Fig. 9.2 Schematic operating theatre setting during the abdominal stage (laparoscopy). (Author: Roberto Quattromani)

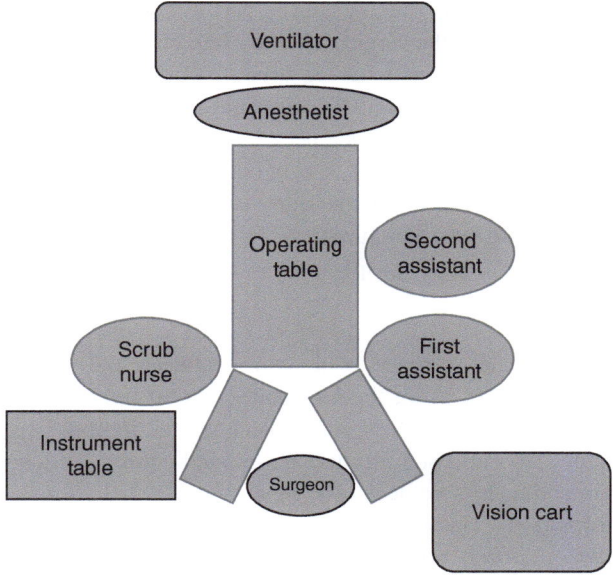

- Face up
- With the right arm to the side
- The left one in extension
- Legs abducted 30–45° from midline

As shown in Fig. 9.2 the surgeons should stand between the open legs (chief) and at the patient's left side (assistants). The scrub nurse resides on the right side with the stand behind, between them and the chief surgeon.

Before starting surgery, the operating table has to be inclined in a reverse Trendelenburg tilt.

9.4   Trocar Positioning

Laparoscopic incisions are made supraumbilical first (i.e., the level between the umbilicus and the xiphoid process is slightly variable and depending on the patient's body constitution), and a Hasson trocar is placed to progressively establish a 12-mmHg pneumoperitoneum.

This procedure has to be run with a 10-mm, 30-degrees inclined camera, optionally supporting the NIR imaging for the intraoperative fluorescence. After the induction of the pneumoperitoneum, the laparoscope insertion allows an accurate inspection of the abdominal cavity and confirmation of the planned surgery.

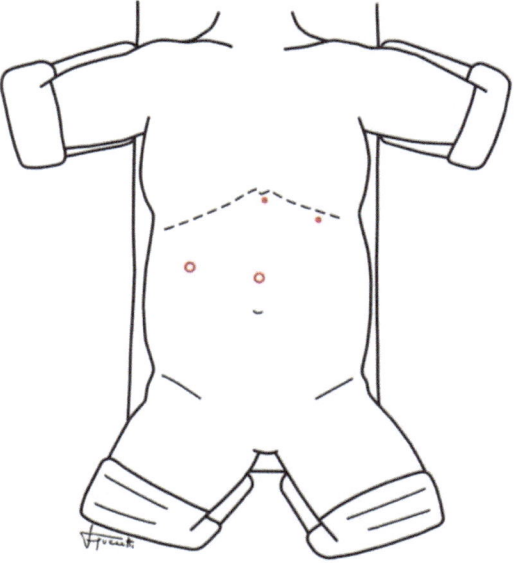

Fig. 9.3 Trocar positioning (laparoscopy). (Author: Francesco Puccetti)

In the absence of findings consistent with an unresectable tumor, three more ports are placed at the following standardized abdominal sites (shown in Fig. 9.3):

- Two 5-mm ports are positioned at the upper and the left subcostal area, respectively. The former allows the assistant to perform a wide exposure of the surgical field by retracting the liver, while the latter is used by the chief surgeon to handle their right-side instrument (energy device, grasper, needle holder, etc.)

- A 5- to 12-mm port is eventually placed at the right flank, on the transverse umbilical line, for the chief surgeon's left hand instrument (10-mm grasper and a 12-mm linear stapler).

The chief surgeon will stand between the patient's legs, using the left hand (12-mm right flank port) for graspers and staplers and the right hand (left subcostal 5-mm port) to handle graspers and energy devices. The laparoscope is held through the Hasson trocar by an assistant, while the other can retract the liver from the upper trocar.

At the end of the operation, trocars have to be removed under visual control (to avoid chances of postoperative port bleedings) and all 5- to 12-mm ports closed with an endoclosure device (Polysorb® 0), while titanium clips/sutures are used for the skin closure.

9.5 Abdominal Lymphadenectomy

An extended lymphadenectomy (12a, 5, 8a, 9, 7, 3, 2, 1, 11p, and 11d) is routinely performed due to the high incidence of lymph node metastases coming with esophageal cancer, especially when the lower or junctional esophagus is involved.

Similar to gastrectomy, lymphadenectomy starts from the upper pancreatic margin and runs through the adventitial surface of the hepatic artery, up to the distal splenic artery lymph node stations.

An energy device performing dissection and sealing for minor vessel and lymphatic ducts, represents the best dissecting instrument for lymphadenectomy since its capacity of lymphatic spillage prevention and the reduction of intra-abdominal liberation of circulating tumor cells.

The only caution to be observed consists of small "bites," meant as the size of individual dissections, leading to a greater accuracy and lower rates of iatrogenic injuries.

The list of lymph node stations is summarized in Table 9.1.

Table 9.1 JCGA Abdominal Lymph-node stations

1	Right paracardial (including those around the esophageal branch of the left gastric artery in front of the right diaphragmatic crus)
2	Left paracardial (including those around the esophageal branch of the left inferior phrenic artery)
3a	Lesser curvature, along the left gastric artery branches
3b	Lesser curvature, along the distal part of right gastric artery and its second branch
4sa	Greater curvature, along the short gastric arteries (perigastric area)
4sb	Greater curvature, along the left gastroepiploic artery (perigastric area)
4d	Greater curvature (second branch and distal part of the right gastroepiploic artery)
5	Suprapyloric (around the right gastric artery and its first branch into the hepatoduodenal ligament)
6	Infrapyloric (around the origin and the proximal part of the right gastroepiploic artery near the gastrocolic trunk of Henle)
7	Left gastric artery (around the tract of the artery between its origin from the celiac trunk and the origin of its ascending branch, i.e., its entrance into the small omentum where it relates to the gastric lesser curvature)
8a	Common hepatic artery, anterosuperior group
8p	Common hepatic artery, posterior group
9	Celiac trunk
10	Splenic hilum: lymph nodes associated with the splenic artery between the hilum and pancreatic tail, lymph nodes at the root of short gastric arteries, and lymph nodes along the left gastroepiploic artery proximal to its first gastric branch
11p	Splenic artery, proximal (from its origin to half its length between its origin and the end of the pancreatic tail)
11d	Splenic artery, distal (from the middle of its length between its origin and the end of the pancreatic tail to the pancreatic tail)

Table 9.1 (continued)

12a	Hepatoduodenal ligament, along the proper hepatic artery in the caudal half between the confluence of the hepatic ducts and the upper margin of the pancreas
12b	Hepatoduodenal ligament, along the biliary tract in the caudal half between the confluence of the hepatic ducts and the upper margin of the pancreas
12p	Hepatoduodenal ligament, in the caudal half of the portal vein between the confluence of the hepatic ducts and the upper border of the pancreas
13	Posterior surface of the pancreatic head (in relation to the posterior pancreatic-duodenal arterial arch and cranial to the duodenal papilla)
14v	Superior mesenteric vein
14a	Root of superior mesenteric artery (between the origin of the superior mesenteric artery, the trunk of Henle on the right and the jejunal vessels caudally)
15	Middle colic vessels
16a1	Aortic hiatus
16a2	Para-aortic from the upper margin of the celiac trunk origin to the lower margin of the left renal vein
16b1	Para-aortic from the lower margin of the left renal vein to the upper margin of the inferior mesenteric artery
16b2	Para-aortic from the superior margin of the origin of the inferior mesenteric artery to the aortic bifurcation
17	Anterior surface of the pancreatic head
18	Lower margin of the pancreatic body
19	Infradiaphragmatic, mainly along the inferior phrenic artery
20	Paraesophageal (esophageal hiatus of the diaphragm)

9.6 The Gastric Conduit

Fashioning the gastric conduit includes different surgical procedures, which are performed with the following aims:

- *Verification of adequate pyloric patency*
  - *Pyloromyotomy and pyloroplasty:* a longitudinal incision is made (with or without the mucosal layer preservation), closed with a transverse discontinued suture with PDS 3-0 stitches.
  - *Preservation of the pyloric (right gastric) artery.*
- *Gastric mobilization and extension*
  - *Kocher maneuver:* the detachment of the duodenum from the retroperitoneum along an avascular surface. It has to be a blunt dissection and can be done through grasping tractions and bipolar cauterization.
  - *Ligation and dissection of left gastric vessels:* the accurate identification of both left gastric vein and artery does allow their ligation with metallic clips and interruption with the energy device.
  - *Gastrolysis:* gastrocolic ligament dissection along the greater curvature is per-formed, by preserving the gastroepiploic artery. Gastric fundus mobilization is then obtained through the ligation of short gastrics and left gastroepiploic vessels. Preserving the right gastroepiploic vessels is mandatory to guarantee a sufficient stomach blood supply.
  - *Conduit shaping:* starting from the Crow's foot, the gastric conduit fashioning is performed through multiple shoots of linear staplers (i.e., Echelon 45-mm 3.8-mm Tri-Staple) along the lesser curvature up to the gastric fundus. The stapler enters the abdomen from the right 12-mm trocar. The gastric conduit needs to be wide enough in order to ensure a proper gastric intraparietal (submucosal) blood supply.
- *Maintenance of an adequate visceral perfusion*
  - *Preservation the gastroepiploic artery.*
  - *Intraoperative fluorescence-mediated angiography:* After the gastrolysis, an intraoperative angiography with ICG will assess the gastroepiploic arcade integrity and the gastric conduit blood perfusion.

9.7 US-Guided Inguinal Nodes ICG Injection

After the abdominal stage, an US-guided ICG injection of bilateral inguinal lymph nodes is performed to spread the ICG dye over the lymphatic system and allow a clear NIR identification of the thoracic duct during the second stage (right thoracoscopy).

9.7.1 Patient and Operator Positioning

A supine position, as shown in Fig. 9.4, involves patient lying:

– Face up
– With the right arm to the side
– The left one in extension
– Adducted legs

The chief surgeon should stand at the patient's right side and the US monitor to the patient's left side, in front of the operator.

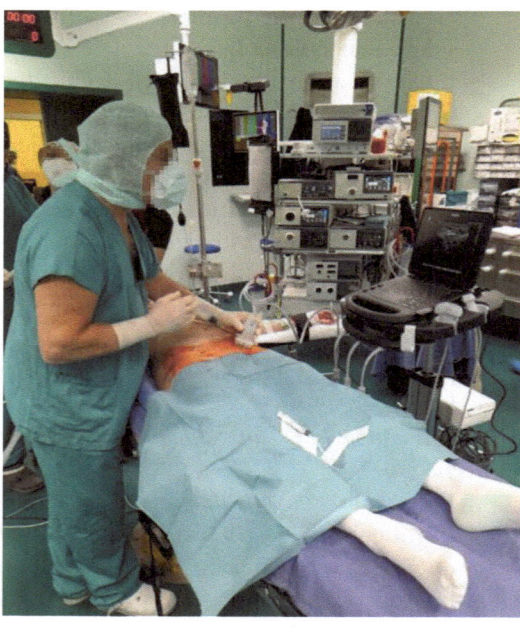

Fig. 9.4 Ultrasound-guided inguinal node ICG injection

9.8 Thoracic Stage (Right Thoracoscopy)

Consecutive sequence of the main stages:

1. **Azygos vein ligation:** to allow the complete exposure of the whole intrathoracic esophagus.
2. **Esophageal dissection:** the mobilization of the esophagus includes the upper mediastinal pleura incision (above the azygos vein) and, inferiorly, the visceral pleura up to the inferior pulmonary ligament and diaphragmatic hiatus
3. **Thoracic duct ligation:** the thoracic duct is identified through NIR imaging between the descending aorta and the lower esophagus, close to the hiatus. Before dissection, double Hem-o-lok ligation has to be performed with ICG fluorescence assistance in order to immediately check for leaks.
4. **Esophagectomy and lymphadenectomy:** a radical resection is mandatory and includes both visceral and lymph node components. It represents the surgical demolition of the thoracic stage.
5. **Preparation for anastomosis fashioning:** before performing the esophagogastric anastomosis, the following steps are necessary: esophageal disconnection with a visceral section above the Azygos vein, purse-string suture to secure the circular stapler anvil, careful intrathoracic pull-up of the gastric conduit, and intraoperative angiography to assess visceral perfusion at the anastomotic site.
6. **Mini-thoracotomy:** a 5- to 6-cm intercostal opening is performed at the medial trocar site for the specimen extraction and circular stapler insertion. The intercostal opening is protected with a single-use wound protector/retractor and a pediatric Finochietto rib retractor is placed.
7. **End-to-side esophagogastric anastomosis:** it is generally performed by means of a 25- to 29-mm-wide circular stapler, according to the esophageal stump caliper. A NG tube is placed

through the anastomosis, under direct vision, and a leak test is performed with methylene blue to assess the anastomosis integrity.

8. ***Paravertebral catheter positioning:*** in the fifth or sixth right intercostal space, under camera vision, for the postoperative pain management. Current scientific evidence does support this technique as the best analgesia due to the minor hemodynamic impact on patient's recovery.

9.9 Thoracic Stage (Right Thoracoscopy), Description

9.9.1 Patient and Operator Positioning

Then, the patient position turns from supine into a lateral position, as shown in Fig. 9.5:

- Left lateral position (semiprone position).
- Left arm abducted perpendicular to the body.
- Right arm bended on the left arm.
- Legs in lower position, adducted (the lower one bended, the upper one straight with a pillow between them).
- Supports on the patient's back and sternum.
- Belts are necessary for fastening head, legs, and arms.

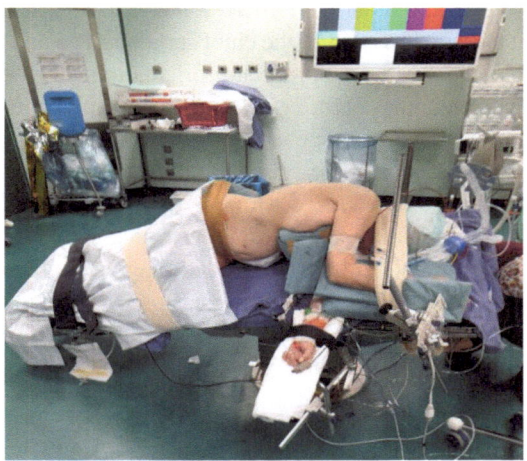

Fig. 9.5 Patient positioning during the thoracic stage

As shown in Fig. 9.6 the surgeons should stand on the left side of the operating table, facing the patient. The scrub nurse resides on the right side with the stand beside.

Before starting surgery, the operating table has to be tilted laterally to the left, to achieve maximal exposure.

9.9.2 Trocar Positioning

The double-lumen endotracheal tube (i.e., Robertshaw) allows the single-lung ventilation (left), with the initial collapse of the right one allowing a safe placement of the trocars, preventing from possible lung injury. The ideal position of the optical trocar is approximately two fingers caudally to the inferior corner of the scapula. An 8-mmHg pneumothorax is established and further three more ports are placed at the following standardized thoracic sites (shown in Fig. 9.7):

- Two 5- to 12-mm ports are placed on the posterior axillary line at the level of the axilla (about the second intercostal space) and medially just above the diaphragm. The latter will host the mini-thoracotomy for the specimen extraction and circular stapler insertion.
- Then a 5-mm port along the posterior axillary line will be placed in the lower part of the ribcage.

9.9.3 Mediastinal Lymphadenectomy

The following node stations are harvested separately: subcarinal (107), main bronchus (109R and L), tracheobronchial (106 tb R), and eventually recurrent laryngeal nerve (106 rec R and L). Esophageal dissection and en bloc lymphadenectomy (upper and medium paraesophageal nodes, stations 105 and 108, respectively) are achieved with adequate traction using an umbilical tape placed around the esophagus.

Thoracic duct dissection is then performed along the aortic adventitia, with en bloc lymph-

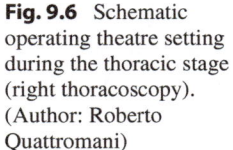 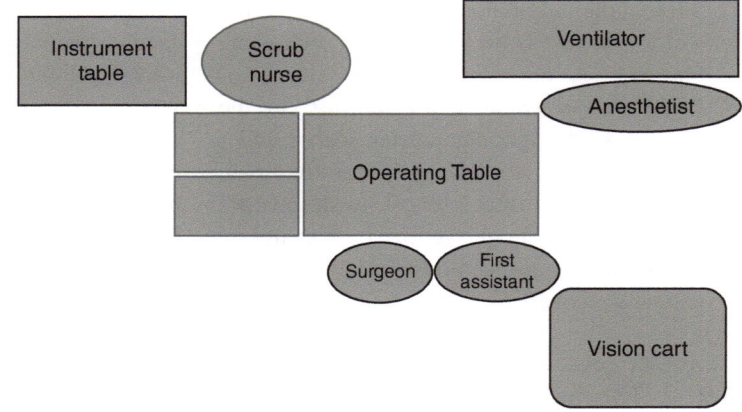

Fig. 9.6 Schematic operating theatre setting during the thoracic stage (right thoracoscopy). (Author: Roberto Quattromani)

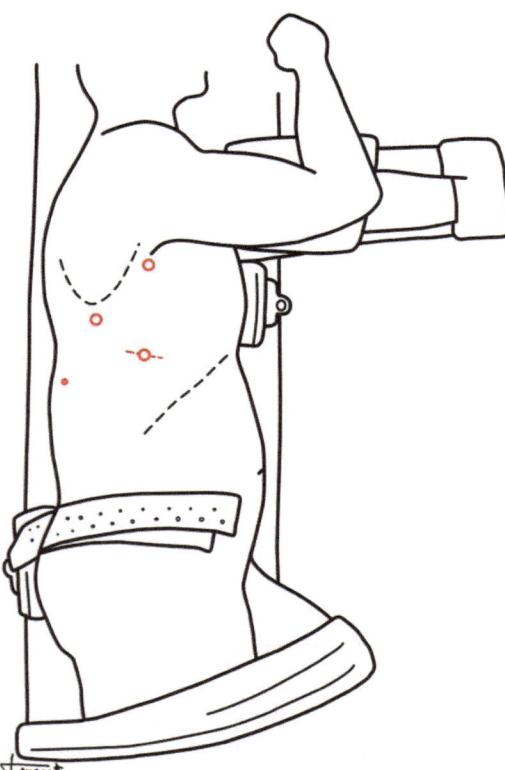

Fig. 9.7 Trocar positioning (right thoracoscopy). (Author: Francesco Puccetti)

adenectomy of the lower paraesophageal stations and posterior mediastinum (110, 111, 112).

Lymphadenectomy is generally performed with the energy device. The bipolar grasper is preferred especially when close to the main airways or vessels.

9.9.4 Intra-thoracic Anastomosis

A purse-string suture securing the anvil into the esophageal stump can be made manually or through a specific forceps. The anastomotic level on the esophageal side has to come above the azygos vein, and the gastric side is chosen in the proximal stomach according to the ICG angiography (better when performed with fluorescence quantification). Through the thoracotomy, the specimen is removed and the conduit eventually prepared to establish the mechanical esophagogastric anastomosis with a circular stapler entering the conduit from a lateral gastrostomy. The stapler and anvil have to be joined intrathoracic under direct vision of the chief surgeon, who double-checks the appropriate orientation of the whole conduit before staplering. After these controls, an end-to-side esophagogastric anastomosis is performed, the stapler carefully removed, and the gastrotomy closed with one or two cartridges of linear stapler. A leak test is performed introducing 60 cc of saline solution with methylene blue through the NG tube. The anastomosis tension can be reduced by suturing the gastric conduit to the upper mediastinal pleura, while the anastomotic mechanical suture is shielded with a wrap of greater omentum.

Table 9.2 JES Thoracic/Mediastinal Lymph-node stations

101	Cervical
102	Cervical paraesophageal
103	Deep cervical LNs
104	Peripharyngeal
105	Supraclavicular and upper mediastinal (upper thoracic paraesophageal LNs)
106 rec	Recurrent nerve LNs L/R
106 pre	Pretracheal LNs
106 tb	Tracheobronchial LNs L/R
107	Subcarinal
108	Middle thoracic paraesophageal
109	Main bronchus L/R
110	Paraesophageal (inferior mediastinum)
111	Supradiaphragmatic (distinct from periesophageal lymph nodes)
112	Posterior mediastinum (distinct from periesophageal lymph nodes)
113	Ligamentum arteriosum LNs
114	Anterior mediastinal LNs

The transhiatal Jackson-Pratt drainage is pulled up and placed beside the gastric tube until the anastomosis.

9.9.4.1 JCGA Abdominal Lymph Node Stations

9.9.4.2 JES Thoracic/Mediastinal Lymph Node Stations (Table 9.2)

9.10 Surgical Instruments Required

Two surgical trolleys are required, one for the minimally invasive surgery (laparoscopy and thoracoscopy) and one for the open surgery instruments, which may be used in case of conversion to laparotomy and/or thoracotomy.

9.10.1 First Instrument Trolley

9.10.1.1 Laparoscopic and Thoracoscopic Instruments
- 1 Hasson trocar

- 5 ports (three 5–12-mm trocar [1 for the abdominal part, 2 more for thoracic stage needed] and two 5 mm for the abdominal stage [only one for thoracic stage needed])
- 1 port with tubing set for the stabilization of the pneumoperitoneum
- 1 port with tubing set for smoke evacuation
- 30° ICG camera with light cable
- 1 laparoscopic 10-mm fenestrated Johann grasping forceps
- 2 laparoscopic 5-mm fenestrated Johann grasping forceps
- 1 bipolar fenestrated forceps
- 1 monopolar cautery hook
- 1 sealing instrument (Thunderbeat)
- 1 laparoscopic needle holder 5 mm
- 2 laparoscopic curved dissecting forceps 5 and 10 mm
- Laparoscopic suction/irrigation system
- 10-mm laparoscopic clip applier (medium reload)
- Hem-o-lok clips with laparoscopic applier of various sizes (large/extra-large)
- Laparoscopic scissors
- Scope warmer
- Laparoscopic linear stapler 45 mm
- Circular stapler (25 or 29 or 31 mm)
- 1 Berci fascial closure device
- 1 purse-string suture forceps 10 mm
- One 10-mm anvil grasper
- One 120-mL endobag
- 1 kangaroo feeding jejunostomy kit
- Skin stapler

9.10.1.2 Open Instruments
- 2 Janach (steel bowls)
- 2 scalpels with stainless steel blade 15 cm length (sizes 11 and 21)
- 2 toothed forceps 16 cm length
- 1 insulated dressing forceps 19 cm length
- 2 dressing forceps 16 cm length
- 2 Farabeuf retractors 12 cm length
- 2 Farabeuf retractors 16 cm length
- 1 Roux retractor 16 cm length
- 1 Mayo curved scissors 18 cm length
- 1 Mayo straight scissors 18 cm length
- 2 curved Kocher clamps 20 cm length

- 2 curved Klemmer clamps 20 cm length
- 2 needle holders 18 cm length
- 2 needle holders 22 cm length
- 2 curved mosquitoes forceps 13 cm length
- 1 monopolar electric scalpel
- 1 suction system
- 1 single-use wound protector/retractor (Alexis)
- 1 pediatric Finochietto retractor

9.10.2 Second Instrument Trolley

9.10.2.1 Open Instruments for Eventual Conversion

- 2 Janach (steel bowls)
- 4 dressing forceps 25 and 30 cm length
- 1 insulated dressing forceps 25 cm length
- 2 Resano forceps 25 cm length
- 2 DeBakey forceps 25 cm length
- 1 bipolar forceps with irrigation system 25 cm length
- Abdominal malleable spatulas, different sizes
- 2 Mikulicz abdominal wall retractors
- 2 Middledorf abdominal wall retractors
- 1 Roux retractor 18 cm
- 1 Allison lung spatula
- 12 curved Klemmer clamps 20, 22, and 25 cm length
- 4 O'Shaughnessy forceps (right angle) 18, 22, and 25 cm length
- 6 Allis forceps 18 and 25 cm length
- 3 Duval forceps 20 cm length
- 2 Duval forceps 25 cm length
- 6 curved mosquito forceps 13 cm length
- 2 curved Kocher clamps 16 cm length
- 4 straight Kocher clamps 16 cm length
- 4 straight Klemmer clamps 16 cm length;
- 4 needle holders 22 and 24 cm length
- 4 Nelson-Metzenbaum dissection scissors 22 and 24 cm length
- 2 bulldog clamps
- 4 vascular clamps
- 3 laparotomic clip applier (small, medium, and large)
- 1 Marberger (Gil Vernet) retractor
- 1 Martin Rochard abdominal retractor

- 1 Balfour static abdominal retractor
- 1 Burford rib spreader

9.10.3 Other Devices

9.10.3.1 ICG (Indocyanine Green)

The indocyanine green dye (IGC) is stocked in 25-mg powder vials, which needs to be reconstituted before EV injection.

- To be used as 2.5 mg/mL concentration.
- Dilute with sterile distilled water, *not* sodium chloride (NaCl 0.9%) solution, as the latter could cause precipitate solution.
- After reconstitution, the solution must be stored in a dark and cool place to avoid rapid deterioration, within 6 h.
- Dose administration is 0.3 mg/kg.

9.11 Surgical Steps and Related Instruments

9.11.1 Abdominal Stage (Laparoscopy)

9.11.1.1 Hasson Technique for Laparoscopic Access

- 1 scalpel (blade 11)
- 2 toothed forceps
- 2 Farabeuf retractors
- 1 Mayo curved scissors
- 2 curved Kocher clamps to grasp fascia
- 2 Polysorb® 0 27 mm 5/8 sutures
- 2 curved Klemmer clamps to grasp parietal peritoneum
- Hasson port
- 2 curved mosquito forceps
- 10 mL syringe filled with Naropin 7.5%
- 1 needle holder

9.11.1.2 Instruments for the Other Port Placement

- 1 scalpel (blade 11)
- 10-mL syringe filled with Naropin 7.5%
- One 5- to 12-mm port
- Two 5-mm ports

- 1 port with tubing set for the stabilization of pneumoperitoneum
- 1 port with tubing set for smoke evacuation

The abdominal laparoscopic part provides the stomach mobilization (gastrolysis), pyloromyotomy with pyloroplasty, lymphadenectomy, and the gastric conduit formation for the subsequent gastric tube transposition into the thorax through the hiatus.

The instruments to be used are as follows:

- For the first assistant:
  - 30° ICG camera with light cable
  - Scope warmer
  - Port tubing set for the stabilization of pneumoperitoneum
- For the second assistant:
  - Laparoscopic Johann forceps 5 mm
- Pyloromyotomy and pyloroplasty:
  - Sealing instrument (Thunderbeat)
  - Monopolar cautery hook
  - Laparoscopic 10-mm Johann forceps
  - Laparoscopic needle holder 5 mm
  - Laparoscopic scissors
- Kocher maneuver, lesser omentum dissection, lymphadenectomy, and gastrolysis:
  - Laparoscopic Johann forceps 10 mm
  - Laparoscopic Johann forceps 5 mm
  - Bipolar fenestrated forceps
  - Monopolar cautery hook
  - Sealing instrument
  - Laparoscopic dissecting forceps curved 5 and 10 mm
  - Laparoscopic suction/irrigation system
- Left gastric vessel ligation:
  - 10-mm laparoscopic clip applier with relative reload medium
  - Sealing instrument
- Gastric tubulization:
  - Linear stapler 45, minimum 5 reload (3.8 mm)
  - Laparoscopic Johann forceps
- If feeding jejunostomy is performed:
  - Laparoscopic Johann forceps
  - Laparoscopic needle holder 5 mm
  - Laparoscopic scissors
  - Kangaroo feeding jejunostomy kit
  - Barbed suture

- Skin suture
- Mayo scissors
- 20-mL syringe
- Drainage placement:
  - Jackson-Pratt drainage 4 × 10 mm
  - Laparoscopic Johann forceps 10 mm
  - Laparotomy needle holder
  - Nonabsorbable skin suture
  - Mayo scissors
- Colopexy:
  - Laparoscopic Johann forceps
  - Laparoscopic needle holder 5 mm
  - Laparoscopic scissors
  - Barbed suture
- 5- to 12-mm port's fascia closure:
  - Berci fascial closure device
  - Absorbable suture
- Skin closure:
  - Skin stapler

9.11.2 Thoracic Stage (Right Thoracoscopy)

9.11.2.1 Port Placement
- 1 scalpel (blade 11)
- Mayo curved scissors
- 10-mL syringe with Naropin 7.5%
- Three 5- to 12-mm ports
- One 5-mm port

The thoracoscopic part provides the complete esophageal mobilization, lymphadenectomy, gastric conduit transposition, and subsequent anastomosis. After that the specimen dissection and retrieval will be performed.

The instruments to be used are as follows:

- For the first assistant:
  - 30° ICG camera with light cable
  - Scope warmer
  - 1 port tubing set for the stabilization of pneumoperitoneum
  - 1 port tubing set for smoke evacuation
  - Laparoscopic Johann forceps 10 mm
  - Laparoscopic Johann forceps 5 mm
- Azygos vein dissection and ligation:
  - Laparoscopic Johann forceps 10 mm
  - Laparoscopic Johann forceps 5 mm

- Monopolar cautery hook
- Sealing instrument
- Laparoscopic curved dissecting forceps
- Laparoscopic suction/irrigation system
- Laparoscopic scissors
- Hem-o-lok clips with laparoscopic applier (large size clips)
- Thoracic duct dissection/ligation and esophageal mobilization:
  - Laparoscopic Johann forceps
  - Monopolar cautery hook
  - Sealing instrument
  - Laparoscopic curved dissecting forceps
  - Laparoscopic suction/irrigation system
  - Laparoscopic scissors
  - Hem-o-lok clips with laparoscopic applier (large size clips)
  - Cotton umbilical tape
- Lymphadenectomy:
  - Hem-o-lok clips with laparoscopic applier (large size clips)
  - 120-mL endobag
  - Laparoscopic suction/irrigation system
  - Sealing instrument
  - Laparoscopic Johann forceps
  - Laparoscopic bipolar forceps
- Proximal esophagus section and purse-string suture:
  - The specific 10-mm purse-string forceps
  - Laparoscopic Johann forceps
  - Laparoscopic needle holder
  - Laparoscopic scissors
  - 2 endoloop
  - Monosoft® 2-0, 60-mm double taper point straight needle, 90 cm length
- Esophagogastric anastomosis:
  - Specific 10-mm anvil grasper
  - Laparoscopic Johann forceps
  - Laparoscopic scissors
  - Linear stapler 45 mm, 2 reload (3.5 mm)
  - Circular stapler (25 or 29 or 31 mm)
- 5- to 12 mm port's fascia closure:
  - 2 Farabeuf retractors
  - Needle holder

- Toothed forceps
- Absorbable suture
- Paravertebral catheter positioning:

  - Specific kit
  - 5-mL syringe
  - Laparotomy needle holder
  - Prolene suture

9.11.2.2 Instruments for Mini-thoracotomy

- 1 scalpel (blade 21)
- 2 toothed forceps 16 cm length
- 2 dressing forceps 16 cm length
- 2 Farabeuf retractors 16 cm length
- 1 Roux retractor 16 cm length
- 1 monopolar electric scalpel
- 1 suction system
- 1 single-use wound protector/retractor
- 1 pediatric Finochietto rib spreader
- 1 needle holder
- Absorbable suture (rib approach and fascia closure)
- Skin stapler

References

1. Morris-Stiff G, Hughes LE. Ivor Lewis (1895-1982)—Welsh pioneer of the right-sided approach to the oesophagus. Dig Surg. 2003;20:546–52; discussion 552–543.
2. DePaula AL, Hashiba K, Ferreira EA, et al. Laparoscopic transhiatal esophagectomy with esophagogastroplasty. Surg Laparosc Endosc. 1995;5:1–5.
3. Swanstrom LL, Hansen P. Laparoscopic total esophagectomy. Arch Surg. 1997;132:943–7; discussion 947–949.
4. Peracchia A, Rosati R, Fumagalli U, et al. Thoracoscopic esophagectomy: are there benefits? Semin Surg Oncol. 1997;13:259–62.
5. Luketich JD, Nguyen NT, Weigel T, et al. Minimally invasive approach to esophagectomy. JSLS. 1998;2:243–7.
6. Watson DI, Davies N, Jamieson GG. Totally endoscopic Ivor Lewis esophagectomy. Surg Endosc. 1999;13:293–7.

Robot-Assisted Minimally Invasive Esophagectomy (RAMIE)

10

S. van der Horst, J. W. van der Berg, J. P. Ruurda, and R. van Hillegersberg

10.1 Demolitive Phase

The demolitive phase in turn consists of two parts: organ resection and lymphadenectomy.

The organ resection can be partial or total: in the first case we will talk about total gastrectomy, while in the second about distal or proximal partial gastrectomy.

10.2 General Information

10.2.1 Operating Theatre Setting

The operating theatre setting for the thoracic phase of an esophagectomy is performed as follows (Fig. 10.1a):

- Operating table in the centre of the theatre
- Vision cart positioned to the right of the patient, at the level of the feet
- Patient cart positioned to the right of the patient, at the level of the shoulders
- Surgeon positioned at the surgical console, trainee positioned at the dual console
- First assistant at the operating table to the left of the patient

S. van der Horst · J. W. van der Berg · J. P. Ruurda · R. van Hillegersberg (✉)
Department of Surgery, University Medical Center Utrecht, Utrecht University, Utrecht, the Netherlands
e-mail: R.vanHillegersberg@umcutrecht.nl

- Instrument nurse to the left of the first assistant
- Serving cart at the left of the patient at the level of the feet

The operating theatre setting for the abdominal phase of an esophagectomy is performed as follows (Fig. 10.1b):

- Operating table in the centre of the theatre
- Vision cart positioned at the feet of the patient
- Patient cart positioned to the right of the patient at the level of the shoulders
- Surgeon positioned at the surgical console, trainee positioned at the dual console
- First assistant at the operating table positioned to the right of the patient
- Instrument nurse positioned to the left of the patient opposite tot the first assistant
- Serving cart at the left of the patient at the level of the feet

10.2.2 Patient Positioning

Patient positioning for the thoracic phase is performed as shown in Fig. 10.2a:

- Left lateral decubitus position tilted towards prone; on bean bag
- Table break at the level of the tip of the scapula

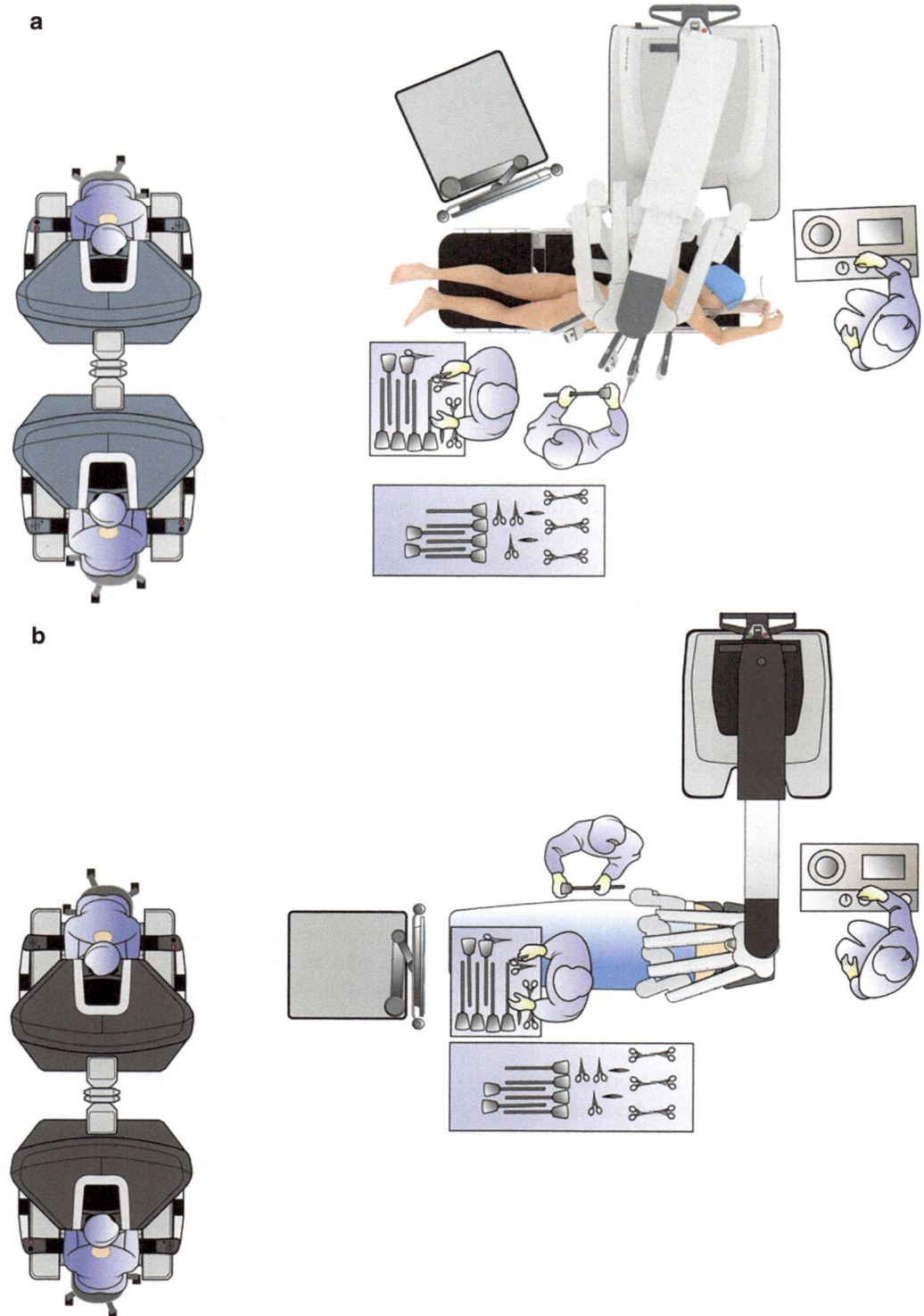

Fig. 10.1 (**a**) Schematic operating theatre setting for thoracic phase esophagectomy. (**b**) Schematic operating theatre setting for abdominal phase esophagectomy

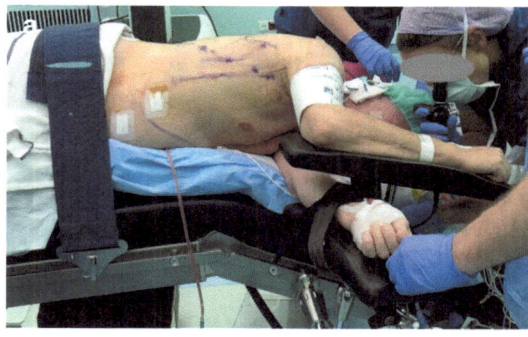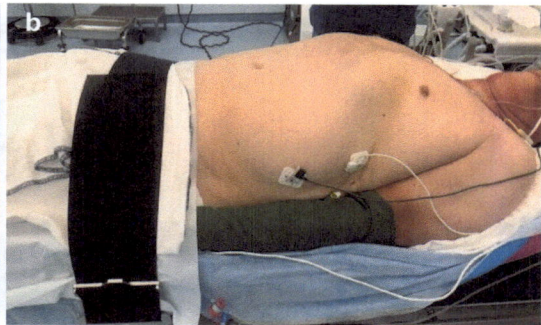

Fig. 10.2 (**a**) Patient positioning for thoracic phase RAMIE. (**b**) Patient positioning abdominal phase RAMIE

- Right arm kept low at 90-degree angle

Patient positioning for the abdominal phase is performed as shown in Fig. 10.2b:

- Supine position on bean bag
- Arms adducted along the body
- Table in reverse Trendelenburg and slight tilt to the right

10.2.3 Port Placement and Robotic Docking

10.2.3.1 Port Placement and Robotic Docking Thoracic Phase

- 1 12-mm port for assistance
- 1 robotic 12-mm port
- 4 robotic 8-mm ports

The thoracic phase starts with single (left) lung ventilation. An 8-mm robotic trocar is inserted in the sixth intercostal space for introduction of the camera and CO_2 insufflation (8 mmHg) is started. The other three robotic 8-mm trocars are inserted in the fourth, eighth, and tenth intercostal space. The 12-mm assistant port is placed in the fifth intercostal space. After extraction of the specimen the 8-mm robotic port in the eighth intercostal space will (Fig. 10.3a).

10.2.3.2 Port Placement and Robotic Docking Abdominal Phase

- 1 10-mm port for open introduction and assistance

- 1 robotic 12 mm port
- 3 robotic 8 mm ports

A 10-mm balloon trocar is placed below the umbilicus. The robotic ports are placed along a transverse line. The position of the robotic ports is depending on the location of the transverse colon, which indicates the height of the transverse line for the robotic ports. Two 8-mm robotic trocars are placed at the left lateral side of the patient; 1 12-mm and 1 8-mm robotic trocar are placed at the right lateral side of the patient (Fig. 10.3b).

Once the ports have been positioned and the patient cart is positioned on the operating table, the arm that accommodates the endoscope (arm 3) is connected after alignment and the camera is pointed at the target anatomy (hiatus in the abdominal phase, left main bronchus just below azygos vein in thoracic phase). Once the targeting is complete, the other arms are docked and the robotic instruments are inserted, after positioning the reducer on the 12-mm port to avoid loss of pneumoperitoneum (arm 1, Cadiere forceps; arm 2, vessel sealer; arm 4, permanent cautery hook).

10.2.4 Surgical Instruments Required

10.2.4.1 Robotic Instruments
- 4 robotic ports (three 8-mm ports and one 12-mm ports)
- 1 port reducer
- 30° robotic endoscope

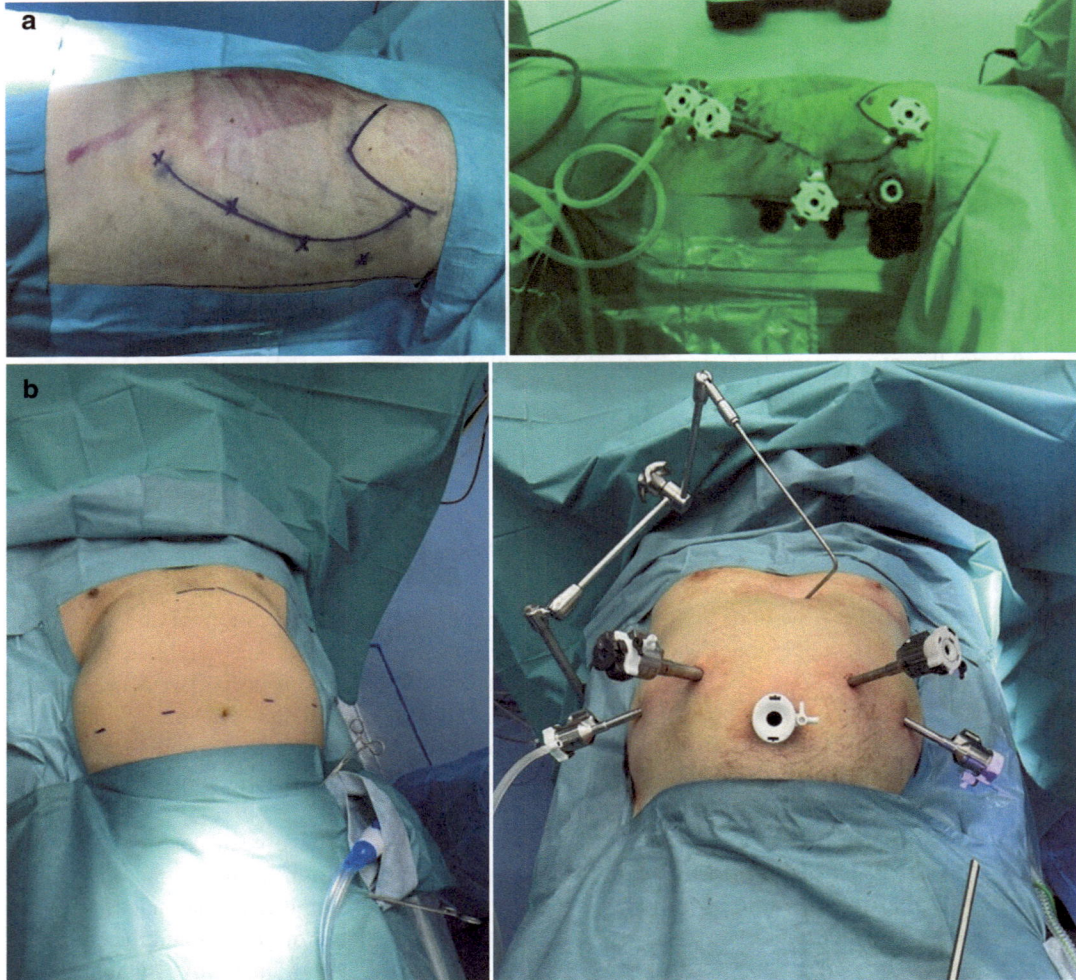

Fig. 10.3 (**a**) Port placement for thoracic phase RAMIE. (**b**) Port placement for abdominal phase

- 1 grasping forceps (Cadiere® forceps)
- 1 monopolar instrument (permanent cautery hook®)
- 1 sealing instrument (Vessel Sealer Extend®)
- 1 stapler (SureForm EndoWrist Stapler® 60 mm)
- 1 needle holder (Large Needle Driver®)
- 1 Hem-o-lok ®clip applier

10.2.4.2 Laparoscopic Instruments
- 1 10-mm balloon trocar (abdominal phase)
- 1 12-mm trocar (robotic phase)
- Laparoscopic scissors
- Laparoscopic grasping forceps
- Laparoscopic suction/irrigation system

10.2.4.3 Open Instruments
- 1 scalpel with stainless steel blade
- 1 Mayo scissors
- 1 Metzenbaum dissection scissors (McKeown)
- 2 toothed forceps large
- 2 toothed forceps small
- Needle driver large
- Needle driver small
- 2 Kocher clamps
- 2 curved Crawford clamps
- 1 Debakey-Semb ligature carrier (McKeown)
- 1 Adson retractor (McKeown)
- 1 Foerster clamp (McKeown)
- 2 Allis clamps (McKeown)
- 2 sharp retraction clamps large (McKeown)

- 1 monopolar electric scalpel
- 1 Alexis port small (Applied medical)
- 1 oesophageal bridle (McKeown)
- 1 shoelace (McKeown)
- 1 ultrasound transducer cover (McKeown)
- Nathanson® liver retractor
- Kidney basin
- 3 bowls
- Suction device open surgery (McKeown)
- Jackson-Pratt® drains
- Gloves size 9
- Small paper ruler

10.2.4.4 Other Devices

ICG (Indocyanine Green)

The indocyanine green fluorescent (IGC) dye is presented in vials of 50 mg of powder for solution for injection.

- Use in concentrations of 2.5 mg/mL.
- Dilute with 20 mL sterile distilled water and *not* sodium chloride (NaCl) as the latter could cause aggregation.
- After preparation, the solution must be stored in a dark and cool place to avoid rapid deterioration of the whitening fluorescence.
- Administer 3 mL (7.5 mg) in bolus over peripheral infuse with 10 mL NaCl flush.
- During ICG angiography: MAP >70 mmHg.

Contraindications for administering ICG: allergy for Jodium/ICG, hyperthyroidism/thyroid adenoma.

10.3 Surgical Procedure

10.3.1 Robot-Assisted Minimally Invasive Esophagectomy: Cervical Anastomosis (McKeown)

A robot-assisted minimally invasive esophagectomy (RAMIE) with cervical anastomosis can basically be divided into three stages: the thoracic phase, the abdominal phase and the cervical phase.

10.3.1.1 Thoracic Phase: McKeown Procedure

The thoracic phase of robot-assisted minimally invasive esophagectomy with cervical anastomosis consists of the following steps:

- Single-lung ventilation
- Introduction of 8-mm robotic trocar with blunt obturator using scalpel and Mayo scissors
- CO_2 insufflation at low pressure (8 mmHg)
- Placement of three extra robotic trocars with blunt obturators and one 12-mm assistance port
- Docking of robot arm 3, alignment and introduction of camera for targeting at the level of the left main bronchus just below the azygos arch
- Docking of the other robot arms
- Introduction of the robotic instruments: arm 1, Cadiere forceps®; arm 2, Vessel Sealer Extend®; arm 4, permanent cautery hook®
- Division of the pulmonary ligament
- Dissection of the anterior parietal pleura of the oesophagus
- Dissection of the oesophagus from the pericardium
- Division of the azygos vein at the level of the aortic arch using Hem-o-lok clips
- Dissection of the upper mediastinal parietal pleura
- Dissection of the proximal oesophagus from the trachea
- Bilateral paratracheal lymph node dissection
- Dissection of the right main bronchial artery with the vessel sealer
- Exposure of the right main bronchus and dissection of the vagus nerve at the level of the lower edge of the right main bronchus
- Dissection of the parietal pleura along the azygos vein from cranially to caudally along the aorta
- Para-aortal dissection of the paraoesophageal lymph nodes and thoracic duct and ligation of aorta-oesophageal branches with the vessel sealer
- Clipping and division of thoracic duct about 5 cm above the diaphragm with Hem-o-lok clips

- Dissection of the oesophagus from the pericardium and pulmonary vein up to the level of the subcarinal lymph nodes
- En bloc dissection of the subcarinal lymph nodes
- Dissection of the oesophagus from the left main bronchus
- Completion of mobilization of the oesophagus at the level of the crus and the thoracic inlet
- Insertion of a Jackson-Pratt drain in the right sinus
- In case of lung injury insertion of a standard chest tube
- Insufflation of the right lung under sight
- Closure of wounds

10.3.1.2 Abdominal and Cervical Phase: McKeown Procedure

The abdominal phase of robot-assisted minimally invasive esophagectomy with cervical anastomosis consists of the following surgical steps:

- Open introduction for placement of a 10-mm balloon trocar subumbilical using scalpel, Kocher clamp and Mayo scissors
- Insufflation of abdomen (12 mmHg) and inspection of the abdomen
- Introduction of three 8-mm robotic trocars and one 12-mm robotic trocar
- Introduction of the Nathanson liver retractor
- Placement of a Jackson-Pratt drain in the left pleural cavity
- Docking of robot arm 3 and, after alignment, introduction of camera for targeting at level of the hiatus
- Docking of the other robot arms
- Introduction of the robotic instruments: arm 1, Cadiere forceps®; arm 2, Vessel Sealer Extend®; arm 4, permanent cautery hook®
- Dissection of the lesser curvature of the stomach following the right crus, with preservation of aberrant hepatic artery if indicated
- Opening of the parietal pleura along the hiatus
- Release of the cranial part of the gastrophrenic ligament
- Dissection of the greater curvature of the stomach with preservation of the right gastro-epiploic artery and vein

- Dissection of the coeliac trunk; dissection of left gastro-epiploic vein with vessel sealer and artery with Hem-o-lok clips
- Separate lymphadenectomy station 8, 9 and 11; extraction in finger of glove
- Creation of gastric tube with robotic stapler green load using ruler to determine the width of the gastric tube
- Dissection of the hiatus and connection with thoracic dissection plane
- Re-attachment of gastric tube to the specimen to prevent torsion of the gastric tube during extraction
- Vertical incision at the left side of the neck
- Mobilization of the oesophagus sparing the laryngeal nerve
- Encircling of the oesophagus with an oesophageal bridle
- Opening of the oesophagus and repositioning of the nasogastric tube
- Placement of a Crawford clamp on the specimen side of the oesophagus, completion of dissection of the oesophagus where after attachment of shoe lace to the specimen side of the oesophagus
- Placement of Allis clamps on all layers of the proximal oesophageal wall in the neck to align al the separate layers of the wall of the oesophagus
- Vertical incision left lateral abdomen 5–7 cm in width for placement of the Alexis wound protector
- Extraction of the specimen and gastric tube
- Placement of ultrasound transducer cover over gastric tube for smooth pass through hiatus and mediastinum, attachment of shoe lace (which is now passing through the mediastinum) to the gastric tube
- Bringing up the gastric tube through the hiatus and mediastinum up to the neck, manually assisted using the shoelace as a guide
- Extraction of the ultrasound transducer through the cervical incision
- Vertical opening of the gastric tube for end to side anastomosis
- Hand-sewn end to side anastomosis between oesophagus and gastric tube
- Extraction of the tip of gastric tube using robotic stapler

- Closure of the hiatus
- Endoscopic identification of Treitz ligament
- Placement of a feeding jejunostomy through the transverse incision
- Closure of the wounds

10.3.2 Robot-Assisted Minimally Invasive Esophagectomy: Intrathoracic Anastomosis (Ivor Lewis)

10.3.2.1 Abdominal Phase: Ivor Lewis Procedure

The abdominal phase of robot-assisted minimally invasive esophagectomy with cervical anastomosis consists of the following surgical steps:

- Open introduction of a 10-mm balloon trocar subumbilical using scalpel, Kocher clamp and Mayo scissors.
- Insufflation of the abdomen (12 mmHg) and inspection of the abdomen.
- Introduction of three 8-mm robotic trocars and one 12-mm robotic trocar.
- Introduction of the Nathanson liver retractor.
- Placement of a Jackson-Pratt drain in the left pleural cavity.
- Docking of robot arm 3, and after alignment, introduction of the camera for targeting at the level of the hiatus.
- Docking of other robot arms.
- Introduction of robotic instruments: arm 1, Cadiere forceps®; arm 2, Vessel Sealer Extend®; arm 4, permanent cautery hook®.
- Dissection of the lesser curvature of the stomach following the right crus, preservation of aberrant hepatic artery if indicated.
- Opening of the parietal pleura along the hiatus.
- Release of the cranial part of gastro-phrenic ligament.
- Dissection of the greater curvature of the stomach with preservation of the right gastro-epiploic artery and vein.
- Dissection of the coeliac trunk; dissection of left gastro-epiploic vein with vessel sealer and artery with Hem-o-lok clips.

- Separate lymphadenectomy station 8, 9 and 11; extraction in finger of glove.
- Creation of the gastric tube with robotic stapler green load, using a ruler to determine the width of the gastric tube.
- Depending on the anatomy gastric tube formation can be performed before coeliac trunk dissection and lymphadenectomy of station 8, 9 and 11.
- Dissection of the hiatus.
- Re-attachment of gastric tube to the specimen and aligning gastric tube and specimen for a smooth pass through the hiatus.
- Endoscopic identification of Treitz ligament.
- Placement of a feeding jejunostomy.
- Closure of the wounds.

10.3.2.2 Thoracic Phase: Ivor Lewis Procedure

The thoracic phase of robot-assisted minimally invasive esophagectomy with cervical anastomosis consists of the following steps:

- Single-lung ventilation
- Introduction of 8-mm robotic trocar with blunt obturator using scalpel and Mayo scissors.
- CO_2 insufflation at low pressure (8 mmHg)
- Placement of three extra robotic trocars with blunt obturators and one 12-mm assistance port
- Docking of robot arm 3, alignment and introduction of camera for targeting at level of left main bronchus just below azygos arch
- Docking of the other robotic arms
- Introduction of robotic instruments: arm 1, Cadiere forceps®; arm 2, Vessel Sealer Extend®; arm 4, permanent cautery hook®
- Division of the pulmonary ligament
- Dissection of the anterior parietal pleura of the oesophagus
- Dissection of the oesophagus from the pericardium
- Division of the azygos vein at the level of the aortic arch using Hem-o-Lok clips
- Dissection of the upper mediastinal parietal pleura
- Dissection of the proximal oesophagus from the trachea

- Bilateral paratracheal lymph node dissection, extraction using finger of glove
- Dissection of the right main bronchial artery with the vessel sealer
- Exposure of the right main bronchus and dissection of the vagus nerve at the level of the lower edge of the right main bronchus
- Dissection of the parietal pleura along the azygos vein from cranially to caudally along the aorta
- Para-aortal dissection of the paraoesophageal lymph nodes and thoracic duct and ligation of aorta-oesophageal branches with the vessel sealer
- Clipping and division of thoracic duct about 5 cm above the diaphragm using Hem-o-lok clips
- Dissection of the oesophagus from the pericardium and pulmonary vein up to the level of the subcarinal lymph nodes
- En bloc dissection of the subcarinal lymph nodes
- Dissection of the oesophagus from the left main bronchus
- Completion of mobilization of the oesophagus at the level of the crus and the thoracic inlet
- Mobilization of specimen through the hiatus into the chest
- Dissection of the oesophagus at the preferred level of the anastomosis
- Placement of laparoscopic clamp at the specimen side of the oesophagus to prevent leakage
- Placement of stitches through the proximal oesophageal wall to align the separate layers of the oesophageal wall
- Extension of the incision up to 3–4 cm in the tenth intercostal space for extraction of the specimen
- Placement of Alexis port
- Placement of 12-mm robotic trocar through the Alexis port
- Administering of ICG to determine the level of anastomosis on gastric tube
- If indicated extraction of the tip of gastric tube using robotic stapler
- Vertical opening of the gastric tube
- Hand-sewn end to side anastomosis between oesophagus and gastric tube

- Placement of enforcement stiches over the anastomosis
- Omental plasty
- Closure of hiatus
- Insertion of a Jackson-Pratt drain in the right sinus
- In case of lung injury insertion of a standard chest tube
- Insufflation of right lung under sight
- Closure of wounds

10.3.3 Lymphadenectomy

Oesophageal lymph node stations are numerous and are distinguished on the basis of their location:

Thoracic lymph node stations	
	Thoracic duct compartment
2R	Upper right paratracheal
2L	Upper left paratracheal
4R	Lower right paratracheal
4L	Lower left paratracheal
5	Aorta-pulmonary window
6	Anterior mediastinum
7	Subcarinal
8M	Mid paraoesophageal
8L	Lower paraoesophageal
9	Pulmonary ligament
10R	Right tracheobronchial
10L	Left tracheobronchial
Abdominal lymph node stations	
1	Right paracardial
2	Left paracardial
3a	Lesser curvature, along the left gastric artery branches
3b	Lesser curvature, along the distal part of right gastric artery and its second branch
7	Left gastric artery (around the tract of the artery between its origin from the coeliac trunk and the origin of its ascending branch, i.e. its entrance into the small omentum where it relates to the gastric lesser curvature)
8a	Common hepatic artery, antero-superior group
8p	Common hepatic artery, posterior group
9	Coeliac trunk
11p	Splenic artery, proximal (from its origin to half its length between its origin and the end of the pancreatic tail)
11d	Splenic artery, distal (from the middle of its length between its origin and the end of the pancreatic tail to the pancreatic tail)

Lymphadenectomy can be performed in three different ways:

- En bloc: all lymph node stations are extracted together with the surgical specimen and sent to the pathological anatomy laboratory for recognition.
- For each station: each lymph node station is removed by the surgeon separately and therefore as different samples.
- Back table: the lymph node stations are removed with the surgical specimen and the surgeon proceeds to recognize and separate the various lymph node stations.

10.3.4 Intraoperative Complications

The most frequent intraoperative complications to manage during a robotic esophagectomy are basically haemorrhage, injuries of parenchymatous or hollow organs (pancreas, spleen, bowel).

Damage of bronchus/trachea

Damage to recurrent nerves

Damage to pulmonary veins

Accidental damage to the aortic branches to the oesophagus or bronchus

In these circumstances, the instrument nurse must have the following instruments available:

- Laparoscopic suction/irrigation system
- 10 × 10 cm gauze to be passed to the assistant at the request of the surgeon
- Robotic small clip applier with titanium clips
- Robotic needle holder and monofilament suture with small-gauge needle to attempt to repair the bleeding vessel or, in case of injury of parenchymatous/hollow organ, needle holder and monofilament/barbed suture to repair it

Laparoscopic Gastrectomy

11

Hogla Aridai Resendiz Aguilar, Rossella Reddavid, and Maurizio Degiuli

11.1 Introduction

Gastrectomy is the partial or total removal of the stomach. The type of gastric resection and the extent of nodal dissection depend on the tumor location, TNM category, and histological subtype [1].

After pneumoperitoneum is established, laparoscopic gastrectomy starts with a general inspection of the liver, pelvis, paracolic gutters, greater and lesser omentum, transverse mesocolon, and the parietal peritoneal surface, looking for metastatic disease, that can modify the therapeutic decision and other conditions such as adherences that can make it difficult to continue the dissection by laparoscopic approach. Some centers routinely collect peritoneal fluid for cytologic examination.

Technically, the stomach can be completely (**total gastrectomy**) or partially resected by laparoscopy (**distal or proximal gastrectomy**). These procedures are characterized by a demoli-

tion phase (represented by the removal of the stomach and the regional lymph nodes), and by a reconstruction phase, when restoring the continuity of the gastrointestinal tract takes place.

11.2 Total Gastrectomy

Total gastrectomy is a challenging procedure, which is mandatory in case of GC located in the upper third of the stomach. The main steps of this procedure are the following:

- *Gastric exposure*: the left lateral segment of the liver is lifted up; different devices or a liver suspension technique can be used for this purpose.
- *Fundus and greater curvature mobilization*: the dissection starts with the division of the gastrocolic ligament about 4 cm far from the gastroepiploic vessel arcade and proceeds along the greater curvature towards the cardias; the left gastroepiploic vessels and then the short gastric vessels are identified and divided. This dissection continues until the angle of His and the diaphragmatic left crus and then proceeds caudally towards the pylorus with the ligation and section of the right gastroepiploic vessels at their origin.
- *Duodenum mobilization*: the hepatoduodenal ligament is divided on the side of the lesser curvature (pars tensa of the lesser omentum).

H. A. Resendiz Aguilar · R. Reddavid
Department of Oncology, University of Turin, San Luigi University Hospital, Orbassano, Italy

M. Degiuli (✉)
Department of Oncology, University of Turin, San Luigi University Hospital, Orbassano, Italy

University of Turin, Turin, Italy
e-mail: maurizio.degiuli@unito.it

The right gastric artery is divided close to its origin from the proper hepatic artery, and then the duodenum is transected close to the pancreas.

- *Lymphadenectomy*: depending mostly on the stage of the disease, a D1, D1+, or D2 lymph node dissection is performed.
- Identification and division of the left gastric vein and of the left gastric artery close to its origin from the celiac axis. The dissection proceeds then towards the phreno-esophageal ligament till the right diaphragmatic crus is identified.
- Completion of gastrectomy with the transection of the esophagus proximal to the gastro-esophageal junction.
- Surgical specimen extraction.

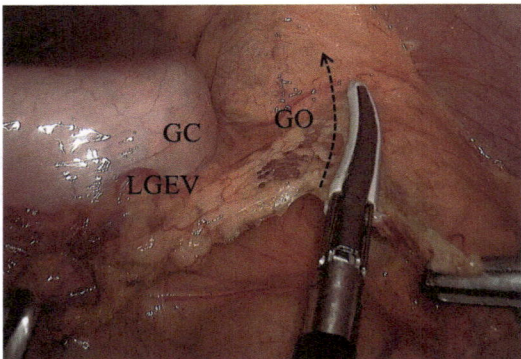

Fig. 11.1 Greater curvature mobilization. *GC* greater curvature, *GO* greater omentum, *LGEV* left gastroepiploic vessels

11.3 Distal Gastrectomy

Distal gastrectomy consists of partial stomach resection including the antrum and the pylorus. Sometimes the mobilization of the stomach fundus and short gastric vessel division could be avoided according to the tumor location. Furthermore, the ascending branch of the left gastric artery could be preserved too. The main steps of this procedure are the following:

- Gastric exposure: the falciform ligament and left lateral segment of the liver are suspended to the abdominal wall to obtain a good exposure of the operative field; many different devices or suspension techniques can be used for this purpose.
- Greater curvature mobilization: the greater omentum is divided and dissected towards the lower pole of the spleen till the point chosen for gastric resection. The left gastro-epiploic vessels should be identified and divided at their origin from the splenic vessels. The branches for the left side of the omentum and short gastric vessels are preserved (Fig. 11.1).
- The dissection of the gastroepiploic ligament proceeds then caudally towards the pylorus. The right gastroepiploic vessels are identified, ligated, and divided at their origin.

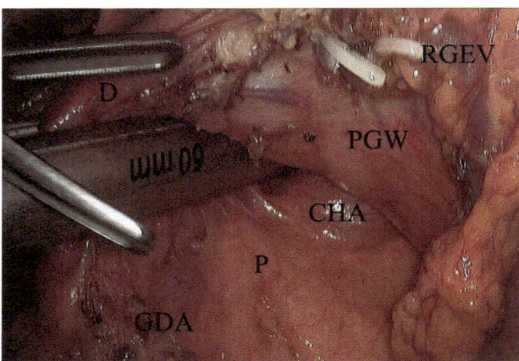

Fig. 11.2 Duodenal transection. *D* duodenum, *P* pancreas, *PGW* posterior gastric wall, *RGEV* right gastric vessels, *GDA* gastroduodenal artery, *CHA* common hepatic artery

- The hepatoduodenal ligament and the posterior wall of the duodenum are dissected and mobilized. The duodenum is mechanically transected with a stapler 0.5 cm far from the head of the pancreas (Fig. 11.2).
- The right gastric vessels are then identified, ligated, and dissected at their origin.
- The left gastric artery is identified and ligated at its origin from the celiac axis.
- The final step is the transection of the stomach following a line defined to ensure a sufficient free resection margin of at least 3 cm in case of T2 or deeper tumors with an expansive growth pattern and of 5 cm in case of those tumors with an infiltrative growth pattern.
- Surgical specimen extraction with dedicated devices.

11.4 Proximal Gastrectomy

Proximal gastrectomy is a type of partial gastrectomy consisting of resection of the upper third of the stomach including the cardia. The body, the antrum, and the pylorus are preserved. This type of resection is recommended as a treatment option for early proximal gastric cancer by Japanese guidelines, due to the fact that lymph node metastasis spread to the distal stomach is rare. This is a function-preserving surgery attempting to increase long-term nutritional outcomes and to reduce gastroesophageal reflux disease.

The surgical steps are as follows:

- Gastric exposure: the left lobe of the liver is retracted using different devices or suspension techniques.
- Partial omentectomy starts from the middle of the gastrocolic ligament, about 4 cm far from the gastroepiploic vessels arcade, towards the lower pole of the spleen. The left gastroepiploic vessels are divided distal to the bifurcation point of their omental branch, and then the dissection continues towards the left side of the esophageal hiatus by dividing the short gastric vessels.
- The lesser omentum is dissected towards the right side of the esophageal hiatus.
- The right gastric artery is isolated and ligated distally close to the stomach.
- Hence, the stomach is transected nearby the gastric angle through a linear stapler. The proximal gastric portion is then retracted to the left side.
- The left gastric artery is divided at its origin from the celiac axis.

- The retroperitoneal attachment of the stomach is dissected up to the diaphragmatic crura; then the phreno-esophageal membrane is dissected, and the vagus nerves are divided leading to the full mobilization of the abdominal esophagus.
- Distal esophagus transection.
- Surgical specimen extraction.

11.5 Lymphadenectomy

The Japanese Gastric Cancer Association [2] defined 33 different regional lymphatic stations. The extent of lymph nodal dissection is sorted by the D-level criteria into D1, D1+, or D2 and is defined according to the type of gastrectomy performed (total, distal, or proximal gastrectomy) (Table 11.1). Each of the D levels has specific indications based on the tumor location, TNM category, and histological subtype.

Some centers systematically perform indocyanine green fluorescence imaging for lymphatic mapping during laparoscopic gastrectomy, especially in case of total gastrectomy [3].

Lymph node dissection can be performed in three different ways:

- En bloc: all lymph node stations are removed together with the surgical specimen.
- For each station: each lymph node station is removed by the surgeon separately.
- Back table: firstly, the lymph node stations are removed together with the surgical specimen, and subsequently, the surgeon proceeds to identify and divide each lymph node station which will be sent separately to the pathologist.

Table 11.1 D-level criteria, the Japanese Gastric Cancer Association

	Total gastrectomy	Distal gastrectomy	Proximal gastrectomy
D0	Lymphadenectomy less than D1	Lymphadenectomy less than D1	Lymphadenectomy less than D1
D1	No. 1–7	No. 1, 3, 4sb, 4d, 5, 6, 7	No. 1, 2, 3a, 4sa, 4sb, 7
D1+	D1+ no. 8a, 9, 11p	D1+ no. 8a, 9	D1+ No. 8a, 9, 11p
D2	D1+ no. 8a, 9, 11p, 11d, 12a	D1+ no. 8a, 9, 11p, 12a	

11.6 Reconstruction After Gastrectomy

The time of reconstruction starts when the frozen section can confirm distal and proximal free resection margins.

To date, several anastomotic methods are described in the literature, each of them having been reported with advantages and disadvantages [4, 5]. All different types of anastomoses are reported as follows according with the type of gastric resection (Table 11.2):

However, the most performed types of anastomoses are Billroth I (B-I), Billroth II (B-II), and Roux-en-Y procedure.

The *Billroth I (B-I)* reconstruction restores the duodenal and jejunal continuity between the remnant proximal stomach and the duodenal stump. Despite the higher frequency of gastritis, esophagitis, and bile reflux, B-I gastroduodenostomy is the only procedure that restores a physiological digestive tract continuity and the first choice after distal gastrectomy in most eastern facilities. B-I is commonly carried out extra- abdominally due to the fact that the intra-abdominal procedure is rather challenging. This type of anastomosis can be performed hand-sewn or employing circular or linear staplers (delta-shaped anastomosis) and fashioned as an end-to-end, end-to-side, or side-to-side anastomosis [6]. The essential steps are reported as follows:

- Completing the mobilization of the duodenum
- Creating a duodenotomy and a gastrotomy to introduce the stapler
- Creating a gastroduodenostomy between the duodenal stump and the stomach wall
- Closing the gastrotomy

Several tests can be made to check the anastomosis' quality (ICG, blue test, endoscopic examination).

The *Billroth II (B-II)* reconstruction provides a jejunal (but not a duodenal) continuity by an end-to-side or a side-to-side gastrojejunal anastomosis (Fig. 11.3). The B-II reconstruction can be fashioned in an antecolic or a retrocolic position and as an isoperistaltic or an antiperistaltic anastomosis. The essential steps are reported as follows:

- Identifying the ileal loop about 40 cm far from the angle of Treitz
- Creating a jejunotomy on the antimesenteric side of this loop and a gastrotomy on the posterior wall of the stomach
- Creating a side-to-side anastomosis by employing a linear stapler or of an end-to-side anastomosis by using a circular stapler
- Closing the gastro-enterotomy created to introduce the stapler with a linear stapler or manually

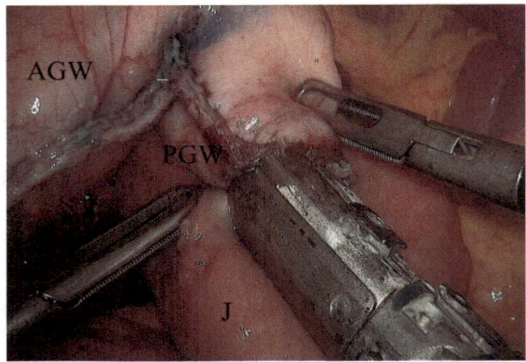

Fig. 11.3 Billroth II gastrojejunostomy. *AGW* anterior gastric wall, *PGW* posterior gastric wall, *J* jejunum

Table 11.2 Reconstruction methods by gastrectomy type

Total gastrectomy	Distal gastrectomy	Proximal gastrectomy
Roux-en-Y esophagojejunostomy	Billroth I gastroduodenostomy	Esophagogastrostomy
Jejunal interposition	Billroth II gastrojejunostomy	Jejunal interposition
Double-tract method	Roux-en-Y gastrojejunostomy	Double-tract method
	Jejunal interposition	

Several tests can be used to check the anastomosis' quality (ICG, blue test, endoscopic examination).

The *Roux-en-Y* reconstruction is characterized by two anastomoses, a gastrojejunal (after distal gastrectomy) or an esophagojejunal (after total gastrectomy) anastomosis using an autonomized jejunal loop and a jejuno-jejunal anastomosis to restore the continuity of the small bowel. Several studies have analyzed the endoscopic findings during patient's follow-up documenting that the Roux-en-Y reconstruction can reduce the incidence of food residues, esophagitis, gastritis, and bile reflux as compared to the B-I and B-II procedures [7]. The essential steps are reported as follows:

- Finding the ligament of Treitz and dividing the jejunum about 40 cm far from it, creating an autonomized Roux-en-Y loop and a biliopancreatic loop.
- Bringing the Roux-en-Y loop up to the esophagus/proximal stomach in an antecolic (above the transverse colon) or a transmesocolic (behind the transverse colon through a mesocolic hole) fashion.
- Creating an esophagojejunal/gastrojejunal anastomosis with the help of a circular (end-to-side anastomosis) or a linear stapler (side-to-side anastomosis). After total gastrectomy, in case of the use of a circular stapler, the anvil is inserted into the esophageal stump using the purse-string instrument or a hand-sewing method. The anvil can be inserted also trans orally with the OrVil™ technique.
- Closing the esophagotomy/gastrostomy with a linear stapler or manually.
- Creating a jejuno-jejunal anastomosis with a linear stapler in previously aligned antimesenteric side of the biliopancreatic and the Roux loops (about 70 cm far from the previous anastomosis).
- Closing the enterotomy with a linear stapler or manually.

Several tests can be made to check the anastomosis' quality (ICG, blue test, endoscopic examination)

Esophagogastrostomy (EGS) is the most popular and classical reconstruction method after proximal gastrectomy because it involves a unique anastomosis site. This procedure is widely used worldwide. It is well documented that the EGS procedure can often lead to severe reflux esophagitis due to resection of the cardiac sphincter. Its essential steps are reported as follows:

- Creating a window on the anterior wall of the gastric remnant
- Creating a window on the posterior wall of the esophagus
- Carrying out an esophagogastrostomy with a linear stapler
- Closing the enterotomy mechanically with a further linear stapler (or manually with an hand-sewn suture)

Double-tract reconstruction (DTR) is based on a conventional Roux-en-Y esophagojejunostomy and consists of an additional gastrojejunostomy, to preserve the duodenal route. It has been proposed and developed to promote a better food passage, reduce the acid reflux, and decrease the rate of anastomotic stricture. Nevertheless, double-tract reconstruction is technically challenging and time-consuming. The essential steps are reported as follows:

- Transecting the jejunum 20–30 cm from the angle of Treitz to obtain an autonomized jejunal loop.
- Creating an esophagojejunostomy on this loop using a circular (the anvil of the stapler is inserted into the esophageal lumen, end-to side anastomosis) or a linear stapler (side-to-side anastomosis).
- Creating a side-to-side mechanical gastrojejunostomy on the same loop, performed at least

20 cm below the previous esophagogastrostomy.

- Closing the common entry hole of the gastrojejunostomy.
- Creating a side-to-side jejuno-jejunostomy as in case of Roux-en-Y reconstruction. The antimesenteric borders of the proximal and distal jejunal loops are approximated 20 cm below the gastrojejunostomy.
- Closing the common entry hole of the jejuno-jejunostomy with a linear stapler or manually.

11.7 Operating Room Setup

The operating room disposition for gastrectomy is described below:

- A split-leg table is positioned in the center of the theatre.
- The laparoscopic column is placed on the left side of the patient.
- Two monitors for the laparoscopic camera are positioned by the side of each patient's shoulder and angled as to provide an optimal view for both the operating surgeon and the assistants.
- The instrument tables are placed at the distal third of the right leg board.
- The scrub nurse is positioned on the right side of the patient.

Positions for the surgeon and assistants can be different according to the local practice; however, it is usually dynamic during surgery.

At the beginning of the procedure, the surgeon stands on the patient's right side and the first assistant on the left side. The second assistant holds the camera between the patient's legs. Subsequently, during the different steps of the procedure, the surgeons can switch places as necessary (Fig. 11.4).

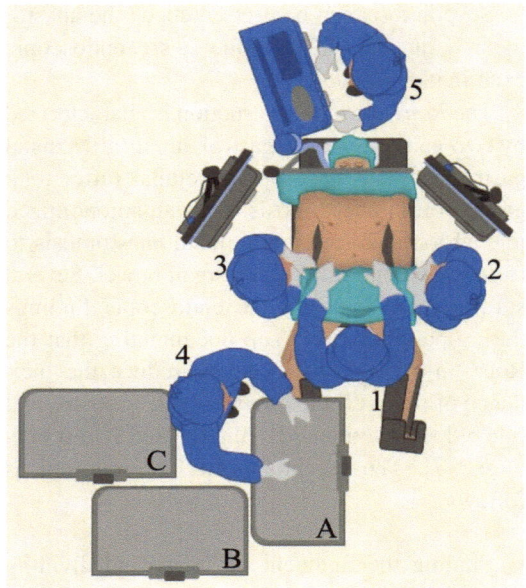

Fig. 11.4 Operating room setup. (**a**) Laparoscopic instruments, (**b**) instruments for open surgery, (**c**) other instruments, (1) camera assistant, (2) first assistant, (3) surgeon, (4) scrub nurse, (5) anesthesiologists

11.8 Patient Positioning

Usually, the patient is placed supine, with the arms extended along the body and secured with safety straps to the table. Patient's legs are split and secured into the footboard to avoid sliding. All pressure points must be padded [8].

Under general anesthesia, the patient is placed in the reverse Trendelenburg position with the head elevated about 15–30°.

11.9 Abdominal Access and Port Placement

Access to the abdominal cavity can be done through:

- Veress needle technique on Palmer's point (left upper quadrant 3 cm below the costal margin, on the midclavicular line)
- Hasson trocar placement under direct open visualization at the supraumbilical region

Pneumoperitoneum is maintained with CO2 insufflation at an intra-abdominal pressure of 12 mmHg.

A total of 5 trocars are usually sufficient to complete surgery. The camera is first inserted through the umbilical trocar of 12 mm. The other ports are inserted under direct vision in the right upper quadrant (5–12 mm), in the left upper quadrant (5–12 mm), and in the right and left flank (5 mm) of the abdomen. A 10-mm 30° camera is employed, and a sixth port is placed in the epigastrium in case of external liver retraction (Fig. 11.5).

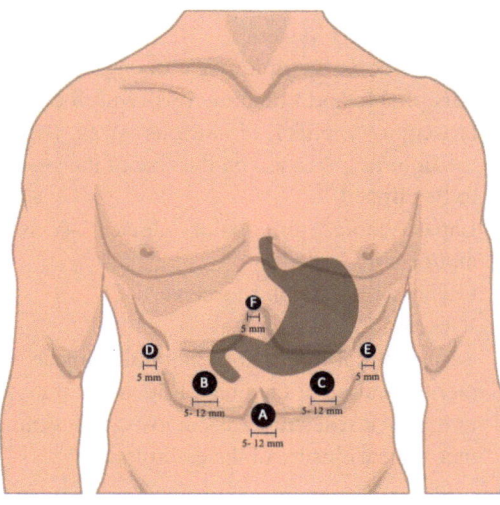

Fig. 11.5 Port placement: (**a**) camera port, (**b–e**) operative ports, (**f**) liver retractor port

11.10 Equipment and Surgical Instruments Required

A conventional laparoscopic column, including a high-definition camera and display systems, a CO_2 insufflator, light source, video and image storage devices, and a basic package for open surgery must be available.

11.10.1 Laparoscopic Instrument

- 5- to 12-mm trocars
- 30° endoscope
- Laparoscopic grasping forceps (Croce-Olmi forceps, Grasper or Johann forceps)
- Laparoscopic suction/irrigation system
- Absorbable and titanium clips (with dedicated laparoscopic applier) of various sizes (small/medium/large)
- Laparoscopic monopolar devices—scissors and or hook
- Laparoscopic bipolar forceps
- Laparoscopic needle holder
- Scope warmer
- Vessel sealing system
- Varieties of intestinal Endo-GIA and circular staplers—on surgeon's request
- A wound protector-retractor for removal of the specimen
- Sutures on surgeon's requests

11.10.2 Open Instrument

- 2 scalpels with stainless steel blade (sizes 11 and 24)
- 1 kidney basin

- 2 Janach (steel bowls)
- 2 anatomical tissue forceps
- 2 toothed forceps
- 4 straight Klemmer forceps
- 4 straight Kocher forceps
- 1 Mayo scissors
- 1 Nelson-Metzenbaum dissection scissors
- 1 foerster clamp
- 4 Backhaus clamps
- 1 Mixter right angle forceps
- 1 curved Bengolea forceps
- 3 Mathieu retractors
- 2 Langenbeck retractors
- 1 monopolar electric scalpel
- 1 wound protector/retractor
- 700-mL endobag

11.11 Other Devices

11.11.1 ICG (Indocyanine Green)

The indocyanine green fluorescent (IGC) dye is presented in vials of 25 mg of powder for solution for injection.

- The ICG should be used in concentrations of 0.5 mg/mL and administered at a dose of 0.05 mg/kg.
- It should be diluted with sterile distilled water and *not* with sodium chloride (NaCl) as the latter could cause aggregation.
- After preparation, the solution must be stored in a dark and cool place to avoid rapid deterioration of the whitening fluorescence.

11.11.2 Surgical Steps and Related Instruments

11.11.2.1 Hasson Technique for Laparoscopic Access
- 1 scalpel (blade 11)
- 2 tissue forceps
- 2 Mathieu retractors
- 1 Nelson-Metzenbaum dissection scissors
- 2 straight Kocher forceps to grasp fascia
- 2 straight Klemmer forceps to grasp parietal peritoneum

11.11.2.2 Veress Technique for Laparoscopic Access
- Scalpel (blade 11)
- Veress needle
- Syringe for saline drop test

11.11.2.3 Port Placement
- Scalpel (blade 11)
- 1 monopolar electric scalpel
- 5 and 5- to12-mm trocars
- Tubing set for the CO_2 insufflation

11.11.2.4 Demolitive Phase
The demolitive phase provides a complete mobilization of the stomach, its transection, and a lymphadenectomy as planned according to tumor location and pathology and TNM stage.

The needed instruments are the following:

- A 30° endoscope and a scope warmer
- Grasping forceps
- Vessel sealing system
- Laparoscopic suction/irrigation system
- Absorbable and titanium clips (with their laparoscopic applier) of various sizes (small/medium/large) based on the size of the vessels to be clipped
- Laparoscopic monopolar device—scissors and/or hook
- Laparoscopic bipolar forceps
- ICG (indocyanine green)
- Sufficient cartridges for Endo-GIA linear stapler to be used at the time of duodenal transection, gastric resection, anastomosis, and eventual mechanical closure of the enterotomies.

11.11.2.5 Reconstructive Phase
During the reconstructive phase, the required instruments are as follows:

- A 30° endoscope and a scope warmer
- Grasping forceps
- Vessel sealing system
- Laparoscopic suction/irrigation system
- Laparoscopic monopolar device—scissors and/or hook
- Laparoscopic bipolar forceps
- Laparoscopic needle holder
- Staplers and sutures on surgeon request

Once the anastomosis and the hemostasias in the surgical field have been completed, the instrumental nurse makes gauze and needle counts.

The specimen is extracted through a Pfannenstiel mini-laparotomy or a periumbilical incision (more indicated in obese patients) using a wound protector/retractor.

During the specimen extraction phase, the required instruments are as follows:

- 1 scalpel (blade 24)
- 1 monopolar electric scalpel
- 2 anatomical/toothed tissue forceps (based on surgeon's requests)
- 3 Mathieu retractors
- 1 Nelson-Metzenbaum dissection scissors
- 2 straight Kocher forceps to grasp the fascia
- 2 straight Klemmer forceps to grasp the parietal peritoneum
- 1 wound protector/retractor to safely extract the specimen
- 1 absorbable suture for peritoneum
- 1 looped/monofilament/braided suture (based on surgeon's request) to perform closure of the fascia
- 1 monofilament/braided suture (based on surgeon's request) to perform suture of the subcutaneous plane
- Titanium skin clips/suture to perform skin closure

11.11.3 Intraoperative Complications

In comparison with open surgery, the incidence of intraoperative complications during laparoscopic procedures appears to be similar, and bleeding and injuries to contiguous organs are the most frequent [9]. In these circumstances, the scrub nurse must have the following instruments available:

- Laparoscopic suction/irrigation system
- 10 × 10 cm gauzes

- Absorbable and titanium clips (with their laparoscopic applier) of various sizes (small/medium/large) based on the size of the vessel needing to be clipped
- Laparoscopic monopolar devices—scissors and/or hook
- Laparoscopic bipolar forceps
- Laparoscopic needle holder and monofilament suture with a small-gauge needle to attempt the direct repair of the bleeding vessel
- Laparoscopic vascular clamp

References

1. Lordick F, et al. Gastric cancer: ESMO clinical practice guideline for diagnosis, treatment and follow-up. Ann Oncol. 2022;33(10):1005–20. https://doi.org/10.1016/j.annonc.2022.07.004.
2. Japanese gastric cancer association. Japanese gastric cancer treatment guidelines 2021 (6th edition). Gastric cancer 2023;26:1–25. https://doi.org/10.1007/s10120-022-01331-8.
3. Chen Q-Y, et al. Safety and efficacy of Indocyanine green tracer-guided lymph node dissection during laparoscopic radical gastrectomy in patients with gastric cancer. JAMA Surg. 2020;155(4):300. https://doi.org/10.1001/jamasurg.2019.6033.
4. Huang CM, Zheng CH. Reconstruction of the digestive tract after laparoscopic gastrectomy for gastric cancer. In: Laparoscopic gastrectomy for gastric cancer; 2015. pp. 309–337. https://doi.org/10.1007/978-94-017-9873-0_8.
5. Inokuchi M, et al. Long-term outcomes of roux-en-Y and Billroth-I reconstruction after laparoscopic distal gastrectomy. Gastric Cancer. 2012;16(1):67–73. https://doi.org/10.1007/s10120-012-0154-5.
6. Zhang S, Fukunaga T. Current status of technique for Billroth-I anastomosis in totally laparoscopic distal gastrectomy for gastric cancer. Mini-invasive Surg. 2019;3:2. https://doi.org/10.20517/2574-1225.2018.64.
7. Lee M-S, et al. What is the best reconstruction method after distal gastrectomy for gastric cancer? Surg Endosc. 2011;26(6):1539–47. https://doi.org/10.1007/s00464-011-2064-8.
8. Lam J, et al. Minimally invasive gastrectomy. In: Minimally invasive surgical techniques for cancers of the gastrointestinal tract; 2019. pp. 85–91. https://doi.org/10.1007/978-3-030-18740-8_9.
9. Etoh T, Chung HY, Kim MC. Intraoperative complications of laparoscopic gastrectomy. In: Laparoscopic gastrectomy for cancer; 2012. pp. 121–122. https://doi.org/10.1007/978-4-431-54003-8_25.

Robotic Gastrectomy

12

Marco Milone, Michele Manigrasso,
Salvatore D'Angelo, Salvatore Aprea,
and Giovanni Domenico De Palma

12.1 Gastrectomy

Gastrectomy can basically be divided into two moments: the demolitive phase and the reconstructive phase.

12.1.1 Demolitive Phase

The demolitive phase in turn consists of two parts: organ resection and lymphadenectomy.

Organ resection can be partial or total: in the first case we will talk about total gastrectomy, while in the second about distal or proximal partial gastrectomy.

12.1.1.1 Total Gastrectomy

Total gastrectomy consists of the following surgical steps:

- Mobilization of gastric greater curvature, through coloepiploic detachment and section of gastrocolic and gastrosplenic ligaments

- Ligation and section of right gastroepiploic vessels, left gastroepiploic vessels, and short gastric vessels along the greater curvature
- Mobilization of the duodenum, through section of the hepatoduodenal ligament on the side of the gastric lesser curvature (*pars tensa* of the lesser omentum)
- Transection of the duodenum below the pylorus
- Lymphadenectomy of the main lymph node stations (D2 lymphadenectomy)
- Identification, ligation, and section of left gastric artery on the lesser curvature
- Completion of gastrectomy by transection of distal esophagus

12.1.1.2 Distal and Proximal Partial Gastrectomy

Distal partial gastrectomy provides the removal of the distal part of the stomach and differs from total gastrectomy in the type of organ section and in the vascular sections that are performed. Therefore, the surgical steps are as follows:

- Mobilization of gastric greater curvature
- Ligation of right and left gastroepiploic vessels with safeguarding of short gastric arteries
- Mobilization of duodenum and its transection below the pylorus
- Identification and ligation of left gastric artery (some authors recommend safeguarding the

M. Milone (✉) · S. D'Angelo · S. Aprea ·
G. D. De Palma
Department of Clinical Medicine and Surgery,
"Federico II" University of Naples, Naples, Italy
e-mail: giovanni.depalma@unina.it

M. Manigrasso
Department of Advanced Biomedical Sciences,
"Federico II" University of Naples, Naples, Italy
e-mail: michele.manigrasso@unina.it

ascending branch of the left gastric artery to ensure adequate vascularization of the residual gastric pouch)

- Transection of the stomach, along its horizontal axis, into the proximal part of it

Proximal partial gastrectomy (or superior polar gastrectomy) consists of removal of the proximal part of the stomach, or of the fundus and part of the body.

The surgical steps are as follows:

- Mobilization of greater curvature at the gastrosplenic ligament
- Section of short gastric arteries and safeguarding of gastroepiploic vessels
- Identification, ligation, and section of left gastric artery at its origin, on the side of the lesser curvature
- Mobilization of the distal esophagus
- Partial mobilization of the duodenum to allow the subsequent esophagogastric anastomosis
- Transection of distal esophagus
- Transection of stomach along its horizontal axis at the level of gastric body

Lymphadenectomy

Gastric lymph node stations are numerous and are distinguished on the basis of their location:

1	Right paracardial (including those around the esophageal branch of the left gastric artery in front of the right diaphragmatic crus)
2	Left paracardial (including those around the esophageal branch of the left inferior phrenic artery)
3a	Lesser curvature, along the left gastric artery branches
3b	Lesser curvature, along the distal part of right gastric artery and its second branch
4sa	Greater curvature, along the short gastric arteries (perigastric area)
4sb	Greater curvature, along the left gastroepiploic artery (perigastric area)
4d	Greater curvature (second branch and distal part of right gastroepiploic artery)
5	Suprapyloric (around the right gastric artery and its first branch into the hepatoduodenal ligament)

6	Infrapyloric (around the origin and the proximal part of the right gastroepiploic artery near the gastrocolic trunk of Henle)
7	Left gastric artery (around the tract of the artery between its origin from the celiac trunk and the origin of its ascending branch, i.e., its entrance into the small omentum where it relates to the gastric lesser curvature)
8a	Common hepatic artery, antero-superior group
8p	Common hepatic artery, posterior group
9	Celiac trunk
10	Splenic hilum: lymph nodes associated with the splenic artery between the hilum and pancreatic tail, lymph nodes at the root of short gastric arteries, and lymph nodes along the left gastroepiploic artery proximal to its first gastric branch
11p	Splenic artery, proximal (from its origin to half its length between its origin and the end of the pancreatic tail)
11d	Splenic artery, distal (from the middle of its length between its origin and the end of the pancreatic tail to the pancreatic tail)
12a	Hepatoduodenal ligament, along the proper hepatic artery in the caudal half between the confluence of the hepatic ducts and the upper margin of the pancreas
12b	Hepatoduodenal ligament, along the biliary tract in the caudal half between the confluence of the hepatic ducts and the upper margin of the pancreas
12p	Hepatoduodenal ligament, in the caudal half of the portal vein between the confluence of the hepatic ducts and the upper border of the pancreas
13	Posterior surface of the pancreatic head (in relation to the posterior pancreatic-duodenal arterial arch and cranial to the duodenal papilla)
14v	Superior mesenteric vein
14a	Root of superior mesenteric artery (between the origin of the superior mesenteric artery, the trunk of Henle on the right, and the jejunal vessels caudally)
15	Middle colic vessels
16a1	Aortic hiatus
16a2	Para-aortic from the upper margin of the celiac trunk origin to the lower margin of the left renal vein
16b1	Para-aortic from the lower margin of the left renal vein to the upper margin of the inferior mesenteric artery
16b2	Para-aortic from the superior margin of the origin of the inferior mesenteric artery to the aortic bifurcation

17	Anterior surface of the pancreatic head
18	Lower margin of the pancreatic body
19	Infradiaphragmatic, mainly along the inferior phrenic artery
20	Paraesophageal (esophageal hiatus of the diaphragm)
110	Paraesophageal (inferior mediastinum)
111	Supradiaphragmatic (distinct from peri-esophageal lymph nodes)
112	Posterior mediastinum (distinct from peri-esophageal lymph nodes)

Lymphadenectomy can be performed in three different ways:

- En bloc: all lymph node stations are extracted together with the surgical specimen and sent to the pathological anatomy laboratory for recognition.
- For each station: each lymph node station is removed by the surgeon separately and therefore as different samples.
- Back table: the lymph node stations are removed with the surgical specimen and the surgeon, with the help of the instrument nurse, proceeds to recognize and separate the various lymph node stations.

12.1.2 Reconstructive Phase

The reconstructive phase involves restoring the continuity of the gastrointestinal tract.

Various types of anastomosis are described in the literature, but those most performed to date and, therefore, the most frequently encountered by an instrument nurse are basically three:

- Billroth I anastomosis
- Billroth II anastomosis
- Roux-en-Y anastomosis

Billroth I anastomosis provides a gastroduodenal anastomosis, which therefore consists of the following surgical times:

- Complete mobilization of the duodenum

- Performing a duodenotomy and a gastrotomy on the posterior wall of the stomach
- End-to-end anastomosis by circular stapler
- Closure of gastrotomy created to introduce the stapler

Billroth II anastomosis, on the other hand, provides an end-to-side or side-to-side gastro-jejunal anastomosis (depending on whether the anastomosis is totally intracorporeal or hand-assisted extracorporeal) and consists of the following surgical times:

- Selection of the ileal loop about 40 cm from the duodenal-jejunal angle of Treitz
- Performing a jejunotomy and a gastrotomy on the posterior wall of the stomach
- Side-to-side anastomosis by linear stapler or end-to-side anastomosis by circular stapler
- Closure of gastro-enterotomy (or gastrotomy) created to introduce the stapler

Roux-en-Y anastomosis instead provides for the execution of a double anastomosis, a gastro-jejunal anastomosis, and a jejuno-jejunal one and consists of the following surgical times:

- Resection of the small intestine about 40 cm from the Treitz ligament, allowing the creation of a double "path": the biliary and the alimentary path
- Anastomosis of the alimentary loop (the intestinal loop that proceeds reaching the ileocecal valve) to the stomach through a side-to-side or end-to-side anastomosis (depending on whether the anastomosis is totally intracorporeal or hand-assisted extracorporeal)
- Anastomosis of the biliary loop (the intestinal loop connected to the duodenal stump) to the alimentary loop about 20–30 cm from the gastro-jejunal anastomosis through a side-to-side or side-to-end anastomosis (also in this case depending on whether the anastomosis is intra- or extracorporeal)
- Closure of gastro-enterotomies created to introduce the staplers

Fig. 12.1 Schematic
operating theatre setting

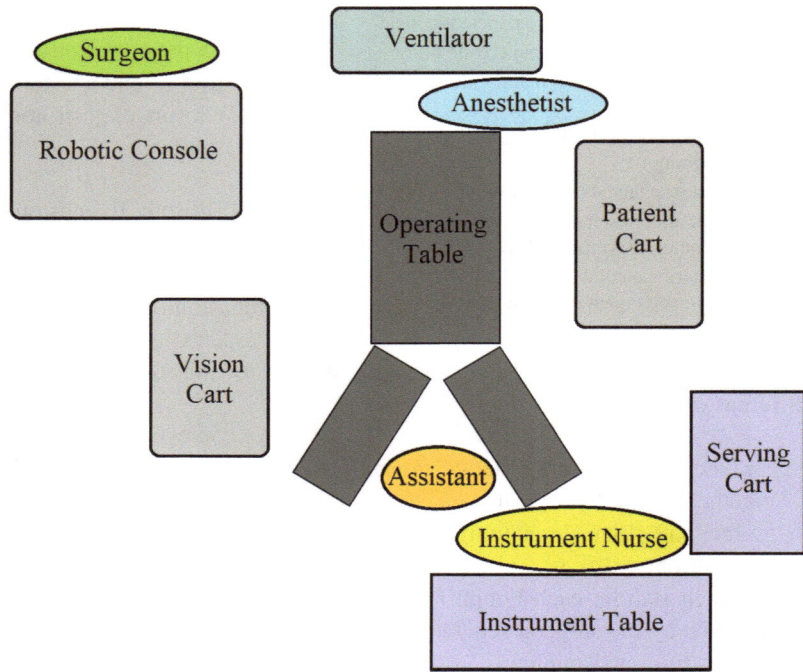

12.2 Operating Theatre Setting

The operating theatre setting for a robotic gastrectomy is performed as follows (Fig. 12.1):

- Operating table in the center of the theatre
- Vision cart positioned to the right of the patient, at the level of the feet
- Patient cart positioned to the left of the patient
- Surgeon positioned at the surgical console
- First assistant at the operating table positioned between the patient's legs
- Instrument nurse to the right of the first assistant
- Serving cart to the right of instrument nurse

12.3 Patient Positioning

Patient positioning is performed as shown in Fig. 12.2:

- Supine position in reverse Trendelenburg with an inclination of about 15° to 20°
- Spread legs
- Arms adducted along the body

The operating table is therefore prepared with a sliding prevent mat (Pink Pad®), or, in its absence, with a leg fixing with bandages to prevent the patient from falling from the operating table.

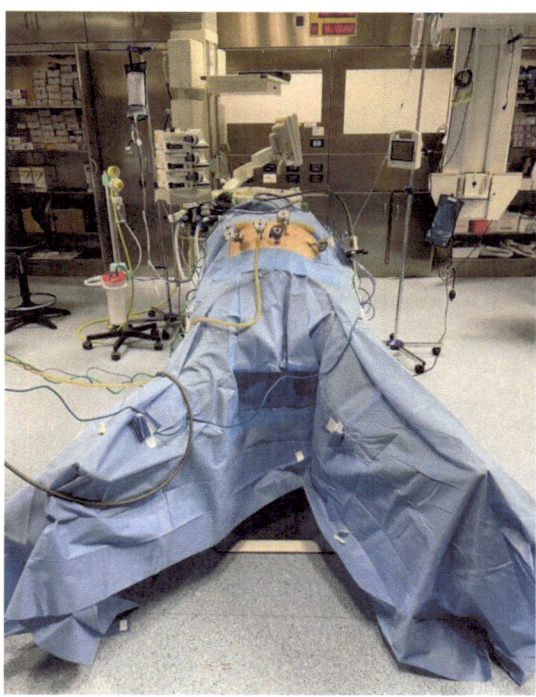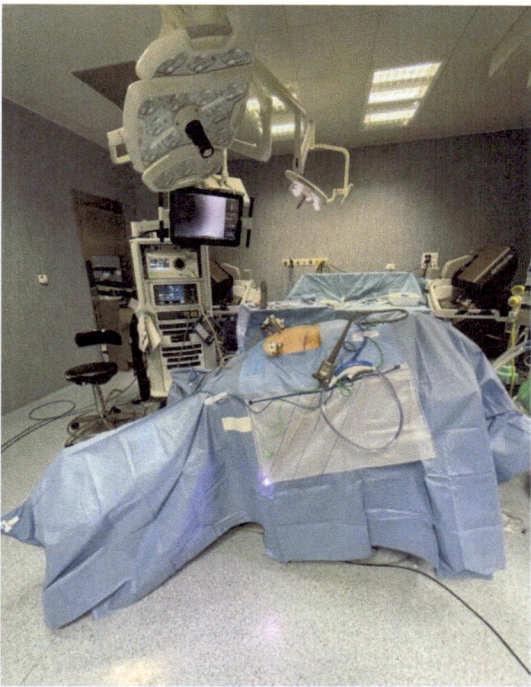

Fig. 12.2 The operating table is prepared with a mat to prevent sliding and the patient cart is directed onto the operating table starting from the patient's left

12.4   Port Placement and Robotic Docking

After the creation of pneumoperitoneum, the following lines are drawn on the abdomen with a sterile marker and ruler:

- Mid-clavicular lines, which joins the midpoint of the clavicle with the anterior-superior iliac spine
- Transverse umbilical line, a transverse line passing through the umbilicus

Port placement in robotic surgery is performed according to a standardized technique, along a transverse line located approximately 4 cm cranially than the transverse umbilical line, as follows (Fig. 12.3):

- Port placement in a straight line at 8 cm from each other.

- The line should pass approximately 4 cm above the transverse umbilical line.
- 8 mm port except for the 12 mm port on the right flank.
- One assistant port or two assistant ports placed caudally than robotic ports according to standardized triangulation.

If the patient is obese and, therefore, the transverse umbilical line is displaced lower than a normal weight patient, the surgeon will position the ports on a transverse line placed more cranially than the transverse umbilical line, considering that the distance between the passing line for ports and target anatomy should not exceed 20 cm.

The "targeting" (the selection through endoscope of the target anatomy) is carried out on the falciform ligament/left lobe of the liver to allow the surgeon at the console to move freely throughout the gastric area.

Fig. 12.3 Port placement to perform a robotic gastrectomy

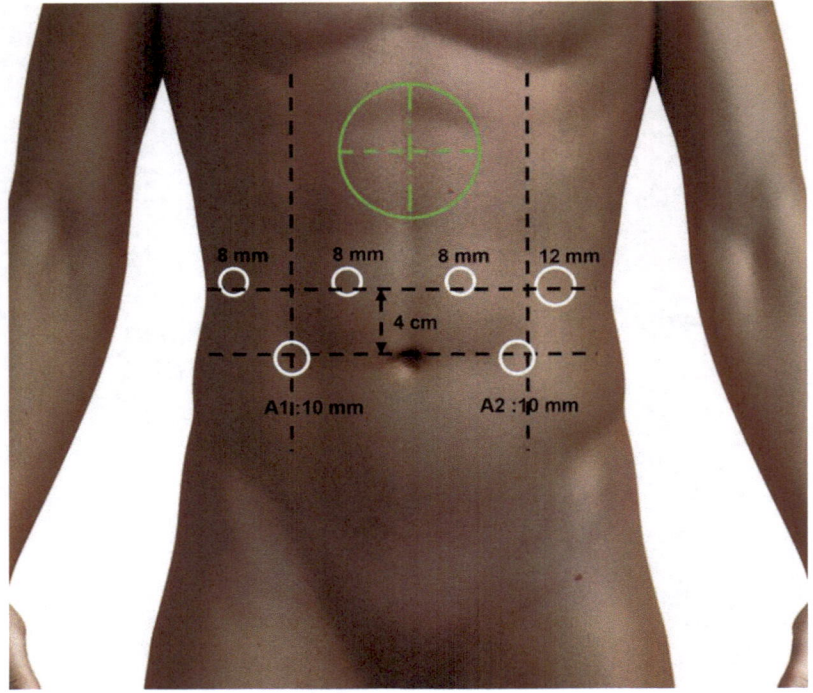

12.5 Surgical Instruments Required

The preparation of the instrument table and the serving cart must be carried out as shown in Fig. 12.4.

Robotic Instruments:
- 4 ports (two 8 mm ports and two 12 mm ports)
- 2 port reducers
- 1 port with tubing set for the stabilization of pneumoperitoneum
- 30° robotic endoscope
- 1 grasping forceps (ProGrasp Forceps® or Cadiere Forceps®)
- 1 bipolar forceps (Fenestrated Bipolar Forceps®)
- 1 monopolar instrument (Permanent Cautery Hook® or Hot Shears®)
- 1 sealing instrument (Vessel Sealer® or Harmonic Ace® 8 mm)
- 1 stapler (SureForm EndoWrist Stapler® 40 mm or 60 mm)
- 1 needle holder (Large Needle Driver®)

Laparoscopic Instrument:
- Laparoscopic grasping forceps (Croce-Olmi forceps, Grasper or Johann forceps)
- Laparoscopic suction/irrigation system
- 2 assistant ports (10 mm)
- 10 mm and 12 mm endoscopic clip applier
- Hem-o-lok clips with laparoscopic applier of various sizes (small/medium/large)
- Laparoscopic scissors
- Scope warmer

Open Instrument:
- 2 scalpels with stainless steel blade (sizes 11 and 24)
- 1 kidney basin
- 2 Janach (steel bowls)
- 2 anatomical tissue forceps
- 2 toothed forceps
- 4 curved Klemmer clamps
- 4 curved Kocher clamps
- 1 Mayo scissors
- 1 Nelson-Metzenbaum dissection scissors
- 1 Foerster clamp
- 4 Backhaus clamps

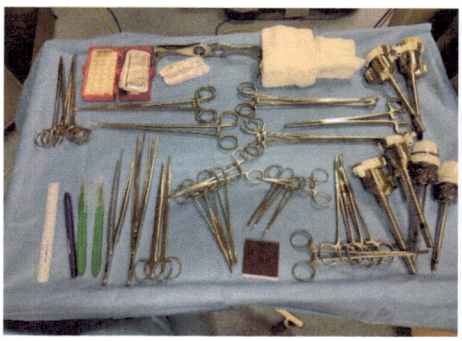 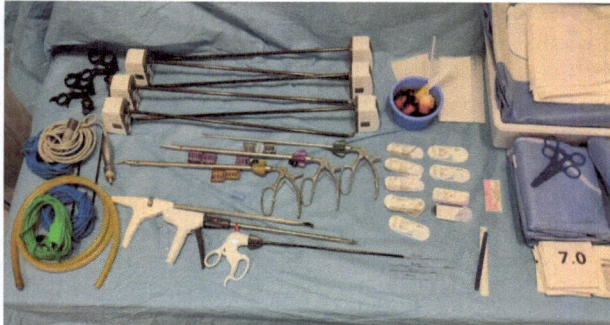

Fig. 12.4 Serving cart (left) and instrument table (right)

- 1 Mixter right angle forceps
- 1 curved Bengolea forceps
- 3 Mathieu retractors
- 2 Langenbeck retractors
- 1 monopolar electric scalpel
- 1 wound protector/retractor
- 700 ml endobag

12.5.1 Other Devices

12.5.1.1   ICG (Indocyanine Green)
The indocyanine green fluorescent (IGC) dye is presented in vials of 25 mg of powder for solution for injection.

- Use in concentrations of 0.5 mg/ml.
- Dilute with sterile distilled water and *not* sodium chloride (NaCl) as the latter could cause aggregation.
- After preparation, the solution must be stored in a dark and cool place to avoid rapid deterioration of the whitening fluorescence.
- For the dosage to be administered, follow the instructions of the anesthetist present in the theatre.

12.6   Surgical Steps and Related Instruments

Hasson Technique for Laparoscopic Access:
- 1 scalpel (blade 11)
- 2 anatomical tissue forceps
- 2 Mathieu retractors

- 1 Nelson-Metzenbaum dissection scissors
- 2 curved Kocher clamps to grasp fascia
- 2 curved Klemmer clamps to grasp parietal peritoneum

Veress Technique for Laparoscopic Access:
- Scalpel (blade 11)
- Veress needle
- Syringe for saline drop test

Port Placement and Robotic Docking:
- Sterile marker and ruler to measure the distance between ports
- 2 robotic 12-mm ports
- 2 robotic 8-mm ports
- 1 port with tubing set for the stabilization of pneumoperitoneum

Once the ports have been positioned and the patient cart positioned on the operating table, the arm that accommodates the endoscope is connected by the instrument nurse and the first assistant at the table performs pointing at the target anatomy. Once the targeting is complete, the other arms are docked and the robotic instruments are inserted by the instrument nurse, after positioning the reducers on the 12-mm ports to avoid loss of pneumoperitoneum.

12.6.1 Demolitive Phase

The demolitive phase provides the complete mobilization of the stomach, its transection, and lymphadenectomy.

The robotic instruments to be used are as follows (based on the surgeon's requests):

- 30° robotic endoscope
- 1 grasping forceps (ProGrasp Forceps® or Cadiere Forceps®)
- 1 bipolar forceps (Fenestrated Bipolar Forceps®)
- 1 monopolar instrument (Permanent Cautery Hook® or Hot Shears®) or, alternatively
- 1 sealing instrument (Vessel Sealer® or Harmonic Ace® 8 mm)
- 1 stapler (SureForm EndoWrist Stapler® 40 mm or 60 mm) to be used at the time of duodenal transection and in the gastric section

The grasping forceps are used by the surgeon during the dissection phases of the planes for the complete mobilization of the stomach, as are the sealing instruments.

The laparoscopic instruments used by the first assistant at the table are as follows:

- Laparoscopic grasping forceps (Croce-Olmi forceps, grasper or Johann forceps)
- Laparoscopic suction/irrigation system
- 10 mm and 12 mm endoscopic clip applier
- Hem-o-lok clips with laparoscopic applier of various sizes (small/medium/large) based on the size of the vase to be clipped
- Laparoscopic scissors

12.6.2 Reconstructive Phase

During the reconstructive phase, the required instruments are as follows:

- 30° robotic endoscope
- 1 grasping forceps (ProGrasp Forceps® or Cadiere Forceps®)
- 1 bipolar forceps (Fenestrated Bipolar Forceps®)
- 1 monopolar instrument (Permanent Cautery Hook® or Hot Shears®) to perform enterotomy and gastrotomy

- 1 stapler (SureForm EndoWrist Stapler® 40 mm or 60 mm) to perform the anastomosis
- 1 needle holder (Large Needle Driver®)
- 1 barbed/monofilament/braided suture (based on the surgeon's requests) to perform closure of gastro-/enterotomies

Once the anastomosis and the revision of the hemostasis have been completed, the instrumental nurse makes gauze and needle counts and the specimen will therefore be extracted.

The specimen is extracted through a Pfannenstiel minilaparotomy or a periumbilical incision (more indicated in obese patients) using a wound protector/retractor.

During the specimen extraction phase, the required instruments are as follows:

- 1 scalpel (blade 24)
- 1 monopolar electric scalpel
- 2 anatomical/toothed tissue forceps (based on the surgeon's requests)
- 3 Mathieu retractors
- 1 Nelson-Metzenbaum dissection scissors
- 2 curved Kocher clamps to grasp fascia
- 2 curved Klemmer clamps to grasp parietal peritoneum
- 1 wound protector/retractor to extract specimen safely
- 1 absorbable suture for peritoneum
- 1 looped/monofilament/braided suture (based on the surgeon's request) to perform closure of fascia
- 1 monofilament/braided suture (based on the surgeon's request) to perform suture of subcutaneous plane
- Titanium skin clips/suture to perform closure of skin

12.7 Intraoperative Complications

The most frequent intraoperative complications to manage during a robotic gastrectomy are basically two: hemorrhage and injuries of parenchymatous organs (pancreas, liver, and more rarely spleen).

In these circumstances, the instrument nurse must have the following instruments available:

- Laparoscopic suction/irrigation system
- 10 cm × 10 cm gauze to be passed to the assistant at the request of the surgeon
- Endoscopic clip applier with titanium clips

- Laparoscopic Hem-o-lok applier, with clips already loaded, if the source of bleeding is clearly visible
- Robotic needle holder and monofilament suture with small-gauge needle to attempt to repair the bleeding vessel or, in case of injury of parenchymatous organ, needle holder, and monofilament/barbed suture to repair it
- Laparoscopic vascular clamp

Part VI

Interventions Protocols in Colorectal Surgery

Laparoscopic Treatment of Inflammatory Bowel Disease

13

J. Meyer and R. J. Davies

13.1 Introduction

Inflammatory bowel disease is a chronic autoimmune disorder of multifactorial aetiology affecting the gastrointestinal tract. The most common forms are Crohn's disease and ulcerative colitis. Crohn's disease causes multifocal transmural inflammation of the entire gastrointestinal tract, which can lead to stricture and/or fistulas/perforation. Ulcerative colitis affects the mucosal layer of both the rectum and the colon, in continuity from the rectum. Patients suffering from inflammatory bowel disease are often affected by weight loss and poor nutrition, which complicate their surgical management. They can also present with extra-intestinal manifestations of the disease.

Preoperative assessment of the disease is key for optimal management and outcomes and usually includes endoscopy and imaging (CT and/or MRI).

Treatment of inflammatory bowel disease is primarily medical and multidisciplinary, and aims at obtaining and maintaining remission. It consists of the correction of nutritional deficiencies and in topical or systemic immunosuppressants (including, among others, corticosteroids and immunomodulatory therapy). Surgery is reserved for patients suffering from complications and/or not responding to medical treatment.

In Crohn's disease, emergency surgery is usually performed for sepsis caused by perforating disease and/or perineal disease. Elective surgery is most often indicated for stricturing disease, usually at the level of the terminal ileum. In these patients, who may undergo several bowel resections during their lifetimes, optimizing nutritional status before surgery and saving bowel length during surgery are key, and the remaining bowel should be systematically measured.

In ulcerative colitis, emergency surgery is indicated in case of severe acute colitis not responding to medical management, toxic megacolon and perforation, as well as severe gastrointestinal haemorrhage. Elective surgery is performed for ulcerative colitis refractory to medical management and for precancerous or cancerous lesions occurring in the lower gastrointestinal tract.

In patients with inflammatory bowel disease needing surgery, laparoscopy should ideally be favoured over laparotomy, but the mode of surgical approach has to be tailored to the patient, the past surgical history and the expertise of the surgeon.

J. Meyer (✉) · R. J. Davies
Cambridge Colorectal Unit, Addenbrooke's Hospital,
Cambridge University Hospitals NHS Foundation
Trust, Cambridge, UK

© The Author(s), under exclusive license to Springer Nature Switzerland AG 2024
M. Milone et al. (eds.), *Scrub Nurse in Minimally Invasive and Robotic General Surgery*,
https://doi.org/10.1007/978-3-031-42257-7_13

13.2   Operating Theatre Setting

The operating theatre setting can depend on local and personal preferences, but should ideally be standardized to optimize access to the abdominal cavity and perineum and to facilitate the task of the theatre team. We propose the following setting in all patients undergoing laparoscopic surgery for inflammatory bowel disease:

Right-sided resections (such as ileocaecal resection for Crohn's disease) and initial laparoscopy (Fig. 13.1):

- Operating table in the centre of the room
- Vision and coagulation tower/stack positioned at the level of the right leg
- Screen positioned at the level of the right flank
- Instrument tables at the level of the left leg
- Surgeon and first assistant on the left side of the patient
- Second assistant (if any) between the legs of the patient

- Scrub nurse at the level of the left leg

Left-sided resections (such as proctectomy for ulcerative colitis) (Fig. 13.2):

- Operating table in the centre of the room
- Vision and coagulation tower/stack positioned at the level of the left leg
- Screen positioned at the level of the left flank
- Instruments tables at the level of the right leg
- Surgeon and first assistant on the right side of the patient
- Second assistant (if any) between the legs of the patient, or on left side close to left shoulder
- Scrub nurse at the level of the right leg

For subtotal colectomy, the theatre setting for left-sided resections can be chosen. During the time for right-sided mobilization, the surgical team will switch sides and look at a second screen added to the right side of the patient.

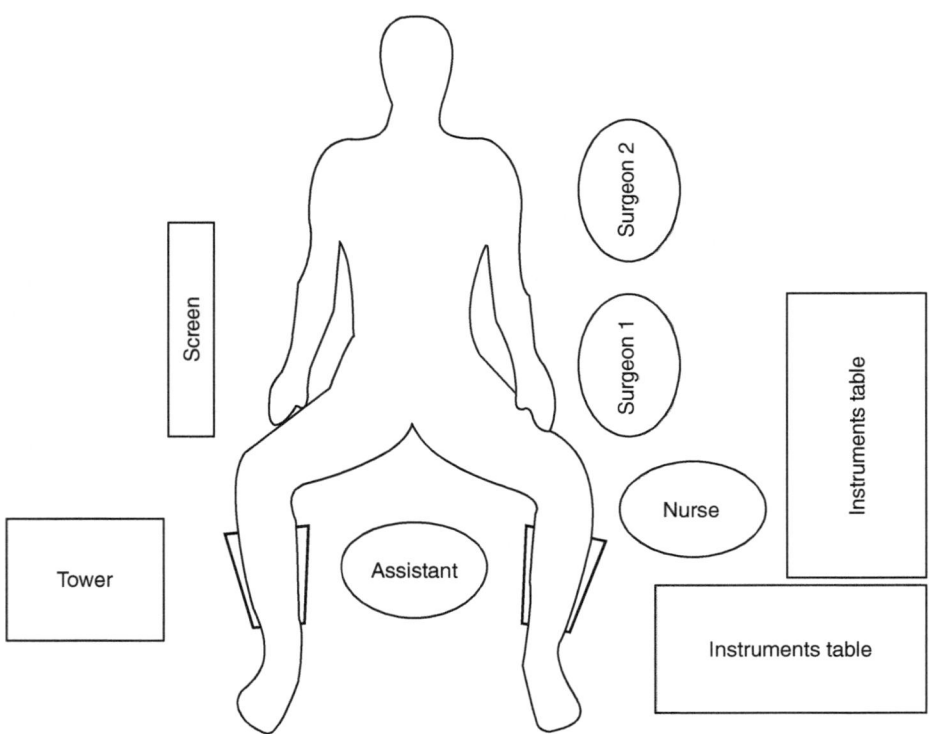

Fig. 13.1 Theatre setting for right-sided resection

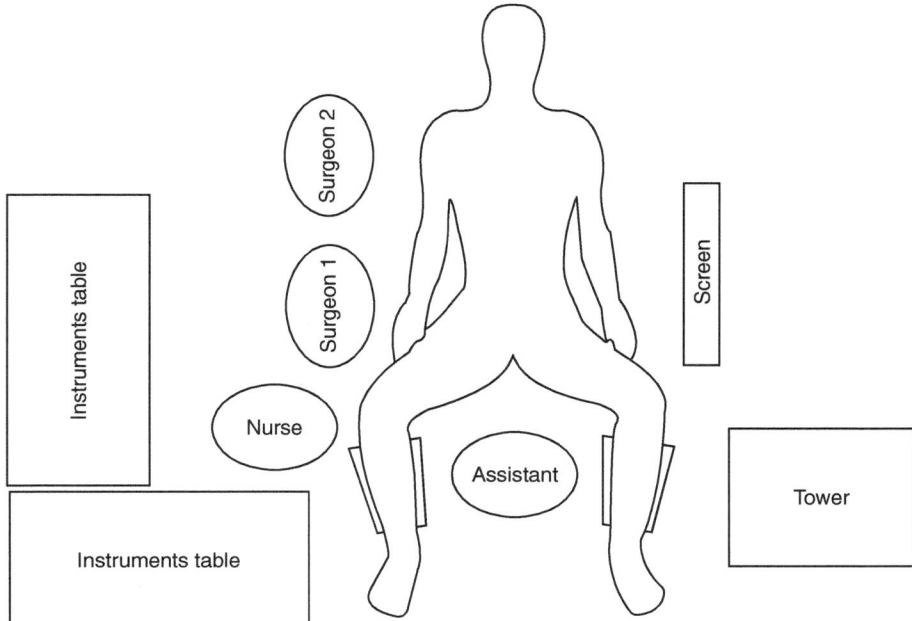

Fig. 13.2 Theatre setting for left-sided/pelvic resection

13.3 Patient Positioning

All patients undergoing laparoscopic surgery for inflammatory bowel disease should ideally be placed as follows:

- In the modified Lloyd–Davies position (gynaecologic position), with thighs kept flat
- Both arms adducted along the body and wrapped
- Equipped with compression anti-thrombosis boots
- On an anti-sliding mat (such as the Pink Pad) or a bean bag
- With a strap across the chest
- With urinary catheter placed

Depending on the surgical procedure or on the step of the surgical procedure, and depending on the anti-sliding mat, the table can be tilted up to 15° on one side and be inclined in Trendelenburg or in reverse Trendelenburg up to 25°. Therefore, the instrument tables should be located at a distance from the patient and not be placed above the legs.

13.4 Required Material

For laparoscopic surgery for inflammatory bowel disease, a standard laparoscopy set should be opened, including the following contents (Fig. 13.3):

- One 30° 10 mm or, ideally 5 mm, camera
- One thermos bottle or warming recipient for the camera
- One light cable
- One diathermy cable, ideally with hand control
- One bipolar cable
- One insufflation cable, ideally for the Airseal system
- One long (42 cm) 5 mm washing and suction device
- One diathermy hook (ideally a disposable one coated with Teflon)
- One bipolar Johann grasper
- One Maryland grasper
- One L-shaped grasper, in two diameters
- One short (34 cm) and one long (42 cm) Microline scissors

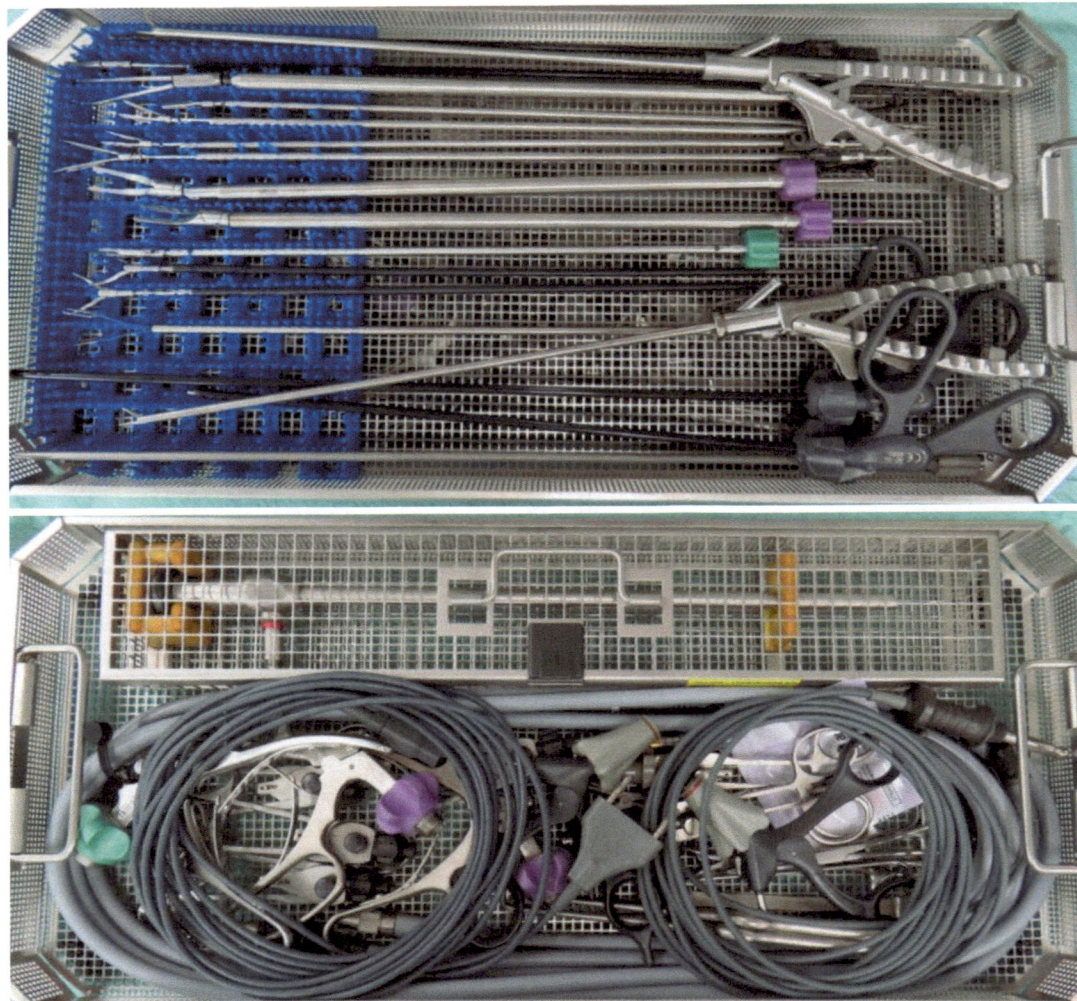

Fig. 13.3 Content of a standard laparoscopy set

- Three atraumatic short-fenestrated (20 mm) Johann graspers
- One atraumatic long-fenestrated (40 mm) Johann grasper
- One green Hem-O-lok clip applier
- One purple Hem-O-lok clip applier
- Two needle holders

In these patients, entry into the abdominal cavity should ideally be performed under direct visual control (not using the Veress needle).

Moreover, parts of the procedure (such as resection and anastomosis) may be performed extracorporeally. Therefore, a basic laparotomy set should also be prepared and included (Fig. 13.4).

The following extra material should be available in the theatre room and used upon surgeon's request:

- One 5 mm vessel sealer device, such as Ligasure (with straight or Maryland tip), Vaillant, Thunderbeat, Ultracision or others

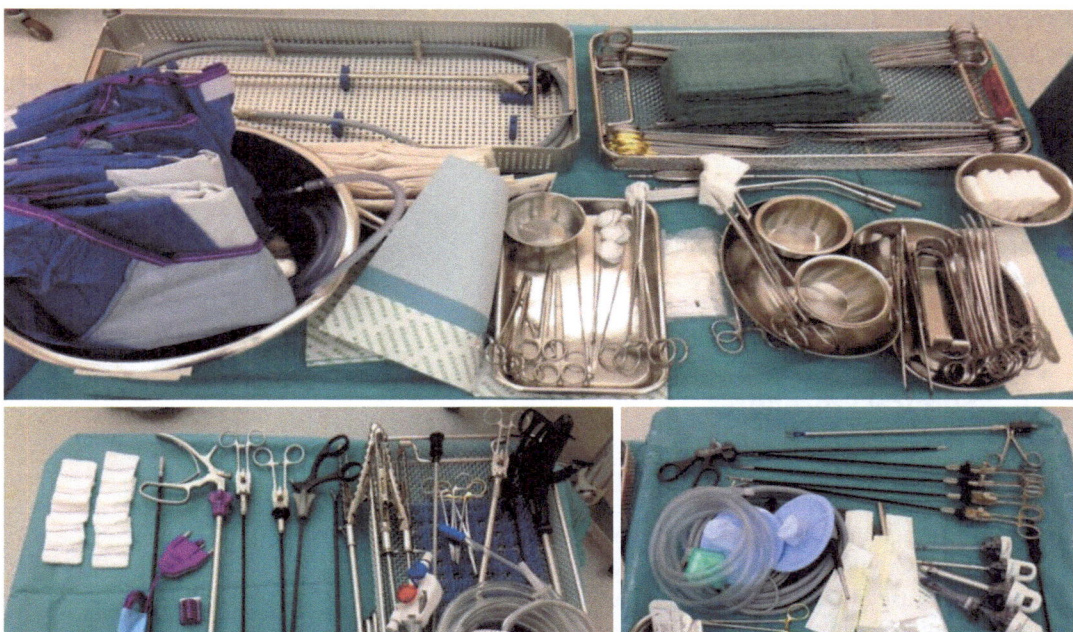

Fig. 13.4 Instrument tables prepared for laparoscopy and including a standard laparoscopy set, a basic laparotomy set and a vessel sealer device

- One straight laparoscopic stapler, motorized or not, such as the EndoPath, Echelon Flex, EndoGIA, Signia or others, with different cartridges for different thicknesses and for controlling vessels
- One straight extracorporeal stapler, such as the Proximate linear cutter (TLC), Proximate linear stapler (TX), GIA stapler or others, with different cartridges for different thicknesses and for controlling vessels
- One gold Hem-O-lok clip applier
- Different Hem-O-lok clips corresponding to the appliers
- Elastic wound retractors (Alexis) for specimen extraction

If rectal resection is planned, the following additional material should be available in the theatre room and be available upon surgeon's request:

- One curved extracorporeal stapler, such as the Echelon Contour curved cutter, with different cartridges for different thicknesses
- Circular rectal sizers of different diameters (usually from 25 to 33 mm)
- Circular staplers of different diameters, motorized or not

The risk of conversion to open surgery should be considered and the required material (large laparotomy set including vascular clamps) should be available (but not opened) in the room.

13.5   Laparoscopic Port Placement

The types and number of ports depend on local preferences and on the planned surgical procedure. Both disposable and reusable ports can be considered.

13.6   Surgical Procedures

13.6.1 Ileocaecal Resection

Ileocaecal resection is usually performed in patients with Crohn's disease, most often for stricturing disease of the terminal ileum, but also for fistulizing/perforating disease.

A 12 mm optical port is inserted at the umbilicus under visual control. Thereafter, two 5 mm ports are inserted in the left iliac fossa and in the suprapubic area, to optimize triangulation of the right iliac fossa. An additional 5 mm port can be placed in the left subcostal area in case the right colon has to be mobilized more distally (Fig. 13.5).

The caecum and the terminal ileum are usually mobilized using a lateral-to-medial or an infero-medial ('bottom-up') approach. In the absence of cancer, proximal control of the ileocolic pedicle is not required. The right ureter and duodenum will be seen and preserved. Once the caecum and right colon is mobile, a small laparotomy (extraction site) is performed and the abdominal wall is protected with a wound protector. The ileocolic vessels are divided where it is technically most straightforward. The mesentery can be controlled using a vessel sealer or with suture ligation. The terminal ileum and the caecum are divided using a linear stapler. An anastomosis can be performed or not, depending on the presence of local sepsis and medication (especially steroids) as well as on the haemodynamic and nutritional status of the patient. Optimally, the small bowel should be explored to exclude any additional stricture or active disease.

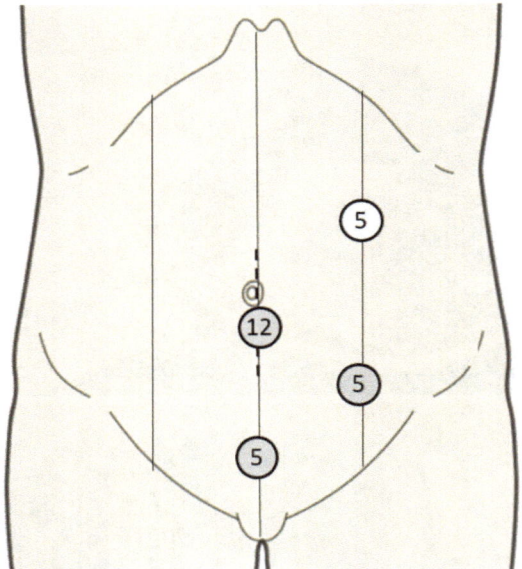

Fig. 13.5 Port placement for ileocaecal resection

13.6.2 Strictureplasty

If a short, fibrotic small bowel stricture is evident, strictureplasty can be performed to avoid a resection and save bowel length. Strictureplasty is usually performed extracorporeally through the extraction site (Figs. 13.6 and 13.7).

13.6.3 Abdomino-Perineal Excision of the Rectum (APER)

Abdomino-perineal excision of the rectum is seldomly performed for Crohn's disease, most often for extensive and refractory anal fistulizing disease or in case of cancer.

A 12 mm optical port is inserted at the umbilicus under visual control. Thereafter, one 12 mm port is inserted in the right iliac fossa, and one 5 mm port is inserted in the right subcostal area. One 5 mm port is inserted in the left flank for assistant-mediated retraction. Additional 5 mm ports can be inserted in the epigastric area for helping splenic flexure mobilization and in the suprapubic area (Fig. 13.8).

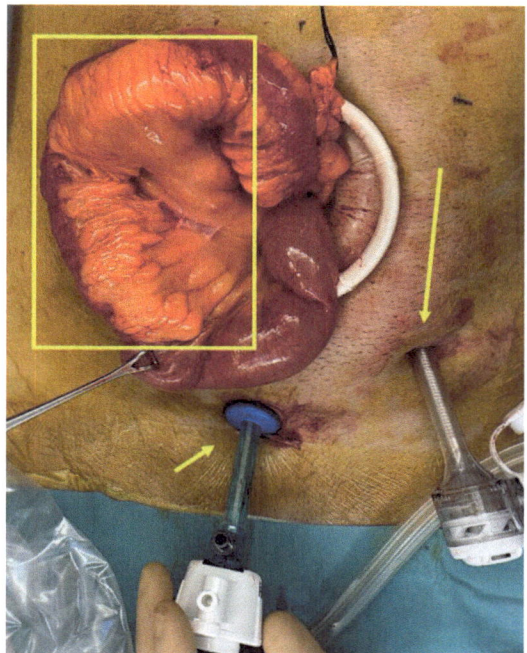

Fig. 13.6 Bowel extraction in a patient with Crohn's disease with stricturing phenotype at the level of the terminal ileum. The yellow square indicates the zone of 'fat wrapping', where the mesentery is progressing towards the anti-mesenteric side of the small bowel, which delineates a zone of chronic transmural inflammation caused by Crohn's disease. This zone was identified as being structured based on preoperative imaging. To mobilize the terminal ileum, a 5 mm balloon port (Applied Medical) was placed in the suprapubic area (short arrow) and a 5 mm AirSeal port (ConMed) was placed in the left iliac fossa (long arrow). Due to the length of the affected segment, the patient underwent resection of the terminal ileum involved using an ileocaecectomy

The descending and sigmoid colon are mobilized using a lateral-to-medial or a medial-to-lateral approach. The left ureter is seen and preserved. Considering that an end stoma is performed, mobilization of the splenic flexure is usually not necessary. In the absence of cancer, proximal control of the root of the inferior mesenteric artery is not required. The procedure continues with mobilization of the rectum, preferentially in the total mesorectum excision plane (to avoid bleeding), avoiding the autonomic nerves, down to the pelvic floor. Thereafter, a perineal approach is performed, resecting the inflamed area and ideally sparing the external anal sphincter by using an intersphincteric perineal dissection (if possible). Perineal closure is performed primarily whenever possible, or rarely using a myocutaneous graft in case of a wide tissue defect.

13.6.4 Subtotal Colectomy

Surgical treatment for ulcerative colitis usually consists of an initial subtotal colectomy and ileostomy, with eventual synchronous or metachronous proctectomy, with or without restoration of intestinal continuity. Restoration of intestinal continuity is most commonly in the form of subsequent proctectomy and ileo-anal pouch, or more uncommonly with an ileo-rectal anastomosis.

For subtotal colectomy, a 12 mm optical port is inserted at the umbilicus under visual control. Thereafter, one 12 mm port is inserted in the right iliac fossa, and four 5 mm ports are inserted in the suprapubic area, in the right and left subcostal areas and in the left iliac fossa. An additional 5 mm port can be inserted in the epigastric area (Fig. 13.9).

The procedure can be started either with the right colon mobilization or with the left colon mobilization. Mobilization of the entire large bowel is usually performed using the lateral-to-medial approach. Once one side is completed, the team has to move to the other side to complete mobilization of the contralateral side. Both ureters and the duodenum will be seen and preserved. In the absence of cancer, the mesocolon is divided close to the bowel. The terminal ileum is divided intracorporeally. Distal division of the large bowel is performed at the distal sigmoid colon, either intracorporeally or through the Pfannenstiel incision.

13.6.5 Ileo-Rectal Anastomosis

If the rectum is preserved and has no or limited inflammation, an ileo-rectal anastomosis can be

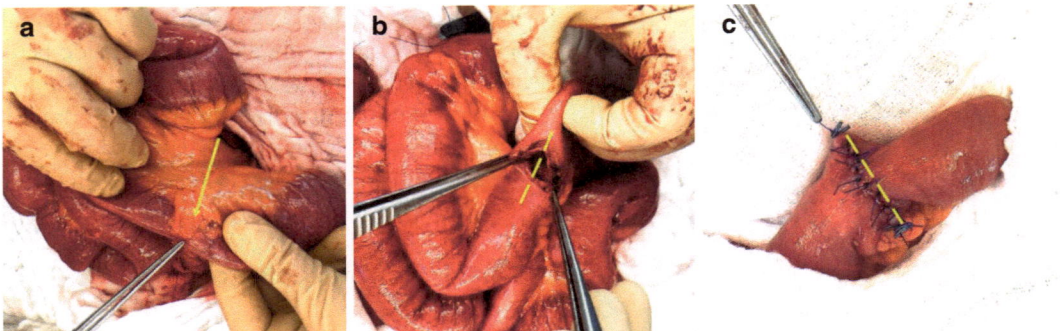

Fig. 13.7 Bowel extraction in a patient with Crohn's disease with stricturing phenotype at the level of the ileum. The stricture was short and is indicated by the arrow (**a**). Fat wrapping can also be seen. Additional zones of strictures were excluded by exploring the bowel lumen using an intraluminal metallic ball. To save bowel length and avoid a resection, a Heineke–Mikulicz strictureplasty was performed (**b** and **c**). The zone of stricture was incised longitudinally and closed axially using separate stitches of slowly resorbable suture (3-0 PDS)

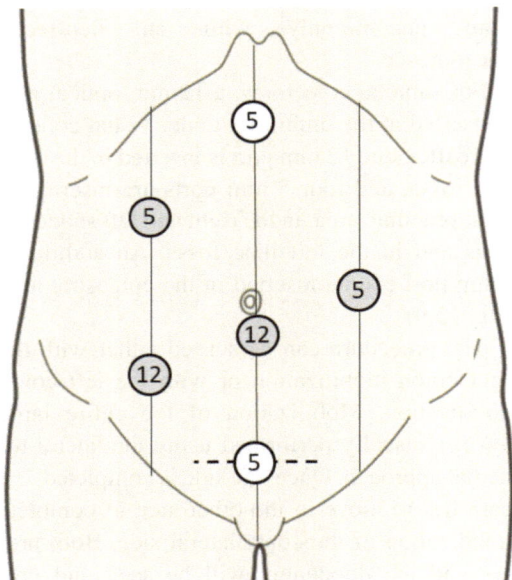

Fig. 13.8 Port placement for abdomino-perineal excision

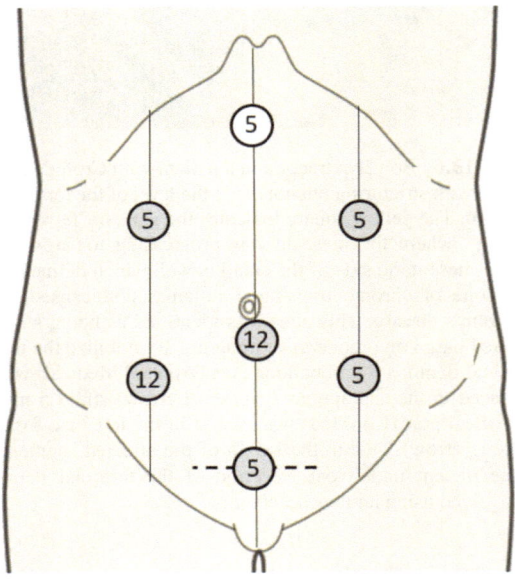

Fig. 13.9 Port placement for subtotal colectomy

13.6.6 Completion Proctectomy, with or Without Ileo-Anal Pouch

considered in some carefully selected and counselled patients. This procedure is usually done in a second step after subtotal colectomy. Briefly, the ileum is exteriorized through the extraction site (midline or Pfannenstiel), the anvil of the circular stapler is inserted and secured with a purse string, and an end-to-end or side-to-end stapled ileo-rectal anastomosis is performed.

Proctectomy can be considered in patients with ulcerative colitis and with inflammation of the rectum, or in case of dysplasia or cancer of the rectum. The procedure is either done at the same time as subtotal colectomy (procto-colectomy), or as a second step (completion proctectomy) as subtotal colectomy is often performed as an emergency procedure.

A 12 mm optical port is inserted at the umbilicus under visual control. Thereafter, one 12 mm port is inserted in the right iliac fossa, and one 5 mm port is inserted in the right subcostal area. One 5 mm port is inserted in the left flank for assistant-mediated retraction. Additional 5 mm ports can be inserted in the epigastric and in the suprapubic area (Fig. 13.10).

Considering that the colon was previously removed (subtotal colectomy), the procedure starts with posterior dissection in the total mesorectal excision (TME) plane, made easier to identify as the inferior mesenteric vessels would normally be preserved at the time of subtotal colectomy. Dissection then proceeds laterally and anteriorly, taking particular care to avoid the autonomic nerves and to mobilize the vagina free in females. If bowel continuity is being restored, the distal rectum is divided at the level of the pelvic floor, usually using a curved stapler with green cartridge or with as few firings with a laparoscopic stapler as possible, with creation of an ileal J-pouch to then go on and perform a pouch–anal (ileo-anal) anastomosis.

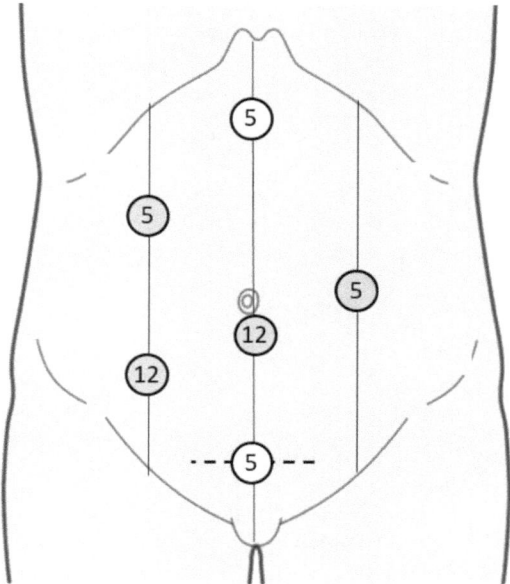

Fig. 13.10 Port placement for completion proctectomy

If intestinal continuity is not being performed, then perineal dissection generally proceeds in the intersphincteric plane without the need for rectal transection, as per the APER section above.

Robotic Treatment of Inflammatory Diseases

14

Francesco Maria Carrano (ORCID)

14.1 Introduction

Inflammatory bowel disease (IBD) is a group of chronic immune-mediated conditions of the bowel that cause severe impairment of patients' quality of life. Crohn's disease (CD) and ulcerative colitis (UC) represent the most cases. Their management is complex, and a multidisciplinary approach that includes medical and surgical consultation is required for optimal treatment results. The discovery of novel therapeutic agents has revolutionized the treatment strategy over the years. Although initially played a minor role, surgeons have become increasingly important in the care team of IBD patients since the early stages of the disease. At the same time, breakthroughs in understanding the physiopathology of the disease in diagnostic tools and surgical equipment have allowed a giant leap in treatment results. While medical therapy remains the first choice for most IBD patients [1], ulcerative colitis can be effectively treated with a proctocolectomy; up to 80% of patients with CD will require surgical treatment during their lifetime for complications [2, 3]. IBD patients also represent a particular population with known operative risk factors, independently of age, often presenting with severe signs of malnutrition and other accessory conditions such as intra-abdominal abscesses, enteroenteric or enterocutaneous fistulae, strictures, and adhesions from previous surgeries. Furthermore, as most diagnoses are made during young adulthood, great attention is given to fertility issues and sexual function, urinary, and bowel continence preservation.

Despite declining surgery rates over the last decades, the global need for surgery in IBD patients is increasing due to the growing number of diagnoses worldwide [4, 5]. Open surgery was the gold standard for emergency and elective surgery in IBD patients for decades. Tactile assessment of the bowel allows the discrimination between healthy tissues from those with active disease, provides a secure feeling when ligating blood vessels and doing hemostasis in swollen and friable Crohn's mesentery, and gives control during the lysis of adhesions. However, with the increasing adoption of minimally invasive surgery (MIS) for IBD cases, data show a positive influence on the reduced formation of adhesions, reduced pain, early bowel function, and shorter hospitalization [3, 6].

For this reason, much attention is given to the role of robotic surgical platforms in improving surgical outcomes for IBD patients.

Two main concepts of robotic surgery exist. The first consists of a monolithic system including all the robotic arms and tools represented by the da Vinci surgical platform (Intuitive Surgical, Inc. Sunnyvale, CA, USA), the current market

F. M. Carrano (✉)
Department of Medical and Surgical Sciences and Translational Medicine, Faculty of Medicine and Psychology, St Andrea Hospital, Sapienza University of Rome, Rome, Italy

© The Author(s), under exclusive license to Springer Nature Switzerland AG 2024
M. Milone et al. (eds.), *Scrub Nurse in Minimally Invasive and Robotic General Surgery*,
https://doi.org/10.1007/978-3-031-42257-7_14

leader. The second is centered on flexibility and scalability, with independent robotic wheeled units that can be deployed independently and possibly moved freely into the operative room. More recent surgical platforms have adopted this second concept. They are represented by Senhance (Asensus Surgical US, Inc., Durham, NC, USA), the Versius (CMR Surgical, Cambridge, UK), and the HUGO RAS System (Medtronic, Minneapolis, MN, USA). Almost all the studies in the literature, at the time of writing, report data coming from da Vinci centers; therefore, in this chapter, we will focus on the primary robotic concept.

We look forward to future studies on novel robotic platforms whose flexibility could provide an even more significant advantage in nonstandard surgical fields like those of a typical IBD patient.

14.2 Robotic Surgery and Crohn's Disease

The MIS approach for the treatment of IBDs, in general, has been slowly adopted, despite initial encouraging results. This was probably due to the increased technical difficulties encountered during surgery because of the severe inflammation, the presence of tenacious strictures, and fistulae predisposed to a high chance of conversion to open. Thanks to technological advancements and the increasing experience with laparoscopy, the MIS approach for Crohn's disease has been demonstrated to be not only feasible and safe but also beneficial for the patient, even in complex and recurrent cases [6]. The use of robotics in CD surgery is in its early stages of adoption and mainly consists of elective ileocolic resections for uncomplicated CD. However, more evidence is surfacing for penetrating complicated CD as well. Data from the literature demonstrate that, despite longer operative times, the robotic approach provides significantly shorter hospital stays, lower ileostomy creation rates, a lower rate of 30-day postoperative complications, and more home discharges compared to open ileocolic resection [7, 8]. Compared to laparoscopy, the

robotic approach has shown comparable length of stay, earlier return of bowel function, and a lower overall complication rate [9].

14.3 Robotic Ileocolic Resection

Performing an ileocolic resection using a robotic approach has several advantages, mostly related to the more accessible construction of an intracorporeal anastomosis. This type of anastomosis has been associated with an earlier return of bowel function [10] and allows the extraction site to be moved off the midline with reduced incisional hernia rates [7]. It also requires a reduced colonic mobilization, which, theoretically, can minimize adhesion formation and the occurrence of duodenal fistulae. In fact, without extensive need for right colonic mobilization, the duodenum remains in the retroperitoneum, protected by the ascending colon and its mesentery.

Using the da Vinci XI robotic platform, the ports are placed straight across the abdomen,

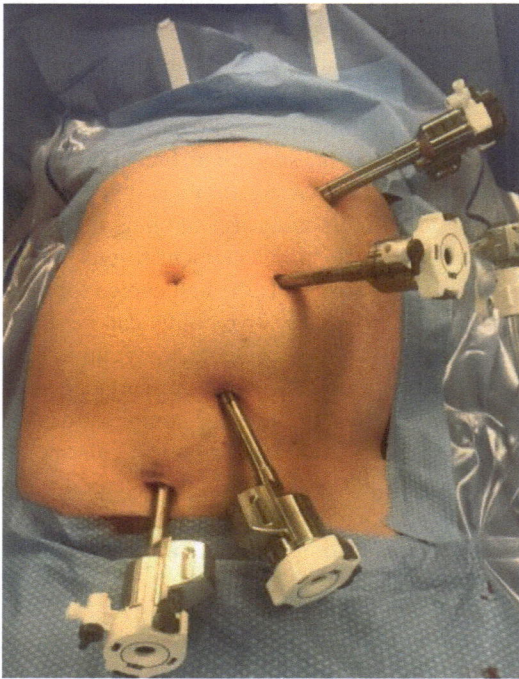

Fig. 14.1 Ports positioning for robotic ileocolic resection using the da Vinci XI. Image from Gunnells et al. [7]

from the left upper quadrant to the suprapubic region (Fig. 14.1).

Unlike oncologic right colectomies, in ileocolic resections for CD, the dissection is undertaken in a lateral to medial fashion without the need for extended lymphadenectomy and ligation at the origin of the ileocolic vessels. The first essential step is to isolate the terminal ileum from the right pelvis and the cecum, which tend to be tenaciously adherent due to inflammation. The high-definition 3D view and the superior dexterity provided by the robotic platform are handy for precise dissection of the various structures, preserving the retroperitoneum intact and reducing the risk of injuries to the right ureter. Once mobilized, the ascending colon and terminal ileum are transected. A standard laparoscopic stapler can be used, or a robotic stapler. The mesentery is then divided, and a side-to-side isoperistaltic ileocolic anastomosis is fashioned using the stapler. The enterotomies used to place the stapler can then be closed with a double-layer continuous barbed wire suture. Finally, the specimen is extracted through a Pfannenstiel incision or other service access sites, according to the surgeon's preference.

Some accessory considerations are to be made. In cases of penetrating CD, multiple bowel segments are typically involved, with the sigmoid colon being the most frequent. If a fistula is present, the inflamed tissue around the fistula tract is excised, and the resulting defect is primarily closed. The robotic approach aids in the ease of suturing the defect closed [7]. In the case of multiple critical ileal strictures, the need for performing strictureplasties typically prevents from completing a procedure only in a minimally invasive fashion. However, initial experiences of totally robotic intracorporeal strictureplasties have been described [11].

During an ileocolic resection for CD, great attention should be given to achieving perfect hemostasis. The mesentery is particularly challenging, as it is typically thickened due to inflammation, fragile, and prone to bleedings that are difficult to control, even with high-energy devices. In case of a bleeding mesentery, hemostasis can be achieved with the interrupted figure-of-eight sutures or U-stitches like in the open setting.

14.4 Robotic Surgery and Ulcerative Colitis

During the past 20 years, the treatment approach to UC has evolved substantially. However, despite significant progress in medical therapy, many patients still do not respond to it; therefore, surgery remains their only treatment opportunity. At the same time, both the surgical strategy and the surgical techniques have changed, with the shift from one-stage procedures to multistage and with the transition from open to laparoscopy, single-port surgery, and transanal approaches. Notwithstanding the growing data supporting the application of robotic techniques to colorectal procedures, data is scarce regarding the use of the da Vinci Xi platform in multi-quadrant surgical settings like extended colonic resections for elective or emergent treatment of UC patients. One possible reason may be the reported longer operating times for robotic surgery and the subsequent need to maintain patients in extreme positions (steep Trendelenburg or anti-Trendelenburg) that may influence the hemodynamic stability of the patient, especially of those requiring emergency treatment for toxic colitis. However, recent reports have shown that, despite longer operating times, the robotic approach seems safe and has outcomes comparable to laparoscopy, without the theoretical need for skilled assistants, even for emergent procedures [12] in hemodynamically stable patients. Robotic proctectomy has been described to be superior to laparoscopy because it offers a stable platform, wristed instruments, and increased magnification in the bony confines of the pelvis.

A word of caution comes from Remzi and colleagues, who have published one of the largest case series of redo surgeries for UC patients. The authors have noted that most patients requiring a redo pelvic pouch for retained rectums, ischemic strictures, and/or pouch twists had their primary operation performed minimally invasively. This occurrence may be due to the learning curve of such minimally invasive procedures or to intrinsic technical limits of the endoscopic staplers in the deep pelvic space. Although Intuitive Sureform robotic staplers represent a tangible upgrade over standard laparoscopic staplers, being capable of monitoring tissue compression before and during firing, making automatic adjustments to optimize the staple line, and providing a 120° cone of articulation, they can reduce but not eliminate the crisscrossing of multiple staple lines during double-stapled anastomosis. At the same time, to achieve a single staple fire, the proper level of transection may be sacrificed to a more proximal level, which then leads to retained rectum and ongoing inflammation from the presence of ongoing proctitis, both being a significant source of morbidity to the patient and a reason why patients with mechanical pouch failures are often misdiagnosed as having CD of the pouch. Pouch twists are also commonly found after minimally invasive procedures due to difficulties finding the correct bowel orientation due to limited visibility [13].

The operation of choice for refractory ulcerative colitis is the ileal pouch-anal anastomosis (IPAA) procedure with a laparoscopic approach. This is usually performed in two stages in the elective setting: first, patients undergo a restorative total proctocolectomy with IPAA and J-pouch and a temporary diverting loop ileostomy; in the second later stage (usually performed 6 to 8 weeks later), the stoma is reversed, and bowel continuity is restored [14].

However, in cases of severe acute colitis requiring urgent or emergent surgical treatment, performing a total restorative proctocolectomy with IPAA is not recommendable due to higher risks of morbidity and mortality. A safer option is performing a subtotal colectomy with end ileostomy without or with a mucous fistula creation (in cases of very severe rectal inflammation). This second option could be considered outside the emergent setting if the patient has severe concerns regarding the associated risk of pelvic nerve damage, infertility, and sexual dysfunction with proctectomy. This is an important consideration, especially in females of childbearing age.

However, retaining the rectal stump is not without consequences. Patients can decrease their quality of life due to persistent symptoms, including ongoing mucous or bloody discharge,

low-grade fevers, and feelings of rectal discomfort or urgency due to ongoing proctitis. Not to be forgotten is the risk of malignancy in the retained rectum, which is as high as 3% compared to 1% in those who undergo IPAA.

In summary, refractory UC can be surgically treated in two primary modalities:

1. Two-stage IPAA: first, MIS total restorative proctocolectomy with IPAA + temporary diverting loop ileostomy, and second, stoma closure.
2. Three-stage IPAA: first, MIS subtotal colectomy with end ileostomy (± mucous fistula); second, laparoscopic completion proctectomy and IPAA; and third, stoma closure.

In this chapter, we will focus on the robotic subtotal colectomy + end ileostomy in a single and double-docking approach and on the completion proctectomy with IPAA.

14.5 Robotic Subtotal Colectomy with End Ileostomy

14.5.1 Single-Docking Approach

The patient is placed in a modified Lloyd-Davis position. According to the Hasson technique, a 12-mm port is placed in the right iliac fossa (Fig. 14.2), and the pneumoperitoneum is insufflated. Three 8-mm ports are then placed in the umbilical region (camera), in the left iliac fossa, and in the right and left upper quadrants. Finally, two 5-mm ports are placed in the right and left flanks, with one using the Airseal device (Conmed, Utica, NY, USA). The procedure can be started from the left or right side of the colon, according to the surgeon's preference (Fig. 14.3). The approach to the vessels can be at their origin (high tie, oncologic approach) in case of known concurrent dysplasia or multiple colonic polyps. Otherwise, vessels can be safely ligated distally (low tie). Also, the choice of the instruments should reflect the surgeon's preference; however, in cases with heavily inflamed tissues such as

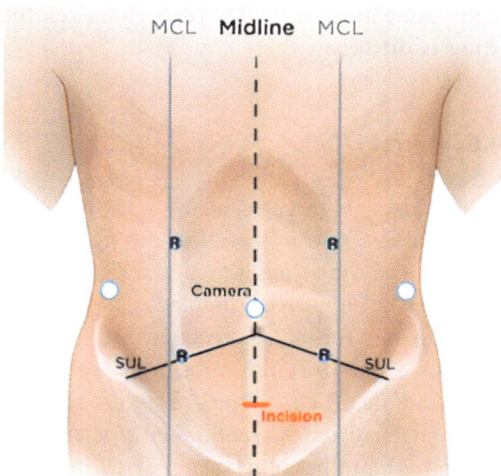

Fig. 14.2 Trocar position for robotic single docking subtotal colectomy. Image modified from Jimenez-Rodriguez et al. [15]

those in the urgent or emergent setting, using the SynchroSeal or the Vessel Sealer Extend could provide better control on the vessels and the mesentery.

We now describe the procedure starting from the right side.

The patient is placed in a 15° Trendelenburg position with a 30° left-side tilt, and the surgical cart (the boom) is positioned between the legs of the patient and docked.

The retroperitoneum is incised with the monopolar curved scissors in the avascular portion of the mesentery between the superior mesenteric artery and the ileocolic vessels. After the retroperitoneal structures, including the third portion of the duodenum and the pancreas, are pushed posteriorly, the ileocolic vessels are isolated and divided with Hem-O-loks. Dissection proceeds along the superior mesenteric vein axis to isolate

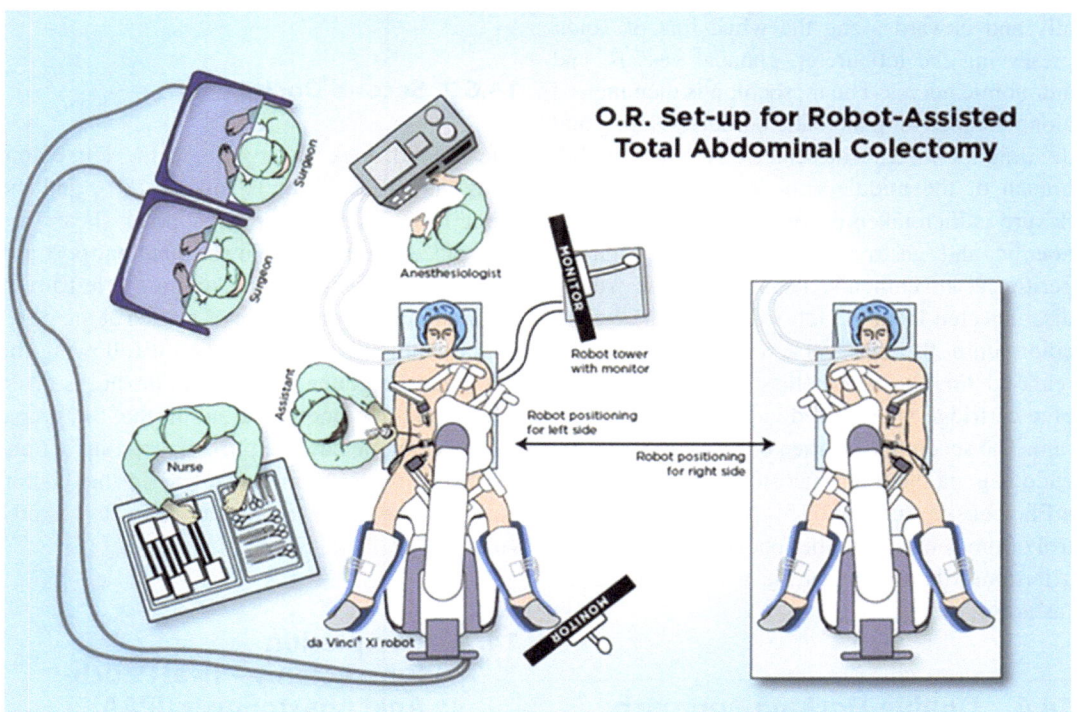

Fig. 14.3 Operating room setup for robotic single-docking subtotal colectomy. Image courtesy of Jimenez-Rodriguez et al. [15]

and divide the right colic artery and vein (when present) and the middle colic artery and vein. The mesentery of the right colon is mobilized from medial to lateral, and the omentum is opened to enter the lesser sac and complete the mobilization of the right colon. At this point, the terminal ileum is divided with the preferred robotic stapler (SureForm or EndoWrist) using a 45 mm blue cartridge.

The robotic arms are then detached from the trocars, the boom is rotated 180° without moving the patient-side cart, and the patient is repositioned with a 30° right-side tilt, with the 15° Trendelenburg position maintained. The robotic arms are then reconnected to the trocars. A peritoneal incision is made below the inferior mesenteric artery downward to the sacral promontory and extended upward to the inferior pancreatic margin. The inferior mesenteric artery and vein are divided while preserving the superior rectal artery. Mesocolic mobilization is continued laterally and upward along the white line of Toldt, preserving the left ureter, gonadal vessels, and autonomic nerves. The mesocolon is then incised along the inferior pancreatic border, isolating and dividing the inferior mesenteric vein and the left branch of the middle colic artery. The splenic flexure is then taken down by dividing the splenocolic and gastrocolic ligaments and lateral peritoneal attachments. The omentum is wholly disconnected from the left side of the transverse colon until the transverse colon is also fully released. Finally, the robotic stapler with a 60 mm blue cartridge is used to divide the superior rectum. The specimen can then be extracted using an endo bag via the future ileostomy site or through a Pfannenstiel incision [15]. After accurate control of the hemostasis, the robot is undocked, and a terminal ileostomy can be made in the usual fashion.

14.6   Double-Docking Approach

The double-docking approach originates from the previous, more extensive experience with the older robotic platforms. The surgical steps are the same as described before. However, the setting is different.

14.6.1   First Dock

The first dock is targeted at the right colon. A 12-mm robotic port is placed in the right lower quadrant, as close as possible to the future ileostomy site. A 5-mm trocar is placed in the right upper quadrant for the laparoscopic assistant. An additional 8-mm working port is placed in the left lower quadrant. The monopolar scissors are used in the right hand and the fenestrated bipolar in the left hand. The right colon is mobilized in a bottom-up approach, from the terminal ileum to the splenic flexure. Once completely mobilized, the terminal ileum is divided with a robotic stapler. The robot is undocked, and a right upper quadrant 5-mm assist port is placed for left colon mobilization.

14.6.2   Second Dock

The second dock is targeted at the left colon. Thus the surgical cart is rotated 180°, and the robot is re-docked. The monopolar shears are now placed in the right lower quadrant port and the fenestrated bipolar forceps in the left lower quadrant port. Mobilization is started at the proximal rectum and extended upward following the left paracolic gutter. The splenic flexure is taken down, and the mobilization of the transverse colon is completed. The proximal rectum is transected using the robotic stapler via the 12-mm port. The specimen can then be extracted as previously described [12].

14.7   Completion Proctectomy + Ileal Pouch-Anal Anastomosis (IPAA)

The patient is placed into a modified lithotomy position with both arms on the sides. The da Vinci is prepared on the patient's left side.

The first step is the dissection of the previously constructed terminal ileostomy. Once mobilized, the small bowel should be exteriorized and pulled towards the pubic bone to verify the reach of the future pouch (with the last 15–20 cm of bowel folded in a J shape, the apex of the future pouch should extend more than 2 cm past the pubic bone). This step is fundamental, as the IPAA should be made without tension. In case of insufficient bowel length, mesenteric lengthening techniques will be required (i.e., stair stepping of the mesentery, high tie of the ileocolic artery, division of the distal branches of the superior mesenteric artery, etc.) before proceeding with the proctectomy. The ileal pouch is then constructed. Approximately 15–20 cm proximal from the distal ileal staple line, two enterotomies are made at the apex of the future pouch and allow the insertion of a 100-mm extracorporeal linear stapler. The J-pouch should be between 15 and 20 cm long; thus, two stapler fires are necessary. The staple line and the blind limb of the pouch are reinforced by oversewing with a nonabsorbable suture. A purse string suture is then placed at the apex of the pouch to accommodate the anvil of a 28- or 29-mm circular stapler. The anvil and pouch are then repositioned in the abdomen, and a 15-mm trocar is placed at the ileostomy site as an additional working port. The pneumoperitoneum is obtained, and four robotic trocars are placed 15 cm from the pubic bone, from the left to the right flank, spaced 6–8 cm apart to avoid any conflict between the robotic arms. A 5 mm assistant port with an AirSeal device is placed in the left upper quadrant. The patient is placed in Trendelenburg, and the robot is docked from the left. The instruments are as follows: hot shears in arm 1, camera in arm 2, fenestrated bipolar in arm 3, and a grasping retractor in arm 4. Arm 3 is used to pull the rectal stump down and out of the pelvis to provide proper counter traction on the anterior structures. The assistant aids the dissection by placing a suction device or grasper lifting anteriorly, at the level of the seminal vesicle or posterior vaginal wall. The proctectomy is performed from right to left, leaving the anterior dissection at last and taking great care in preserving the superior hypogas-

tric nerves and the ureters. The dissection can be performed in a "close rectal" fashion, preserving the mesorectal layer or following the total mesorectal excision principles in case of oncologic concerns. Once the levator ani plane is reached, the rectum is transected just above the anorectal junction (verified by digital rectal examination) with a single fire of a 60 mm SureForm stapler (in a wide pelvis) or with two shots of a 45-mm SureForm stapler using a blue cartridge. The specimen is placed in an endo bag for later extraction through the previous ileostomy site. Under robotic control, the pouch and the anvil are brought towards the pelvis, and a 28- or 29 mm circular stapler is introduced transanally to complete the IPAA. An air-leak test of the anastomosis should be performed routinely, as well as a check of proper vascularization using Firefly fluorescence imaging mode with indocyanine green. Direct visual inspection of the pouch via endoscope is also very useful to exclude any defects of the pouch. At this point, the specimen is extracted, and a diverting loop ileostomy is constructed. A 19-F Jackson-Pratt flat-type drain is then placed into the pelvis [16].

References

1. Bemelman WA, collaborators SE. Evolving role of IBD surgery. J Crohns Colitis. 2018;12(8):1005–7.
2. Koltun WA. The future of surgical management of inflammatory bowel disease. Dis Colon Rectum. 2008;51(6):813–7.
3. Lightner AL, Pemberton JH, Dozois EJ, Larson DW, Cima RR, Mathis KL, Pardi DS, Andrew RE, Koltun WA, Sagar P, Hahnloser D. The surgical management of inflammatory bowel disease. Curr Probl Surg. 2017;54(4):172–250. https://doi.org/10.1067/j.cpsurg.2017.02.006. Epub 2017 Feb 21
4. Soop M, Spinelli A. What is at the cutting edge of IBD? Proceedings of the European Crohn's and Colitis Organisation 2018 Congress from a Surgical Perspective. Dis Colon Rectum. 2018;61(8):879–82.
5. Burisch J, Munkholm P. The epidemiology of inflammatory bowel disease. Scand J Gastroenterol. 2015;50(8):942–51. https://doi.org/10.3109/0036552 1.2015.1014407.
6. Abdalla S, Abd El Aziz MA, Calini G, Saeed H, Merchea A, Shawki S, Behm KT, Larson DW. Perioperative outcomes of minimally invasive ileocolic resection for complicated Crohn dis-

ease: results from a referral center retrospective cohort. Surgery. 2022;172(2):522–9. https://doi.org/10.1016/j.surg.2022.01.046.

7. Gunnells D, Cannon J. Robotic surgery in Crohn's disease. Clin Colon Rectal Surg. 2021;34(5):286–91. https://doi.org/10.1055/s-0041-1729862.

8. Raskin ER, Gorrepati ML, Mehendale S, Gaertner WB. Robotic-assisted ileocolic resection for Crohn's disease: outcomes from an early national experience. J Robot Surg. 2019;13(3):429–34. https://doi.org/10.1007/s11701-018-0887-1.

9. Aydinli HH, Anderson M, Hambrecht A, Bernstein MA, Grucela AL. Robotic ileocolic resection with intracorporeal anastomosis for Crohn's disease. J Robot Surg. 2021;15(3):465–72. https://doi.org/10.1007/s11701-020-01125-z.

10. Calini G, Abdalla S, Abd El Aziz MA, Saeed HA, D'Angelo AD, Behm KT, Shawki S, Mathis KL, Larson DW. Intracorporeal versus extracorporeal anastomosis for robotic ileocolic resection in Crohn's disease. J Robot Surg. 2022;16(3):601–9. https://doi.org/10.1007/s11701-021-01283-8.

11. Scaringi S, Giudici F, Zambonin D, Ficari F, Bechi P. Totally robotic intracorporeal side-to-side isoperistaltic strictureplasty for Crohn's disease. J Minim Access Surg. 2018;14(4):341–4. https://doi.org/10.4103/jmas.JMAS_212_17.

12. Anderson M, Lynn P, Aydinli HH, Schwartzberg D, Bernstein M, Grucela A. Early experience with urgent robotic subtotal colectomy for severe acute ulcerative colitis has comparable perioperative outcomes to laparoscopic surgery. J Robot Surg. 2020;14(2):249–53. https://doi.org/10.1007/s11701-019-00968-5.

13. Schwartzberg DM, Remzi FH. The role of laparoscopic, robotic, and open surgery in uncomplicated and complicated inflammatory Bowel disease. Gastrointest Endosc Clin N Am. 2019;29(3):563–76. https://doi.org/10.1016/j.giec.2019.02.012.

14. Mège D, Figueiredo MN, Manceau G, Maggiori L, Bouhnik Y, Panis Y. Three-stage laparoscopic ileal pouch-anal anastomosis is the best approach for high-risk patients with inflammatory Bowel disease: an analysis of 185 consecutive patients. J Crohns Colitis. 2016;10(8):898–904.

15. Jimenez-Rodriguez RM, Quezada-Diaz F, Tchack M, Pappou E, Wei IH, Smith JJ, Nash GM, Guillem JG, Paty PB, Weiser MR, Garcia-Aguilar J. Use of the Xi robotic platform for total abdominal colectomy: a step forward in minimally invasive colorectal surgery. Surg Endosc. 2019;33(3):966–71. https://doi.org/10.1007/s00464-018-6529-x.

16. Lightner AL, Kelley SR, Larson DW. Robotic platform for an IPAA. Dis Colon Rectum. 2018;61(7):869–74. https://doi.org/10.1097/DCR.0000000000001125.

Laparoscopic Appendectomy

N. Vettoretto and E. Botteri

15.1 Surgical Technique

15.1.1 Introduction

Laparoscopic appendectomy (LA) was first described more than 40 years ago, but has become the gold standard only for pre-menopausal women in which diagnostic advantages have always been demonstrated [1]. Nowadays, together with the increasing spread of laparoscopy for most abdominal surgeries, LA has become more and more diffuse, in comparison with traditional open appendectomy [2]. Still, in 2012, less than 30% of all appendectomies was performed laparoscopically [3]. Problems related to emergency conditions, night- or weekend time, slightly longer operating time, and insufficient experience especially for younger surgeons on-call justify these rates. Ten years after, our feeling and hope is that these rates are higher in all surgical wards, both hub and spoke, community or university hospitals.

15.1.2 Technique

1. Access to the peritoneal cavity: The pneumoperitoneum can be established either by means of "open" access (Hasson technique) or by "closed" technique (direct insertion of the trocar or, more commonly, by the use of a Veress needle and an optical trocar). In the former a small (2-cm) incision is practiced in the umbilicus (better if preceded by cutaneous infiltration with a long-lasting anesthetic). Blunt dissection with scissors and forceps shows the linea alba fascia which is again infiltrated with anesthetic and incised with the use of Kocher clamps. Blunt dissection is then conducted through the preperitoneum until access to the peritoneal cavity is obtained. At this point the fascia is suspended with absorbable sutures which are meant to be used in the end for the closure and in the meanwhile are assured to the Hasson trocar to keep it in site and guarantee the sealing for the pneumoperitoneum. As for the closed techniques the most used is the Veress needle, a blunt-tipped needle which can be inserted in the Palmer site (left hypocondrium, where the possibility of vascular and visceral injury is lower); after the pneumoperitoneum is established, a visual 10/12 mm trocar (blunt trocar with a transparent tip with the camera inserted within) is placed in the umbilical region, after a 2-cm incision of the skin. Direct trocar insertion consists instead in a "semi-open" technique in which the parietal skin aside the umbilicus is

N. Vettoretto (✉) · E. Botteri
Montichiari Surgery, ASST Spedali Civili, Brescia, Italy

M. Milone et al. (eds.), *Scrub Nurse in Minimally Invasive and Robotic General Surgery*,
https://doi.org/10.1007/978-3-031-42257-7_15

lifted up after an incision of the skin and sometimes of the fascia and a semi-blunt trocar is inserted in a caudal direction "blindly." Neither of these techniques has proven better than the other, and it depends mainly on the surgeons' attitude and experience. Pneumoperitoneum must be established slowly, starting with a 4 l/min flow to reach a mean intraperitoneal pressure of 12–14 mmHg. We standardized the trocar access preemptive anesthetic injection as it proved to reduce significantly postoperative pain in most laparoscopic surgery, also in appendectomy [4].

2. Explorative laparoscopy: The first momentum of the operation is the so-called explorative laparoscopy. After the camera has been inserted in the peritoneum, a first look is given to ascertain direct or indirect signs of a complicated appendicitis, which might be free fluid, inflammatory masses, inflammation of the peritoneum, or adhesions. After this, two other trocars must be placed in order to manipulate the viscera and complete the exploration. These can be put in different positions but are generally located below the umbilical line. Exploration starts generally in the cecal area by bluntly moving the omentum which can have inflammatory adhesions with the appendix. The position of the organ might vary from the subcostal region to the deep pelvis. If the appendicitis is mild and cannot justify the symptoms, we must continue exploration and search for other causes. First, we aim at seeing thoroughly the pelvis and the reproductive organs especially in the female and eventually call for a gynecologic consultation if needed. Then we explore the terminal ileum to look for a Meckel's diverticulum [5].

3. Dissection of the mesenteriolum: Once established appendicitis the next step is the dissection of the mesenteriolum. It has to be exposed with an adequate lifting of the appendix (with or without a previous peritoneal dissection if the appendix is located retrocecally or subserosally). Dissection can be performed either near the organ or at the base of the appendix.

The latter needs more caution in hemostasis as the appendicular artery is dissected at its origin. Energy devices (Fig. 15.1a), clips (Fig. 15.1b), or sutures can be used but mostly bipolar energy is enough to achieve the correct hemostasis [6]. Dissection is extended until the appendicular base is clearly seen (Fig. 15.1c).

4. Closure of the stump: Once the appendix base has been cleared, we must section the stump after closing it. A maneuver to be done is a gentle squeezing of the base in order to displace eventual fecaliths. Closure methods comprise the stapler (Fig. 15.2b), suture (or endoloop) (Fig. 15.2a), or reabsorbable clips (Hem-o-lok) (Fig. 15.1). Neither method carries advantages over the other except for differences in cost [7]. Guidelines suggest the use of staplers (higher cost) only in case of gangrenous appendicular base. Attention must be paid to the remnant as it does not have to exceed the 1–2 cm in length (in order to prevent stump inflammation). In our experience, with the use of endoloops, one is enough, but in case of securing the stump with two endoloops, be careful to put the second in the same place as the first, not to create ischemic areas in between the two sutures.

5. Extraction of the specimen: the appendix must then be retrieved from the abdomen in a safe way, taking care not to contaminate the abdominal wall or the rest of the abdomen with fecal material. In the classical three-trocar technique, the specimen can be retrieved in an endobag (Fig. 15.3) or through a 10/12 mm trocar (by removing the valve mechanism), under endoscopic vision.

6. Wash and drain: There is debate over the need for peritoneal lavage [8]. In order to be efficacious, ex vivo studies suggest that 6–8lt of sterile saline are needed to reduce significantly the bacterial charge in case of diffuse peritonitis. This obviously takes time, changes of decubitus and a peristaltic pump with a warmer for the injected liquids. In case of localized peritonitis or phlegmonous appendicitis without fecal

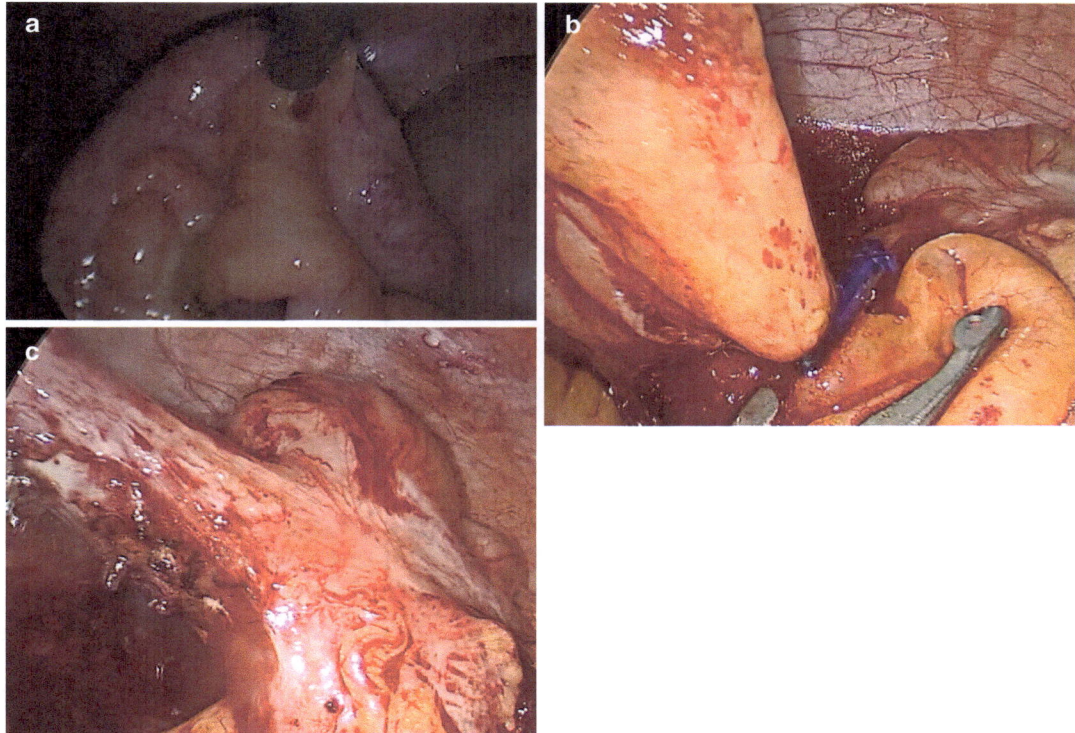

Fig. 15.1 (**a**) Mesenteriolum dissection carried out by monopolar hook. (**b**) Mesenteriolum vascular closure with Hem-o-lok® clip. (**c**) Mesenteriolum dissection completed unto the appendicular base

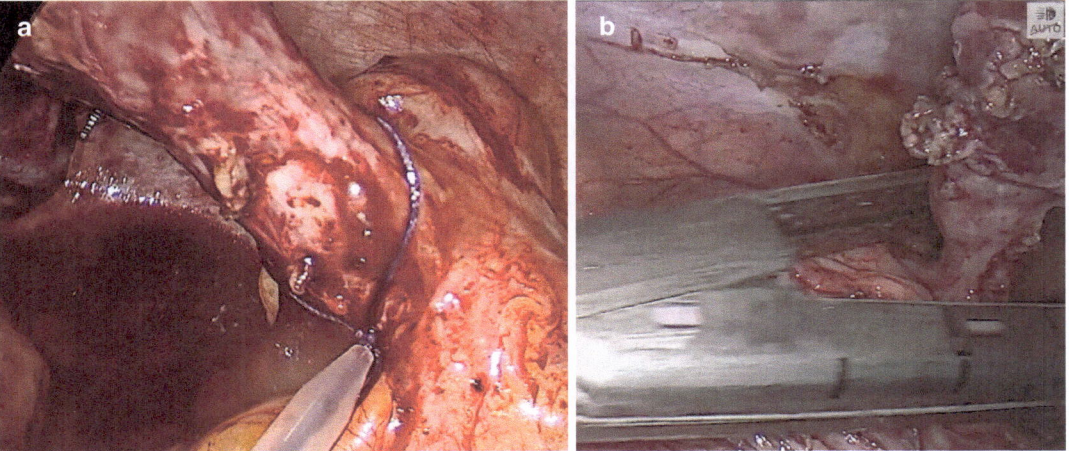

Fig. 15.2 (**a**) Stump closure with endoloop. (**b**) Stump closure with stapler

contamination, a simple aspiration of liquids might prove enough without lavage. If the washing is necessary and the full amount of liquid to use is not fully accomplished, we suggest to put a drain in the pelvis for the first day. The drain is also suggested in case of complicated appendicitis with abscess or gangrene.

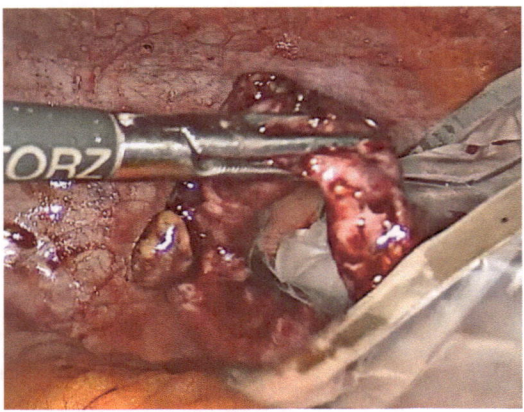

Fig. 15.3 Surgical specimen retrieved with endobag

7. Closure of the accesses: Every laparoscopic access, especially if 10–12 mm and located below the umbilicus, must be closed with fascial sutures in order to prevent trocar-site hernias. This can be done from the outside (open technique) or from the inside (with a needle retriever or with other systems).

15.2 Operating Theatre Setting

– Setting: The OR is settled as for every laparoscopic operation, with an instruments' cart for laparoscopy and one settled for an emergency conversion to open surgery. Conversion of a laparoscopic appendectomy is below 10% (depending on the surgeons' expertise) and usually performed for difficult anatomy, excessive adhesions, or technical problems which cannot be solved by laparoscopic means, and a large umbilico-pubic median laparotomy is generally needed. The monitors and the column are generally put to the right of the patient, while the energy machine can be placed in the lower left side, together with the aspirator.
– Vision systems (2D, 3D, 4K, fluorescence): In recent times improved vision systems for laparoscopy are having an increasing importance in laparoscopic surgery and also in appendectomy. The traditional 2D monitors

can be replaced by 3D visions (used with polarized glasses worn by the surgeons and the scrub nurse) or by 4 K larger monitors up to 55 inches, offering a clearer view and an increased precision for surgeons [9]. Recently, indocyanine green (ICG) injection and visualization with dedicated cameras have gained importance in laparoscopic surgery, especially in the colorectal and upper GI surgery; its use in appendicitis (intraoperative endovenous injection of ICG to ascertain the vascularization of the stump with the aim to reduce postoperative abscesses) has not yet been published but some studies are ongoing [10].

15.3 Patient and Trocar Positioning

– Patient's positioning: Patient is set supine, with his/her right arm externalized (for anesthetist's use) and the left arm along the body. Trendelenburg position and left tilting are generally needed, and the patient must be protected from decubitus lesions, incorrect arm and shoulder positioning, and skin burns from monopolar energy.
– Operator positioning: After the induction of the pneumoperitoneum (in which the leading surgeon and its aid stand on opposite sides of the patient), both surgeons (operator and assistant) stand on the left of the patient, generally the assistant being cephalad. The scrub nurse is also on the left of the patient and of the operating surgeon but he/she can also stand on the right of the patient in case the OR is equipped with double monitors. The anesthetist's team is near the head of the patient.
– Three-port technique (Fig. 15.4): The classical laparoscopic operation is done with three ports. One is the camera port and is generally positioned in the umbilicus (T1). The operator's right hand (T2) is generally positioned in the left flank and the auxiliary trocar (T3) in

Fig. 15.4 OR setting and standard trocar position

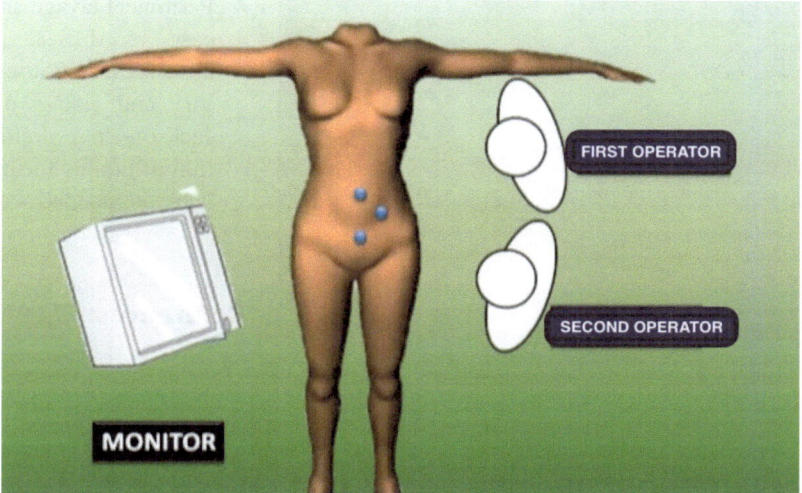

the left iliac fossa. T2 or T3 might be both 0/12 mm, 5, and 10/12 or both 5 mm depending on the surgeons' experience. Endobag use or clip positioning requires a 10/12 trocar unless a 5 mm camera is used, even if 5 mm commercial devices exist but are not so diffuse at present. The choice between disposable or multiple-use trocars is up to the surgeons' experience and availability, as long as the blunt-tip trocars are used (blade trocars might be more hazardous for trocar site bleeding). Another position of the two operating port sites has been purposed in order to improve the aesthetic results by choosing a double suprapubic access together with the camera trocar in the umbilicus.

– Single-port technique: Noncomplicated appendicitis can be treated with a single-port technique with similar results in terms of pain and overall complications – aesthetic results of this technique are particularly appreciated by young patients [11]. Commercial or handmade devices for single-access surgery are disposable, even if we are used to the cheap and self-made "glove-port" technique (Fig. 15.5) [12]. The decision about whether to perform single or multiport surgery is taken after the positioning of the camera port and

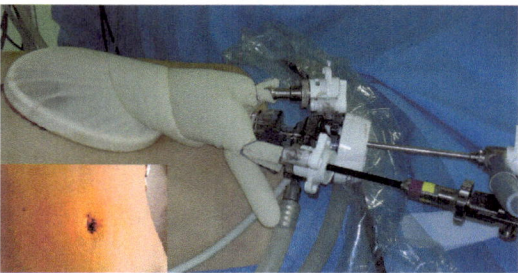

Fig. 15.5 "Glove port" for single-port appendectomy and aesthetic result

explorative laparoscopy. We prefer to limit this indication to young patients with uncomplicated appendicitis and without the need for a drain. The access for this operation might be limited to a 2-cm cut of the fascia and the operating time is similar when the surgeon's experience in single-port surgery is acquired.

– Other techniques (miniports, transvaginal, laparoscopically assisted): Standard multiport appendectomy can be done with the use of dedicated mini-instruments (3–5 mm) and there are disposable or multiuse sets dedicated to this surgery. Optical trocar and extraction site (usually located in the umbilicus) remains larger than 5 mm. In Germany a large series of transvaginal (NOTES) appendectomies have

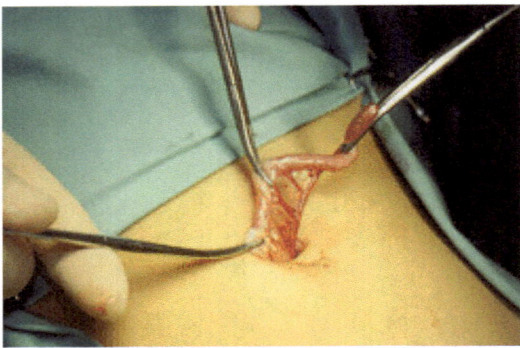

Fig. 15.6 Pediatric trans-umbilical appendectomy (TULA)

been published with the use of various techniques (flexible endoscopic camera, dedicated articulated instruments) with interesting results in terms of patients' satisfaction but it is still an experimental technique, performed in a few centers [13]. Pediatric surgeons once used a "laparoscopically assisted" technique based on the laparoscopic grasping and extraction of the appendix and an open appendectomy performed through the umbilical incision, but this technique has almost been abandoned (Fig. 15.6).

15.4 Adopted Instruments During the Procedure

– Standard instrumentation: Verress needle (for the closed technique, or open surgery instrumentation for the open Hasson access), blunt-tip trocars (3), 10 mm camera, two endoscopic atraumatic forceps (Johann or similar), endoscopic suction/lavage device, endoscopic clip applier, endoscopic suture device or endoloop, monopolar hook or scissors, bipolar forceps, endobag, endoscopic grasper, dissection forceps (i.e., angle droit).
– Dissection instruments: Energy devices like radiofrequency, ultrasound, or mixed might be required.
– Devices for stump closure: Endoloop, Hem-o-lok, or endo-GIA might be used for the stump closure.

– Peritoneal lavage and intraoperative swabs: In case of diffuse peritonitis, gangrene, or abscesses, a peritoneal lavage might be necessary and also a drain (Redon, laminar, or Jackson-Pratt drains). Intraoperative collection of liquids for laboratory culture or swabs is recommended.

References

1. Vettoretto N, Gobbi S, Corradi A, Belli F, Piccolo D, Pernazza G, Mannino L. Italian Association of Hospital Surgeons (Associazione dei Chirurghi Ospedalieri Italiani). Consensus conference on laparoscopic appendectomy: development of guidelines. Color Dis. 2011;13(7):748–54.
2. Di Saverio S, Podda M, De Simone B, Ceresoli M, Augustin G, Gori A, Boermeester M, Sartelli M, Coccolini F, Tarasconi A, De' Angelis N, Weber DG, Tolonen M, Birindelli A, Biffl W, Moore EE, Kelly M, Soreide K, Kashuk J, Ten Broek R, Gomes CA, Sugrue M, Davies RJ, Damaskos D, Leppäniemi A, Kirkpatrick A, Peitzman AB, Fraga GP, Maier RV, Coimbra R, Chiarugi M, Sganga G, Pisanu A, De' Angelis GL, Tan E, Van Goor H, Pata F, Di Carlo I, Chiara O, Litvin A, Campanile FC, Sakakushev B, Tomadze G, Demetrashvili Z, Latifi R, Abu-Zidan F, Romeo O, Segovia-Lohse H, Baiocchi G, Costa D, Rizoli S, Balogh ZJ, Bendinelli C, Scalea T, Ivatury R, Velmahos G, Andersson R, Kluger Y, Ansaloni L, Catena F. Diagnosis and treatment of acute appendicitis: 2020 update of the WSES Jerusalem guidelines. World J Emerg Surg. 2020;15(1):27.
3. Vettoretto N, Agresta F, Presenti L, Morino M. Evidence-based laparoscopic appendectomy practice requires national database studies. Surg Endosc. 2013;27(7):2652–3.
4. Molfino S, Botteri E, Baggi P, Totaro L, Huscher M, Baiocchi GL, Portolani N, Vettoretto N. Pain control in laparoscopic surgery: a case-control study between transversus abdominis plane-block and trocar-site anesthesia. Updat Surg. 2019;71(4):717–22.
5. Agresta F, Ansaloni L, Baiocchi GL, Bergamini C, Campanile FC, Carlucci M, Cocorullo G, Corradi A, Franzato B, Lupo M, Mandalà V, Mirabella A, Pernazza G, Piccoli M, Staudacher C, Vettoretto N, Zago M, Lettieri E, Levati A, Pietrini D, Scaglione M, De Masi S, De Placido G, Francucci M, Rasi M, Fingerhut A, Uranüs S, Garattini S. Laparoscopic approach to acute abdomen from the Consensus Development Conference of the Società Italiana di Chirurgia Endoscopica e nuove tecnologie (SICE), Associazione Chirurghi Ospedalieri Italiani (ACOI), Società Italiana di Chirurgia (SIC), Società Italiana di Chirurgia d'Urgenza e del Trauma (SICUT), Società Italiana di Chirurgia nell'Ospedalità Privata (SICOP),

and the European Association for Endoscopic Surgery (EAES). Surg Endosc. 2012;26(8):2134–64.

6. Botteri E, Podda M, Arezzo A, Vettoretto N, Sartori A, Agrusa A, Allaix ME, Anania G, Brachet Contul R, Caracino V, Cassinotti E, Cuccurullo D, D'Ambrosio G, Milone M, Muttillo I, Petz WL, Pisano M, Guerrieri M, Silecchia G, Agresta F. Current status on the adoption of high energy devices in Italy: an Italian Society for Endoscopic Surgery and New Technologies (SICE) national survey. Surg Endosc. 2021;35(11):6201–11.

7. Lasek A, Wysocki M, Mavrikis J, Myśliwiec P, Bobowicz M, Dowgiałło-Wnukiewicz N, Kenig J, Stefura T, Walędziak M, Pędziwiatr M, Pol-LA (Polish Laparoscopic Appendectomy) Collaborative Study Group. Comparison of stump closure techniques during laparoscopic appendectomies for complicated appendicitis—results from Pol-LA (Polish laparoscopic appendectomy) multicenter large cohort study. Acta Chir Belg. 2020;120(2):116–23.

8. Burini G, Cianci MC, Coccetta M, Spizzirri A, Di Saverio S, Coletta R, Sapienza P, Mingoli A, Cirocchi R, Morabito A. Aspiration versus peritoneal lavage in appendicitis: a meta-analysis. World J Emerg Surg. 2021;16(1):44.

9. Botteri E, Ortenzi M, Alemanno G, Giordano A, Travaglio E, Turolo C, Castiglioni S, Treppiedi E, Rosso E, Gattolin A, Caracino V, Prosperi P, Valeri A, Guerrieri M, Vettoretto N. Laparoscopic appendectomy performed by junior SUrgeonS: impact of 3D visualization on surgical outcome. Randomized multicentre clinical trial. (LAPSUS TRIAL). Surg Endosc. 2021;35(2):710–7.

10. Vettoretto N, Foglia E, Ferrario L, Gerardi C, Molteni B, Nocco U, Lettieri E, Molfino S, Baiocchi GL, Elmore U, Rosati R, Currò G, Cassinotti E, Boni L, Cirocchi R, Marano A, Petz WL, Arezzo A, Bonino MA, Davini F, Biondi A, Anania G, Agresta F, Silecchia G. Could fluorescence-guided surgery be an efficient and sustainable option? A SICE (Italian Society of Endoscopic Surgery) health technology assessment summary. Surg Endosc. 2020;34(7):3270–84.

11. Vettoretto N, Cirocchi R, Randolph J, Morino M. Acute appendicitis can be treated with single-incision laparoscopy: a systematic review of randomized controlled trials. Color Dis. 2015;17(4):281–9.

12. Di Saverio S, Mandrioli M, Birindelli A, Biscardi A, Di Donato L, Gomes CA, Piccinini A, Vettoretto N, Agresta F, Tugnoli G, Jovine E. Single-incision laparoscopic appendectomy with a low-cost technique and surgical-glove port: "How To Do It" with comparison of the outcomes and costs in a consecutive single-operator series of 45 cases. J Am Coll Surg. 2016;222(3):e15–30.

13. Magdeburg R, Kähler G. Neue Wege in der operativen Behandlung der akuten Appendizitis? [New ways in the surgery of acute appendicitis?]. Zentralbl Chir. 2013;138(3):284–8.

Robotic Appendectomy

16

Diego Coletta ⓘ and Alberto Patriti ⓘ

16.1 Introduction

The most common disease that leads to removal of the appendix is inflammation. Other diseases that lead to removal of the appendix include neoplastic changes, as carcinoid tumors, mucinous cystadenocarcinomas, colonic-type adenocarcinomas, and rare tumors [1] usually requiring right colectomy, extended multiorgan resections, and peritonectomy. Laparoscopic appendectomy represents the gold standard of surgical treatment for acute appendicitis. Robot-assisted surgery is not indicated to perform appendectomy as a single procedure due to high costs [2] and the absence of advantages in terms of pain and length of stay, over the pure laparoscopic approach. No evidence comparing the two different approaches exists. In general surgery no studies reported a description of the appendectomy technique by using the robotic system. Some authors report robot-assisted appendectomies during oncological, gynecological, and urological procedures

[3–5]. Thus, the trocar placement and the surgical instrument adopted are those of pelvic surgery or right colectomy. We aimed to explain how to perform a robotic appendectomy as a single procedure.

16.1.1 Appendectomy

Appendectomy consists of the following surgical steps:

- Exposure of the cecum, appendix, and distal ileal loop.
- Ligation and section of appendicular vessels.
- Ligation and transection of the appendix.
- Specimen extraction.
- Closure of port wounds.

16.2 Operating Theatre Setting

The operating theatre setting for a robotic appendectomy is performed as follows (Fig. 16.1):

- Operating table in the center of the theatre.
- Vision cart positioned on the right of the patient, at the level of the feet.
- Patient cart positioned to the right of the patient.
- Surgeon positioned at the surgical console.

D. Coletta
Department of General Surgery, San Salvatore Hospital, AST Pesaro-Urbino, Pesaro, Italy

Department of Surgical Sciences, Policlinico Umberto I University Hospital, Sapienza University of Rome, Rome, Italy

A. Patriti (✉)
Department of General Surgery, San Salvatore Hospital, AST Pesaro-Urbino, Pesaro, Italy

© The Author(s), under exclusive license to Springer Nature Switzerland AG 2024
M. Milone et al. (eds.), *Scrub Nurse in Minimally Invasive and Robotic General Surgery*,
https://doi.org/10.1007/978-3-031-42257-7_16

Fig. 16.1 Schematic
operating theatre setting

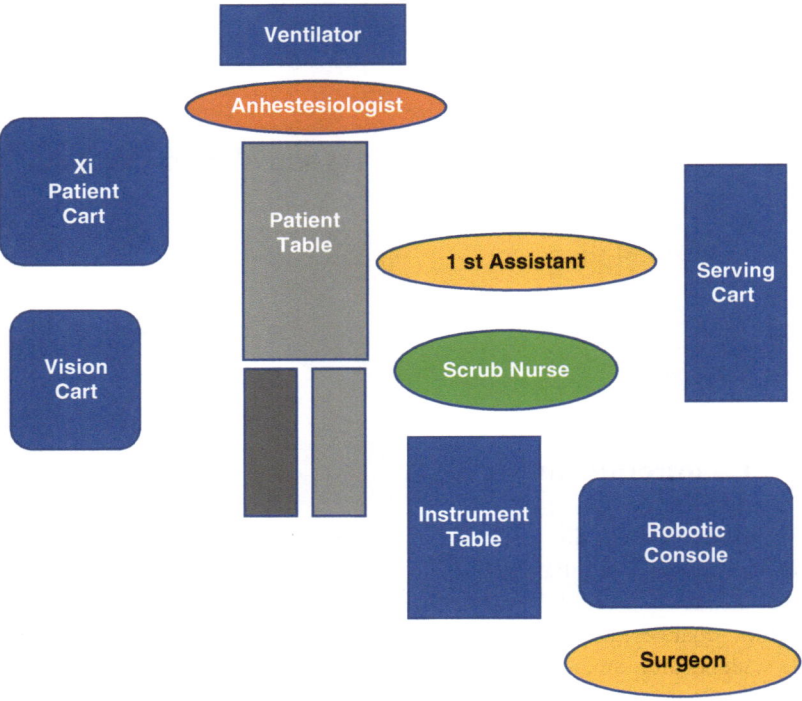

- First assistant at the operating table positioned on the left of the patient.
- Instrument nurse to the legs of the patient.
- Serving cart on the left of the scrub nurse.

16.3   Patient Positioning

Patient positioning is performed as shown in Fig. 16.2:

- Supine position in Trendelenburg with an inclination of about 15° to 20°.
- Left rotation.
- Arms adducted along the body.

The operating table is therefore prepared with a sliding prevent mat or, in its absence, with a leg fixing with bandages to prevent the patient from falling from the operating table.

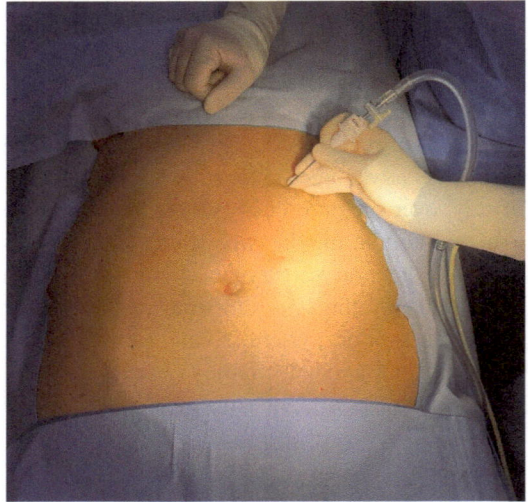

Fig. 16.2 Creation of pneumoperitoneum by the Veress technique

16.4 Port Placement and Robotic Docking

The first step is the creation of pneumoperitoneum by inserting a Veress needle at the Palmer point (Fig. 16.2).

- First robotic 8 mm trocar placement is performed according to a standardized blind Veress-assisted technique, approximately 2 cm to the left of the umbilicus along to the transverse umbilical line.
- The following two or three 8 mm trocars could be placed in a straight line at 8 cm from each other.
- In case of use of a robotic stapler, a 12 mm trocar is needed.
- One assistant 5 mm or 12 mm port is placed caudally than the robotic trocar according to standardized triangulation (Fig. 16.3).

The "targeting" (the selection through endoscope of the target anatomy) is carried out on the right iliac fossa or on the pelvis.

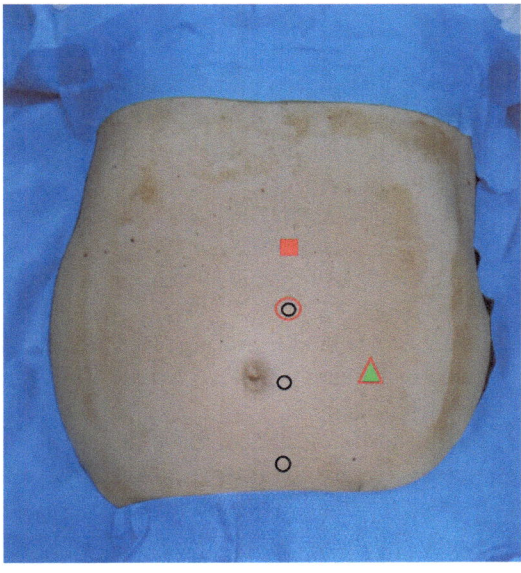

Fig. 16.3 Port placement to perform a robotic appendectomyBlack circle, robotic 8 mm trocar; red circle, robotic 12 mm trocar; red square, third robotic 8 mm or 12 mm trocar; green triangle, 5 mm assistant trocar; red triangle, 12 mm assistant trocar

16.5 Surgical Instruments Required

16.5.1 Robotic Instruments

- 4 ports (two or three 8 mm ports and one 12 mm port)
- 1 port reducer
- 1 port with tubing set for the creation and stabilization of pneumoperitoneum
- 30° robotic endoscope
- 1 grasping forceps (ProGrasp Forceps® or Cadiere Forceps® or Tip-Up Forceps®)
- 1 bipolar forceps (Fenestrated Bipolar Forceps® or Maryland Bipolar Forceps®)
- 1 monopolar instrument (Permanent Cautery Hook® or Hot Shears®)
- 1 sealing instrument (Vessel Sealer®)
- 1 stapler (SureForm EndoWrist Stapler® 40 mm)
- 1 needle holder (Large Needle Driver®).

16.5.2 Laparoscopic Instrument

- Laparoscopic grasping forceps (Croce-Olmi forceps, Grasper or Johann forceps).
- Laparoscopic suction/irrigation system.
- 1 assistant port (5 or 12 mm)
- 5 mm and 10 mm endoscopic clip applier
- Hem-o-lok clips with laparoscopic applier of various sizes (small/medium).
- Laparoscopic scissors.
- Laparoscopic stapler 45 mm (white charge).
- Endoloop.
- Absorbable suture 2/0–3/0 length 10–12 cm (Vicryl®, PDS®).
- Absorbable wound closure device suture 2/0, 3/0 (V-Loc®, Stratafix®).
- Endobag (small).
- Berci forceps.
- Scope warmer.

16.5.3 Open Instrument

- 2 scalpels with stainless steel blade (sizes 11 and 22)

- 2 Janach (steel bowls)
- 2 anatomical tissue forceps
- 2 toothed forceps
- 4 curved Klemmer clamps
- 4 curved Kocher clamps
- 1 Mayo scissors
- 1 Nelson-Metzenbaum dissection scissors
- 4 Backhaus clamps
- 1 Mixter right angle forceps
- 2 Mathieu retractors
- 2 Farabeuf retractors
- 1 monopolar electric scalpel
- Absorbable suture (Vicryl® 0 or 1).
- Absorbable suture 3/0 (Vicryl Rapide®).
- Abdominal drain (Blake®).

16.6 Surgical Steps and Related Instruments

Veress Technique for Laparoscopic Access
- Scalpel (blade 11).
- Veress needle.
- Syringe for saline and drop test.

Port Placement and Robotic Docking
- 2 robotic 8 mm ports
- 1 or 2 robotic 8 mm ports or 12 mm port with reducer
- Tubing set for the stabilization of pneumoperitoneum.
- 1 robotic 5 mm or 12 mm assistant port.

Once the ports have been positioned and the patient cart positioned on the operating table, the arm that accommodates the endoscope is connected by the scrub nurse and the first assistant at the table to perform the targeting. Once the targeting is complete, the other arms are docked and the robotic instruments are inserted by the scrub nurse and first assistant, after positioning the reducers on the 12 mm ports to avoid loss of pneumoperitoneum.

16.6.1 Exposure of the Cecum, Appendix, and Distal Ileal Loop

This first phase provides the complete visualization of the cecum, appendix, and distal ileal loop.

The robotic instruments to be used are as follows (based on the surgeon's requests, the number, and the size of robotic trocars):

- 30° robotic endoscope
- 1 grasping forceps (ProGrasp Forceps® or Cadiere Forceps®)
- 1 bipolar forceps (Fenestrated Bipolar Forceps®)
- 1 monopolar instrument (Permanent Cautery Hook®).

16.6.2 Ligation and Section of Appendicular Vessels

This phase provides the complete dissection and ligation of appendicular vessels.

The robotic instruments to be used are as follows (based on the surgeon's requests, the number and the size of robotic trocars):

- 30° robotic endoscope
- 1 grasping forceps (ProGrasp Forceps® or Cadiere Forceps®)
- 1 bipolar forceps (Fenestrated Bipolar Forceps®)
- 1 monopolar instrument (Permanent Cautery Hook®) or alternatively
- 1 sealing instrument (Vessel Sealer®) or alternatively
- 1 robotic needle driver (Large Needle Driver)
- Absorbable suture 2/0–3/0 length 10–12 cm (Vicryl®, PDS®).
- 5 mm and 10 mm endoscopic clip applier
- Hem-o-lok clips with laparoscopic applier of various sizes (small/medium).
- Laparoscopic scissors.

16.6.3 Ligation and Transection of the Appendix

This phase provides the complete dissection, ligation, and transection of the appendix.

The robotic instruments to be used are the following (based on the surgeon's requests, the number and the size of robotic trocars):

- 30° robotic endoscope
- 1 grasping forceps (ProGrasp Forceps® or Cadiere Forceps®)
- 1 bipolar forceps (Fenestrated Bipolar Forceps®)
- 1 monopolar instrument (Permanent Cautery Hook®) or alternatively
- 1 sealing instrument (Vessel Sealer®) or alternatively
- 1 robotic needle driver (Large Needle Driver)
- Absorbable suture 2/0–3/0 length 10–12 cm (Vicryl®, PDS®).
- 5 mm and 10 mm endoscopic clip applier
- Hem-o-lok clips with laparoscopic applier of various sizes (small/medium).
- Laparoscopic scissors.
- 1 robotic stapler (SureForm EndoWrist Stapler® 40 mm).

The appendix is dissected and ligated at the base with absorbable suture or with Hem-o-lok and then transected with laparoscopic scissors. Alternatively, the appendectomy could be performed by the Vessel Sealer or by robotic stapler directly.

Sometimes the appendicular stump could be reinforced by an absorbable suture V-Loc 3/0.

16.6.4 Specimen Extraction

This phase provides the specimen extraction from the assistant trocar or robotic 12 mm trocar.

The required instruments are as follows:

- Endobag.

At the end of the procedure a Blake drain could be placed in the pelvis of the right iliac fossa (based on the surgeon's request and the intraoperative findings).

16.6.5 Closure of Port Wounds

- Laparoscopic bipolar forceps.
- Berci forceps.
- Absorbable suture (Vicryl® 0 or 1).
- 1 absorbable suture (based on the surgeon's request) to perform closure of fascia
- 1 absorbable suture to perform closure of the skin.

The port wounds could be cauterized with laparoscopic bipolar forceps (for 5 and 8 mm ports) or sutured with Berci forceps.

16.7 Intraoperative Complications

The most frequent intraoperative complications to manage during a robotic appendectomy are basically two: hemorrhage and injuries to the bowel.

In these circumstances, the instrument nurse must have the following instruments available:

- Laparoscopic suction/irrigation system.
- 10 cm × 10 cm gauze to be passed to the assistant at the request of the surgeon
- Endoscopic clip applier with titanium clips.
- Laparoscopic Hem-o-lok® applier, with clips already loaded, if the source of bleeding is clearly visible.
- Robotic needle holder and absorbable suture with a small-gauge needle to attempt to repair the bleeding vessel or, in case of injury of bowel segments, needle holder and absorbable suture to repair it (Vicryl®, PDS®, V-Loc®, Stratafix®).

References

1. McGory ML, Maggard MA, Kang H, O'Connell JB, Ko CY. Malignancies of the appendix: beyond case series reports. Dis Colon Rectum. 2005;48(12):2264–71. https://doi.org/10.1007/s10350-005-0196-4.

2. Alqahtani A, Albassam A, Zamakhshary M, Shoukri M, Altokhais T, Aljazairi A, Alzahim A, Mallik M, Alshehri A. Robot-assisted pediatric surgery: how far can we go? World J Surg. 2010;34(5):975–8. https://doi.org/10.1007/s00268-010-0431-6.

3. Orcutt ST, Anaya DA, Malafa M. Minimally invasive appendectomy for resection of appendiceal mucocele: case series and review of the literature. Int J Surg Case Rep. 2017;37:13–6. https://doi.org/10.1016/j.ijscr.2017.05.027.

4. Akl MN, Magrina JF, Kho RM, Magtibay PM. Robotic appendectomy in gynaecological surgery: technique and pathological findings. Int J Med Robot. 2008;4(3):210–3. https://doi.org/10.1002/rcs.

5. Hüttenbrink C, Hatiboglu G, Simpfendörfer T, Radtke JP, Becker R, Teber D, Hadaschik B, Pahernik S, Hohenfellner M. Incidental appendectomy during robotic laparoscopic prostatectomy-safe and worth to perform? Langenbeck's Arch Surg. 2018;403(2):265–9. https://doi.org/10.1007/s00423-017-1630-5.

Right Hemicolectomy

Gabriele Anania, Francesco Marchetti, Alberto Campagnaro, Nicola Tamburini, and Giuseppe Resta

17.1 Introduction

The right hemicolectomy and the extended right hemycolectomy procedures can be delineated into a demolitive phase a reconstructive phase. The extent of resection required for malignant disease depends on the tumor margin and the need for adequate oncologic lymphadenectomy as defined by the blood supply. Guidelines for colorectal cancer recommend a 5-cm margin, both proximally and distally, for adequate tumor resection and a minimum of 12 lymph nodes for complete lymphadenectomy [1].

G. Anania (✉) · F. Marchetti · A. Campagnaro
Unit of General Surgery, S. Anna University Hospital of Ferrara, Cona, FE, Italy

Department of Medical Science, University of Ferrara, Ferrara, Italy
e-mail: gabriele.anania@unife.it; mrcfnc1@unife.it; cmplrt@unife.it

N. Tamburini
Unit of Thoracic Surgery, S. Anna University Hospital of Ferrara, Cona, FE, Italy
e-mail: n.tamburini@ospfe.it; g.resta@ospfe.it

G. Resta
Unit of General Surgery, S. Anna University Hospital of Ferrara, Cona, FE, Italy
e-mail: g.resta@ospfe.it

17.2 Demolitive Phase

Right hemicolectomy consists of the following surgical steps [2]:

- Mobilization of the hepatic flexure through the section of the hepatocolic ligament
- Detachment of the peritoneal reflection laterally to the ascending colon and separation of the cecum and ascending colon from the posterior Toldt and Gerota fascia and the duodenal plane
- Clearance of omentum and fat on both sides of the transverse colon at the level selected for transection
- Clearance of the terminal ileum at the level of last or second-last ileal loop
- Fan-shaped excision of the mesentery of the ileum and the right colon, ligation, and sectioning of ileocolic vessels, right colic vessels (if present), and right-hand branches of middle colic vessels
- Transection of the transverse colon and of the distal ileum

17.3 Widened Right Hemicolectomy

In some cases, such as with neoplasms of the first third of the transverse colon or affecting the transverse colon itself, some surgeons, to avoid

© The Author(s), under exclusive license to Springer Nature Switzerland AG 2024
M. Milone et al. (eds.), *Scrub Nurse in Minimally Invasive and Robotic General Surgery*,
https://doi.org/10.1007/978-3-031-42257-7_17

Right colectomy for malignancy

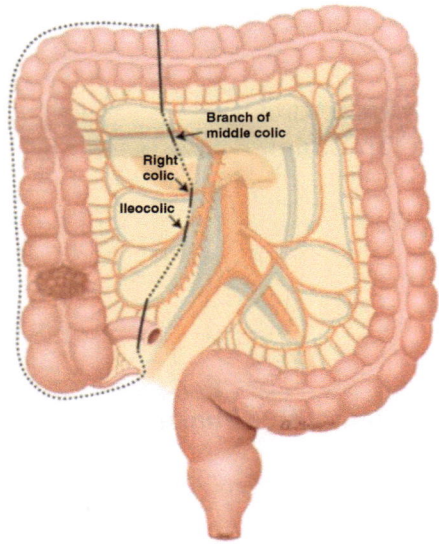

This figure illustrates the extent of a right colectomy. For malignant lesions, the resection involves isolating and dividing the ileocolic vessels, right colic vessels, and either the right or hepatic branch of the middle colic artery and vein at their origins.

Extended right colectomy for malignancy

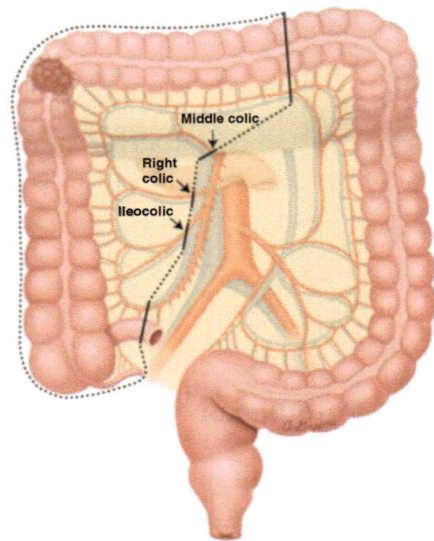

This figure depicts the boundaries of an extended right hemicolectomy, which includes the resection of the distal transverse colon and sometimes the splenic flexure, and, for cancer, involves ligating the ileocolic, right colic, and middle colic vessels at their origin.

Fig. 17.1 Right hemicolectomy for malignancy on the right and extended right hemicolectomy on the left [3]

problems related to vascular deficiency, prefer to widen the right hemicolectomy to the transverse colon, rather than performing a transverse colon resection. This procedure is identical to the right hemicolectomy, but the middle colic vessels are sectioned and the resection is extended up to the splenic flexure (Fig. 17.1).

17.4 Lymphadenectomy

Lymphadenectomy is carried out by descending as far as possible along the course of the right colic and ileocolic vessels and including their mesentery, which hosts the lymphatic stations draining this region.

Right colic lymph node stations are numerous and are distinguished based on their location (Fig. 17.2) [4]:

- Pericolic lymph nodes: lymph nodes along the marginal arteries and near the bowel wall (201, 211, 221)

- Intermediate lymph nodes: lymph nodes along the ileocolic, right colic, and middle colic arteries (ileocolic nodes [202], right colic nodes [212], right middle colic nodes [222-rt])
- Main lymph nodes: Lymph nodes at the origin of the ileocolic, right colic, and middle colic arteries (ileocolic root nodes [203], right colic root nodes [213], middle colic root nodes [223])

Based on the extent of the lymphadenectomy the resection can be classified as follows:

- D1: complete pericolic/perirectal lymph node dissection
- D2: complete pericolic/perirectal and intermediate lymph node dissection
- D3: pericolic/perirectal, intermediate, and main lymph node dissection

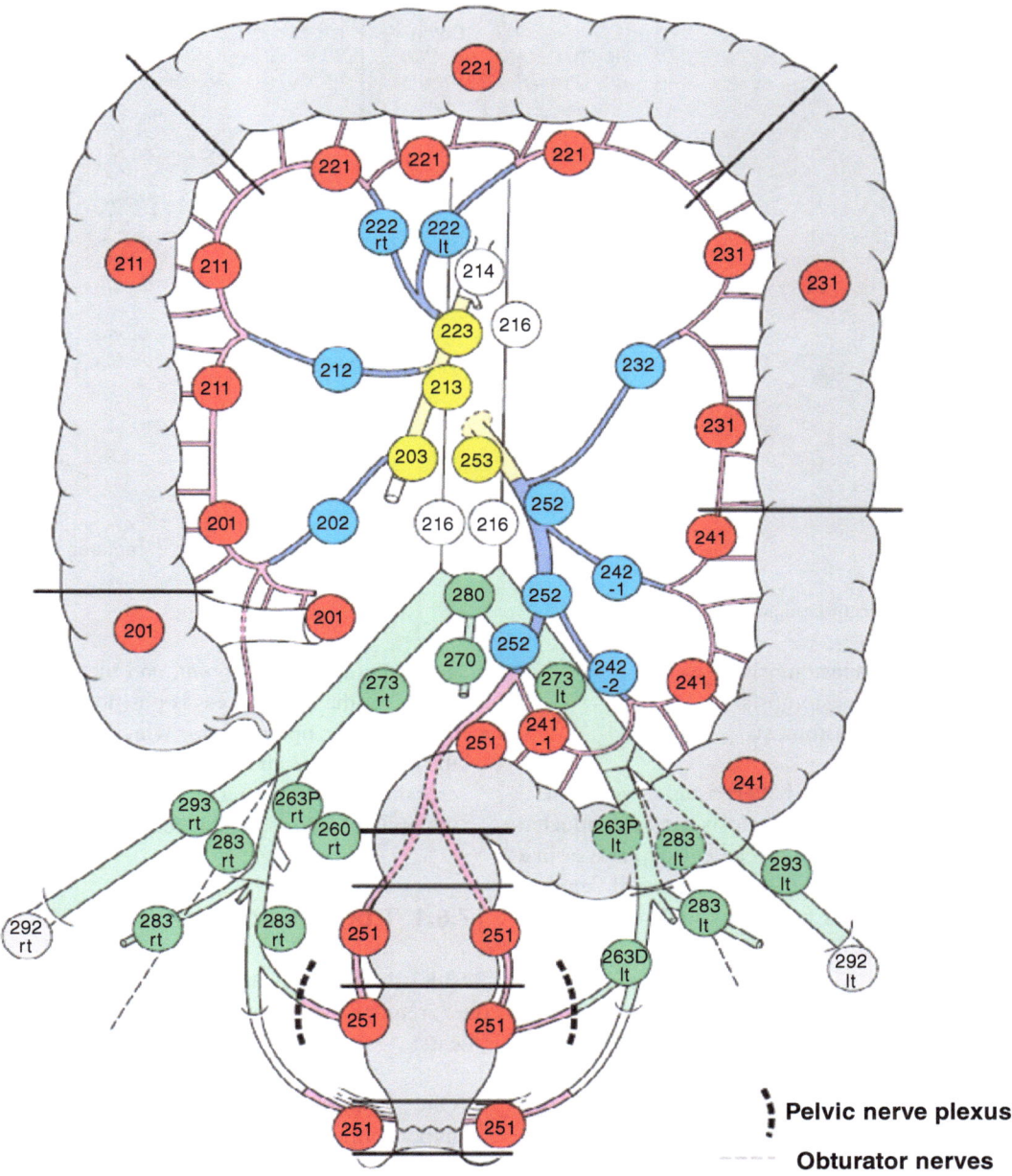

Fig. 17.2 Lymph node colon stations [4]

17.5 Reconstructive Phase

The reconstructive phase involves restoring the continuity of the gastrointestinal tract through the anastomosis of the terminal ileum to the transverse colon [2].

The anatomical continuity of the gastrointestinal tube can be conducted with many different techniques:

- Side-to-side anastomosis (the most commonly used)

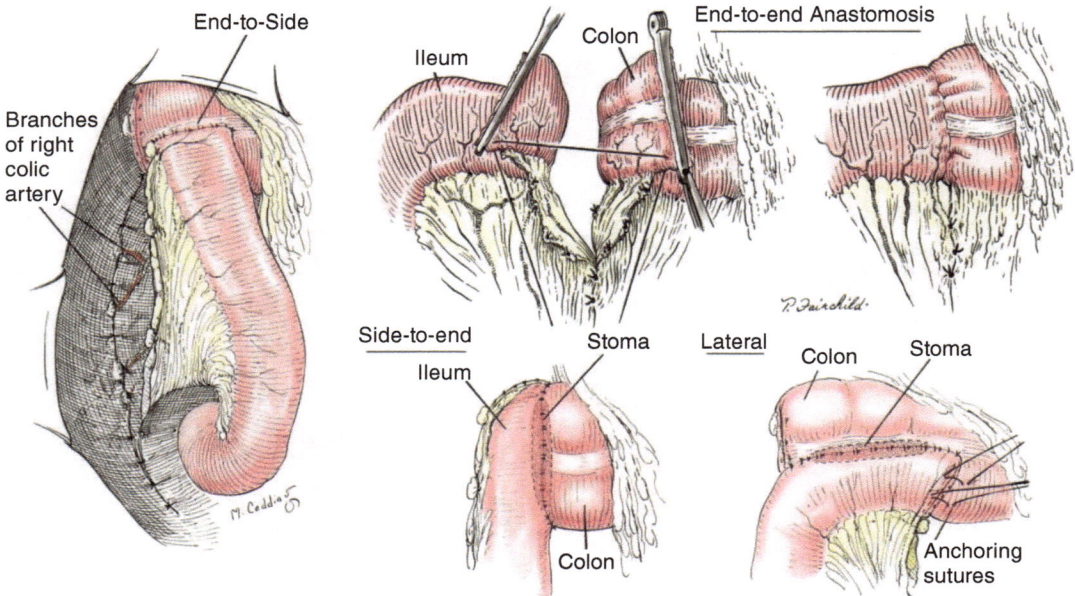

Fig. 17.3 Different techniques for anastomosis [2]

- end-to-side anastomosis
- side-to-end anastomosis
- end-to-end anastomosis

See Fig. 17.3 for a better visual description.

In addition, the anastomosis can be conducted in a manual (without mechanical staplers) or in a mechanical fashion (with mechanical staplers creating the bowel continuity and resecting the enterotomies).

17.6 Laparoscopic Procedure

The access to the abdominal cavity and the positioning of the optic trocar can be achieved with three main techniques:

- Open laparoscopy, in which the surgeon creates a minilaparotomy of about 2–3 cm, generally periumbilical, and inserts a 12-mm trocar for the optic device
- Verress needle technique, in which the pneumoperitoneum is created before accessing the abdominal cavity through a mini-incision,

generally at Palmer's point, and then the first trocar for the optic access is positioned
- Visual trocar optic access, which consists of the access to the abdominal cavity by visually crossing the abdominal wall layers, guided by the optic positioned inside the trocar

17.6.1 Trocar Position

Besides the optic trocar, the laparoscopic procedure requires the positioning of three more trocars:

- One 12-mm operative trocar in the left hypocondrium
- One 5-mm trocar in the left iliac fossa
- One 5-mm trocar in the right lumbar

However, the positions of the trocars depend on the surgeon's choice, always with the purpose to allow a better triangulation in order to improve the access to the operative area (Fig. 17.4).

The demolitive phase is identical to open surgery but the dissection of the mesentery from the

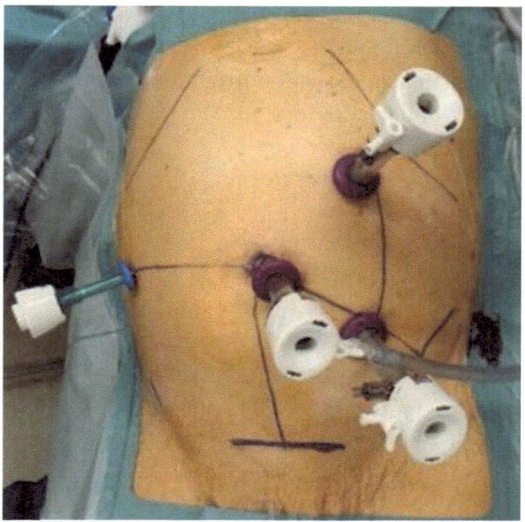

Fig. 17.4 Trocar position [5]

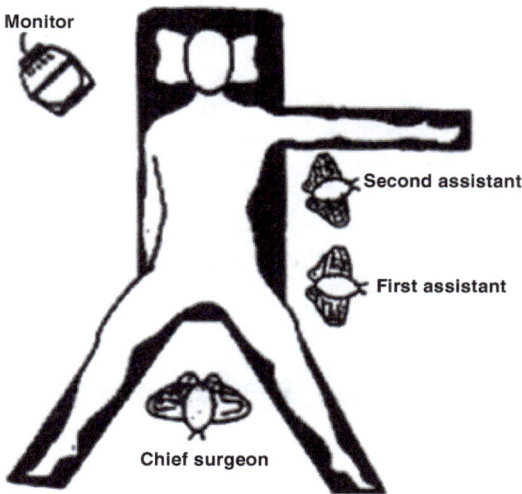

Fig. 17.5 Patient positioning [7]

retroperitoneum is conducted in medial-to-lateral direction.

For what it concerns, the anastomosis can be executed in two ways:

- Extracorporeal, which means that at the moment of the creation of the anastomosis, a laparotomy is created in order to complete the procedure in the same way as an open procedure
- Intracorporeal, which consists of the creation of enterotomies on both the distal ileum and colon, creation of the anastomosis through a mechanical stapler, and closure of the enterotomies by intracorporeal suturing [6]

17.7 Positioning

Patient positioning is performed as shown in Fig. 17.5:

- Supine position in reverse Trendelenburg with an inclination of about 15–20° and inclined to the left side with an inclination of about 20–25°.
- Spread legs.

- Right arm adducted along the body and left arm wide abducted.
- The operating table is therefore prepared with a mat to prevent sliding and with a leg fixed with bandages to prevent the patient from falling off the operating table.

17.8 Surgical Instruments and Surgical Cart

The preparation of the instrument table and the serving cart must be carried out as shown in Figs. 17.6 and 17.7.

17.8.1 Open Instruments

- 2 scalpels with stainless steel blade (sizes 15 and 24)
- 1 kidney basin
- 2 Janach (steel bowls)
- 2 anatomical tissue forceps
- 2 toothed forceps
- 6 curved Klemmer clamps
- 6 curved Kocher clamps
- 1 Mayo scissors
- 1 Nelson-Metzenbaum dissection scissors

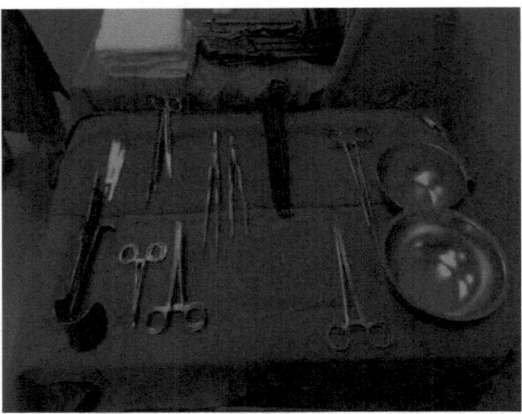

Fig. 17.6 Serving cart

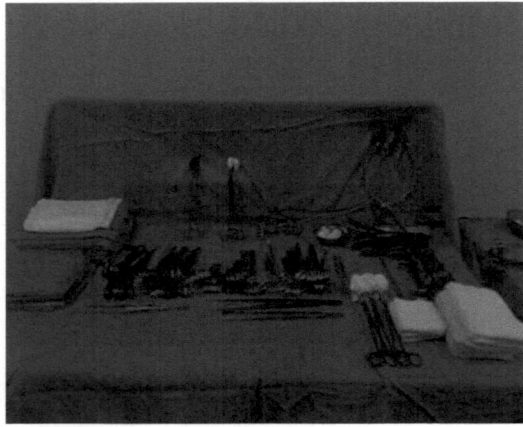

Fig. 17.7 Instrument table

- 1 Foerster clamp
- 4 Backhaus clamps
- 1 Mixter right angle forceps
- 1 curved Bengolea forceps
- 2 Mathieu retractors
- 2 Langenbeck retractors
- 1 monopolar electric scalpel
- 1 needle holder
- 1 wire passers
- 1 wound protector/retractor

17.8.2 Laparoscopic instruments

- Laparoscopic grasping forceps (Croce-Olmi forceps, Grasper or Johann forceps)

- Energy cutting and sealing device (ultrasound or radiofrequency)
- Laparoscopic suction/irrigation system
- 30° optic endoscope
- 1 bipolar forceps
- 1 monopolar instrument
- 1 stapler
- 1 needle holder
- 2 × 5 mm ports
- 2 × 12 mm ports
- 10-mm and 12-mm endoscopic clip applier
- Hem-o-lok clips with laparoscopic applier of various sizes (small/medium/large)
- Laparoscopic scissors
- Scope warmer

17.9 ICG (Indocyanine Green) Optic System

The indocyanine green (IGC) fluorescent dye is presented in vials of 25 mg of powder for solution for injection.

- Use in concentrations of 0.5 mg/ml.
- Dilute with sterile distilled water and *not* sodium chloride (NaCl) as the latter could cause aggregation.
- After preparation, the solution must be stored in a dark and cool place to avoid rapid deterioration of the whitening fluorescence.
- For the dosage to be administered, follow the instructions of the anesthetist present in the theatre.

17.10 Surgical Steps and Related Instruments

Open laparoscopy technique for laparoscopic access:

- 1 scalpel (blade 15)
- 2 anatomical tissue forceps
- 2 S retractors
- 2 curved Kocher clamps to grasp fascia
- 2 curved Klemmer clamps to dissect the abdominal layers and to grasp parietal peritoneum

Veress technique for laparoscopic access:

- 1 scalpel (blade 15)
- 1 Veress needle
- 1 syringe for saline drop test

Port placement:

- 1 scalpel (blade 15)
- 2 × 12 mm ports
- 2 × 5 mm ports

17.10.1 Demolitive Phase

The demolitive phase provides the complete mobilization of the distal ileum, of the ascending colon, and of the first third of the transverse colon, their transection, and lymphadenectomy.

The open instruments to be used are as follows (based on the surgeon's requests):

- 1 retractor or 1 Alexis device
- 2 anatomical forceps
- 1 dissection scissors
- 1 wire passers
- 2 curved Kelly clamps
- 1 bipolar forceps
- 1 monopolar instrument (electrical scalpel) or, alternatively
- 1 cutting and sealing instrument
- 1 stapler to be used at the time of ileal and colon transection

The forceps and wire passers are used by the surgeon during the dissection phases of the planes for the complete mobilization of the ascending colon, as are the sealing instruments.

The laparoscopic instruments used at the table are as follows:

- 30° laparoscopic endoscope
- Laparoscopic grasping forceps (Croce-Olmi forceps, Grasper or Johann forceps)
- Laparoscopic suction/irrigation system

- Laparoscopic bipolar forceps
- 10-mm and 12-mm endoscopic clip applier
- Hem-o-lok clips with laparoscopic applier of various sizes (small/medium/large) based on the size of the vase to be clipped
- 1 cutting and sealing instrument
- 1 mechanical stapler with various sizes of length and suture paces depending on the surgeon's request and on the tract of bowel that needs to be transected
- Laparoscopic scissors

17.10.2 Reconstructive Phase

For the open procedure, the instruments needed are the same as the ones needed for the demolitive phase, with the addition of the following:

- 3 Allis forceps
- 2 intestinal clamps

During the laparoscopic reconstructive phase, the required instruments are as follows:

- 30° laparoscopic endoscope
- Laparoscopic grasping forceps (Croce-Olmi forceps, Grasper or Johann forceps)
- Laparoscopic bipolar forceps
- 1 monopolar instrument (crochet or scissors) to perform enterotomies
- 1 stapler to perform the anastomosis
- 1 laparoscopic needle holder
- 1 barbed/monofilament/braided suture (based on the surgeon's requests) to perform closure of enterotomies

Once the anastomosis and the revision of the hemostasis have been completed, the instrumental nurse makes gauze and needle counts and the specimen will therefore be extracted.

The specimen is extracted through a Pfannenstiel minilaparotomy or a periumbilical incision (more indicated in obese patients) using a wound protector/retractor.

During the specimen extraction phase, the required instruments are as follows:

- 1 scalpel (blade 24)
- 1 monopolar electric scalpel
- 2 anatomical/toothed tissue forceps (based on the surgeon's requests)
- 3 Mathieu retractors
- 1 Nelson-Metzenbaum dissection scissors
- 2 curved Kocher clamps to grasp fascia
- 2 curved Klemmer clamps to grasp parietal peritoneum
- 1 wound protector/retractor to extract specimen safely
- 1 absorbable suture for peritoneum
- 1 looped/monofilament/braided suture (based on the surgeon's request) to perform closure of fascia
- 1 monofilament/braided suture (based on the surgeon's request) to perform suture of subcutaneous plane
- Titanium skin clips/suture to perform closure of skin

17.11 Complete Mesocolic Excision

Complete mesocolic excision (CME) is a new technique for colon cancer surgery, on which there is a large literature debate. The idea of complete mesocolic excision (CME) is based on the huge results in terms of increased survival rate and disease-free survival obtained by the TME (total mesorectal excision) for rectal cancer. The original CME technique, for colon cancer, emphasized the following [8]:

1. Meticulous dissection between the mesocolon and retroperitoneum along the Toldt fascia and retrieval of the specimen as one unbreached mesocolon package.
2. Central vascular ligation (CVL, central ligation of the main arteries and veins at their roots, SMA, and SMV) to clear all locoregional lymph nodes.
3. Adequate proximal and distal margins should be obtained.

Central ligation of main supplying vessels reduces a risk of residual metastatic lymph nodes and enables accurate staging and prognostication. Some studies observe that D3 lymphadenectomy for T3 and T4 colon cancer was superior to D2 lymphadenectomy in terms of overall survival. Survival benefit was also seen in patients without lymph node metastasis. They postulated that removal of micrometastasis in the main nodes may improve survival [9]. About proximal and distal resection margins, there are no objective data. Mesocolic fat is more prominent around major vessels and that creates a bulky vascular pedicle. Although there is some difference, CME technique favors the 10-cm rule for proximal and distal margins. Epicolic and paracolic node metastases occur along the marginal artery, and thereafter, tumor spreads to the intermediate and apical lymph nodes along the main supplying artery. Thus, sufficient proximal and distal margins are needed to remove the mesocolon containing lymph nodes and thereby improve oncologic outcomes [10, 11].

17.11.1 CME with CVL for Right-Sided Colon Cancer

For laparoscopic right-side colon cancer CME, one 10-mm port is utilized for a camera at the umbilicus and three working ports [8]:

- 5-mm or 12-mm port on the left.
- 5-mm port on the left lower quadrant.
- 5-mm port on the right quadrant.
- Another 5-mm port at the right upper quadrant is utilized in difficult cases.

After placement of the trocars, the patient is placed in a Trendelenburg with the right side up position.

A medial to lateral dissection is advocated in most cases, but when the origin of ileocolic pedicles is not clearly identified, the dissection is alternated with lateral to medial fashion. The terminal ileum and the ascending colon are dissected off through the embryological plane.

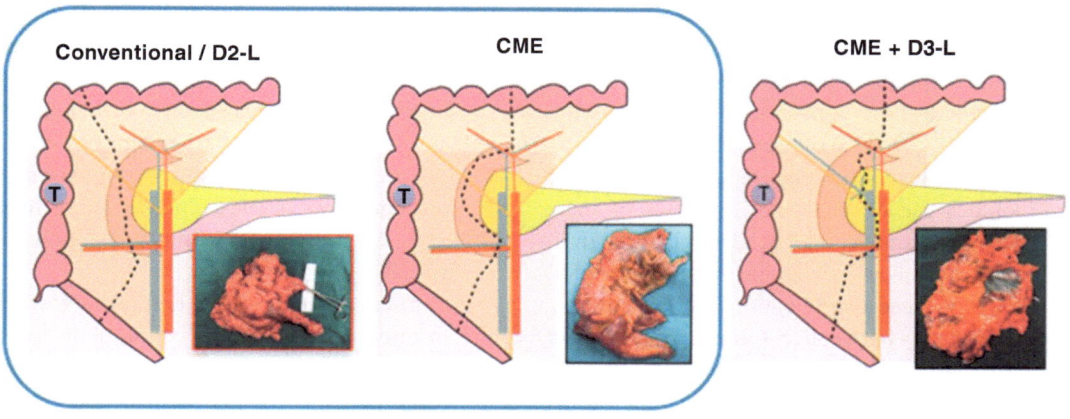

CONTROL GROUP (CLASSIC)

Fig. 17.8 Conventional CME dissection and CME+D3 dissection [12]

Dissection between the mesocolon and Gerota's fascia continues to the duodenum and head of the pancreas. Once the ileocolic vessels are identified, the mesocolon package containing lymph nodes is cleared along the vessels while exposing the ventral side of the SMV and SMA. The ileocolic vessels are ligated at the root of the SMV and SMA, and the dissection continues cephalad to the right colic vessels, the gastrocolic trunk of Henle, and the middle colic vessels. The right colic vessels, if present, are skeletonized and transected at the root. Then, the middle colic vessels are identified and skeletonized at the roots of the SMA and SMV. Tumor-specific CME is performed according to the tumor location. For cecal and proximal ascending colon cancers, right hemicolectomy is performed, and the right branches of the middle colic artery and vein are ligated. For hepatic flexure and proximal transverse colon cancers, extended right hemicolectomy is performed and the roots of the middle colic artery and vein are ligated. Omentectomy is performed just below the gastroepiploic vessels and, unless infiltrated by the tumor, the right gastroepiploic vessels are preserved (Fig. 17.8).

17.12 Right Hemicolectomy Complications

The main complications of right hemicolectomy include the following [13]:

- Injury to the right ureter or right gonadal vessels
- Small bowel and duodenal injury
- Major vessel injury
- Gastric injury
- Early postoperative small bowel obstruction
- Surgical site infection
- Anastomotic leaking and bleeding

There are several critical structures that must not be damaged during the colectomy:

- Injury to the right ureter or right gonadal vessels—when incising the lateral peritoneal attachments of the cecum and ascending colon, the operating surgeon must be keenly aware of the location of the right ureter and right gonadal vessels. Injury to these structures are avoided by dissecting anteromedial to them within the areolar plane along the white line of Toldt. The incidence of intraoperative ureteral injury with open or laparoscopic colorectal surgery ranges from <1% to 8% [14]. Only 20–30% of ureteral injuries are recognized during the operation [15]. Repair includes use of a stent or, in cases of more extensive damage, advanced surgical repair.

- Small bowel and duodenal injury—the incidence of these complications during colorectal surgery is between less than 1% and 3% for open and laparoscopic techniques [16, 17]. The risk of an inadvertent enterotomy increases with previous abdominal surgery, while injury to the duodenum is most likely to occur during right colon mobilization. An unrecognized enterotomy can lead to peritonitis in the first few postoperative days, necessitating prompt surgical intervention, and an intra-abdominal abscess or an enterocutaneous fistula in the later postoperative period. Missed duodenal injuries can have disastrous consequences, including free perforation or the development of difficult duodenal fistulas, and are associated with high rates of mortality:
  - The therapeutic approach varies with the type and extent of injury.
  - Veress needle injury to the small bowel can be managed conservatively.
  - A trocar injury to the small bowel requires primary operative repair, either laparoscopically or open. Full-thickness small bowel enterotomies are repaired in one or two layers. In contrast, a segmental resection with a primary anastomosis should be performed if multiple enterotomies occur in a short segment or the small bowel mesentery is compromised.
  - Serosal tears are repaired with imbricating seromuscular sutures.
  - Technically, the most challenging repair is an enterotomy of the duodenum. A primary repair should not compromise the duodenal lumen. If a primary repair cannot be safely performed, a duodenal to jejunal anastomosis is performed.

- Major vessel injury—during an open or laparoscopic colectomy, this complication is rare, but the following types of injury can occur:
  - Injuries can occur with traction on mesenteric vessels during mobilization of the bowel.
  - A Veress needle used during laparoscopic resections rarely causes major hemorrhage and is treated by simple ligation of vessels.
  - A trocar can cause fatal hemorrhage when inserted into the aorta or common iliac vessels; this occurs in fewer than 1% of laparoscopic cases. A vessel lacerated by a trocar usually requires immediate conversion to an open procedure for control of the bleeding vessel; however, there have been reports of successful laparoscopic management of major vascular injuries sustained during colectomy [18].
  - Venous bleeding during ligation of the middle colic vessels. The surgeon must avoid excessive upward traction as this may cause avulsion of a large collateral branch between the middle colic vein and inferior pancreaticoduodenal vein.
  - Inadvertent ligation of the superior mesenteric artery: the superior mesenteric artery (SMA) must not be mistaken for the right colic artery. Ligation of the SMA will result in bowel infarction.

- Gastric injury—injuries to the stomach occur in fewer than 1% of colectomies and are more likely to occur during dissection of dense adhesions, excessive use of electrocautery, and/or failure to develop an adequate plane.

- Early postoperative small bowel obstruction—it is the most frequent complication in the early postoperative period after colorectal surgery that occurs in 1.2–8%. Inflammatory peritoneal adhesions account for the majority of cases. Immediate reoperation for early postoperative SBO should be avoided because of both the high rate of spontaneous resolution and the intense inflammatory response within the abdominal cavity in the perioperative period (from 10 days to 6 weeks). Indications for surgery should be limited to unresolved obstruction after prolonged nasogastric tube drainage, high-grade SBO, or suspected ischemic small bowel [19].

- Surgical site infection—colorectal operations are clean-contaminated procedures with an inherent risk of gross contamination of the peritoneal cavity and incision that can result in a surgical site infection (SSI). In general, laparoscopic colon surgery is associated with a lower SSI rate (4.1%) than open colon surgery (7.9%) [20]. Management of an SSI depends upon the site of the infection. An intra-abdominal SSI can be treated by percutaneous catheter drainage or operative drainage in most cases [21].
- Anastomotic complication—intestinal anastomotic complications are associated with an increased patient mortality and morbidity. The most common complications are as follows:
  - Minor bleeding (usually within 24 h): minor bleeding is defined as bleeding that does not require blood transfusion and/or intervention (endoscopic, angiographic, or surgical). It is usually manifested by the self-limited passage of dark blood with the patient's first few bowel movements. It is hypothesized that anastomotic bleeding occurs secondary to inadequate clearance of the mesentery prior to division and/or stapling of the bowel, or due to bleeding diathesis. Careful inspection of the stapler line, inspection of the linear staple line prior to closure of the enterotomy, suture ligation of bleeding points, and reinforcement of the anastomosis with an absorbable suture are the main options to reduce minor bleeding [13].
  - Major bleeding is defined as one or more of the following: hemodynamic instability, and blood transfusion, and an emergency procedure is warranted (e.g., endoscopic, angiographic, surgical). There is no significant association between the risk of bleeding and the technique of performing the anastomosis (hand-sewn versus stapled colocolic anastomoses) [22]. The management of patients with anastomotic bleeding should follow the same principles as the management of patients with lower gastrointestinal bleeding from other causes. Surgical intervention should be reserved for unstable patients or those who fail conservative measures [23] (blood transfusion, endoscopic procedure).
  - Dehiscence and leaks: the overall incidence of anastomotic dehiscence and subsequent leaks is 2–7% when performed by experienced surgeons (1–3% for the ileocolic anastomosis). Most anastomotic leaks usually become apparent between five and seven days postoperatively; 12% occurs after postoperative day 30 [24]. To define an anastomotic leak, we can use clinical signs, radiographic findings, and intraoperative findings [25, 26]. The clinical signs include pain, fever, tachycardia, peritonitis, feculent, or purulent drainage. Radiographic signs, usually during CT scan, are fluid collections and gas-containing collections. Otherwise, the intraoperative findings include gross enteric spillage and anastomotic disruption.

    The most important risk factors associated with anastomosis leaking are as follows: anastomosis ischemia, obesity, male sex, ASA score III–V, emergency surgery, prolonged operative surgery, hand-sewn ileocolic anastomosis, denutrition (hypoalbuminemia, alcohol intake, weight loss), postoperative corticosteroids, and postoperative NSAIDs (reduction in prostaglandin-mediated collagen deposition) [27].

    Once an anastomotic leak has been recognized, patients should receive intravenous fluid resuscitation and broad-spectrum antibiotics. Further management is dictated by the clinical scenario and, if patient stability permits, radiologic investigation to localize the leak and determine its severity. Management strategies include observation, bowel rest, percutaneous drainage, colonic stenting, surgical revision, diversion, or drainage [28].

References

1. Salvatore L. et al. Linee guida: Tumori del colon AIOM 2021; 2021
2. Robert M. Zollinger Jr, E. Christopher Ellison. Zollinger's Atlas of surgical operations
3. Andrea C. Bafford. Right and extended right colectomy: open technique. In: Uptodate. 2021st ed. Available from: https://www.uptodate.com/contents/right-and-extended-right-colectomy-open-technique?search=right%20emiocolecthomy&source=search_result&selectedTitle=1~150&usage_type=default&display_rank=1
4. Japanese Society for Cancer of the Colon and Rectum. Japanese Classification of colorectal, appendiceal, and anal carcinoma. 3d English Edition (Secondary Publication). J Anus Rectum Colon. 2019;3(4):175–95.
5. Aniello Santoro G, Novello S, Grossi U, Zucchella M, Kazemi Nava A, Zanus G. Laparoscopic right colectomy. Intracorporeal anastomosis is associated with better outcome. In: Vannelli A, editor. Colorectal cancer. IntechOpen; 2021. [cited 2022 Sep 8]. Available from: https://www.intechopen.com/books/colorectal-cancer/laparoscopic-right-colectomy-intracorporeal-anastomosis-is-associated-with-better-outcome.
6. Anania G, Agresta F, Artioli E, Rubino S, Resta G, Vettoretto N, et al. Laparoscopic right hemicolectomy: the SICE (Società Italiana di Chirurgia Endoscopica e Nuove Tecnologie) network prospective trial on 1225 cases comparing intra corporeal versus extra corporeal ileo-colic side-to-side anastomosis. Surg Endosc. 2020;34(11):4788–800.
7. Yang X, Wu Q, Jin C, He W, Wang M, Yang T, et al. A novel hand-assisted laparoscopic versus conventional laparoscopic right hemicolectomy for right colon cancer: study protocol for a randomized controlled trial. Trials. 2017;18(1):355.
8. Kim NK, Kim YW, Han YD, Cho MS, Hur H, Min BS, et al. Complete mesocolic excision and central vascular ligation for colon cancer: Principle, anatomy, surgical technique, and outcomes. Surg Oncol. 2016;25(3):252–62.
9. Kotake K, Mizuguchi T, Moritani K, Wada O, Ozawa H, Oki I, et al. Impact of D3 lymph node dissection on survival for patients with T3 and T4 colon cancer. Int J Colorectal Dis. 2014;29(7):847–52.
10. Søndenaa K, Quirke P, Hohenberger W, Sugihara K, Kobayashi H, Kessler H, et al. The rationale behind complete mesocolic excision (CME) and a central vascular ligation for colon cancer in open and laparoscopic surgery: proceedings of a consensus conference. Int J Colorectal Dis. 2014;29(4):419–28.
11. Park IJ, Choi GS, Kang BM, Lim KH, Jun SH. Lymph node metastasis patterns in right-sided colon cancers:
is segmental resection of these tumors oncologically safe? Ann Surg Oncol. 2009;16(6):1501–6.
12. Balciscueta Z, Balciscueta I, Uribe N, Pellino G, Frasson M, García-Granero E, et al. D3-lymphadenectomy enhances oncological clearance in patients with right colon cancer. Results of a meta-analysis. Eur J Surg Oncol. 2021;47(7):1541–51.
13. Boushey R. Management of anastomotic complications of colorectal surgery. In: Uptodate. 2021st ed; 2021.
14. Halabi WJ, Jafari MD, Nguyen VQ, Carmichael JC, Mills S, Pigazzi A, et al. Ureteral injuries in colorectal surgery: an analysis of trends, outcomes, and risk factors over a 10-year period in the United States. Dis Colon Rectum. 2014;57(2):179–86.
15. Selzman AA, Spirnak JP. Iatrogenic ureteral injuries: a 20-year experience in treating 165 injuries. J Urol. 1996;155(3):878–81.
16. Rose J, Schneider C, Yildirim C, Geers P, Scheidbach H, Köckerling F. Complications in laparoscopic colorectal surgery: results of a multicentre trial. Tech Coloproctol. 2004;8(Suppl. 1):S25–8.
17. Franko J, O'Connell BG, Mehall JR, Harper SG, Nejman JH, Zebley DM, et al. The influence of prior abdominal operations on conversion and complication rates in laparoscopic colorectal surgery. JSLS. 2006;10(2):169–75.
18. Jafari MD, Pigazzi A. Techniques for laparoscopic repair of major intraoperative vascular injury: case reports and review of literature. Surg Endosc. 2013;27(8):3021–7.
19. Shin JY, Hong KH. Risk factors for early postoperative small-bowel obstruction after colectomy in colorectal cancer. World J Surg. 2008;32(10):2287–92.
20. Caroff DA, Chan C, Kleinman K, Calderwood MS, Wolf R, Wick EC, et al. Association of open approach vs laparoscopic approach with risk of surgical site infection after colon surgery. JAMA Netw Open. 2019;2(10):e1913570.
21. Cinat ME, Wilson SE, Din AM. Determinants for successful percutaneous image-guided drainage of intra-abdominal abscess. Arch Surg Chic Ill 1960. 2002;137(7):845–9.
22. Neutzling CB, Lustosa SAS, Proenca IM, da Silva EMK, Matos D. Stapled versus handsewn methods for colorectal anastomosis surgery. Cochrane Database Syst Rev. 2012;2:CD003144.
23. Martínez-Serrano MA, Parés D, Pera M, Pascual M, Courtier R, Egea MJG, et al. Management of lower gastrointestinal bleeding after colorectal resection and stapled anastomosis. Tech Coloproctol. 2009;13(1):49–53.
24. Hyman N, Manchester TL, Osler T, Burns B, Cataldo PA. Anastomotic leaks after intestinal anastomosis: it's later than you think. Ann Surg. 2007;245(2):254–8.

25. Lipska MA, Bissett IP, Parry BR, Merrie AEH. Anastomotic leakage after lower gastrointestinal anastomosis: men are at a higher risk. ANZ J Surg. 2006;76(7):579–85.

26. Law WI, Chu KW, Ho JW, Chan CW. Risk factors for anastomotic leakage after low anterior resection with total mesorectal excision. Am J Surg. 2000;179(2):92–6.

27. Modasi A, Pace D, Godwin M, Smith C, Curtis B. NSAID administration post colorectal surgery increases anastomotic leak rate: systematic review/meta-analysis. Surg Endosc. 2019;33(3):879–85.

28. Phitayakorn R, Delaney CP, Reynolds HL, Champagne BJ, Heriot AG, Neary P, et al. Standardized algorithms for management of anastomotic leaks and related abdominal and pelvic abscesses after colorectal surgery. World J Surg. 2008;32(6):1147–56.

Robotic Treatment of Left Colon Tumors

18

Riccardo Piagnerelli, Ludovico Carbone, and Franco Roviello

18.1 Technical Notes

Once the pneumoperitoneum is established with a Verress needle, we assess the absence of peritoneal carcinomatosis, ascites, and presence of liver metastasis (intraoperative ultrasound liver scan can be useful). The endoscopic dye tattoo on the colic wall is evaluated.

In a slight Trendelenburg position with right tilt, the entire small bowel is retracted in the right lateral quadrants.

The operating room table inclination should be adapted to patient's anatomic conditions (visceral fat, bowel distention).

The Xi robotic patient cart is docked in a lateral docking from the patient's left side.

The inferior mesenteric vein is identified at the Treitz ligament.

The Toldt fascia must be incised under the vein and the dissection is carried out in between the two layers of the Toldt's fascia towards the parieto-colic peritoneal reflection leaving the inferior pancreatic margin under the dissection plane (Figs. 18.1 and 18.2).

Once the inferior mesenteric vein (IMV) is freed from the mesocolic peritoneum, it can be

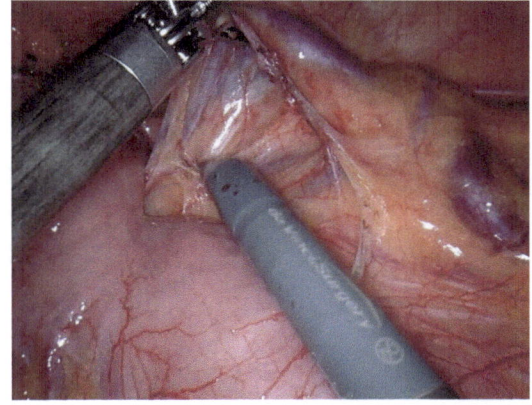

Fig. 18.1 Mesocolic window creation

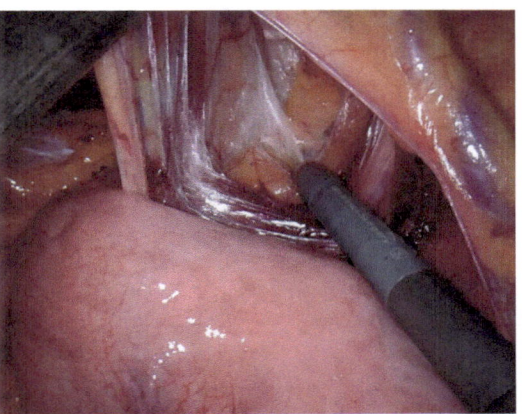

Fig. 18.2 Toldt's fascia division

R. Piagnerelli · L. Carbone · F. Roviello (✉)
Department of Medicine Surgery and Neuroscience,
Unit of General Surgery and Surgical Oncology,
University of Siena, Siena, Italy
e-mail: franco.roviello@unisi.it

sectioned between clips at the inferior pancreatic border (Fig. 18.3).

The robotic fourth arm, when employed, ensures a stable mesocolon retraction. It is useful to leave in this avascular plane a 5-cm gauze as a landmark.

Now the dissection is carried out on the same plane down to the left lower quadrant.

A stable cranial and uplifted retraction of the sigmoid colon exposes the *"Bacon's axilla,"* the angle between the inferior mesenteric artery (IMA) and the aorta. The middle tissue is incised and the Toldt's fascia is divided between its leaves (Fig. 18.4). Attention is paid to let down the left ureter and gonadal vessels preserving the hypogastric plexus [1] (Fig. 18.5).

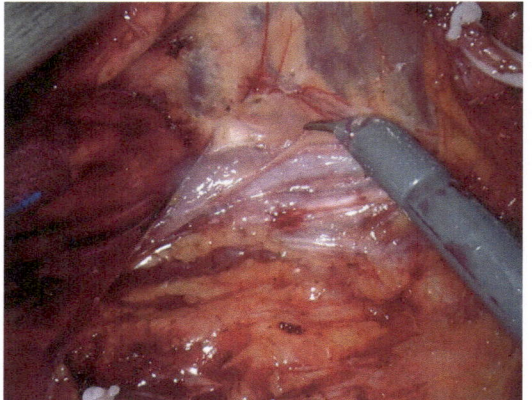

Fig. 18.5 Ureteral and Gonadal vessel plan

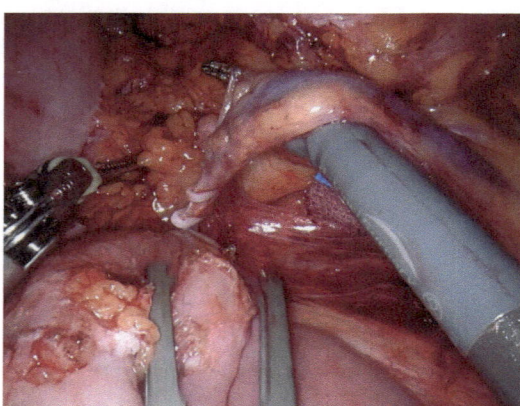

Fig. 18.3 Superior mesenteric vein ligation

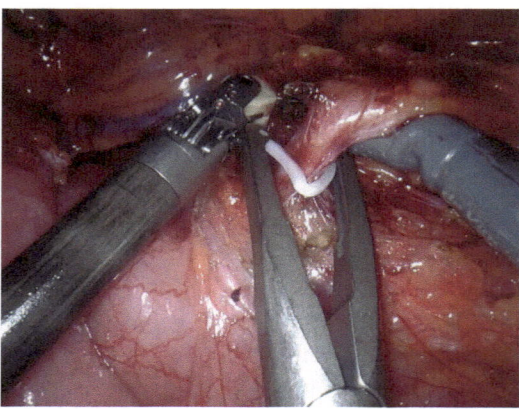

Fig. 18.6 Inferior mesenteric vein ligation

Once the mesocolic tent is achieved, the IMA can be sectioned between clips and the two mesocolic tents can be joined (Fig. 18.6).

For colonic malignancies, the IMA should be sectioned next to its origin from the aorta. Although some studies underline how a low ligation of IMA (right after the origin of left colic artery) high node dissection could achieve the same oncological outcomes, the high ligation is mandatory for a tension-free anastomosis [2, 3].

Splenic flexure mobilization is achieved by dividing the gastrocolic ligament (Fig. 18.7). That maneuver is achieved by lifting up the stomach with the robotic arms and the colon downward with the aim of the assistant clinch. Once the Bouchet's area is exposed, the gastrocolic ligament can be incised in medial to lateral direc-

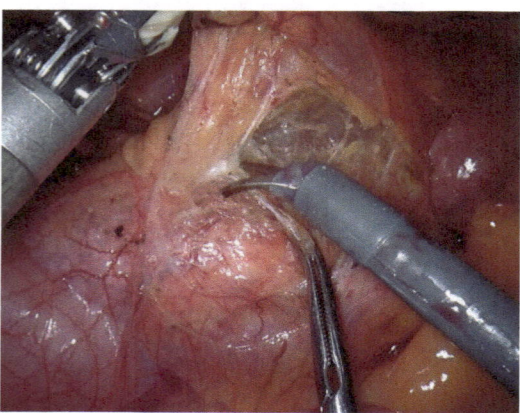

Fig. 18.4 Finding of Bacon's axilla

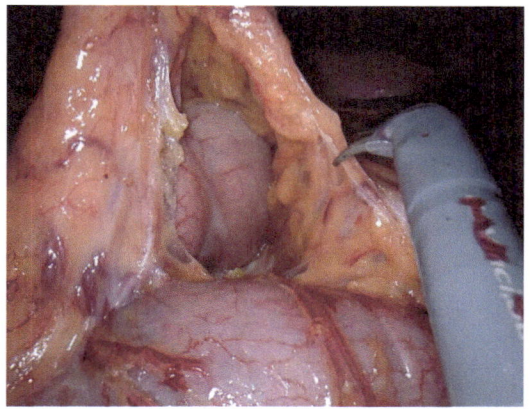

Fig. 18.7   Colo-epiploic ligament dissection

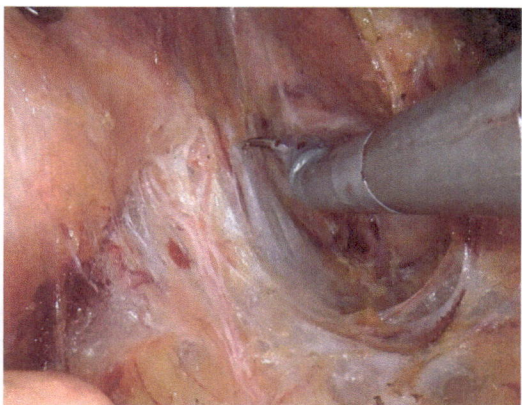

Fig. 18.9   Hypogastric nerve preservation

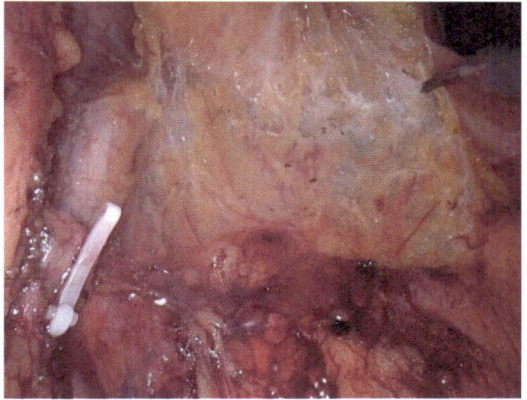

Fig. 18.8   Posterior rectal dissection

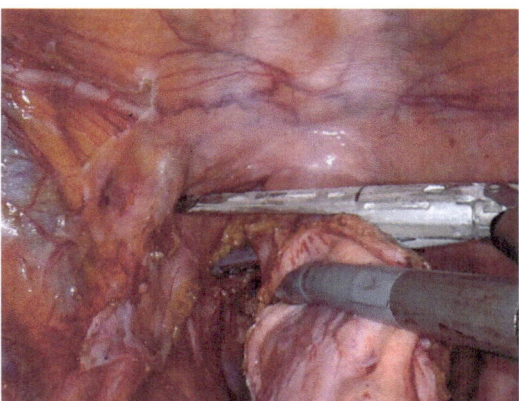

Fig. 18.10   Rectal stump stapling

tion. The phrenicocolic, the splenocolic, and the parietocolic ligaments are incised.

The complete mobilization of the colon is achieved by incising the pancreatic colic ligament.

In order to complete a full mobilization of the distal colon, the dissection must be furthered caudally till the distal peritoneal reflection (Douglas' pouch in woman).

In Trendelenburg position with right tilt, posterior dissection is carried out prolonging the line of peritoneal incision caudally on the left and right side of the proximal rectum (Fig. 18.8). The left and right hypogastric nerves are now visible under the Waldeyer's fascia on the posterior floor of the surgical field (Fig. 18.9).

Once the rectum is fully dissected, an endo-stapler or a robotic stapler (SureForm) can be used for the transection. The stapler must be placed perpendicularly across the rectum because an angled stapled line could create zones of isch-emia of the rectal stump (Figs. 18.10 and 18.11).

The specimen extraction is carried out per-forming a small incision medially to the left arcu-ate line in the left lower quadrant [4, 5].

The use of a wall protector is mandatory to avoid abdominal wall contamination or, worse, seeding by cancer. Once the specimen is extracted, the left colectomy can be completed. The level of the proximal colonic section depends on the distance from the tumor and on the mobi-lized colon vascularization. The vascularization

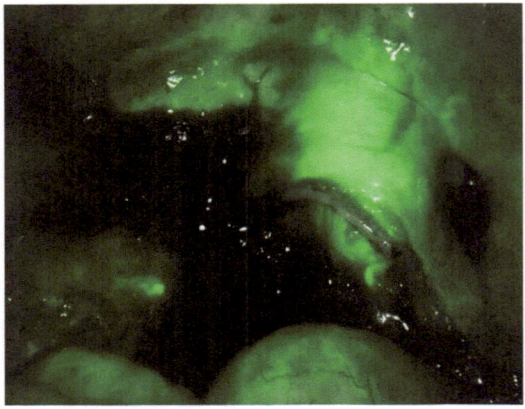

Fig. 18.11 Indocyanine green rectal stump vascularization check

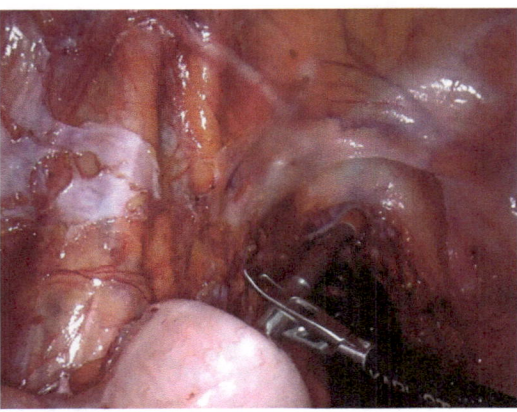

Fig. 18.13 Colorectal T-T anastomosis (Knight-Griffen)

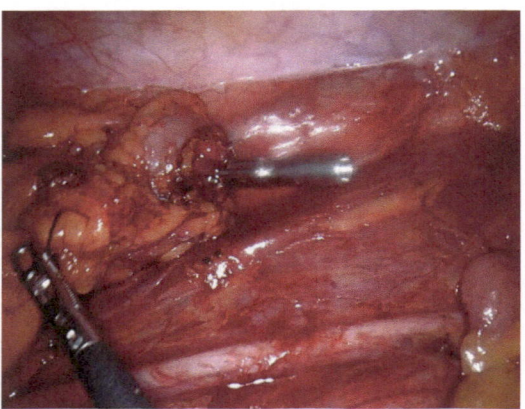

Fig. 18.12 Proximal colon stump anvil placement

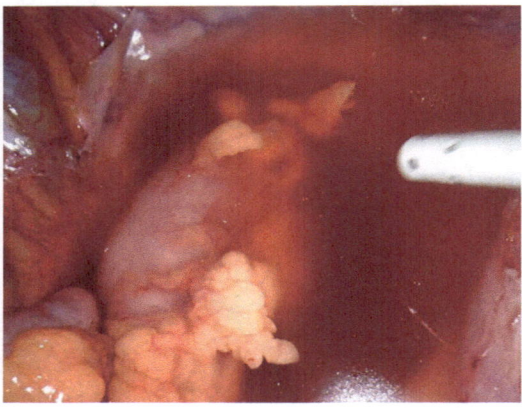

Fig. 18.14 Hydro-pneumatic anastomotic test

is assured by the Drummond's marginal artery that must be identified and preserved [6].

After the transection the anvil of a circular stapler is secured to the colon with a Mikulicz running suture (Fig. 18.12). The colon is now reintroduced in the abdominal cavity and an end-to-end anastomosis is carried out according to the Knight-Griffen technique (Fig. 18.13) [7].

A hydro-pneumatic test can be conducted in order to check anastomotic air leak (Fig. 18.14).

A silicon drain is finally placed in the left flank next to the anastomosis (Fig. 18.15).

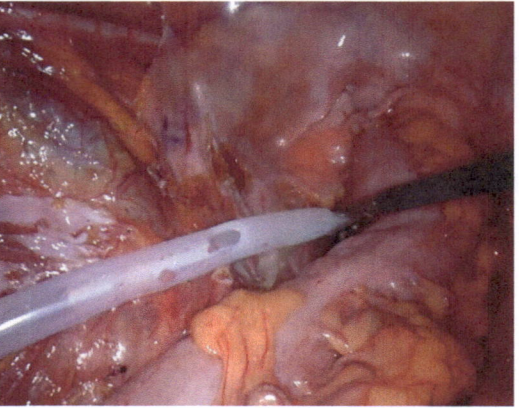

Fig. 18.15 Peri-anastomotic drain placement

18.2   Operating Room Setup

The robotic cart is positioned in the patient's left flank; the vision cart stays on cart's left side.

The anesthesiologist equipment stays at the patient's head.

The first assistant stays on the patient's right flank.

The scrub nurse stays on the first assistant's right side, next to the two Mayo's surgical tables.

18.3   Patient Positioning

The patient lies in a supine position with both arms tucked along the body, and the legs are placed in Allen-type support; the right Allen-type support should allow the hyperextension of the leg in order to avoid conflicts with instruments placed in the right lower quadrant. The splenic flexure mobilization and IMV and IMA ligation are achieved with a 15° Trendelenburg position with 15–20° tilt-right inclination. Rectal dissection is carried out with a 30–35° Trendelenburg position with the same tilt-right angle.

18.4   Port Placement (da Vinci Xi)

Four robotic trocars and one assistant 10–12 mm port are needed.

Correct port placement is achieved drawing a line from the mid of the inguinal ligament to where the left midclavicular line crosses (MCL) over the left costal margin.

Place port 2 (camera port) at the crossing of this line with the midline.

Place ports 1, 3, and 4 at a distance of 8 cm to other ports of this line.

Place the assistant port as far away as possible from the da Vinci ports and lateral to the right MCL.

Ports may be shifted according to the habitus of the patient and visceral anatomy. The *da Vinci* port distance should range between 6 and 10 cm.

Surgeons should consider a right shift of the above cited trocar line or a double docking if the working space extends beyond the splenic flexure in another quadrant.

18.5   Equipment and Surgical Instruments

Robotic surgical drape kit.

Robotic fenestrated bipolar forceps.

Robotic monopolar scissors or monopolar hook.

Robotic Cadière forceps.

Robotic 30° scope.

Robotic clip applier (optional).

Robotic stapler +12 mm robotic trocar (optional).

2 energy wires (monopolar + bipolar).

Robotic vessel sealer (optional).

18.6   Laparoscopic Instruments

1 Verress needle.

1 CO_2 tube.

2 Croce-Olmi/Cadiere forceps.

1 suction/irrigation system.

1 clip appliers.

1 circular wound protector/retractor.

1 US laparoscopic probe + US unit (optional)

18.7   Open Instruments

1 Backhaus clamp.

4 Kocher clamps.

2 Klemmer clamps.

2 Farabeuf retractors.

1 Scalpel n.11.

References

1. Fiori E, Crocetti D, Lamazza A, DE Felice F, Scotti GB, Sterpetti AV, Mingoli A, Sapienza P, DE Toma G. Defecatory dysfunction after colon cancer resection: the role of inferior mesenteric artery tie. Anticancer Res. 2020;40:2969–74.
2. Yin T-C, Chen Y-C, Su W-C, Chen P-J, Chang T-K, Huang C-W, Tsai H-L, Wang J-Y. Low liga-

tion plus high dissection versus high ligation of the inferior mesenteric artery in sigmoid colon and rectal cancer surgery: a meta-analysis. Front Oncol. 2021;11:774782.

3. Park SS, Park B, Park EY, Park SC, Kim MJ, Sohn DK, Oh JH. Outcomes of high versus low ligation of the inferior mesenteric artery with lymph node dissection for distal sigmoid colon or rectal cancer. Surg Today. 2020;50:560–8.

4. Al Dhaheri M, Ibrahim M, Al-Yahri O, Amer I, Khawar M, Al-Naimi N, Ahmed AA, Nada MA, Parvaiz A. Choice of specimen's extraction site affects wound morbidity in laparoscopic colorectal cancer surgery. Langenbeck's Arch Surg. 2022;407:3561–5.

5. Williams GL, Beaton C, Codd R, Stephenson BM. Avoiding extraction site herniation after laparoscopic right colectomy. Tech Coloproctol. 2012;16:385–8.

6. Skinner D, Wehrle CJ, Van Fossen K (2022) Anatomy, abdomen and pelvis, inferior mesenteric artery.

7. Celoria G, Falco E, Nardini A, Stefani R, Gadducci G, Di Alesio L. The Knight-Griffen technique in colorectal surgery. Minerva Chir. 1993;48:1411–4.

8. Vasudevan V, Reusche R, Wallace H, Kaza S. Clinical outcomes and cost-benefit analysis comparing laparoscopic and robotic colorectal surgeries. Surg Endosc. 2016;30:5490–3.

9. Solaini L, Bocchino A, Avanzolini A, Annunziata D, Cavaliere D, Ercolani G. Robotic versus laparoscopic left colectomy: a systematic review and meta-analysis. Int J Color Dis. 2022;37:1497–507.

10. Bertani E, Chiappa A, Ubiali P, Cossu ML, Arnone P, Andreoni B. Robotic colectomy: is it necessary? Minerva Chir. 2013;68:445–56.

11. Addison P, Agnew JL, Martz J. Robotic colorectal surgery. Surg Clin North Am. 2020;100:337–60.

Laparoscopic Left Hemicolectomy and Rectal Resection

19

Monica Ortenzi and Mario Guerrieri

19.1 Introduction

Laparoscopic colectomy was first described in the early 1990s. The first randomized study comparing the open and minimally invasive techniques demonstrated less blood loss, earlier recovery of bowel function, reduced postoperative stay, and a shorter length of stay favoring the laparoscopic procedures [1–5].

Because of the inflammatory nature of most benign conditions prompting colectomy, there was some hesitation regarding the feasibility of a laparoscopic approach for malignant diseases or for conditions implying a greater inflammation. However, with the increase of the available evidence supporting the safety and feasibility of laparoscopy, a broadening of the initial indications of these minimally invasive techniques was witnessed [1–5].

For example, as far as data evaluating laparoscopic sigmoid colectomy in patients with diverticulitis were accumulating [6–10], laparoscopic left colonic resection was increasingly applied to these conditions. The first studies demonstrated that laparoscopic left or sigmoid colectomy is possible in patients with diverticular disease with an increased operative time compared to open

surgery, a decreased length of stay, and a decreased complication profile [1–5].

As for laparoscopy applied to rectal cancer, nowadays, laparoscopic low anterior resection for rectal cancer is one of the more challenging minimally invasive colorectal procedures to master. The confined and narrow spaces of the pelvis often limit visualization, exposure, and access. Additionally, it is imperative to maintain proper planes of dissection to achieve a sound oncologic resection. Straying from the embryologic planes may result in a field obscured with nuisance bleeding and injury to critical structures [1–5].

It is therefore essential to approach each case in a stepwise fashion with a clear understanding of the anatomical considerations as well as the precise location of the tumor [1–5].

19.2 Benefits of Laparoscopic Surgery and Preoperative Workup

The benefits of laparoscopy include reduced postoperative pain, earlier return of bowel function, shorter length of stay, and fewer wound complications (e.g., wound infection). With modern techniques and newer technologies, there is rarely a case that cannot be approached using laparoscopic technique [1–5].

The major debates regard the feasibility and safety of laparoscopic resection in more chal-

M. Ortenzi (✉) · M. Guerrieri
Clinica di Chirurgia Generale e d'Urgenza, Università Politecnica delle Marche, Ancona, Italy

lenging patients including elderly patients, with multiple medical morbidities, extreme obesity, or prior open abdominal procedures.

An adequate preoperative workup is essential to correctly plan the procedure and in the decision-making during the operation.

This is particularly true for rectal resections for malignant rectal diseases. In the absence of locally advanced disease or a threatened circumferential resection margin (CRM), upper rectal tumors, and select mid-rectal tumors, can be treated like colon cancers via upfront surgical resection, avoiding the risk of the increased morbidity usually observed in lower resections.

However, the anatomical distinction between upper/mid-rectum and the lower rectum can be sometimes difficult. If the tumor is large enough, to be detected by CT or MRI, the radiology imaging could provide reliable anatomic landmarks, such as the distance from the values of Houston or the sacral promontory, even preoperatively. Intraoperatively, the top of the rectum can be identified by where the tenias play and the epiploic appendages disappear. Drawing an imaginary line drawn between the top of the sacral promontory and the bottom of the pubic symphysis could help too in the delineation between the sigmoid colon and the rectum.

Additionally, sometimes, the exact intraluminal margins of the tumor could not be easily detected and, for this reason, advocating the help of an intraoperative rectoscopy, could be useful to properly locate the distal transection margin. Additionally, performing a rigid proctoscopy preoperatively could constitute a much more reliable assessment of "true" distance of the tumor from the anal, thus helping to choose between the procedures to perform to resect it.

Nevertheless, it also allows the surgeon to exact the circumferential location of the tumor, thus knowing which structures could be potentially involved during the dissection and transection steps and have to be accurately taken care of and preserved (e.g., the vagina in case of an anterior location of the tumor).

19.3 Laparoscopic Left Colectomies and Rectal Resection Setup

19.3.1 Operative Room Setup

Careful positioning of the video screens, insufflator, and light sources is required to maximize access to the abdomen, facilitate the assumption of ergonomic positions for all the components of the surgical team, and, eventually, minimize entanglement of cables.

The position of the primary view screen might vary according to the surgeon's preference and the available equipment; however, it is generally on the left side of the patient. If a subsidiary screen is available, it will be paced on the other side to allow a good view of the operative field to the assistant surgeon.

Some operating rooms are equipped with ceiling-mounted booms that carry the equipment, making the whole setup simpler and more adaptable to the needs of the operative team.

As a general rule, however, when setting up the operative room, it is important to keep in mind that the surgeon and camera assistant will both need to be on the opposite sides of the patient, facing the left colon, and the bank of equipment needs to be able to move between the patient's hip and shoulder in order to maintain the desirable straight line between the surgeon's hands, operative site, and screen, as this helps to minimize surgeon fatigue and provide an optimal view of the operative field to all the surgical team.

The most common laparoscopic approach is multiport surgery with the placement of four or five ports. Reduced port techniques, such as single-port laparoscopic surgery, have been described.

Single-port laparoscopic surgery can be performed, but anatomical constraints of the lower pelvic anatomy result in less-than-ideal exposure and access with this approach. Another approach, which can be especially useful in the morbidly obese, is a hand-assisted technique via either a

Pfannenstiel or lower midline approach. The patient is secured to safely enable steep Trendelenburg and right-side elevation throughout the procedure. This should be ensured by a preoperative "Trendelenburg test."

The choice of the energy device to perform the operation could influence the operating room setup as well. Both monopolar cautery and high-energy devices, as bipolar vessel sealer or ultrasonic devices, could be used, mostly according to the preferences of the operating surgeon, as our energy sources. These instruments should be tested and placed on the field at the beginning of the operation. A colonoscope could be used during the procedure and should be available and ready to be used if needed.

19.3.2 Patient Positioning

*P*atients are positioned in a modified lithotomy position on a split-leg table. A bean bag might be used, or in alternative, shoulder support should be placed in order to avoid the patient to slip while in a Trendelenburg position. The arms are tucked at the sides and surrounded by foam padding and, possibly, an inflated bean bag. The arms and chest could be additionally wrapped circumferentially with silk tape to assure a better affixing to the table.

The legs are split with the buttock well exposed at the bottom of the table to allow for trans-anal access, and then the legs are secured in place with Velcro straps. Patients are given antibiotic prophylaxis, less than 1 hour before surgical incision, according to the existing local and international guidelines, and compression devices could be applied to prevent deep venous thrombosis prophylaxis.

The Foley catheter is placed before the sterile drapes are positioned.

19.3.2.1 General Operating Room Setup

- Patient supine.
- Both arms tuck.
- Modified lithotomy or split-leg position.
- Surgeon and assist on the patient's right side.

- Scrub nurse and sterile instrument table on the patient's left side.
- Monitor angled at the left shoulder and left lower extremity.

19.4 Operative Technique

19.4.1 Laparoscopic Left/Sigmoid Resection

19.4.1.1 Port Placement

Generally, a 12 mm Hassan port is placed in the umbilicus, while 5 mm (or 10 mm, according to the preferences) ports are placed in the right upper quadrant, the right lower quadrant, and the left lower quadrant. Extraction could be performed either through a small Pfannenstiel incision, via an extension of the Hassan port site or a left McBurney incision.

If the hand-assisted approach is chosen, at the beginning of the operation, either an 8-cm lower midline incision or a Pfannenstiel incision 2 cm above the pubis for the hand port is made. The hand device is then placed into the incision, and then three 5 mm trocars are placed in the left lateral, right lateral, and umbilical positions.

The trocars are placed always under direct vision or with the help of the hand inside the abdomen in case of a hand-assisted procedure, with the aim to avoid bowel injuries during this phase.

General Port Position
- 5 (or 10/12) mm camera port at the umbilicus
- 5 (or 10) mm ports in the right upper quadrant (RUQ) and right lower quadrant (RLQ)
- Optional 5 mm port in the left lower quadrant (LLQ) or subxiphoid Pfannenstiel incision for extraction.

Instruments
- Atraumatic bowel graspers.
- Energy devices:
  - Monopolar energy devices include the L or J hook, spatula, or scissors with cautery.
  - High-energy devices (bipolar device or ultrasonic devices).

- Wound protector.
- Clips.
- Staplers.

19.4.1.2 Operative Technique: Left/ Sigmoid Colectomies

Several ways to approach the left colon have been described and there is still ongoing debate about whether the performance of some of the surgical steps could be recommended routinely or only in selected occasions (e.g., the mobilization of the splenic flexure).

In our practice, we usually use a medial to lateral approach to mobilize the left/sigmoid colon. In order to have a good exposure of the left colon, at the beginning of the procedure, the omentum is gently lifted over the transverse colon, and the small bowel is moved toward the right quadrants even with the help of a right tilt of the operating table. Then the mesentery lateral to the inferior mesenteric vein (IMV), between the left colic and first sigmoidal branches, thus exposed, is grasped and lifted.

An incision of this mesentery is performed laterally to the IMV, and the IMV is isolated and divided at the inferior boarder of the pancreas. Clips could be used to assure a better hemostasis. Then the distal transverse mesocolon is freed from the inferior boarder of the pancreas. The dissection continues between the left colon mesentery and Gerota's fascia until the lateral wall is reached. The gonadal vessels are usually visualized below with Gerota's fascia.

The left ureter is typically under the inferior mesenteric artery (IMA) pedicle and it should be visualized in order to carry out a safe dissection, without harming it. If a sigmoidectomy is being performed, the first one or two sigmoid branches are identified, isolated, and divided with the bipolar vessel sealer, and clips could be placed if considered safer. Otherwise, in standard left hemicolectomies, for oncological reasons, the IMA should be isolated and cut, usually after the positioning of hemostatic clips on the remaining pedicle, in order to retrieve a larger number of lymph nodes.

The mobilization of the left colon then continues, medially to laterally, in a plane overlying

Gerota's fascia until reaching the left pelvic sidewall, inferiorly, into the upper retrorectal space, and the splenic flexure, superiorly.

If the surgeon decides to proceed with the mobilization of the splenic flexure, the lateral attachments of the splenic flexure are divided.

This might be particularly useful when additional length of the proximal colon is needed to perform the anastomosis in a tension-free fashion, especially in lower resection as described in the next paragraph.

The best way to accomplish the lateral dissection is to have the assistant to gently retract the proximal colon medially to expose and stretch the peritoneal refection. The surgeon uses an atraumatic instrument to push the colon medially for countertraction, thus putting the peritoneal attachments on tension (e.g., phreno-colic ligament, spleno-colic ligament). Like this, the division of this attachment will be efficiently conducted all the way up to the splenic flexure, medially to Gerota's fascia. This technique is continued entering the lesser sac by dissecting the small omentum close to the distal transverse colon. This type of dissection would allow us to fully mobilize the splenic flexure.

The omentum is taken off of the distal transverse colon allowing the splenic flexure to be approached from a medial direction. During this step of the procedure, the assistant surgeon might need to move to the area between the legs of the patient to provide a better assistance.

At this point, the colon should be assessed for reach down to the proximal rectum before transecting it. For the distal transection margin, the mesentery can be taken up to the edge of the colon. A laparoscopic stapler is inserted and used to transect the colon inside the abdomen.

At this point, the bowel can be exteriorized, and the specimen can be brought out through the hand port (in the case of hand assisted) or through an extraction site, using a small wound protector to ease specimen extraction and to protect the wound from contamination. The proximal transection is completed via the extraction site. The anvil of a circular stapler is placed in the proximal colon before it is returned to the abdomen. The stapled circular colorectal anastomosis can be performed while under laparoscopic view (or in some cases through the wound directly if a Pfannenstiel or lower midline incision is used).

It is critical to ensure that there are no twists in the proximal colon or the mesentery and that the small bowel is not trapped under the left colon mesentery before the stapler is fired.

In either approach, the omentum is brought down over the small bowel and colon to an anatomical position. Following the anastomosis, air leak testing is performed with colonoscopy, and the mucosa could be examined for perfusion. The anastomosis may be reinforced with a few additional sutures depending upon the surgeon's preference.

A drain might be placed in the pelvis according to the preferences and choices of the operating surgeon.

19.4.2 Laparoscopic Anterior Rectal Resection

The techniques to approach rectal resection might vary depending on several factors related to patient characteristics (e.g., gender), size, and site of the tumor. To simplify the procedure in this section the technique of laparoscopic anterior rectal resection for mid-upper rectal cancer will be described.

19.4.2.1 Port Placement

The general rules of trocar positioning are similar to those previously described, with some slightly different possible variations. In the fashioning of an ileostomy, for example, the 10 mm RLQ trocar can be placed in correspondence to the predetermined ileostomy site.

The same option for the extraction site previously presented exists also in rectal resections, and usually they are chosen according to the surgeon's preferences. Some surgeons prefer to perform the Pfannenstiel incision also to have direct access to the anastomosis in cases in which repair of an anastomotic defect is required.

19.4.2.2 Operative Steps

Planes of the Mesorectum
Both medial-to-lateral and lateral-to-medial approaches could be used during the laparoscopic procedure.

The first part of the procedure is similar to that previously described for left hemicolectomies. The additional steps regard the management of the rectal dissection.

Once the dissection extends to the pelvis, the medial side of the mesentery is exposed by elevating the rectosigmoid with a bowel grasper to identify the thin base near the sacral promontory. The peritoneum is carefully scored and the avascular presacral plane is identified and carefully dissected.

The left ureter and gonadal vessels are exposed at a very early stage and should be carefully identified in order to carry on a safe dissection. Care should be taken also not to injure the nerves in the deeper plane. Dissection continues laterally in the retroperitoneal plane toward the line of Toldt (which is usually whiter than the surrounding tissue), inferiorly to the level of the sacral promontory and superiorly toward the base of the IMA.

The plane between the retroperitoneal structures posteriorly and the mesorectum anteriorly is then developed. Dissection derived from the CO_2 insufflation could help to identify this avascular plane; after infiltrating into the tissues, they appear as white fibers, also called "angel's hair."

The procedure continues with the dissection of the IMA. Once the vascular pedicle has been adequately skeletonized, and the surgeon has ensured that the left retroperitoneal structures at risk (i.e., ureter, gonadal vein) are lateral, the vessel can be divided. The artery can be cut at several levels: a low ligation indicates that the division of the artery is made to preserve the left colic (LCA) and/or sigmoid indicates that none of the previously named vessels are preserved.

The surgeon then continues the mesenteric transection up to the site of planned proximal colonic division, which can be immediately performed via endoscopic stapler or, alternatively, it can be performed later through the extraction site.

To gain more length and to be able to perform a tension-free anastomosis, we usually perform the splenic flexure mobilization with the previously described technique.

Pelvic Dissection and Division of the Rectum

Dissection continues in the presacral mesorectal plane from the sacral promontory toward the retrosacral fascia. Care is taken to maintain the correct dissection plane identified by the avascular alveolar tissue while keeping the investing fascia of the mesorectum intact. Now the assistant is required to grasp the sigmoid, while the surgeon lifts the rectum with a blunt instrument and dissects in the posterior plane up and over the sacral promontory into the pelvis. The lateral stalks of the rectum are divided with bipolar energy devices. Next, the anterior reflection of the peritoneum is divided and the rectum is carefully dissected from the anterior pelvic strictures (seminal vesicles in a man and vagina in a woman).

We usually begin with the division of the mesentery circumferentially to the rectum, taking care not to injure the rectal wall. Once the rectal wall is well visible circumferentially, a linear stapler is placed through the 12 mm RLQ port, and the rectal wall is stapled and divided. A second staple cartridge load is often necessary to complete the rectal division.

Alternatively, some surgeons could decide to use the Pfannenstiel extraction incision and perform division of the bowel and mesentery under direct nonlaparoscopic access. However, in our opinion, this should be reserved for large bulky tumor or in the presence of difficult anatomical conditions (e.g., narrow pelvis). The most important aspect of this step is to maintain adequate distal and circumferential resection margins. A distal margin is considered properly transected when it ensures a distance of at least 2 cm from the distal margin of the tumor. Performing an intraoperative rectoscopy (either rigid or flexible) could be helpful to properly locate this margin.

Specimen Extraction and Anastomosis

We usually perform a small left McBurney incision for our extraction site. We are used to protect the wound with specifically designed wound protectors that can allow to reestablish the pneumoperitoneum after the transection step leaving them in place and without the need to close the incision.

Generally, we also transect the colon and place and secure the anvil of the circular stapler into the proximal end of the colon externally through this incision. We usually perform the end-to-end anastomosis under direct laparoscopic vision, after having reestablished the pneumoperitoneum.

The assistant then moves between the leg of the patient and places the circular stapler through the anum. The stapler is opened inside the abdomen and opens the stapler aiming anteriorly to the rectal staple line, trying to avoid the crossing of the two mechanical sutures (the one from the linear stapler and the one from the circular stapler). The anvil is then attached to the head of the stapler, which is closed actuated. An air leak test could be performed after the circular stapler is extracted. The patient is put in an anti-Trendelenburg position and the pelvis is filled with saline, submerging the anastomosis. The assistant, with the help of either a flexible or rigid proctoscope, inflates the rectum and the operating surgeon assesses for the presence of any bubbling from the anastomosis, indicating a potential discontinuity of the circumferential staple line.

A drain could be left in place according to the preferences of the operating surgeon.

Generally, for upper and mid-rectal tumors, in a patient that did not underwent neoadjuvant chemoradiotherapy, we do not perform a diverting loop ileostomy unless there show specific characteristics that could be considered as risk factors for altered anastomotic healing and, consequently, for postoperative anastomotic leak.

References

1. Han J, Min BS. Laparoscopic-assisted radical left hemicolectomy for colon cancer. J Vis Surg. 2016;2:148. https://doi.org/10.21037/jovs.2016.08.05.

2. Shen MY, Leow YC, Chen WTL. Laparoscopic Left Hemicolectomy. In: Lomanto D, Chen WTL, Fuentes MB, editors. Mastering endo-laparoscopic and thoracoscopic surgery. Singapore: Springer; 2023. https://doi.org/10.1007/978-981-19-3755-2_70.

3. Ammendola M, Filice F, Battaglia C, Romano R, Manti F, Minici R, de'Angelis N, Memeo R, Laganà D, Navarra G, Montemurro S, Currò G. Left hemicolectomy and low anterior resection in colorectal cancer patients: Knight-Griffen vs. transanal purse-string suture anastomosis with no-coil placement. Front Surg. 2023;10:1093347. https://doi.org/10.3389/fsurg.2023.1093347.

4. Solaini L, Bocchino A, Avanzolini A, Annunziata D, Cavaliere D, Ercolani G. Robotic versus laparoscopic left colectomy: a systematic review and meta-analysis. Int J Color Dis. 2022;37(7):1497–507. https://doi.org/10.1007/s00384-022-04194-8.

5. Hajibandeh S, Hajibandeh S, Hussain I, Zubairu A, Akbar F, Maw A. Comparison of extended right hemicolectomy, left hemicolectomy and segmental colectomy for splenic flexure colon cancer: a systematic review and meta-analysis. Color Dis. 2020;22(12):1885–907. https://doi.org/10.1111/codi.15292.

6. Zhang Y, Liu C, Nistala KRY, Chong CS. Open versus laparoscopic Hartmann's procedure: a systematic review and meta-analysis. Int J Color Dis. 2022;37(12):2421–30. https://doi.org/10.1007/s00384-022-04285-6.

7. Chavrier D, Alves A, Menahem B. Is laparoscopy a reliable alternative to laparotomy in Hartmann's reversal? An updated meta-analysis. Tech Coloproctol. 2022;26(4):239–52. https://doi.org/10.1007/s10151-021-02560-2.

8. Celentano V, Giglio MC, Bucci L. Laparoscopic versus open Hartmann's reversal: a systematic review and meta-analysis. Int J Color Dis. 2015;30(12):1603–15. https://doi.org/10.1007/s00384-015-2325-4.

9. Lin H, Zhuang Z, Huang X, Li Y. The role of emergency laparoscopic surgery for complicated diverticular disease: A systematic review and meta-analysis. Medicine (Baltimore). 2020;99(40):e22421. https://doi.org/10.1097/MD.0000000000022421.

10. Abraha I, Binda GA, Montedori A, Arezzo A, Cirocchi R. Laparoscopic versus open resection for sigmoid diverticulitis. Cochrane Database Syst Rev. 2017;11(11):CD009277. https://doi.org/10.1002/14651858.CD009277.pub2.

Luca Montesarchio [ID], Antonio Sciuto [ID],
Annamaria Mottola, Felice De Stasio,
and Felice Pirozzi [ID]

Colorectal cancer is the third most common cancer worldwide, and rectal cancer accounts for over one-third of cases. Surgical management of colorectal cancer involves resection of the affected bowel segment with a tumor-free margin, ligation of the major vascular pedicle feeding the tumor along with its lymphatics, and en bloc resection of any involved adjacent organs [1–3].

Depending upon the clinical stage, size, and location of the tumor, a rectal cancer can be treated with either local or radical excision. A local excision is usually performed transanally, while a radical excision is carried out through an abdominal or a combined abdominoperineal approach. Rectal cancers invading adjacent organs may require a multivisceral resection [4–6].

Anterior resection is the most common procedure for the radical excision of rectal or rectosigmoid cancer and involves removal of the sigmoid colon and rectum through an abdominal approach. A *low anterior resection* (LAR) is defined as one that entails resection of the rectum (or proctectomy) below the peritoneal reflection. Rectal resection also involves the removal of the perirectal adipose tissue—which is called mesorectum and contains the blood and lymphatic supply to the rectum—to prevent spread of cancer and its recurrence. Excision of the mesorectum may be complete or partial based on the location of the tumor; accordingly, the procedure is called *total mesorectal excision* (TME) for tumors of the middle and low rectum, or *partial mesorectal excision* (PME) for tumors of the upper rectum and rectosigmoid junction. After resection, intestinal continuity is reestablished with a *colorectal anastomosis* between the descending colon and the distal end of the rectum. A *temporary diverting stoma* is often performed to protect anastomosis, especially after low anterior resection which carries a high risk of anastomotic leakage. For temporary diversion, loop ileostomy is generally preferred over loop colostomy. If intestinal continuity cannot be reestablished (e.g., seriously incontinent patient, technical reasons), an end colostomy is performed after rectal resection (*Hartmann procedure*). In selected patients in whom a standard LAR would not achieve an adequate distal margin, *proctectomy with inter-*

L. Montesarchio · A. Mottola · F. De Stasio ·
F. Pirozzi (✉)
Department of General Surgery, Santa Maria delle
Grazie Hospital, Pozzuoli, NA, Italy
e-mail: luca.montesarchio@aslnapoli2nord.it;
annamaria.mottola@aslnapoli2nord.it; felice.
destasio@aslnapoli2nord.it;
felice.pirozzi@aslnapoli2nord.it

A. Sciuto
Department of General Surgery, Santa Maria delle
Grazie Hospital, Pozzuoli, NA, Italy

Department of Electrical Engineering and
Information Technology, University of Naples
Federico II, Naples, Italy
e-mail: antonio.sciuto@aslnapoli2nord.it

sphincteric resection may be performed. This procedure extends the distal margin by removing the internal sphincter partially or completely and is conducted through an abdominal and a perineal approach. Intestinal continuity is reestablished with an anastomosis between the descending colon and the anus (*coloanal anastomosis*). When the tumor involves or is too close to the external anal sphincter, or in patients in whom an intersphincteric is not possible (e.g., unfavorable body habitus, preoperative incontinence), an *abdominoperineal resection* or *Miles' procedure* is indicated. This procedure involves complete excision of the rectum and anus by dissection through the abdomen and perineum, with suture closure of the perineum and creation of a permanent colostomy [7, 8].

The screening campaigns and technological innovation, along with more effective preoperative neoadjuvant treatments, have considerably increased the rate of sphincter-saving surgery for low rectal cancer and improved functional and oncological outcomes.

Rectal surgery, especially low in a narrow pelvis, is one of the abdominal surgeries that has benefited most from the use of a robotic approach. This is mainly due to a three-dimensional magnified view, articulated instruments without tremor, and a stable camera platform. In this chapter, anterior resection of the rectum, proctectomy with intersphincteric resection, and abdominoperineal resection carried out using the da Vinci Xi robotic platform are described [7, 8].

20.1 Surgical Technique

20.1.1 Anterior Resection of the Rectum with Colorectal Anastomosis

This procedure involves an abdominal and a pelvic phase. Each of these phases entails a specific arrangement of the robotic arms. Bowel continuity is restored through a mechanical colorectal anastomosis, and a temporary diverting ileostomy is often performed, especially for LAR.

20.1.1.1 Abdominal Phase
The abdominal phase involves mobilization of the left colon and ligation of the inferior mesenteric vessels. The surgical steps are as follows:

- Coloepiploic detachment.
- Identification of the inferior mesenteric vein and medial-to-lateral dissection along an avascular plane between the Toldt's and Gerota's fasciae, taking care to avoid injury to the retroperitoneal structures (ureter, gonadal vessels, nerves).
- Identification and division of the inferior mesenteric artery.
- Division of the inferior mesenteric vein and detachment of the transverse mesocolon from the lower edge of the pancreas.
- Splenic flexure mobilization and division of the lateral attachments of the descending and sigmoid colon.

20.1.1.2 Pelvic Phase
The pelvic phase requires redocking of the robot and involves mobilization of the sigmoid colon and rectum, bowel transection, and fashioning of a mechanical colorectal anastomosis. The surgical steps are as follows:

- Complete mobilization of the sigmoid colon, avoiding injury to the ureter.
- In female patients, retraction of the uterine fundus to the anterior abdominal wall.
- Dissection of the rectum along with the mesorectum to a level of 5 cm below the lower margin of the tumor (PME) or down to the pelvic floor (TME), taking care to avoid injury to the autonomic nerves.
- Transection of the rectum.
- Robot undocking and extraction of the bowel through a Pfannenstiel incision.
- Division of the mesentery of the descending colon and indocyanine green (ICG) fluorescence test to assess blood supply to the chosen transection line of the colon.
- Transection of the descending colon and preparation of the colonic stump for anastomosis.
- Reestablishment of pneumoperitoneum, robot redocking, and fashioning of a mechanical

colorectal anastomosis using the double-stapling Knight-Griffen technique (a colonic J-pouch or side-to-end anastomosis may be performed).

- Air-leak test to identify any anastomotic leak and doughnut inspection;
- Closure of the mesenteric defect to prevent internal hernias.
- Placement of an abdominal drain.
- Fashioning of a diverting ileostomy if needed.
- Closure of abdominal incisions and opening of the ileostomy.

20.1.2 Intersphincteric Proctectomy with Coloanal Anastomosis

This procedure involves an abdominal phase, a pelvic phase, and a perineal phase. The order of these phases may differ, and the resected bowel may be removed through the abdomen or anus. Bowel continuity is restored through a hand-sewn coloanal anastomosis, and a temporary diverting ileostomy is usually performed.

20.1.2.1 Abdominal Phase

The abdominal phase involves mobilization of the left colon and ligation of the inferior mesenteric vessels. The surgical steps are as follows:

- Coloepiploic detachment.
- Identification of the inferior mesenteric vein and medial-to-lateral dissection along an avascular plane between the Toldt's and Gerota's fasciae, taking care to avoid injury to the retroperitoneal structures (ureter, gonadal vessels, nerves).
- Identification and division of the inferior mesenteric artery.
- Division of the inferior mesenteric vein and detachment of the transverse mesocolon from the lower edge of the pancreas.
- Splenic flexure mobilization and division of the lateral parietal attachments of the descending and sigmoid colon.

20.1.2.2 Pelvic Phase

The pelvic phase requires redocking of the robot and involves mobilization of the sigmoid colon and rectum down to the pelvic floor. The surgical steps are as follows:

- Complete mobilization of the sigmoid colon, avoiding injury to the ureter.
- In female patients, retraction of the uterine fundus to the anterior abdominal wall.
- Dissection of the rectum along with the mesorectum down to the pelvic floor (TME), taking care to avoid injury to the autonomic nerves.

20.1.2.3 Perineal Phase

This phase requires undocking of the robot and involves resection of the internal anal sphincter and performing a coloanal anastomosis. The surgical steps are as follows:

- Exposing the mucosa of the anal canal and closing the lumen with a purse-string suture.
- Circumferentially incising the mucosa of the anal canal and the internal sphincter.
- Dissecting the intersphincteric plane until the pelvic floor is reached and the already dissected pelvic portion of the rectum is found.
- Extraction of the bowel through the anus and division of the descending colon after ICG test.
- Performing a hand-sewn coloanal anastomosis.

If an intersphincteric proctectomy is planned before surgery, perineal dissection may be performed first during the operation, while transanal bowel division and coloanal anastomosis are performed after the robotic mesorectal dissection has been completed.

The operation ends with the following steps which complete the pelvic phase:

- Closure of the mesenteric defect
- Placement of an abdominal drain.
- Fashioning of a diverting ileostomy if needed.
- Closure of abdominal incisions and maturation of the ileostomy.

If the surgical specimen is removed through the abdomen instead of the anus, following perineal dissection and robotic mesorectal excision, the robot is undocked, and the bowel is exteriorized through a Pfannenstiel incision. The mesentery of the descending colon is divided, and an indocyanine green fluorescence test is made to assess blood supply to the chosen transection line of the colon. Then, the descending colon is transected and reinserted into the abdomen, and pneumoperitoneum is reestablished. The descending colon is exteriorized through the anus. Closure of the mesenteric defect, placement of a drain, and fashioning of a diverting ileostomy are performed. A coloanal anastomosis is performed, thus completing the perineal phase. Finally, abdominal incisions are closed, and the ileostomy is matured.

20.1.3 Abdominoperineal Resection or Miles' Procedure

This procedure includes an abdominal phase, a pelvic phase, and a perineal phase. After complete removal of the rectum and the anus, intestinal continuity is not reestablished, and a permanent end colostomy is performed.

20.1.3.1 Abdominal Phase
The abdominal phase involves mobilization of the left colon and ligation of the inferior mesenteric vessels. The surgical steps are as follows:

- Identification of the inferior mesenteric vein and medial-to-lateral dissection along an avascular plane between the Toldt's and Gerota's fasciae, taking care to avoid injury to the retroperitoneal structures (ureter, gonadal vessels, nerves).
- Identification and division of the inferior mesenteric artery.
- Division of the inferior mesenteric vein.
- Division of the lateral attachments of the descending colon.

20.1.3.2 Pelvic Phase
The pelvic phase requires redocking of the robot and involves mobilization of the sigmoid colon and rectum down to the pelvic floor. The surgical steps are as follows:

- Complete mobilization of the sigmoid colon, avoiding injury to the ureter.
- In female patients, retraction of the uterine fundus to the anterior abdominal wall.
- Dissection of the rectum along with the mesorectum down to the pelvic floor (TME), taking care to avoid injury to the autonomic nerves.
- Division of the mesentery of the descending colon and indocyanine green fluorescence test to assess blood supply to the chosen transection line of the colon.
- Transection of the descending colon.

20.1.3.3 Perineal Phase
The perineal phase requires undocking of the robot and involves excision of the anus, the anal sphincters, and the distal rectum as well as closure of the perineum. The surgical steps are as follows:

- Closure of the anus with a purse-string suture and circumferential perineal incision around the anus.
- Dissection of the subcutaneous adipose tissue including the external sphincter and section of the anococcygeal ligament.
- Division of the levator ani muscle.
- Removal of the surgical specimen through the perineal wound.
- Layered closure of the perineal wound with absorbable sutures or reconstruction with a biological mesh (or a myocutaneous flap) for large defects.

Following the perineal phase, the robot is redocked, the pelvic floor peritoneum is closed, and a drain is placed. Alternatively, a Dufour catheter with saline-filled balloon is used to occupy the pelvis and prevent small bowel obstruction. Finally, after robotic undocking, abdominal incisions are closed, and an end colostomy is performed.

Fig. 20.1 Schematic view of the operating room setup

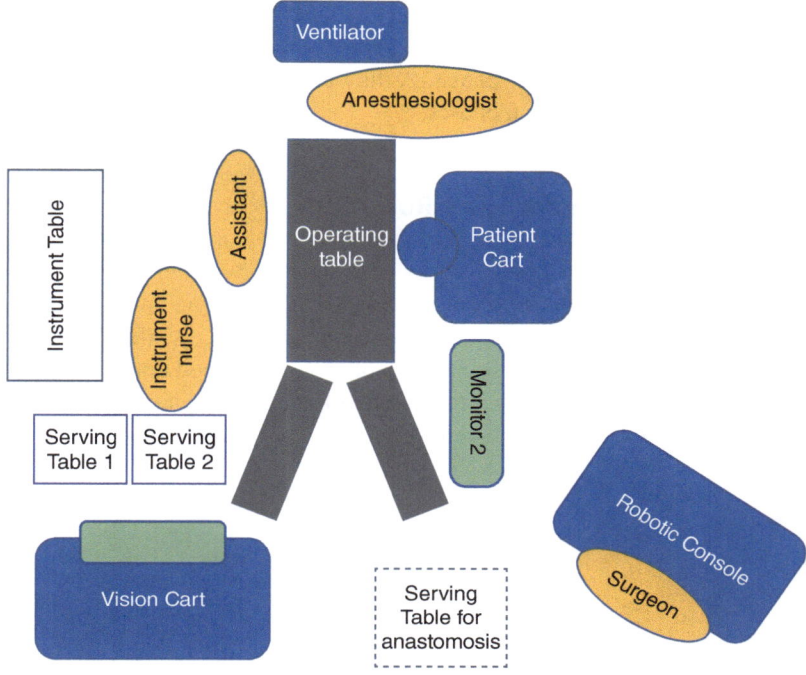

20.2 Operating Theatre Setting

The operating theatre for all the above surgeries is set up as follows (Fig. 20.1):

- Operating table in the center of the theatre.
- Vision cart positioned to the right of the patient, at the level of the feet.
- Supplementary monitor to the left of the patient, at the level of the leg.
- Patient cart to the left of the patient.
- Surgeon at the robotic console.
- First assistant to the right of the patient.
- Instrument nurse to the right of the first assistant.
- Serving table to the right of instrument nurse.

20.3 Patient Positioning

Surgery is performed under general anesthesia. An orogastric tube and a Foley catheter are inserted. The patient is positioned as shown in Fig. 20.2:

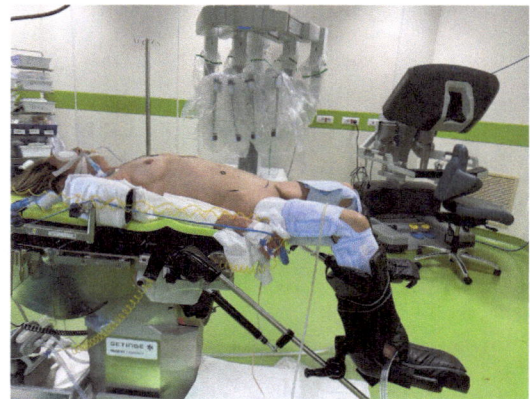

Fig. 20.2 Patient position

- Supine.
- Both arms alongside the body.
- Legs apart on Allen stirrups.

A viscoelastic mat (CarePad®) is placed on the operating table to prevent the patient sliding throughout surgical procedures and to reduce the risk of pressure injuries. A lateral support is also placed at the level of the right shoulder.

The patient is rotated to the right and 15–20° Trendelenburg during the abdominal phase or 20–30° during the pelvic phase. A lithotomy position is used for perineal phases.

20.4 Port Placement and Robotic Docking

A 12-mmHg pneumoperitoneum is achieved by using a Veress needle through a small incision in the left upper quadrant. Subsequently, a sterile marker and ruler may be used for drawing bone reliefs and port sites on the patient skin.

Five robotic ports and one assistant port (AirSeal® Access Port) are used. Three 8-mm and one 12-mm robotic ports are placed at least 8 cm from each other, along a straight line directed from the epigastrium to the anterior superior iliac spine, in the right side of the abdomen. The 12-mm port is in the right iliac fossa. The assistant port is placed in the right subcostal region, 5–10 cm away from the robotic ports (Fig. 20.3).

The port A2 is placed first after a saline drop test, while the remaining working ports are placed under direct vision. A sterile staff member docks the arm subsequently used for the endoscope (arm 3) to the endoscope port (A3)

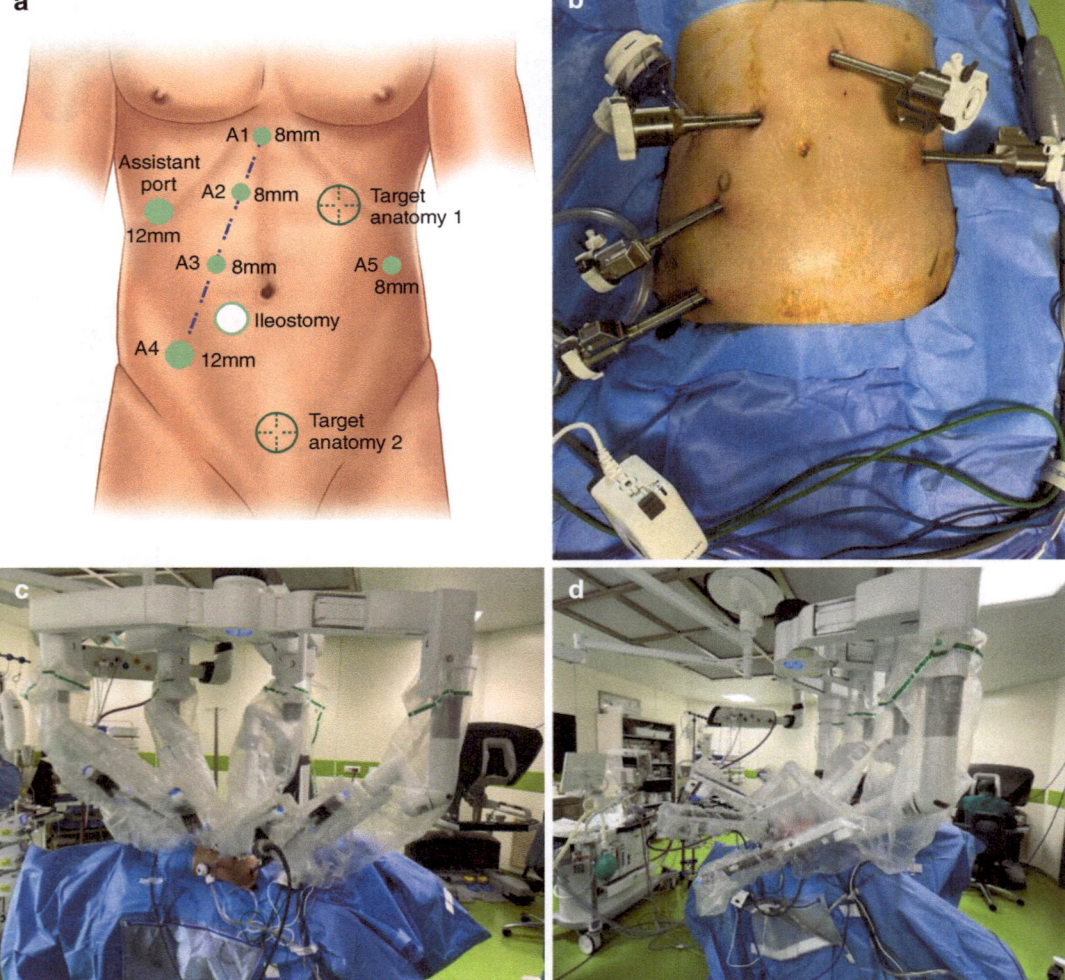

Fig. 20.3 Port placement (**a**, **b**). Robotic docking during the abdominal (**c**) and pelvic (**d**) phase

and then installs the endoscope onto the port. Next, the endoscope is inserted to point the target anatomy which is the splenic flexure of the colon in the abdominal phase. Once targeting—the selection of the target anatomy through the endoscope—is complete, and the endoscope is aligned with the target anatomy, the rest of the arms can be docked and positioned, leaving a fist-width space between the arms and between the patient and the arms. Next, instruments may be inserted, after positioning a reducer on the 12-mm port to avoid loss of pneumoperitoneum.

When passing from the abdominal phase to the pelvic phase, an 8-mm robotic port (A5) is placed in the left flank, and redocking of the patient cart is performed. Targeting is done toward the pelvis, and the robotic arm no. 1 is docked to the port A5.

20.5 Surgical Instruments

The instrument table and the serving cart may be set up as shown in Fig. 20.4. The instruments may vary according to the surgeon's habits and the composition of the surgical containers.

Robotic Instruments:
- 5 robotic ports (four 8-mm ports and one 12-mm port)
- 1 port reducer
- A 30° robotic endoscope.
- 1 grasping forceps (Tip-Up Fenestrated Forceps®)
- 1 bipolar forceps (Fenestrated Force Bipolar Forceps®)
- 1 monopolar instrument (Permanent Cautery Hook®)

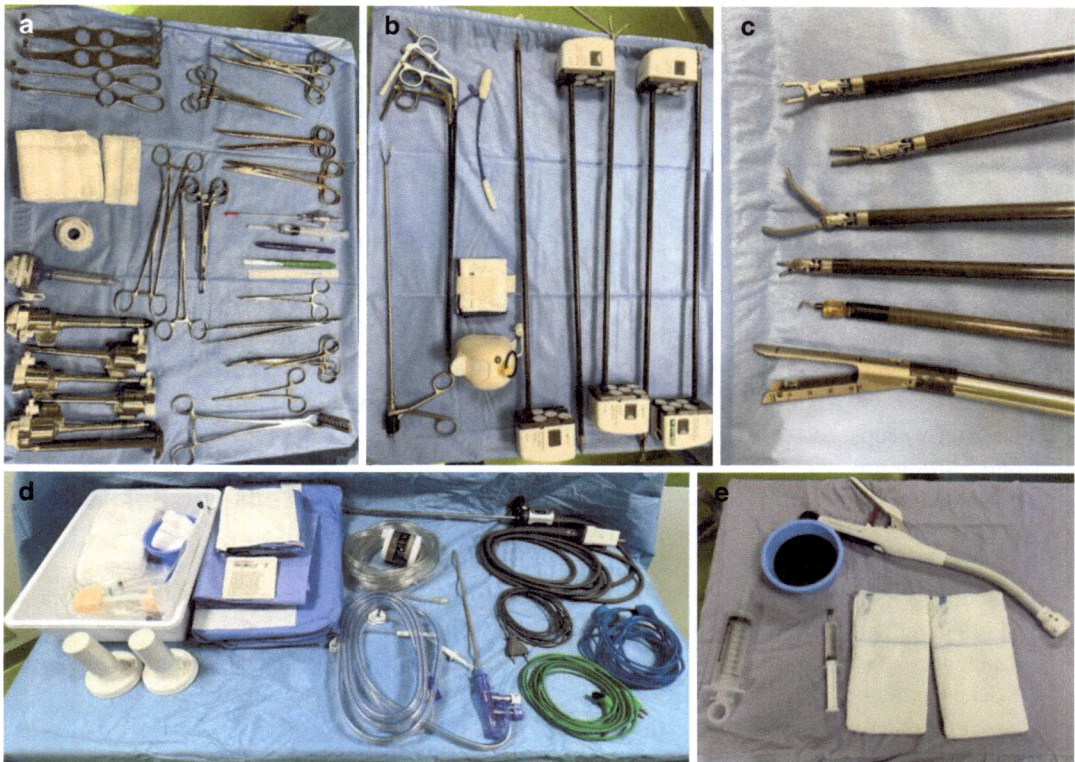

Fig. 20.4 Serving tables (**a**, **b**), tip of the robotic instruments (**c**), instrument table (**d**), serving table for anastomosis (**e**)

- 1 sealing instrument (Vessel Sealer® or Syncrosil®, 8 mm)
- 1 linear stapler (SureForm™ Stapler®, 45 mm)
- 1 clip applier (Medium-Large Clip Applier® with Hem-o-lok® ligating clips)
- 1 needle holder with suture cutter (Large SutureCut™ Needle Driver®)

Laparoscopic Instruments:
- One 12-mm assistant port (AirSeal® Access Port) with insufflation tubing.
- 3 grasping forceps (Johann forceps)
- 1 bipolar forceps
- 1 suction/irrigation system (Dolphin evo®)
- 1 Fibrin glue (Tisseel® or Evicel®) applicator if needed
- 1 linear stapler if needed
- 1 infrared laparoscope if needed.

Laparoscopic scissors (or energy devices) are required if adhesiolysis is performed before robotic docking.

Open Instruments:
- 1 scalpel (no. 11 blade)
- 3 curved Klemmer clamps
- 2 straight Klemmer clamp
- 3 curved Kocher clamps
- 2 straight Kocher clamps
- 1 Mixter forceps
- 2 anatomical tissue forceps
- 2 needle holders
- 2 Nelson-Metzenbaum dissection scissors
- 1 Mayo scissors
- 2 Foerster forceps
- 1 purse-string forceps
- 3 Allis clamps
- 1 curved enterostat
- 1 straight enterostat
- 4 Backhaus clamps
- 2 Mathieu retractors
- 2 Langenbeck retractors
- 2 Kocher retractors if needed
- 1 wound protector/retractor if needed
- 1 Lone Star™ Retractor System if needed
- 1 monopolar electric scalpel
- 1 bipolar forceps if needed
- 1 ultrasonic device (HARMONIC® 1100 Ultrasonic Shears) if needed

20.5.1 Instruments for Mechanical Colorectal Anastomosis

- 1 circular stapler (EEA™ Circular Stapler with Tri-Staple™ Technology or ECHELON CIRCULAR™ Powered Stapler)
- 1 basin
- A 0.9% sodium chloride solution dyed with methylene blue.
- A 100-ml syringe.
- A prefilled syringe with lubricating gel.

Other Devices:
- Sterile surgical gloves, gowns, and drapes.
- Sterile gauzes (5 × 30 cm and 10 × 20 cm gauzes, laparotomy gauzes).
- Sterile marker and ruler.
- Antiseptic solution (nex Clorex 2% Chlorhexidine/70% Alcohol Prep Applicator).
- 1 Veress needle
- A 10 ml syringe filled with 2 mL of saline.
- 1 endoscope cleaning device (Clearify™ Visualization System)
- 1 Biosynthetic mesh (GORE® BIO-A® Tissue Reinforcement), if needed.
- 1 vial of ICG (intravenous injection of a ICG solution of 2.5 mg/mL)
- Absorbable sutures (0 Coated Vicryl™ *Plus* with 5/8 and 1/2 circle needle; 3-0 Coated Vicryl™ *Plus*; 3-0 barbed sutures if needed; 3-0 Coated Vicryl™ Rapide).
- Nonabsorbable sutures (double armed, straight needle 2-0 Prolene™ if needed, silk suture).
- 1 sharp disposal and needle counter box.

20.6 Surgical Steps and Related Instruments

The technique for access to the abdominal cavity as well as port placement, robotic docking, and closure of abdominal incisions IS the same for all the surgical procedures described above.

Veress-Assisted Technique for Access to the Abdominal Cavity:
- Scalpel (no. 11 blade).
- Veress needle.
- Syringe for saline drop test.

Port Placement and Robotic Docking:

- Sterile marker and ruler to measure the distance between the ports.
- Scalpel (no. 11 blade).
- One 12-mm robotic port with port reducer.
- Four 8-mm robotic ports.
- One 12-mm assistant port (AirSeal® Access Port) with insufflation tubing.
- 30° robotic endoscope.

The instruments needed to perform anterior resection of the rectum, proctectomy with intersphincteric resection, and abdominoperineal resection are as follows:

20.6.1 Anterior Resection of the Rectum with Colorectal Anastomosis

20.6.1.1 Abdominal Phase

This phase is basically the same (except for the coloepiploic detachment) whether an anterior resection, an intersphincteric resection, or a Miles' procedure is performed.

The robotic instruments used by the surgeon at the surgical console are as follows:

- 30° robotic endoscope
- Grasping forceps (Tip-Up Fenestrated Forceps®).
- Bipolar forceps (Fenestrated Force Bipolar Forceps®).
- Monopolar instrument (Permanent Cautery Hook®).
- Sealing instrument (Vessel Sealer® or Syncrosil®, 8 mm).
- Clip applier (Medium-Large Clip Applier® with Hem-o-lok® ligating clips).

The energy devices are used for dissection and hemostasis, while the clip applier is used for vessel ligation.

The laparoscopic instruments used by the first assistant at the operating table are as follows:

- Grasping forceps (Johann forceps).
- Suction/irrigation system (Dolphin evo®).

Grasping forceps are used to assist in exposing surgical structures and for passing and withdrawing gauzes. The suction irrigation system is employed to keep the abdominal cavity clear of liquids and blood.

20.6.1.2 Pelvic Phase

The robotic instruments used by the surgeon at the surgical console are the following:

- 30° robotic endoscope
- Grasping forceps (TipUp Fenestrated Forceps®).
- Bipolar forceps (Force Fenestrated Bipolar Forceps®).
- Monopolar instrument (Permanent Cautery Hook®).
- Sealing instrument (Vessel Sealer® or Syncrosil®, 8 mm).
- Clip applier (Medium-Large Clip Applier® with Hem-o-lok® ligating clips).
- Needle holder with suture cutter (Large SutureCut™ Needle Driver®).
- Linear stapler (SureForm™ Stapler®, 45 mm).

Partial or total mesorectal excision and hemostasis are performed by using the energy devices, especially the monopolar cautery hook. A clip applier may be used for division of the mesentery of the descending colon, while a needle holder is employed to suture the uterine fundus to the anterior abdominal wall by using a straight needle monofilament thread and to place any reinforcement sutures on the colorectal anastomosis.

The laparoscopic instruments used by the first assistant at the table are as follows:

- Grasping forceps (Johann forceps).
- Suction/irrigation system (Dolphin evo®).
- Fibrin glue (Tisseel® or Evicel®) applicator.

The latter is used for closure of the mesenteric defect.

Other instruments and devices are used as follows:

- Specimen extraction through a Pfannenstiel incision, preparation of the bowel for anastomosis, and temporary closure of the incision:
  - Scalpel (no. 11 blade).
  - Monopolar electric scalpel.
  - Anatomical tissue forceps.
  - Mathieu retractors.
  - Langenbeck retractors.
  - Wound protector/retractor.
  - Foerster forceps.
  - Curved Klemmer clamps.
  - Nelson-Metzenbaum dissection scissors.
  - 3-0 needle-free Vicryl® thread
  - A vial of ICG.
  - Purse-string forceps.
  - Needle holder.
  - Straight needle, double armed 2-0 polypropylene suture.
  - Curved enterostat.
  - Allis clamps.
  - Anvil of the circular stapler.
  - Straight Klemmer clamp (for grasping the anvil);
  - Laparoscopic bipolar forceps.
  - Laparotomy gauzes.
  - Straight enterostat.
- Performing mechanical colorectal anastomosis and placing a pelvic drain:
  - Circular stapler (EEA™ Circular Stapler with Tri-Staple™ Technology or ECHELON CIRCULAR™ Powered Stapler).
  - Straight Klemmer clamp.
  - Basin.
  - 0.9% sodium chloride solution dyed with methylene blue
  - A 100-ml syringe.
  - A prefilled syringe with lubricating gel.
  - Laparoscopic gauzes.
  - Scalpel (no. 11 blade) or monopolar electric scalpel.
  - Penrose drain.
  - Needle holder.
  - Anatomical forceps.
  - Silk suture.
  - Mayo scissors.

20.6.2 Intersphincteric Proctectomy with Coloanal Anastomosis

20.6.2.1 Abdominal Phase

The robotic instruments used by the surgeon at the surgical console are as follows:

- 30° robotic endoscope.
- Grasping forceps (Tip-Up Fenestrated Forceps®).
- Bipolar forceps (Fenestrated Force Bipolar Forceps®).
- Monopolar instrument (Permanent Cautery Hook®).
- Sealing instrument (Vessel Sealer® or Syncrosil®, 8 mm).
- Clip applier (Medium-Large Clip Applier® with Hem-o-lok® ligating clips).

The laparoscopic instruments used by the first assistant at the operating table are the following:

- Grasping forceps (Johann forceps).
- Suction/irrigation system (Dolphin evo®).

20.6.2.2 Pelvic Phase

The robotic instruments used by the surgeon at the surgical console are as follows:

- 30° robotic endoscope.
- Grasping forceps (TipUp Fenestrated Forceps®).
- Bipolar forceps (Force Fenestrated Bipolar Forceps®).
- Monopolar instrument (Permanent Cautery Hook® to perform enterotomy and gastrotomy.
- Sealing instrument (Vessel Sealer® or Syncrosil®, 8 mm).
- Needle holder with suture cutter (Large SutureCut™ Needle Driver®).

The laparoscopic instruments used by the first assistant at the table are as follows:

- Grasping forceps (Johann forceps).
- Suction/irrigation system (Dolphin evo®).
- Fibrin glue (Tisseel® or Evicel®) applicator.

Other instruments and devices are used as follows:

- Placement of a pelvic drain:
  - Scalpel (no. 11 blade) or monopolar electric scalpel.
  - Penrose drain.
  - Needle holder.
  - Anatomical forceps.
  - Silk suture.
  - Mayo scissors.
- If transabdominal extraction of the specimen is required, a Pfannenstiel incision is made, the descending colon is transected, and the incision is temporarily closed:
  - Scalpel (no. 11 blade).
  - Monopolar electric scalpel.
  - Anatomical tissue forceps.
  - Mathieu retractors.
  - Langenbeck retractors.
  - Wound protector/retractor.
  - Foerster forceps.
  - Curved Klemmer clamps.
  - Nelson-Metzenbaum dissection scissors.
  - 3-0 needle-free Vicryl® thread
  - Laparoscopic bipolar forceps.
  - A vial of ICG.
  - Laparoscopic linear stapler.
  - Laparotomy gauzes.
  - Straight enterostat.

20.6.2.3   Perineal Phase
- Lone Star Retractor System.
- Needle holder.
- Anatomical tissue forceps.
- Silk suture.
- Curved Kocher clamps.
- Monopolar electric scalpel.
- Bipolar forceps.
- Ultrasonic device (HARMONIC® 1100 Ultrasonic Shears).
- Mathieu retractors.
- Foerster forceps.
- Curved Klemmer clamps.

- Nelson-Metzenbaum dissection scissors.
- 3-0 needle-free Vicryl® thread
- Straight enterostat.
- Allis clamps.
- Scalpel (no. 11 blade).
- A vial of ICG.
- Infrared laparoscope.
- Absorbable sutures (3-0 Coated Vicryl™ Plus).
- Mayo scissors.

Instruments may vary if transabdominal extraction of the specimen has been performed.

20.6.3 Abdominoperineal Resection or Miles' Procedure

20.6.3.1   Abdominal Phase
The robotic instruments used by the surgeon at the surgical console are as follows:

- 30° robotic endoscope
- Grasping forceps (Tip-Up Fenestrated Forceps®).
- Bipolar forceps (Fenestrated Force Bipolar Forceps®).
- Monopolar instrument (Permanent Cautery Hook®).
- Sealing instrument (Vessel Sealer® or Syncrosil®, 8 mm).
- Clip applier (Medium-Large Clip Applier® with Hem-o-lok® ligating clips).

The laparoscopic instruments used by the first assistant at the operating table are the following:

- Grasping forceps (Johann forceps).
- Suction/irrigation system (Dolphin evo®).

20.6.3.2   Pelvic Phase
The robotic instruments used by the surgeon at the surgical console are as follows:

- 30° robotic endoscope
- Grasping forceps (TipUp Fenestrated Forceps®).

- Bipolar forceps (Force Fenestrated Bipolar Forceps®).
- Monopolar instrument (Permanent Cautery Hook®).
- Sealing instrument (Vessel Sealer® or Syncrosil®, 8 mm).
- Clip applier (Medium-Large Clip Applier® with Hem-o-lok® ligating clips).
- Linear stapler (SureForm™ Stapler®, 45 mm).

The laparoscopic instruments used by the first assistant at the table are as follows:

- Grasping forceps (Johann forceps).
- Suction/irrigation system (Dolphin evo®).

Other instruments and devices are used:

- A vial of ICG.
- Barbed 3-0 suture.
- Scalpel (no. 11 blade) or monopolar electric scalpel.
- Penrose drain.
- Needle holder.
- Anatomical tissue forceps.
- Silk suture.
- Mayo scissors.
- Dufour catheter.
- A saline-filled syringe.

A barbed suture is used to close the pelvic floor peritoneum. Alternatively, a Dufour catheter with saline-filled balloon is used to occupy the pelvis.

20.6.3.3 Perineal Phase
- Needle holder.
- Anatomical tissue forceps.
- Silk suture.
- Kocher clamps.
- Lone Star Retractor System.
- Monopolar electric scalpel.
- Ultrasonic device (HARMONIC® 1100 Ultrasonic Shears).
- Bipolar forceps.
- Mathieu retractors.
- Kocher retractors.
- Foerster forceps.

- Curved Klemmer clamps.
- Absorbable sutures (0 Coated Vicryl™ *Plus* with 1/2 circle needle; 3-0 Coated Vicryl™ *Plus*).
- Mayo scissors.
- Biosynthetic mesh (GORE® BIO-A® Tissue Reinforcement), if needed.
- Redon drain.
- Silk sutures.

20.6.4 Closure of Abdominal Incisions

- Laparoscopic bipolar forceps.
- Langenbeck retractors.
- Needle holder.
- Anatomical tissue forceps.
- Curved Klemmer forceps.
- Absorbable sutures (0 Coated Vicryl™ *Plus* with 5/8 circle needle; 3-0 Coated Vicryl™ Rapide).
- Mayo scissors.

Laparoscopic bipolar forceps are used to control or prevent bleeding from the port sites. Fascial closure is performed at the 12-mm port sites by using Langenbeck retractors and 0 absorbable sutures with 5/8 circle needle, while skin incisions are closed with 3-0 absorbable sutures.

20.6.5 Ileostomy or Colostomy

A loop ileostomy may be performed in the right flank/iliac fossa following anterior rectal resection or proctectomy with coloanal anastomosis, while an end colostomy is performed in the left flank/iliac fossa following abdominoperineal resection or Hartmann procedure. An ileal loop or the descending colon is extracted through an opening in the abdominal wall. After the abdominal incision IS closed, the ileostomy or colostomy is matured; the bowel lumen is opened, and the bowel wall is sutured to the skin.

The following instruments and devices are used:

- Straight Kocher forceps.
- Monopolar electric scalpel.
- Langenbeck retractors.
- Mathieu retractors.
- Anatomical tissue forceps.
- Curved Klemmer forceps.
- Nelson-Metzenbaum dissection scissors.
- Foerster forceps.
- Allis clamps.
- Laparoscopic bipolar forceps.
- Needle holder.
- Absorbable sutures (3-0 Coated Vicryl™).
- Mayo scissors.

End colostomy may also be performed using a circular stapler.

20.7 Intraoperative Complications

The most frequent intraoperative complications during a rectal resection are bleeding from vascular or spleen injuries, bowel tears, injury to the urinary tract (ureter, bladder, urethra), and issues with the colorectal anastomosis.

When bleeding occurs, the following instruments should be promptly available:

- Laparoscopic suction/irrigation system.
- Gauzes to be passed by the first assistant.
- Bipolar forceps (robotic and/or laparoscopic forceps).
- Robotic sealing instruments.
- Robotic clip applier with a clip already loaded.
- Laparoscopic grasping forceps (or vascular clamps).
- Robotic needle driver with small caliber sutures.
- Topical hemostatic agents (e.g., Floseal, Hemopatch).

Injuries to small vessels are usually controlled with a sealing instrument or bipolar forceps, while bleeding from larger vessels can be controlled with clip ligation or direct repair with nonabsorbable monofilament. Life-threatening hemorrhages due to injury to major vessels may require prompt conversion to open surgery and rarely reconstruction with patches.

Injuries to the urinary tract most frequently affect the ureter and occur by section, ligation, or thermal damage. Ureteral section is repaired by an end-to-end anastomosis with absorbable interrupted stitches, on the guide of a ureteral stent, while in the event of accidental ligation, the obstruction is removed, and a stent is placed. When a thermal damage is recognized intraoperatively, it can be treated by placing a stent. Bladder injuries are managed by closing the breach with absorbable sutures and leaving a urinary catheter in place. Injection of methylene blue dye, either intravenous or through a bladder catheter, may help in detecting ureteral and bladder injuries. Urethral lesions almost exclusively occur during the perineal phase of abdominoperineal resection in males and are repaired by direct suture or end-to-end anastomosis in the event of complete section.

Bowel tears are usually repaired by fine absorbable sutures, and only rarely resection of the affected bowel is required. Issues with colorectal anastomosis usually include a positive air leak test that indicates an anastomotic defect. This can be treated by a direct suture (either transabdominally or transanally) with absorbable threads, a derivative stoma (if not already performed), or a redo anastomosis (colorectal or coloanal).

References

1. Fleshman J, Birnbaum E, Hunt S, Mutch M, Kodner I, Safar B. Atlas of surgical techniques for colon, rectum and anus. St. Louis: Saunders Elsevier; 2012.
2. Wexner SD, Fleshman JW. Colon and rectal surgery: anorectal operations. 2nd ed. Lippincott Williams and Wilkins; 2018.
3. De Manzini N. Rectal cancer: strategy and surgical techniques. 1st ed. Milano: Springer Milano; 2013.
4. Formisano G, Marano A, Bianchi PP, Spinoglio G. Challenges with robotic low anterior resection. Minerva Chir. 2015;70(5):341–54.
5. Crippa J, Grass F, Dozois EJ, Mathis KL, Merchea A, Colibaseanu DT, et al. Robotic surgery for rectal cancer provides advantageous outcomes over laparoscopic approach: results from a large retrospective cohort. Ann Surg. 2021;274(6):e1218–22.

6. Grass JK, Chen CC, Melling N, Lingala B, Kemper M, Scognamiglio P, et al. Robotic rectal resection preserves anorectal function: systematic review and meta-analysis. Int J Med Robot. 2021;17(6):e2329.
7. Mykoniatis I, Siddiqi NN, Khan JS. Robotic low anterior resection. Dis Colon Rectum. 2021;64(2):e32–3.
8. Moghadamyeghaneh Z, Phelan M, Smith BR, Stamos MJ. Outcomes of open, laparoscopic, and robotic abdominoperineal resections in patients with rectal cancer. Dis Colon Rectum. 2015;58(12):1123–9.

Laparoscopic Transanal Treatment of Rectal Tumours

21

Antonino Spinelli and Francesca Di Candido

Natural orifice transluminal endoscopic surgery (NOTES) represents one of the most significant surgical innovations since the introduction of laparoscopy. Parks first described in 1966 the first transanal submucosal excision of a rectal lesion. Transanal endoscopic microsurgery (TEM) was first introduced in 1983 to perform endoluminal local excision of rectal lesions through a closed multiport system, using high-definition visualization, carbon dioxide (CO_2) insufflation, and adapted instrumentation [1–4]. TEM platform was subsequently adapted for conventional laparoscopy although the high costs and steep-learning curve gradually reduced its use. Whiteford et al. first performed a natural orifice transanal endoscopic rectosigmoid resection in a human cadaver, followed by Atallah and colleagues who demonstrated the feasibility and safety of transanal minimally invasive surgery (TAMIS) [5–10]. The transanal approach significantly reduces the potential morbidity associated with abdominal laparoscopic approach (such as impaired urinary and sexual function, rate of permanent

stoma and need for conversion to open approach) without compromising oncological outcomes. Moreover, total mesorectal excision (TME) is a technically demanding procedure which can be significantly influenced by the anatomy of the patient, tumour characteristics, and previous neo-adjuvant therapy. Therefore, transanal TME (taTME) increases the quality of abdominal TME and the fulfilment of a complete mesorectal excision with negative circumferential margins. According to both the National Comprehensive Cancer Network (NCCN) and American Society of Colon and Rectal Surgeons (ASCRS) practice guidelines, transanal local excision, either directly or via a minimally invasive approach, is indicated as curative procedure for early-stage and low-risk T1N0 rectal cancer. Criteria for low risk include tumour size <3 cm, well- to moderately differentiated lesion, location within 8 cm from the anal verge, involvement <30% of the rectal circumference, and the absence of nodal involvement [11–15]. Local excision can also be considered for palliation in patients who are poor candidates for surgery. TME remains the gold-standard surgical approach in combination with neoadjuvant therapy for locally advanced stage II and III rectal cancer [11–15].

Here, we will discuss the two main laparoscopic transanal procedures for rectal lesions: TAMIS and taTME.

A. Spinelli (✉)
Department of Biomedical Sciences, Humanitas University, Milan, Italy

Division of Colon and Rectal Surgery, IRCCS Humanitas Research Hospital, Milan, Italy
e-mail: antonino.spinelli@hunimed.it

F. Di Candido
General Surgery Unit, Ospedale per gli Infermi—AUSL Romagna, Faenza, Ravenna, Italy

© The Author(s), under exclusive license to Springer Nature Switzerland AG 2024
M. Milone et al. (eds.), *Scrub Nurse in Minimally Invasive and Robotic General Surgery*,
https://doi.org/10.1007/978-3-031-42257-7_21

21.1 Transanal Minimally Invasive Surgery (TAMIS)

Transanal minimally invasive surgery (TAMIS) was developed as a hybrid between TEM and Single Incision Laparoscopic Surgery (SILS) by Atallah in 2010. This technique offers a 360-degree view and allows for more distal rectal lesions whose excision is not feasible through TEM platform. TAMIS is performed using direct visualization of the lesion and significantly improved visualization of all lesions within the rectum by using traditional laparoscopic equipment.

21.1.1 Pre-operative Phase and Patient Positioning

All patients should be prepared by standard protocols for colorectal surgery, although there are differences in the details of pre-surgical preparation. Pre-operative bowel preparation is required, but the type depends on the surgeon's preference. The most commonly performed preparation is complete mechanical bowel preparation; however, distal bowel preparation through enemas is also performed. Pre-operative stoma siting should be addressed in the preassessment clinic in the case of unforeseen operative or technical events. Deep vein thrombosis (DVT) is a major complication after colorectal cancer surgery; therefore, prophylaxis with low-molecular-weight heparin is commonly used. Patient is administered general endotracheal anaesthesia with pharmacologic paralysis to decrease bowel movement and reduce discomfort due to gas insufflation during the procedure. Spinal anaesthesia has been evaluated as adequate for TAMIS only in one study and therefore is not a routine procedure. A second-generation cephalosporin and metronidazole are administered parenterally 30 min before incision. Surgery is performed in dorsal lithotomy position, regardless of the location of the lesion. Prone jack-knife could be considered for anteriorly located lesions, as well as lateral decubitus position. Arms should be adducted along the body. The operating table is prepared with a sliding prevent mat (Pink Pad®), or, in its absence, with a leg fixing with bandages to prevent the patient from falling from the operating table.

21.1.2 Operating Theatre Setting

The operating theatre setting for TAMIS procedure is performed as follows:

- Operating table in the centre of the theatre.
- Laparoscopic tower positioned to the right of the patient.
- Screen positioned at the head of the operating table.
- Surgeon positioned between the patient's legs and first assistant on his/her left.
- Scrub nurse behind and on the right of the surgeon.
- Serving cart to the right of instrument nurse.

21.1.3 Surgical Equipment

The GelPOINT Path™ (Applied Medical, Rancho Santa Margarita, CA) and SILS Port™ (Covidien, Mansfield, MA) are the most used surgical devices for transanal access in TAMIS, which are placed transanally with a designated channel to provide gas insufflation for pneumorectum. The GelPOINT Path™ is equipped with an access channel that allows enhanced exposure and suture ties to fix the correct position, a cap to provide triangulation of laparoscopic instrumentation, and self-retaining sleeves to accommodate standard and angled instrumentation (Fig. 21.1).

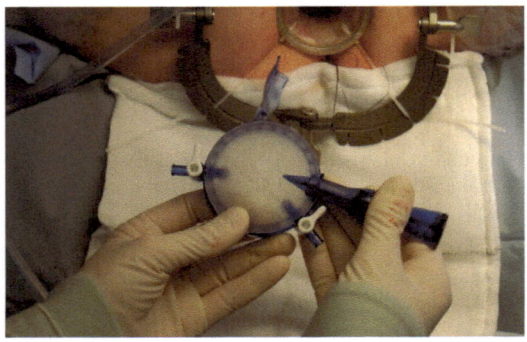

Fig. 21.1 GelPOINT™ path set-up

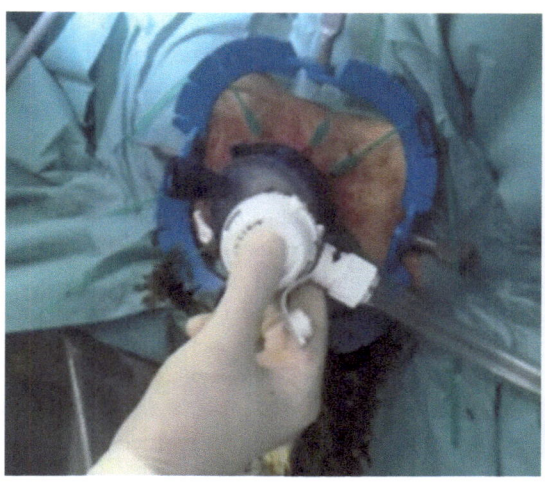 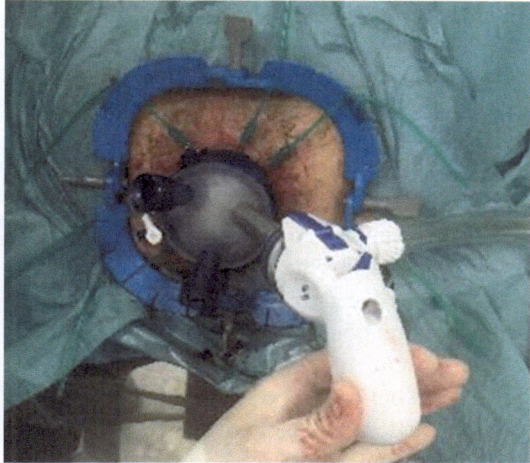

Fig. 21.2 GelPOINT Path™ and AirSeal Insufflation System™

Two ports plus AirSeal are inserted in the platform as far as possible, one to each other, to facilitate triangulation using Applied triangle. Pneumorectum is maintained with CO_2 insufflation with flow set to 40 L/min and pressure set to >15 mmHg (range, 8–20 mmHg). Alternatively, a valveless trocar system (AirSeal Insufflation System™, ConMed, Inc. Utica, NY) provides smoke evacuation and high flow (Fig. 21.2).

A 30-degree 10 mm laparoscope is required to provide optimal visualization during dissection which can be performed through a hook-monopolar electrocautery or advanced bipolar energy devices, according to the surgeon's preference. This apparatus can be connected to a standard suction irrigator to reduce free fluid and smoke during the procedure. Laparoscopic standard instruments, such as grasping forceps (Croce-Olmi forceps, Maryland graspers, or Johann forceps), may be used for retraction. Once dissection is completed, the defect could be closed through an interrupted suture with knot-tying facilitated by laparoscopic knot pushers or, alternatively, continuous V-Loc™ (Covidien, Mansfield, MA) 3-0 absorbable suture using standard needle holders. Laparoscopic suture clips or linear staplers can also be used for large rectal wall defects although there is a relevant risk of rectal stenosis or stricture; therefore, its use depends on the surgeon's preference.

21.1.4 Surgical Steps

Benign lesions can be resected in the submucosal plane with negative resection margins of at least 5 mm. In submucosal dissection procedures, the submucosal plane is elevated by injection of adrenaline/mannitol/blue dye, and dissection is conducted by monopolar hook diathermy on the muscularis propria layer. Full-thickness excision of malignant lesions should be performed with the aim of achieving a 1-cm clear margin and no fragmentation. Pudendal nerve block (lidocaine 1% or bupivacaine 0.25% solution with adrenaline 20 ml) can further relax the sphincter muscle and offers additional analgesia up to 12 h postoperatively. After a dilating digital rectal examination, the GelPOINT Path™ device equipped with ports is gently inserted and fixed, and then the insufflator unit is turned on.

The margin of clearance should be clearly defined with coagulation dots all around the lesion. The dissection may be started from the proximal margin first or in a distal-to-proximal manner, minimizing any errors in orientation. The device should remain perpendicular to the tumour to not compromise deep margins and avoid coning in on the specimen. After the specimen has been extracted, the wound bed should be washed with a suction irrigation device and accurate haemostasis should be ensured.

For benign lesions, submucosal resection can be laid open, whereas full-thickness resection defects should be closed to achieve a watertight closure, if possible. Selected cases, such as resection of posterior rectal lesion, can be left open although this matter is still controversial. Both running and interrupted techniques can be used, typically using an absorbable suture, as previously said. During the closure, the endoluminal pressure is reduced to 10–12 mmHg to allow tissue approximation.

The specimen should be handled with care and pinned out on a rigid support to preserve orientation and relationship between the normal margin and tumour.

21.1.5 Intraoperative Complications

The most common complications during TAMIS are bleeding and peritoneal violation. Intraoperative bleeding is associated with larger tumour size. Bleeding may occur in case of too deep dissection into the perirectal fat or mesorectum which contains large vessels. The bleeding point can be successfully controlled by compression with the tip of an instrument and then grasped with a forceps and coagulated. Peritoneal violation is associated with the anterior and lateral location of the lesion. The defect should be closed as soon as possible because of the loss of the pneumorectum. If there is a suspicion of faecal soiling in the abdominal cavity, peritoneal lavage should be considered with concomitant leak test for the closure site.

21.2 Transanal Total Mesorectal Excision (TaTME)

Achieving a complete mesorectal excision is crucial in rectal cancer surgery and significantly impacts oncological outcomes. Operating in the deep pelvis is significantly challenging and minimally invasive techniques have reliably overcome these difficulties. However, transabdominal approach is associated with relevant potential morbidities and risk of conversion to an open approach, especially when not performed in high-volume centres. Furthermore, the need for multiple firings of linear stapling devices in low rectal division has been associated with an increase in the surgical morbidity of the procedure. The transanal approach to TME was conceived to overcome anatomical challenges in rectal surgery and was first performed by Sylla et al. in 2010 after several iterations in animal models. TaTME can be performed for both benign and malignant lesions where accurate dissection of the mid-rectum and low rectum is required and when failure to proceed through transabdominal approach occurs. Conditions in which TaTME can be considered the preferred procedures include:

- Male sex.
- Rectal cancer with distance from the anal verge <12 cm.
- Marrow and deep pelvis.
- BMI >30 kg/m^2 and visceral obesity.
- Neoadjuvant therapy.
- Prostate hypertrophy.
- Impalpable low primary tumour.
- Tumour diameter > 4 cm.

Subsequently, indications have been expanded to other fields, such as proctectomy for inflammatory bowel disease (IBD) and management of chronic pelvic sepsis. Technical challenges of the transanal approach are partly due to the unfamiliar view of the anatomy from below which increases difficulty in identifying correct tissue planes. Moreover, several reports of urethral injuries that occurred during the procedure have highlighted the importance of optimal training prior to embarking on this technique in order to promote its safe implementation. The TaTME approach allows a more precise definition of the distal resection margin, bottom-up dissection, and end-to-end anastomosis without the need for multiple firings of a linear stapler. The surgery may be started transabdominally, transanally, or simultaneously with double surgical teams (Cecil approach) according to the surgeons' preferences and available resources.

21.2.1 Pre-operative Phase and Patient Positioning

Oral antibiotics plus mechanical bowel preparation should be administered in all patients. Potential stoma sites are marked the day before surgery. Intravenous antibiotic prophylaxis is injected 30 min before skin incision according to the same protocol used for TAMIS. Low-molecular-weight heparin is administered in prophylactic doses to avoid DVT. General endotracheal anaesthesia should be administered with deep neuromuscular blockage to achieve appropriate rectal distension and maintain adequate pneumoperitoneum. A urinary catheter should be inserted, and a rectal enema with diluted iodine solution should be performed. Patient is placed in the modified-lithotomy position with adjustable stirrups and in a steep-Trendelenburg position. As for TAMIS procedure, the operating table should be provided with a sliding prevent mat (Pink Pad®).

21.2.2 Operating Theatre Setting

The operating theatre setting for TaTME procedure is performed as follows (teams for Cecil approach):

- Operating table in the centre of the theatre.
- Laparoscopic tower positioned to the right of the patient.
- Two screens: one for the abdominal team positioned to the left of the patient and one for the transanal team positioned at the head of the patient.
- Abdominal team: surgeon and first assistant on the right of the patient and second assistant on the left of the patient.
- Transanal team: surgeon positioned between the patient's legs and first assistant on his/her left.
- Two scrub nurses who both stand on the right of each surgeon.
- Two serving carts to the right of instrument nurses.

21.2.3 Surgical Equipment

Self-retaining anal retractors (Lonestar™, Cooper Surgical, Trumbull, CT, USA) and anal dilators are used to introduce the transanal platform minimizing trauma (Fig. 21.3). The GelPOINT Path™ is the most used device for transanal access also when TaTME is performed. The set-up of the device, the position of the ports and gas pressure to maintain pneumorectum through AirSeal Insufflation System™ are the same as those used for TAMIS (Fig. 21.3).

A 30-degree 10 mm laparoscope is required to provide adequate visualization. A 0-polypropylene suture with a 26-mm rounded needle is used to construct a purse-string closure of the rectal lumen distal to the tumour. The rectal stump should be washed with iodine solution during the closure of the purse-string. The transection of the rectal wall may be performed with a monopolar hook, whereas laparoscopic standard instru-

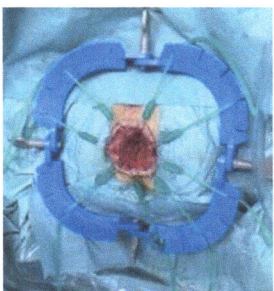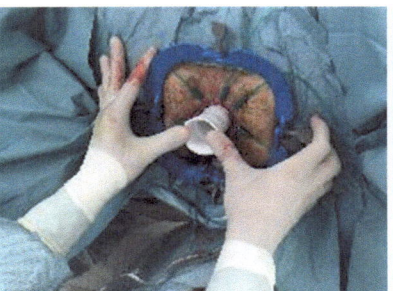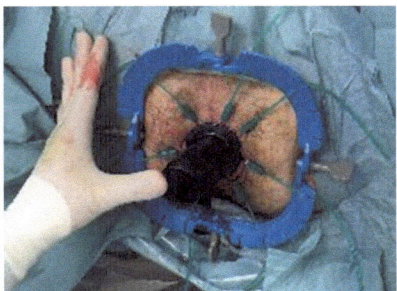

Fig. 21.3 Lonestar™ positioning and anal dilatation

ments, such as grasping forceps (Croce-Olmi forceps, Maryland graspers or Johann forceps), may be used for retraction. Before communication of both fields, a second purse-string is made with 2-0 polydioxanone in the free open edge of the distal stump. At the end of the procedure, a hand-sewn coloanal or a stapled side-to-end or end-to-end anastomosis may be performed. For the stapled technique, the anvil is inserted inside the proximal colon by the abdominal team and a silastic tube is required to ease the manipulation of the anvil and reach the anus. Alternatively, the anvil may be inserted by the transanal team. Several staplers with different diameter may be used, although the most common is a 31-mm Autosuture EEA™ haemorrhoid and prolapse DST series stapler (Medtronic, Minneapolis, MN). The platform may be reinserted to verify completeness of the anastomosis. Additional stitches may be required if a leak is found. For the end-to-end hand-sewn technique, anastomosis is performed with simple stitches of 3-0 polyglycolic acid.

21.2.4 Surgical Steps

The anus is opened using Lonestar™ anal retractor, so the dentate line is clearly viewed. Pudendal nerve block may be performed as before TAMIS to increase sphincter relaxation. After a careful anal dilatation, the GelPOINT Path™ platform is inserted and secured in the right position with two stitches. Distal sigmoid colon should be temporarily clamped by the abdominal team, and then pneumorectum is initiated for a target pressure of 12–15 mmHg. The transanal team performs a purse-string suture to close the rectal lumen distal to the tumour. This suture should be located at the same distance from the device in the entire circumference, with equal depth in every bite, avoiding incorporating surrounding structures such as the vagina. The purse-string is generally started in the anterior wall and continued clockwise until complete closure. During and after the closure, the rectal stump should be flushed with iodine solution to wash out any malignant cells (Fig. 21.4).

Once the purse-string is made, both teams may start working simultaneously. Transanal pressure must be higher than abdominal pressure until the "rendez-vous" phase (the moment when abdominal and transanal team reach the peritoneal reflection) to maintain adequate rectal distention.

The dissection line is marked by tattooing the rectal mucosa with an electric hook distal to the mucosal folds. Full-thickness rectal transection is performed in a progressive and circumferential manner, avoiding a cone shape to ensure the completeness of the mesorectum. A second purse-string is performed in the free open edge of the distal stump when proximity to the abdominal team is perceived. This suture will be tied to the stapler rod when performing the anastomosis. Once the "rendez-vous" moment has been

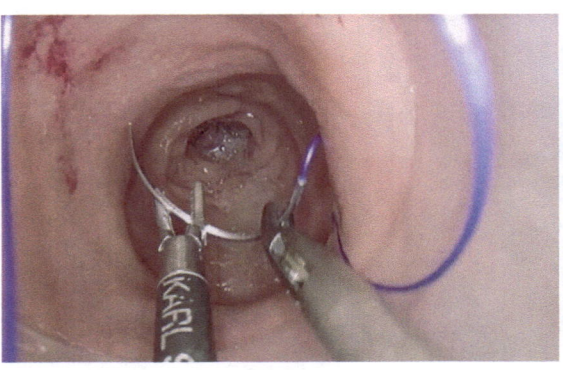 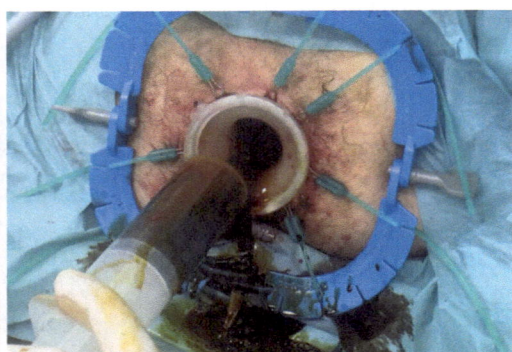

Fig. 21.4 Purse-string creation and rectal wash-out

reached, the two teams continue working together until colon and rectum are completely free. The specimen may be extracted transabdominally through a Pfannenstiel incision, or transanally, except in cases of bulky tumours or narrow pelvis.

The anastomotic configuration depends on the tumour distance from the anal verge and the resulting stump length. If the end-to-end stapled technique is preferred, the anvil is inserted in the proximal colon, extracted through the anus, then the distal purse-string suture is closed and tied to the rod of the circular stapler. The anvil and rod of the circular stapler are connected, and the stapler is fired. If the end-to-end hand-sewn technique is preferred, a colotomy should be created in the antimesenteric border of the proximal colon, and then four stitches are made to the rectal stump and passed through the colon. Colon is descended in the pelvis without tension or twisting and anastomosis is completed with simple stitches. The completeness of the anastomosis should be verified through air-leak test.

21.2.5 Intraoperative Complications

The most common intraoperative event during TaTME is failure of the purse-string with leakage, requiring a repeated purse-string. If rectal dissection is performed too widely on the pelvic side wall, serious injuries to the hypogastric nerves might occur, as well as urethral, bladder, and vaginal injuries, and rectal perforation, which all require proper treatment. Dissecting too posteriorly will result in the dissection being behind the presacral fascia with a significant risk of bleeding from presacral veins requiring quick and effective haemostasis. Laparoscopic suction/irrigation system, endoscopic clip applier with titanium clips, Hem-o-lok applier with clips loaded, and laparoscopic vascular clamps should be available. A needle holder with proper suture should be provided to repair bleeding vessels (when visible) or parenchymatous organs.

References

1. Parks AG. Benign tumours of the rectum. In: Rob C, Smith R, Morgan CN, editors. Abdomen and rectum and anus, Operative surgery, vol. 10. London, Butterworths; 1966. p. 541–8.
2. Buess G, Theiss R, Hutterer F, Pichlmaier H, Pelz C, Holfeld T, Said S, Isselhard W. Die transanale endoskopische Rektumoperation—Erprobung einer neuen Methode im Tierversuch [Transanal endoscopic surgery of the rectum—testing a new method in animal experiments]. Leber Magen Darm. 1983;13(2):73–7.
3. Whiteford MH, Denk PM, Swanström LL. Feasibility of radical sigmoid colectomy performed as natural orifice translumenal endoscopic surgery (NOTES) using transanal endoscopic microsurgery. Surg Endosc. 2007;21(10):1870–4. https://doi.org/10.1007/s00464-007-9552-x.
4. Atallah S, Albert M, Larach S. Transanal minimally invasive surgery: a giant leap forward. Surg Endosc. 2010;24:2200–5.
5. Benson AB, Venook AP, Al-Hawary MM, Cederquist L, Chen YJ, Ciombor KK, Cohen S, Cooper HS, Deming D, Engstrom PF, Grem JL, Grothey A, Hochster HS, Hoffe S, Hunt S, Kamel A, Kirilcuk N, Krishnamurthi S, Messersmith WA, Meyerhardt J, Mulcahy MF, Murphy JD, Nurkin S, Saltz L, Sharma S, Shibata D, Skibber JM, Sofocleous CT, Stoffel EM, Stotsky-Himelfarb E, Willett CG, Wuthrick E, Gregory KM, Gurski L, Freedman-Cass DA. Rectal cancer, version 2.2018, NCCN Clinical Practice Guidelines in Oncology. J Natl Compr Canc Netw. 2018;16(7):874–901. https://doi.org/10.6004/jnccn.2018.0061.
6. You YN, Hardiman KM, Bafford A, Poylin V, Francone TD, Davis K, Paquette IM, Steele SR, Feingold DL, On Behalf of the Clinical Practice Guidelines Committee of the American Society of Colon and Rectal Surgeons. The American Society of Colon and Rectal Surgeons Clinical Practice Guidelines for the management of rectal cancer. Dis Colon Rectum. 2020;63(9):1191–222. https://doi.org/10.1097/DCR.0000000000001762.
7. Atallah S, Albert M, Larach S. Transanal minimally invasive surgery: a giant leap forward. Surg Endosc. 2010;24(9):2200–5. https://doi.org/10.1007/s00464-010-0927-z.
8. Lee TG, Lee SJ. Transanal single-port microsurgery for rectal tumors: minimal invasive surgery under spinal anesthesia. Surg Endosc. 2014;28(1):271–80. https://doi.org/10.1007/s00464-013-3184-0.
9. Keller DS, Tahilramani RN, Flores-Gonzalez JR, et al. Transanal minimally invasive surgery: review of indications and outcomes from 75 consecutive patients. J Am Coll Surg. 2016;222(5):814–22.

10. Motson RW, Whiteford MH, Hompes R, Albert M, Miles WF, Expert Group. Current status of transanal total mesorectal excision (TaTME) following the Second International Consensus Conference. Color Dis. 2016;18(1):13–8. https://doi.org/10.1111/codi.13131.

11. Ito M, Sugito M, Kobayashi A, Nishizawa Y, Tsunoda Y, Saito N. Relationship between multiple numbers of stapler firings during rectal division and anastomotic leakage after laparoscopic rectal resection. Int J Color Dis. 2008;23(7):703–7. https://doi.org/10.1007/s00384-008-0470-8.

12. Sylla P, Rattner DW, Delgado S, Lacy AM. NOTES transanal rectal cancer resection using transanal endoscopic microsurgery and laparoscopic assistance. Surg Endosc. 2010;24(5):1205–10. https://doi.org/10.1007/s00464-010-0965-6.

13. Francis N, Penna M, Mackenzie H, Carter F, Hompes R, International TaTME Educational Collaborative Group. Consensus on structured training curriculum for transanal total mesorectal excision (TaTME). Surg Endosc. 2017;31(7):2711–9. https://doi.org/10.1007/s00464-017-5562-5.

14. Arroyave MC, DeLacy FB, Lacy AM. Transanal total mesorectal excision (TaTME) for rectal cancer: step by step description of the surgical technique for a two-teams approach. Eur J Surg Oncol. 2017;43(2):502–5. https://doi.org/10.1016/j.ejso.2016.10.024.

15. Penna M, Hompes R, Arnold S, Wynn G, Austin R, Warusavitarne J, Moran B, Hanna GB, Mortensen NJ, Tekkis PP, TaTME Registry Collaborative. Transanal total mesorectal excision: International Registry Results of the first 720 cases. Ann Surg. 2017;266(1):111–7. https://doi.org/10.1097/SLA.0000000000001948.

Robotic Transanal Treatment of Rectal Tumours

22

Alberto Arezzo, Filippo Pepe, and Mario Morino

22.1 Clinical Need and Indication for Transanal Surgery

There is no such field in oncological surgery where technological, minimally invasive, and robotic innovations are as meaningful as that of rectal cancer. The whole history of its treatment could be summarised as research towards a less-invasive and more organ-preserving strategy maintaining the same oncological results of traditional treatment. Indeed, the gold standard treatments of rectal cancer, the anterior rectal resection with Transanal Mesorectal Excision (TME), and Abdominal Perineal Resection (APR), despite their laparoscopic or robotic-assisted feasibility, are still burdened by high morbidity outcomes. The main complications include faecal and urinary incontinence, the need for an ostomy and sexual dysfunctions, among others [1].

For a long time, transanal local excision seemed appropriate for benign anorectal polyps up to high-grade dysplasia as there were many doubts concerning a high risk of local recurrence for anorectal cancer. Recently, the application was enlarged to pT1 sm 1 tumours as a curative solution due to their low probability of spreading [2, 3].

Lately, there is always more evidence that local excision of higher grade rectal cancer in selected patients who underwent neoadjuvant chemo- and radiotherapy (nCRT) did not increase the risk of local recurrences and distant metastasis. As shown in PARTTLE and GRECCAR 2 trials, among others, the current nCRT protocols could lead to an excellent local response that, when achieved, would allow local excision to achieve the same oncological results as the traditional surgery, even in T2N0 rectal cancer [4, 5].

Implementing transanal excision to the detriment of abdominal procedures for rectal cancer, if oncologically safe, would increase patients' compliance and quality of life and could even reduce their management's direct or indirect cost.

Luckily, many countries around the world are increasing screening programmes for colorectal disease, which has led to an increase in benign polyps and early rectal cancer diagnoses.

All the above reasons led to the clinical urgency to implement the local excision indication and technical feasibility.

Alberto Arezzo and Filippo Pepe contributed equally to this work.

A. Arezzo (✉) · F. Pepe · M. Morino
Department of Surgical Sciences, University of Turin, Torino, Italy
e-mail: alberto.arezzo@unito.it;
Filippo.pepe@unito.it

22.2 From Transanal Excision to Transanal Endoscopic Microsurgery (TEM) to Transanal Minimally Invasive Surgery (TAMIS)

Up to 1983, when Professor Gerard Buess presented his studies about TEM (Transanal Endoscopic Microsurgery), only a few transanal local excisions were performed, given the limited visibility and reach provided by conventional instruments [6].

Conventional transanal excision was limited to small-size tumours (<4 cm), involving less than 50% of the bowel circumference within 6–8 cm from the anal margin.

The TEM platform (manufactured by Richard Wolf GmbH, Knittlingen, Germany) and the similar TEO (Transanal Endoscopic Operation manufactured by Karl Storz, Tuttlingen, Germany) for the first time offered the possibility of extending the local excision even to larger lesions up to 20 cm from the anal margin, performing the procedure under magnified vision exponentially improving the surgical precision.

TEM (Fig. 22.1) and TEO (Fig. 22.2) are rigid platforms that make possible the transanal introduction of digital videoscope, laparoscopic-type surgical instrument and, above all, the insufflation of CO_2 to achieve an operative pneumo-rectum.

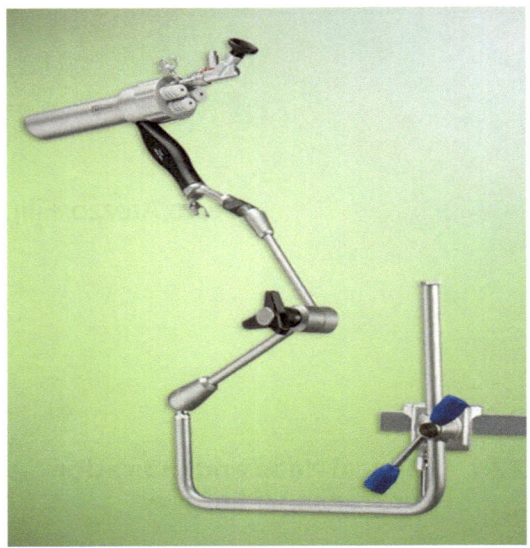

Fig. 22.2 TEO platform

They are composed of a rigid steel rectoscope with a diameter of 4 cm and a length of 7, 15, or 20 cm. It has an articulated arm that can be fixed to the operating table. The distal tip of the rectoscope is bevelled downward to simplify operating on lesions in a dependent position, even if a straight version is available according to the surgeon's preferences. The setup could be complex, especially when first performed, and could take up to 20 min by an unexpert surgeon, but thanks to the anchoring system, no assistants are required for the procedure [7].

However, despite 40 years having passed since their introduction and although there has been an increase in indications for local excision, their diffusion struggles to take hold due to the long learning curve of the procedure, a lack of dexterity in surgical movement (a triangulation of the instruments is unachievable), and the need for expensive specialised devices.

TAMIS was introduced to overcome this in 2009, adapting a port usually used for Single Incision Laparoscopic Surgery (SILS). TAMIS is based on using SILS ™ ports (Covidien, Mansfield, MA, USA) "hooked" onto the anorectal ring to maintain the pneumo-rectum and transanally introduce standard laparoscopic instruments (Fig. 22.3). TAMIS ports are more

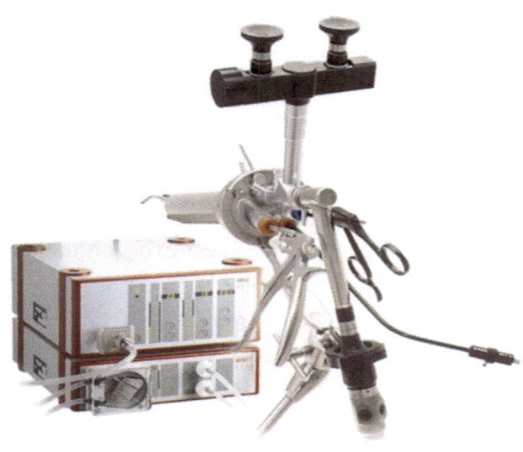

Fig. 22.1 TEM platform

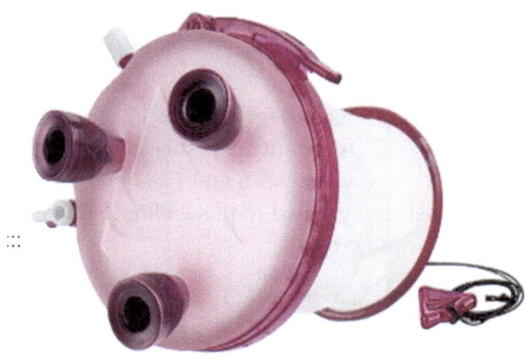

Fig. 22.3 SILS port for TAMIS

flexible than TEM/TEO and make the usage of more familiar tools possible. It takes a medium setup time of 5 min. Still, it requires the presence of an assistant steering the videoscope. Even if it allows achieving a higher degree of freedom, it fails to overcome the technical limitations of the previous technology. Some trials show that suturing large residual parietal defects after full-thickness excision is more technically challenging and time demanding with TAMIS compared to TEM. TAMIS also has some technical limitations due to the lack of a rigid structure that only allows the excision of lesions between 3 and 12 cm from the anal verge.

Unfortunately, it is known that the results with TEM/TEO and TAMIS depend very much on the surgeon's experience. While the excision can be achieved safely, the procedures remain technically challenging [8].

22.3 Road Towards a Robotic Transanal Surgery

The introduction of TAMIS marked a key point for the future of transanal surgery. Although it has failed in its primary purpose by not proving itself superior to already existing technologies, it has awakened interest in the field of transanal surgery.

The narrow spaces typical of this surgery and the limitations of previous technologies seem to be the perfect field for introducing robotic platforms to improve surgical precision, simplify the

most complex surgical gesture and reach more and more distal lesions from the anal verge.

For that reason, starting in the 2010s, the existing robotic platforms began to be used in transanal surgery, leading the way to the birth of entirely new and dedicated technologies beginning in the 2020s [9].

22.3.1 Da Vinci Single-Port (SP) Robotic Platform and SP rTAMIS

A few years after the introduction of TAMIS, attempts were made to apply the existing robotic technology of da Vinci Si. Still, the dimension of the platform and the multiport-designed arms did not apply well when working in the narrow space of transanal surgery.

It was only in 2018 that the da Vinci Single-Port (SP) robotic platform (Intuitive Surgical, Sunnyvale, CA, USA), a flexible system initially designed for single-port surgery, was introduced [10, 11, 12].

The da Vinci SP is composed of a remote console and a display similar to the existing da Vinci XI and a single C-Shape arm with a single robotic port of 25 mm in diameter (Fig. 22.4). The single-port arm has four built-in operative channels allowing the introduction of a 3D digital camera and three other instruments. The instruments are composed of two joints: an elbow joint that opens in the cavity, making an angle to maintain triangulation and a wrist joint with 7 DoF (Fig. 22.5). The system has the possibility of making a 360 rotation of all the instruments and the camera, allowing more freedom of vision in narrow space.

Those features make the platform a fantastic piece of technology theoretically applicable in endoluminal surgery, and since its introduction, trials have been made to test that. The application of da Vinci SP using Gel port for its introduction through the anorectum marked the born of SP rTAMIS. The main advantages of this platform are the increasing precision in the dissection and the increased dexterity in suturing due to the tridimensional view and the wrist motion of the instrument. According to some authors, the con-

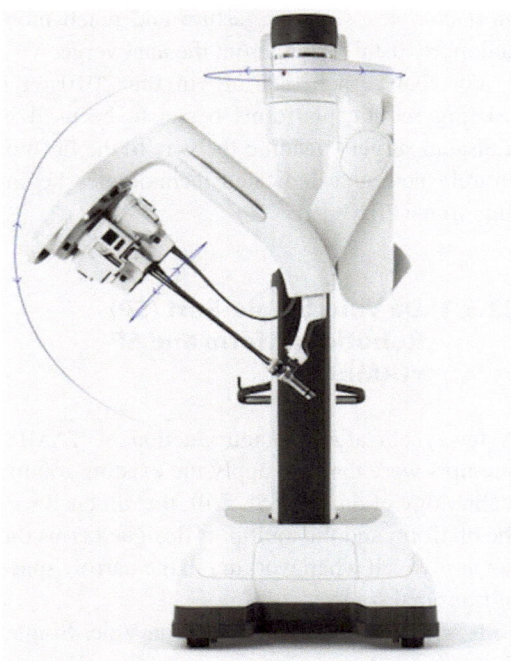

Fig. 22.4 DaVinci SP platform

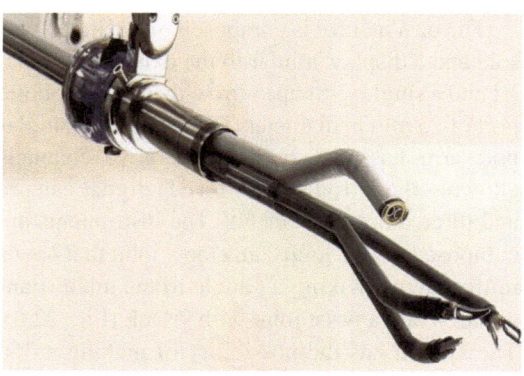

Fig. 22.5 The DaVinci SP operative channel and instruments

trol system is intuitive, and docking time seems to be short (5–8 min). The main disadvantages of the platform are related to the fact that the platform was initially designed for single-port surgery and not the endoluminal application. The fundamental elbow joint requires too much space

to "open up" the elbow joints inside a narrow space like the anorectum leading to multiple collisions of the instrument.

Some years have passed since the first trials described the feasibility of this platform for transanal surgery, and still, no FDA or CE certification has been granted to this technology.

22.3.2 The Flex Robotic System (Medrobotics, Raynham, Massachusetts, USA)

Initially designed for oral endoluminal surgery, the Medrobotics Flex robotic is the first system available on the market, with complete FDA and CE certification obtained in 2017 (Fig. 22.6).

The system is composed of a robotic endoscope and some flexible mechanical instruments with 5–6 DoF (Fig. 22.7). The system utilises a highly articulated multi-linked endoscope that can be piloted through natural endoluminal orifices until the lesion is reached. Then the scope can become rigid to establish a stable surgical platform that allows the insertion of flexible mechanical instruments through two 3.5 mm operating ports for dissecting and suturing. The system includes an insufflation system to establish the pneumo-rectum and an operational console with haptic controllers, joystick type, and a magnified 3D HD display to give surgeons a clear view of the navigation path and surgical site. The first results of this technology are encouraging. The currently existing platform is composed of a 17-cm long endoscope that is also the distal limit of the lesion that can be reached, but the project aims to reach lesions above the recto-sigmoid junction. A new platform version with a 35-cm long scope and instruments is currently being tested. Subsequent goals of a complete robotic platform, even regarding the instrument, are currently on standby due to the economic world crisis due to the Sars-Cov2 worldwide situation [13].

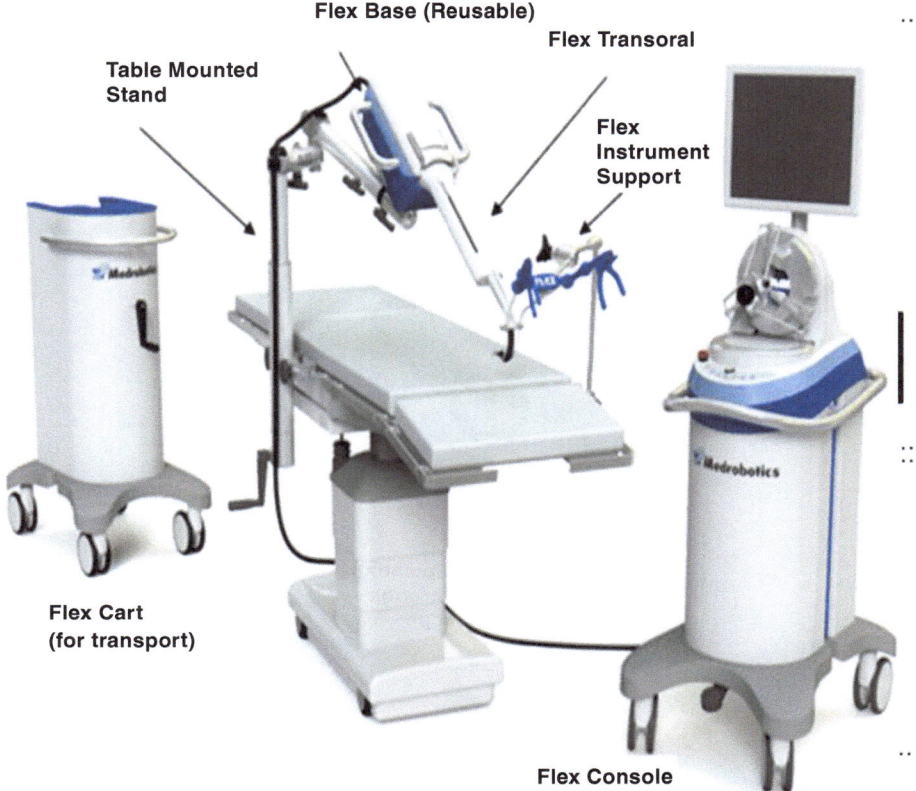

Fig. 22.6 The flex robotic system

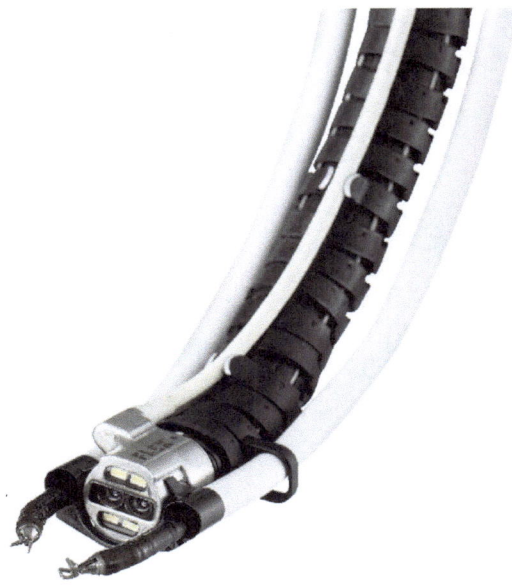

Fig. 22.7 The robotic endoscope of the flex robotics system

22.3.3 EndoLuminal Surgical System (ELS) by ColubrisMX (Houston, TX, USA)

EndoLuminal Surgical System by Colubris (Fig. 22.8) instead is based on a specularly opposite technology to the Flex Robotic. The platform is designed explicitly for transanal surgery, with the potential to reach targets that range 55 cm from the anal verge and potentially further.

It is composed of a surgical console and a bedside operating platform that can be attached to a specific overtube called the Colubriscope. The Colubriscope is a 22 mm flexible overtube with six operative channels composed of a 6 mm mechanical videoscope channel, two 6 mm channels for fully robotic instruments, a 3 mm operative channel for the bedside assistant and two 3 mm insufflation channels. The surgical platform is composed of a double joystick controller

Fig. 22.8 EndoLuminal surgical system by Colubris

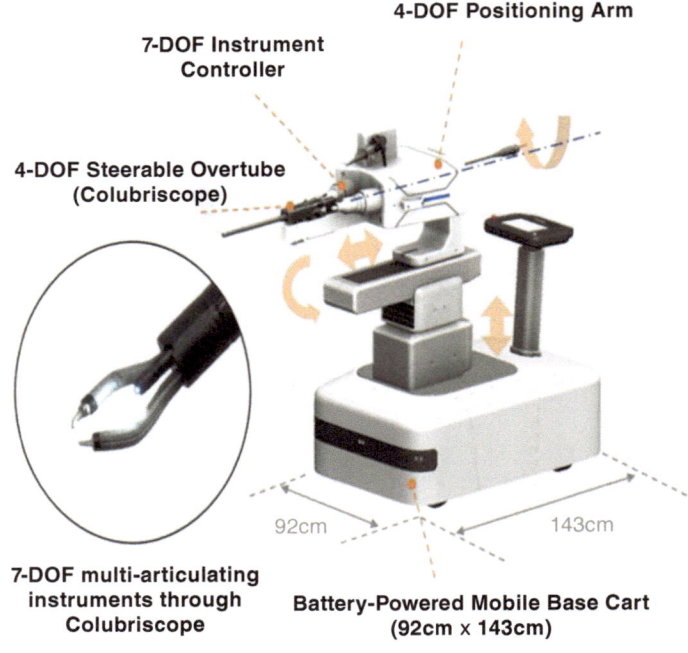

7-DOF multi-articulating instruments through Colubriscope

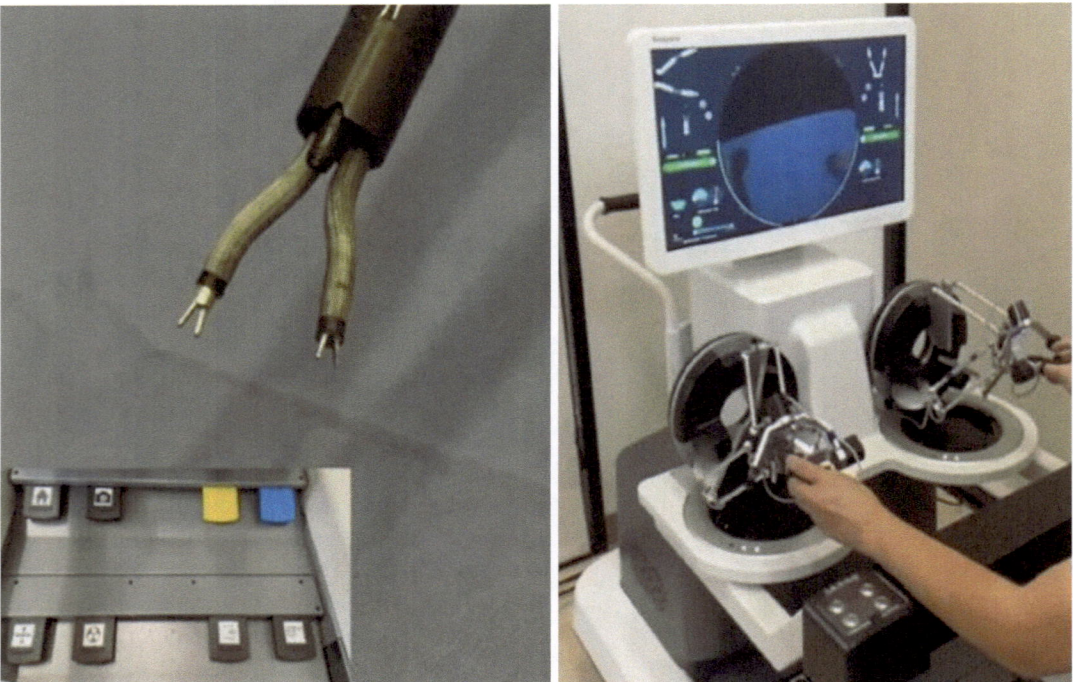

Fig. 22.9 The EndoLuminal surgical system: the colubriscope and the surgical console

moving the robotic instruments and a pedal board that allows steering of the Colubriscope and the videoscope (Fig. 22.9). Lots of instruments are available, all with 6 or 7 DoF. The platform still needs approvals, but it seems that all the cadaveric and preclinical work is completed. The main advantage of the technology is, without a doubt, its ability to reach lesions up to 55 cm distal from the anal verge. However, the system still lacks dexterity, and even for the authors, the platform seems suitable only for partial thickness disc excision.

22.3.4 Precision Robotics (Hong Kong, Hong Kong)

A promising prototype, born with the ambitious intention to overcome intuitive technology, is that made by Precision Robotics. The company is currently developing two types of robotics platforms, one for single-port surgery and one specifically designed for transanal application.

The system is composed of a surgical console with a 3D HD monitor and a single C-shape arm able to control a 5 mm videoscope and two 4 mm instruments with 8–9 DoF. The transanal platform enabled the robotic arm to connect directly to a 4 cm diameter rectoscope. Two dimensions of rectoscope are available to reach lesions closer or further away from the anal verge, similar to TEM/TEO. Future ambitions are achieving surgical movement automation of complex manoeuvres like knot tying. The first impressions suggest the platform has impressive dexterity and surgical precision with an intuitive control system. Precision Robotics still lacks certification allowing its clinical testing.

22.4 Conclusions

Transanal surgery has always been a critical topic in coloproctology. Even if the introduction of TEM was a kind of revolution in that field, the technology failed to spread properly due to some intrinsic difficulty of the technique. Firstly, it may have happened because it was introduced before the advent of laparoscopy when surgeons were not used to performing a video-assisted procedure, and later because of the lack of dexterity due to the parallelism of the instruments and the narrow space of the anorectal cavity, requires a long learning curve even for an expert laparo-

scopic surgeon. Despite an increasing number of indications, these led most surgeons to prefer still more invasive abdominal approaches to the detriment of transanal surgery.

The application of robotics in this field, adding the advantage of motion scaling, ergonomics, multiple degrees of freedom, and improved dexterity, could finally overcome the limitations of the technique originally invented by Buess and help it spread properly.

Robotic platforms in surgery are always burdened by doubt regarding the economic aspects. Indeed, the advent of robotics could be associated with an increase in cost. Still, medical history also proves that when a clear clinical benefit is reached, cost becomes a secondary interest, at least in Western countries.

The above-described platforms and other existing prototypes could permit more patients to benefit from the advantages of minimally invasive endoluminal surgery. A lot of research is still to be done. Still, suppose it is focused on making it easier for surgeons to perform some high-quality complete local excision and reduce postoperative complications by augmenting surgical precision and dexterity. In that case, considerable clinical benefits will not be hard to demonstrate in the future.

References

1. Downing A, Glaser AW, Finan PJ, Wright P, Thomas JD, Gilbert A, Corner J, Richards M, Morris EJA, Sebag-Montefiore D. Functional outcomes and health-related quality of life after curative treatment for rectal cancer: a population-level study in England. Int J Radiat Oncol Biol Phys. 2019;103(5):1132–42. https://doi.org/10.1016/J.IJROBP.2018.12.005.
2. Lezoche E, Baldarelli M, Lezoche G, Paganini AM, Gesuita R, Guerrieri M. A randomised clinical trial of endoluminal locoregional resection versus laparoscopic total mesorectal excision for T2 rectal cancer after neoadjuvant therapy. Br J Surg. 2012;99(9):1211–8. https://doi.org/10.1002/BJS.8821.
3. Giesen LJX, Olthof PB, Elferink MAG, van Westreenen HL, Beets GL, Verhoef C, Dekker JWT. Changes in rectal cancer treatment after the introduction of a national screening program; increasing use of less invasive strategies within a national cohort. Eur J Surg Oncol. 2022;48(5):1117–22. https://doi.org/10.1016/J.EJSO.2021.11.132.

4. Nicolle C, Rouen F, Rullier E, Rouanet P, Tuech J-J, Valverde A, Lelong B, Rivoire M, Faucheron J-L, Jafari M, Portier G, Meunier B, Sileznieff I, Prudhomme M, Marchal F, Pocard M, Pezet D, Rullier A, Vendrely V, et al. Organ preservation for rectal cancer (GRECCAR 2): a prospective, randomised, open-label, multicentre, phase 3 trial. Articles Lancet. 2017;390:469–79. https://doi.org/10.1016/S0140-6736(17)31056-5.

5. Arezzo A, lo Secco G, Passera R, Esposito L, Guerrieri M, Ortenzi M, Bujko K, Perez RO, Habr-Gama A, Stipa F, Picchio M, Restivo A, Zorcolo L, Coco C, Rizzo G, Mistrangelo M, Morino M. Individual participant data pooled-analysis of risk factors for recurrence after neoadjuvant radiotherapy and transanal local excision of rectal cancer: the PARTTLE study. Tech Coloproctol. 2019;23(9):831–42. https://doi.org/10.1007/s10151-019-02049-z.

6. Buess G, Theiss R, Gunther M, Hutterer F, Pichlmaier H. Transanal endoscopic microsurgery. Leber Magen Darm. 1985;15(6):271–9.

7. Buess G, Kipfmüller K, Hack D, Grüßner R, Heintz A, Junginger T. The technique of transanal endoscopic microsurgery. Surg Endosc. 1988;2(2):71–5. https://doi.org/10.1007/BF00704356.

8. Saclarides TJ. The history of transanal endoscopic surgery. Semin Colon Rectal Surg. 2015;26(1):2–5. https://doi.org/10.1053/j.scrs.2014.10.002.

9. Atallah S, Albert M, Larach S. Transanal minimally invasive surgery: a giant leap forward. Surg Endosc. 2010;24(9):2200–5. https://doi.org/10.1007/S00464-010-0927-Z.

10. Rimonda R, Arezzo A, Arolfo S, Salvai A, Morino M. TransAnal Minimally Invasive Surgery (TAMIS) with SILS™ Port versus Transanal Endoscopic Microsurgery (TEM): a comparative experimental study. Surg Endosc. 2013;27(10):3762–8. https://doi.org/10.1007/S00464-013-2962-Z/FIGURES/4.

11. Atallah S, Sanchez A, Bianchi E, Larach SW. Envisioning the future of colorectal surgery: preclinical assessment and detailed description of an endoluminal robotic system (ColubrisMX ELS). Tech Coloproctol. 2021;25(11):1199–207. https://doi.org/10.1007/s10151-021-02481-0.

12. Marks JH, Kunkel E, Salem JF, Martin C, Anderson B, Agarwal S. First clinical experience with single-port robotic transanal minimally invasive surgery (SP rTAMIS) for benign rectal neoplasms. Tech Coloproctol. 2021;25(1):117–24. https://doi.org/10.1007/s10151-020-02358-8.

13. Morino M, Forcignanò E, Arezzo A. Early clinical adoption of a flexible robotic endoscope for local excision of rectal lesions. Br J Surg. 2021;108(9):e296. https://doi.org/10.1093/bjs/znab193. NLM (Medline)

Part VII

Interventions Protocols in Endocrino-metabolic Surgery

Minimally Invasive Treatment of Thyroid Diseases

23

Barbara Mullineris, Sofia Esposito, Daniele Liguori, Umberto Filippi, and Micaela Piccoli

23.1 Introduction

Thyroidectomy consists in the total removal of the thyroid gland; partial removal, on the other hand, is called lobectomy, and if the isthmus is included the correct definition is lobo-isthmusectomy.

Central neck dissection with the removal of lymph nodes and/or lateral neck dissection is performed following ATA indications [1].

In the last 10 years, minimally invasive approaches have increased their applications in neck surgery, and the robotic approach has rapidly spread. The robotic gasless trans-axillary approach and the transoral approach are the more diffuse techniques in this field. In this chapter, the trans-axillary approach is described [2, 3].

23.2 Procedure

The procedure is divided into three steps:

Step 1: Flap or working space—a trans-axillary subcutaneous tunnel is created.
Step 2: Docking time—robotic cart positioning in the operative field and trocars connection to the robotic arms.
Step 3: Console time—procedure on the gland (thyroidectomy, lobo-isthmusectomy, lymphectomy).

23.3 Equipment and Surgical Instruments Required [4]

23.3.1 Step 1: Working Space

A 5 cm incision is performed in the axilla and a subplatysmal skin flap is created over the anterior surface of the major pectoralis muscle till the anterior neck area. The sternocleidomastoid muscle (SCM) is identified and the sternal branch is lifted up with an external retractor, the so-called Modena Retractor (CEATEC R Medizintechnik) that is used from the beginning of flap dissection. Finally, the Modena Retractor is positioned beneath both the sternal branch of the SCM and the strap muscles and the thyroid are discovered. Three robotic instruments are introduced in the incision; the fourth robotic arm is reserved for

B. Mullineris · S. Esposito · M. Piccoli (✉)
General, Emergency and New Technologies Surgery Unit, Baggiovara General Hospital, AOU Modena, Modena, Italy
e-mail: mullineris.barbara@aou.mo.it;
esposito.sofia@aou.mo.it;
piccoli.micaela@aou.mo.it; m.piccoli@ausl.mo.it

D. Liguori · U. Filippi
Department of Anaesthesia and Intensive Care, Baggiovara General Hospital, AOU Modena, Modena, Italy
e-mail: daniele.liguori@aou.mo.it;
filippi.umberto@aou.mo.it

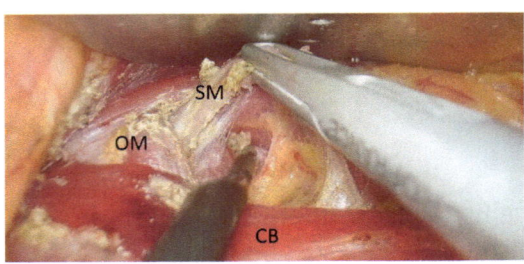

Fig. 23.1 Working space-*OM* omojodeum muscle, *CB* clavicular branch of sternocleidomastoideum muscle, *SM* strap muscles

total thyroidectomy or for nodules larger than 4 cm and is inserted through an independent incision at the inferior part of the axilla incision. This step is performed with laparoscopic instruments [5] (Fig. 23.1).

A conventional laparoscopic column, including a high-definition camera and display system, light source, video and image storage devices, and a basic package for open surgery must be available.

Laparoscopic Instruments
- 30° Endoscope.
- Laparoscopic grasping forceps (Johann forceps).
- Laparoscopic suction/irrigation system.
- Titanium clips (with dedicated laparoscopic applier) of various sizes (small/medium).
- Laparoscopic monopolar devices—hook.
- Laparoscopic bipolar forceps.
- Scope warmer.
- Sutures on surgeon's requests.

Open Instruments
- Modena Retractor.
- 25 cm × 25 cm gauzes.
- 1 monopolar electric scalpel with different lengths (short and long tips).
- 1 scalpel with a stainless-steel blade (sizes 10).
- 2 toothed forceps (18 cm).
- 2 retractors Farabeuf–Haken.
- Kelly forceps (24 cm) with a 12 mm swab on the tip.

- Suction system.
- Modena Retractor blade of various sizes (small/medium/large).
- Suction system connected to the external blade of the Modena Retractor.
- 1 anatomical tissue forceps of 30 cm to position the Modena Retractor during the surgical procedure.
- 1 Mayo scissors of 30 cm.
- Flexible blade of 25 cm.
- 8 mm robotic trocars (3 or 4 on request).
- External flat retractor.

23.3.2 Step 2: Docking Time

We describe the procedure using the DaVinci Xi robotic system (Intuitive, Sunnyvale, CA). The robotic cart is positioned near the operative field, and the surgeon at the operating table directs the maneuver. Three or four robotic arms are used. If it is planned to use three robotic arms, all of them are introduced through the axillary incision; if the fourth is planned or required during the surgical procedure, it is introduced through an independent incision at the inferior part of the axillary incision, but it is always prepared on the field. If we consider the right approach as described in the figure (Fig. 23.2) two 8 mm trocars are connected respectively with arm 1 and 3 and the third 8 mm trocar, holding the camera is connected to second robotic arm, the fourth arm is prepared on the field. We are going to illustrate a three-arm procedure; nevertheless, the fourth arm can be added at any time if necessary.

Robotic Instruments
- Robotic Prograsp 8 mm (used only for total thyroidectomy or for nodules more than 4 cm in diameter).
- Robotic Ultracision© Ethicon 8 mm.
- Robotic bipolar Maryland 8 mm.
- Robotic 30° endoscope 8 mm.
- Scope warmer.

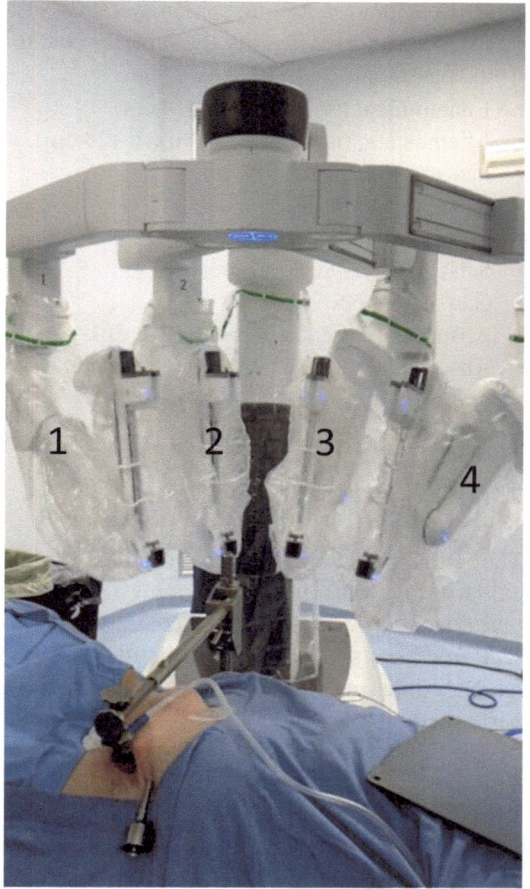

Fig. 23.2 Docking

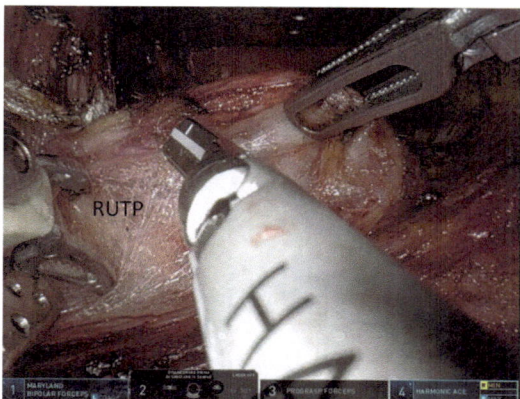

Fig. 23.3 RUTP: Right Upper thyroid pole

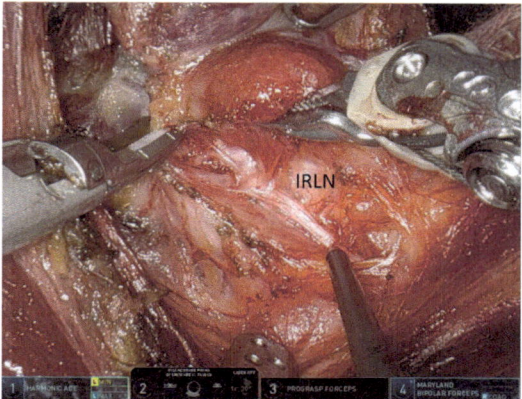

Fig. 23.4 IRLN: inferior right laryngeal nerve

23.3.3 Step 3: Console Time

The operation proceeds with the first surgeon sitting at the robotic console and the assistant at the operating table. All vessel dissections are performed using the harmonic device. The middle thyroid vein is identified and dissected. The upper pole of the thyroid is drawn downward and medially. The superior thyroid pole is approached medially, and the distal branches of the superior pole are closed near the thyroid gland, in order to avoid injuries to the superior laryngeal nerve. The robotic arms and robotic instruments used for this step are represented in Fig. 23.3. The inferior thyroid artery (ITA) and the inferior laryngeal nerve (ILN) are identified. Correct identification of the ILN is achieved with intermittent intraoperative nerve monitoring (IONM) [6] (Fig. 23.4). Superior and inferior parathyroid glands are then identified, and the thyroid lobe is dissected from the trachea and resected with the isthmus. The specimen is extracted through the axillary incision. Contralateral lobectomy, if planned, is performed using medial traction of the thyroid. The upper pole is the first step; afterward, it is time to identify the ILN with the so-called swing technique. The camera moves from arm 2 to arm 3 to arm 4 to follow the correct path of the nerve and then returns to arm 2 at the end of the procedure (Fig. 23.5). The contralateral lobe is extracted through the same axillary incision. Venous bleeding is checked with the Valsalva maneuver. A closed suction drain is positioned

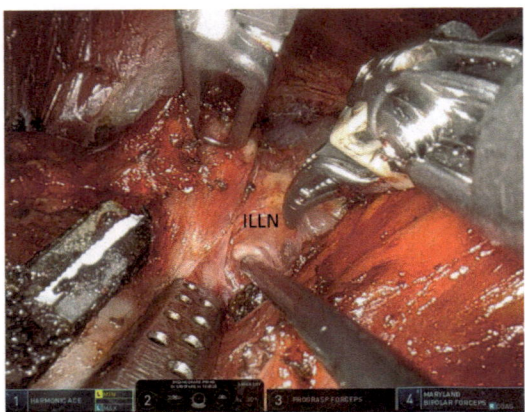

Fig. 23.5 ILLN: inferior left laryngeal nerve with a right access

through a separate incision under the axillary skin incision. De-docking is performed, and the scrub nurse completes gauze and needle counts. The wound is cosmetically closed [7, 8].

23.3.3.1   Instruments Used

- Robotic Prograsp 8 mm (used only for total thyroidectomy or for lobo-isthmusectomy if nodules are more than 4 cm in diameter).
- Robotic Ultracision© Ethicon 8 mm.
- Robotic bipolar Maryland 8 mm.
- Robotic 30° endoscope 8 mm.
- Laparoscopic grasping forceps (Johann forceps).
- 12 mm swab.
- Titanium clips (with dedicated laparoscopic applier) of various sizes (small/medium).
- Laparoscopic suction/irrigation system.
- IONM (avalanche system).
- External flat retractor.

23.3.4   Extraction of the Specimen, Drain Insertion, and Suture: Instruments

- Needle holder CT-ORO Mayo-Hegar 20 cm.
- Laparoscopic grasping forceps (Johann forceps).

- Laparoscopic suction/irrigation system.
- Braided suture to identify the superior pole for the pathologist.
- 1 anatomical tissue forceps (18 cm).
- 1 hemostatic tissue forceps Mixter (23 cm).
- Jackson-Pratt drain 7 mm.
- Nonabsorbable suture 2/0.
- Nonabsorbable silk suture 2/0.
- Scissor Mayo-Stille 17 cm.
- Gauze 25 cm × 25 cm.
- Absorbable thread *Lactomer* 9–1, 3/0.
- Absorbable thread *Polyglytone* 4/0 neddle 3/8 circle 19 mm.

23.3.5   Operating Room Setup

The setting of the operative room (OR) for trans-axillary robotic lobo-isthmusectomy or for total thyroidectomy with or without central neck dissection depends on the side of the malignant or larger nodule since the axillary incision is always performed on this side.

The operating room disposition for right lobo-isthmusectomy or total thyroidectomy with a right axillary access is described below (Fig. 23.6). When a left lobo-isthmusectomy is planned, the operating room is positioned in a specular way.

23.3.6   Right Lobo-isthmusectomy/ Total Thyroidectomy with a Right Axillary Access

- The operating table is positioned in the center of the theatre.
- The laparoscopic column is placed on the left side of the patient.
- Robotic vision cart is placed on the left side of the patient, near the feet.
- Robotic patient cart is placed on the left side of the patient, near the head.
- First surgeon at the console; if foreseen a second console, this is for a surgeon in training.

Fig. 23.6 Operating room set-up

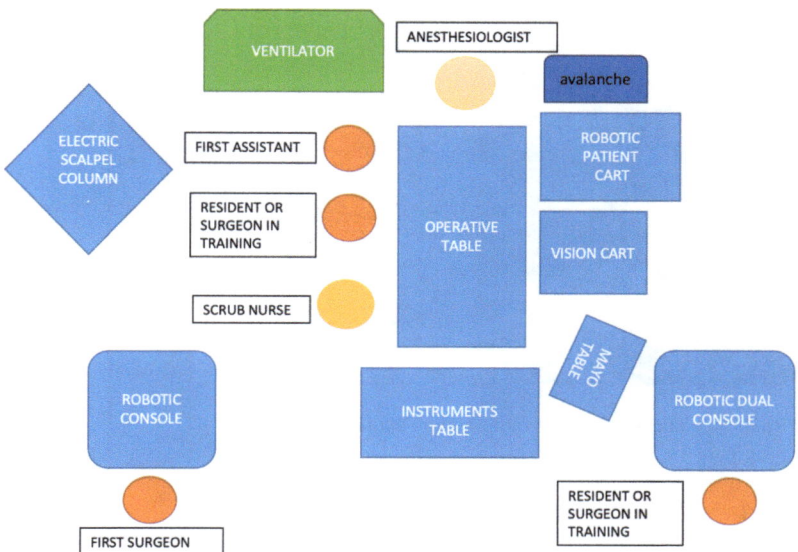

- Assistant surgeon at the operating table, on the patient's right side, with the resident on his left.
- The scrub nurse is positioned on the right side of the patient and on the right side of the resident.
- Mayo table is on the right side of the scrub nurse.

The first step is the creation of the working space, and the resident holds the laparoscopic camera. A laparoscopic 4 K high-definition system with a 60″ monitor is used.

23.3.7 Patient Positioning

The patient is under general anesthesia, and the position is described in Figs. 23.7, 23.8 and 23.9.

- Neck is slightly extended.
- The arm on the axillary access side is raised upon the head and positioned in a way that minimizes the distance from the axilla to the anterior neck.
- The contralateral arm, with venous access, is placed along the body and secured with safety straps to the table. Another support is placed near the head to avoid any lateral movements during the procedure.

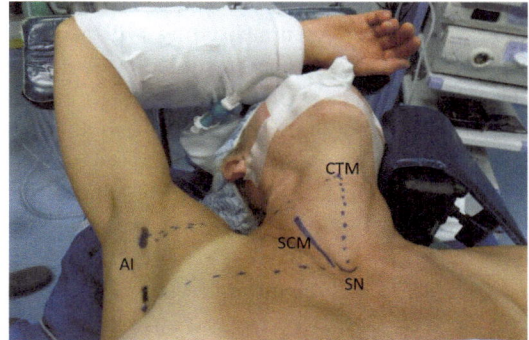

Fig. 23.7 The extended arm is flexed approximately 90° at the elbow with the forearm resting over the forehead. *AI* axillary incision, *SCM* sternocleidomastoid muscle, *SN* sternal notch, *CTM* cricothyroid membrane

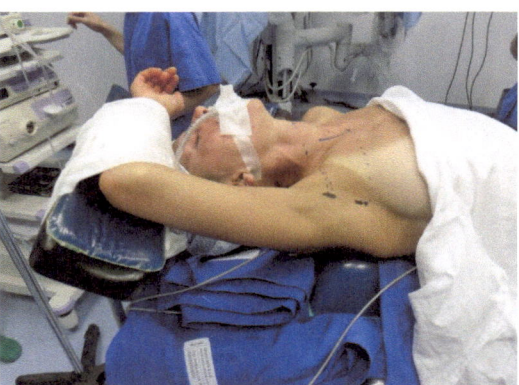

Fig. 23.8 A rubber pad is placed under the shoulder blades

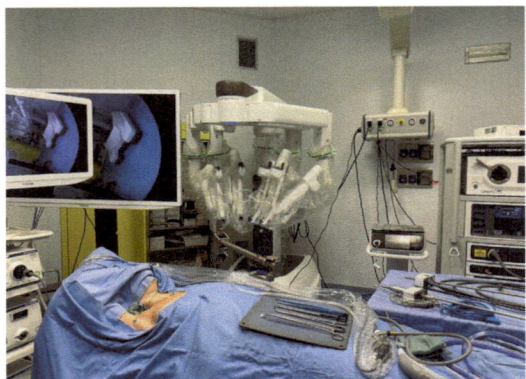

Fig. 23.9 Patient position for a right trans-axillary access

23.4 Modena Retractor˚

The retractor will be mounted at the operating table on the robotic cart side and can be approximately adjusted. Accurate setting will be done from the operating side. The surgeon can change the following adjustments: vertical height of pillar, horizontal depth of boom tube, and angle of blade. The surgeon can choose between six different sizes of blades. Blades are available in two different lengths and in three different widths. The retractor has special features: approximate adjustment of height through quick fastener at robotic cart side, accurate setting can be done from operating side, blades are easily changeable but safely locked, and automatic adaption to operation field due to rotation of boom and blades (Fig. 23.10).

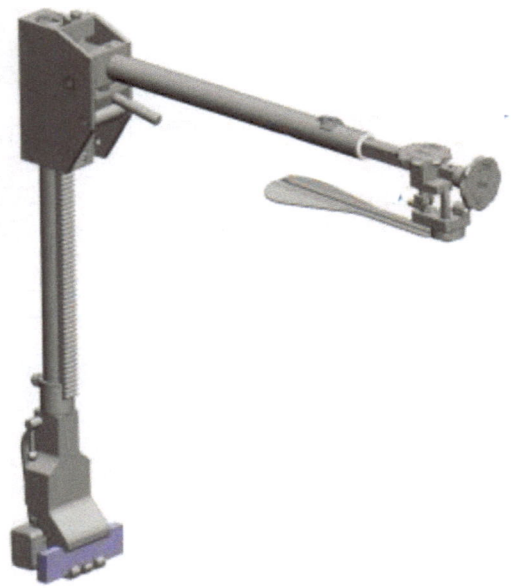

Fig. 23.10 Modena Retractor″ (CEATEC® Medizintechnik)

23.5 Other Devices

23.5.1 ICG (Indocyanine Green)

The indocyanine green fluorescent dye (IGC) is presented in vials of 25 mg of powder for solution for injection:

- The IGC should be administered at a dose of 10 mg to see the activity of the parathyroid gland after thyroidectomy.
- It should be diluted with sterile distilled water and NOT with sodium chloride (NaCl) as the latter could cause aggregation.
- After preparation, the solution must be stored in a dark and cool place to avoid rapid deterioration of the whitening fluorescence.

23.5.2 Intraoperative Complications

During the trans-axillary robotic procedure, one major complication is the bleeding of the main vessels (middle thyroid vein or internal jugular vein).

In these circumstances, the scrub nurse must have the following instruments available:

- Laparoscopic suction/irrigation system.
- 10 cm × 10 cm gauzes.
- Absorbable and titanium clips (with their laparoscopic applier) of various sizes (small/medium/large) based on the size of the vessel needing to be clipped.
- Laparoscopic monopolar devices—scissors and/or hook.
- Laparoscopic bipolar forceps.
- Robotic needle holder and monofilament suture with a small gauge needle to attempt the direct repair of the bleeding vessel.
- 2 laparoscopic grasping forceps (Johann forceps).

References

1. Haugen BR, Alexander EK, Bible KC, Doherty GM, Mandel SJ, Nikiforov YE, Pacini F, Randolph GW, Sawka AM, Schlumberger M, Schuff KG, Sherman SI, Sosa JA, Steward DL, Tuttle RM, Wartofsky L. 2015 American Thyroid Association Management Guidelines for Adult Patients with Thyroid Nodules and Differentiated Thyroid Cancer: The American Thyroid Association Guidelines Task Force on thyroid nodules and differentiated thyroid cancer. Thyroid. 2016;26(1):1–133. https://doi.org/10.1089/thy.2015.0020.

2. Piccoli M, Mullineris B, Gozzo D, Colli G, Pecchini F, Nigro C, Rochira V. Evolution strategies in transaxillary robotic thyroidectomy: considerations on the first 449 cases performed. J Laparoendosc Adv Surg Tech A. 2019;29(4):433–40. https://doi.org/10.1089/lap.2019.0021.

3. Piccoli M, Mullineris B, Santi D, Gozzo D. Advances in robotic transaxillary thyroidectomy in Europe. Curr Surg Rep. 2017;5(8):17. https://doi.org/10.1007/s40137-017-0180-7.

4. Lusuardi R. Sala Operatoria Strumentazione. Edizioni Idelson-Gnocchi; 2021.

5. Al Kadah B, Piccoli M, Mullineris B, Colli G, Janssen M, Siemer S, Schick B. Modifications of transaxillary approach in endoscopic da Vinci-assisted thyroid and parathyroid gland surgery. J Robot Surg. 2015;9(1):37–44. https://doi.org/10.1007/s11701-014-0486-8.

6. Crowther JE, Ali DB, Bamford J, Kang SW, Kandil E. Intraoperative neuromonitoring during thyroid surgery: the effect of surgical positioning. Surg Innov. 2019;26(1):77–81. https://doi.org/10.1177/1553350618799786.

7. Piccoli M, Mullineris B, Gozzo D, Smerieri N, Nigro C. Transaxillary thyroidectomy and parathyroidectomy robotic surgery. In: Spinoglio G, editor. Current applications and new trends. Italia: Springer-Verlag; 2015. p. 15–22. ISBN: 978-88-470-5713-5.

8. Spinoglio G. Robotic surgery-current application and new trends-updates in surgery. Springer; 2015. https://doi.org/10.1007/978-88470-5714-2.

Minimally Invasive Treatment of Adrenal Diseases

24

Carlo Bergamini and Alessio Giordano

24.1 Definition of Adrenalectomy

Adrenalectomy consists of the removal of the adrenal gland, together with the surrounding fat of the adrenal lodge, either with an anterior (trans-peritoneal) or posterior (trans-retroperitoneal) approach. Adrenalectomy can be performed either by open surgery or by minimally invasive (the so-called laparoscopic/retro-peritoneoscopic) procedures [1, 2].

24.2 Indications and Contraindications to Adrenalectomy

Adrenalectomy is indicated in the case of such adrenal tumors:

- Secreting adenoma
  - Aldosteronoma (Conn's syndrome)
  - Cortisol-producing adenoma (ACTH non-dependent Cushing syndrome)

- Bilateral cortical adrenal hyperplasia (ACTH-dependent Cushing syndrome):
    Recurrence of pituitary disease after the resection of pituitary gland surgery.
    Residual hypercortisolism after pituitary gland surgery
    Nonresponder to medical therapy after hypophysectomy
    ACTH-dependent extra-adrenal tumor of unidentified or non-surgically treatable site
  - Pheochromocytoma or other chromaffin cell tumor
- Incidentaloma
  - Secreting (see secreting adenoma)
  - Non-secreting
    Non-secreting adenoma with
    - 3.5–4 cm in diameter
    - Annual growth > 1 cm
    Other histotypes (cysts, myelolipoma, unusual tumors) with
    - Progressive or rapid growth
    - Compression signs to adjacent organs
- Adrenocortical cancer
  - Stages I–III
  - Stage IV only when functioning (usually virilizing syndrome) for debulking purposes
- Metastasis, with the following criteria:
  - Solitary
  - Monoliteral

C. Bergamini (✉)
Emergency Surgery Unit, University Hospital of Careggi, Florence, Italy

A. Giordano
Department of Surgery, General Surgery Unit, Hospital of S. Stefano, Prato, Italy

- Non-locally extended
- Surgical resectable with R0
• Originating from one of the following possible primary malignancies that is surgically resectable
    Kidney
    Lung
    Breast
    Melanoma
    Gastro-intestinal tract

On the contrary, the adrenal surgery is contraindicated in the following cases:

• Incidentaloma.
    - Non-secreting
        Non-functioning adenoma
        • Diameter < 3.5–4 cm
        • Annual growth < 1 cm
        Other unusual histotypes (e.g., myelolipoma, cysts) without
        • Progressive or rapid growth
        • Compression signs to adjacent organs
• Adrenocortical carcinoma IV stage, with no functioning signs
• Metastases with the following feature:
    - Multiple
    - Bilateral
    - Locally extended
    - Non-surgically resectable with R0
    - Originating from a diffuse or nonresectable primitive malignancy
• General or anesthesiologic contraindications

24.3 Minimally Invasive Adrenalectomy (MIA): Advantages, Indications, Contraindications, and Possible Complications

24.3.1 Advantages

The success of the laparoscopic approach to the adrenal gland, which has been increasingly supplanting the "open" way, depends upon the general advantages that this technique offers, both

intra- and post-operatively, compared to the laparotomy technique [3, 4]. In addition, various specific advantages of laparoscopic adrenal surgery are recognizable, such as the possibility to perform the intervention with:

• Minimal dissection of neighboring organs despite the depth of the surgical field, especially for lateral access and on the left.
• No necessity to retract the surrounding structures, particularly in the posterior way.
• No necessity for two incisions in the case of a one-time simultaneous bilateral adrenalectomy.

24.3.2 Indications and Contraindications

Below the indications and contraindication to laparoscopic adrenalectomy are reported [5]:

• Absolute indications:
    - Small functionally active benign tumors, such as
        Aldosteronoma
        Cushing's syndrome caused by
        • Cortisol-producing adrenal adenoma (ACTH-independent Cushing's syndrome)
        • Bilateral hyperplasia (ACTH dependent or independent), when indicated for adrenal surgery (see previous paragraph)
    - Small non-functioning incidentalomas, up to 6 cm in diameter
    - Small tumors of suspected malignant nature (for morphological/radiological criteria) without certain signs of adjacent organ infiltration
• Relative indication/contraindications:
    - Related to the kind of tumor
        Benign tumors of conspicuous size (> 6–8 cm), functioning or non-functioning
        Adrenal tumors of any size, primary or secondary, that have sure morphological/radiological signs of malignancy

Tumors located in glands that are quite friable, or not easy to distinguish from the retroperitoneal fat (as occurs in certain ACTH-dependent hyperplasia) due to the risk of tumor spillage

Neo-vascularized tumors (such as pheochromocytomas) in which there is a high risk of bleeding

Myelolipomas due to their usual big dimensions

– Related to the kind of patient

Obese patients

Patients with previous surgical interventions, which have caused multiple adhesions, or with interventions that have already involved the operative field (nephrectomy, duodenum-pancreatectomy)

Unfavorable laparoscopic chamber due to the low abdomen/tumor diameter ratio

- Absolute contraindications

– General for laparoscopy (coagulopathies, severe and advanced cardio-pulmonary diseases, and any other condition that precludes the safety of general anesthesia after CO_2 insufflation in the abdomen)

– Oncological

Malignant tumors with certain preoperative signs of infiltration of the adjacent organs or tissues

A few notes are to be added to the upon-reported laparoscopic criteria. As regards the tumor dimension, it should be noted that it is still controversial what is the exact cut-off of the tumor size beyond which it is no longer possible (or advisable) to perform laparoscopic adrenalectomy. The literature defines giant adrenal tumors (GAT) as adrenal masses larger than 6 cm. GAT are considered rare, with an incidence ranging from 8.6% to 38.6% of all adrenal tumors. The size is an important variable in predicting malignancy; in fact, if the lesions are smaller than 4 cm, the risk of malignancy is approximately 2%, while for lesions of 4–6 cm, the risk of malignancy is 6%, and for lesions of 6 cm the

risk of malignancy is 25% (10–53%). At the moment, there is no evidence that suggests that a laparoscopic approach is contraindicated for GAT because size is only a predictor factor of malignancy.

However, it is currently thought that the dimensional cut-off for laparoscopic may be influenced by other factors such as:

- The anatomical characteristics of the patient (e.g., obesity, distensibility of the wall, type of fat distribution, anatomical anomalies of the adrenal region).
- The other pathological features of the tumor (beyond the size) such as its shape and its relationship to the large vessels or other critical anatomical structures of the gland, such as the consistency structure, the possibility to be recognized from the retroperitoneal (as occurs in the syndrome of ACTH-dependent Cushing), the presence of neo-vascularization, as it occurs in the case of pheochromocytomas.
- The width of the laparoscopic chamber, which represents the volume within which the laparoscopic instruments are free to be held and moved. This factor, largely determined by the anatomy of the patient and the tumor, is currently considered the main determinant for the feasibility of the adrenal laparoscopy.
- A possible incomplete resection or capsular disruption that increases the risk of local recurrence and intra-abdominal neoplastic dissemination.
- Finally, the experience and technical expertise of the surgical team, quantifiable in the number of annual interventions.

On the other side, the indication of MIA in the case of primary adrenal malignancy is even more controversial. If the tumor appears preoperatively certainly invasive of the adjacent structures, almost all the authors agree that the treatment of choice is the "open" approach. However, in the case of even high suspicion of primary malignancy (adrenocortical carcinoma) but without signs of infiltration toward the adjacent tissues, laparoscopic access is still advisable only for expert teams, with a low threshold of conversion in case of any difficulty that may expose to the risk of tumor capsule damage. Conversely, a more accredited indication of laparoscopy is represented by adrenal metastases, in case they are not of conspicuous dimensions, and they are fully confined within the anatomical boundaries of the gland.

In conclusion, most of the adrenal tumors can be laparoscopically excised, as they are represented by benign and relatively small lesions. The only diseases that cannot be approached with this method, albeit with some reservations, are currently considered benign tumors > 8–10 cm or malignant tumors which has been locally spread.

24.3.3 Possible Complications

Various types of complications may occur during a laparoscopic adrenalectomy. Overall, they can be divided into nonspecific, which may occur in every laparoscopic procedure, and specific to this kind of minimally invasive surgery. Below we report and comment on the most relevant:

- Nonspecific
  - Lower incidence compared to "open" surgery: paralytic ileus, respiratory problems, and urinary and wound infections
  - Same incidence of "open" surgery: thromboembolic disease
- Specific
  - Hemorrhage
    Intra-operative, due to:
    - Rupture of the adrenal gland vessels, capsule, or parenchyma.
    - Injury of the spleen or splenic vessels (left)
    - Rupture of the liver capsule
    - Direct injury of the inferior vena cava
    Post-operative, due to:
    - Hematoma of the adrenal lodge (from glandular residues or from small vessels of the lodge)
    - Intramuscular or subcutaneous hematoma (from the trocar site)

- Accidental opening of the peritoneum (posterior extra-peritoneal route)
- Accidental opening of the pleura (especially for lateral access)
- Lesion of the adrenal capsule with tumor spillage
- Hypertensive crisis from manipulation of adrenal tissue in the presence of pheochromocytoma, with possible acute heart failure, stroke, and acute renal failure

With the advent of laparoscopy, some of the traditional complications of abdominal surgery such as paralytic ileus, respiratory problems (broncho-pneumonic foci, atelectasis, pleural effusion, respiratory failure), urinary infections, and wound complications (infections, dehiscence, hernia) are significantly reduced. This is due to the reduced invasiveness which also allows for an earlier mobilization of the patient and a prompter resumption of normal activities. On the contrary, thrombo-embolic disease has an incidence comparable to that associated with tradiional surgery due to the high endo-abdominal pressures that are developed in this type of surgery due to the insufflation of CO_2. Concerning the specific complications, intra- and post-operative hemorrhages are the most frequent, being responsible for about two-third of the global complications. In the intra-operative setting, the lesion of large vessels is the main cause of laparotomic conversion. This often happens on the right, where the clips on the middle adrenal vein can more easily dislodge due to the short course of the vessel. Even in the post-operative phase, bleeding is the most frequent complication of this procedure. Adrenal hematomas can result from surface bleeding from the glandular residue left in place in the case of partial adrenalectomy. The positive pressure of the pneumo-peritoneum present during surgery could be the cause why this bleeding occurs in the post-operative phase. Their treatment is usually conservative. Bleeding from trocar accesses usually causes well-controlled subcutaneous and intramuscular hemorrhagic infarctions, but sometimes they can cause more massive hemorrhages which may require even early post-operative re-laparoscopies or re-laparotomies. Hypertensive complications in the case of pheochromocytomas are particularly life-threatening since they may lead also to pulmonary edema or even fatal cerebral hemorrhages. Their management requires an expert and dedicated anesthesiologic team.

In conclusion, the complications of laparoscopic adrenalectomy do not differ much from those of open surgery. However, the less invasive surgery, the reduced manipulation of the gland, and the pre-operative selection of patients, as well as the increase in the experience of the multi-disciplinary, team may significantly reduce their incidence.

24.4 Operative Technique of MIA: Trans-Peritoneal Flank Approach

The trans-peritoneal flank approach is the most widely used technique for the MIA. The following are the several advantages and a few limits.

- Advantage:
  - Access to the adrenal lodge at the level of the superior retroperitoneum is easier, especially on the left
  - On the right, there is no need to mobilize the duodenum and the right colonic flexure
  - The retraction of the adjacent organs is facilitated by the gravity that occurs in this position

- Limits
  - It is not possible to have a surgical approach to the contralateral gland at the same time; therefore, in the case of bilateral adrenalectomy, the patient must be repositioned

24.4.1 Patient and Operator Disposition

The patient is positioned in lateral decubitus, with the side corresponding to the gland to be operated on facing upward. The patient's side is "broken" by alternately lowering the trunk and the lower limbs in order to widen the space located between the anterior superior iliac spine and the costal arch, where the trocars will be positioned. The lateral position of about 50–60 ° for the right adrenalectomy and of 70–80° for the left, associated with the position of the operating table in anti-Trendelenburg of about 10–20°, facilitates the exposure of the retroperitoneum. Indeed, the viscera that are placed anteriorly (duodenal-pancreatic block and right colonic flexure for right adrenalectomy and, after mobilization, spleno-pancreatic block and splenic colic flexure on the left) are displaced "for gravity" (Fig. 24.1).

The surgeon places himself laterally in front of the patient, on the opposite side to that of the adrenal gland to be removed. The first and second operators are on the same side, respectively, to the right and to the left of the operator. If two or more monitors are available, to avoid excessive

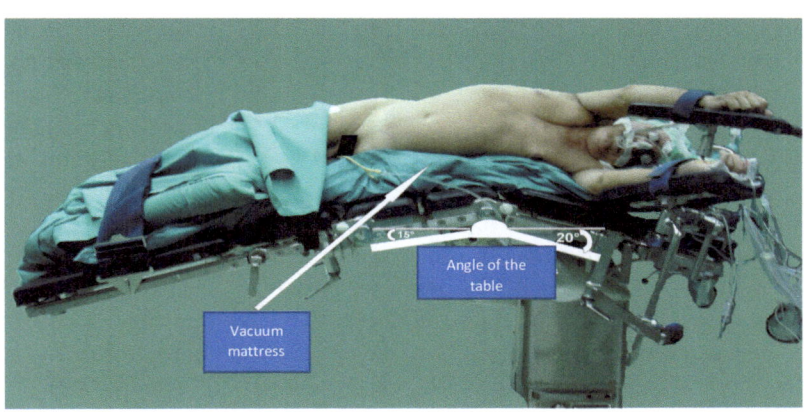

Fig. 24.1 Position of the patients in the case of right adrenalectomy. To be noted the lateral position and the the stability of the position is ensured by various positioning and restraint devices

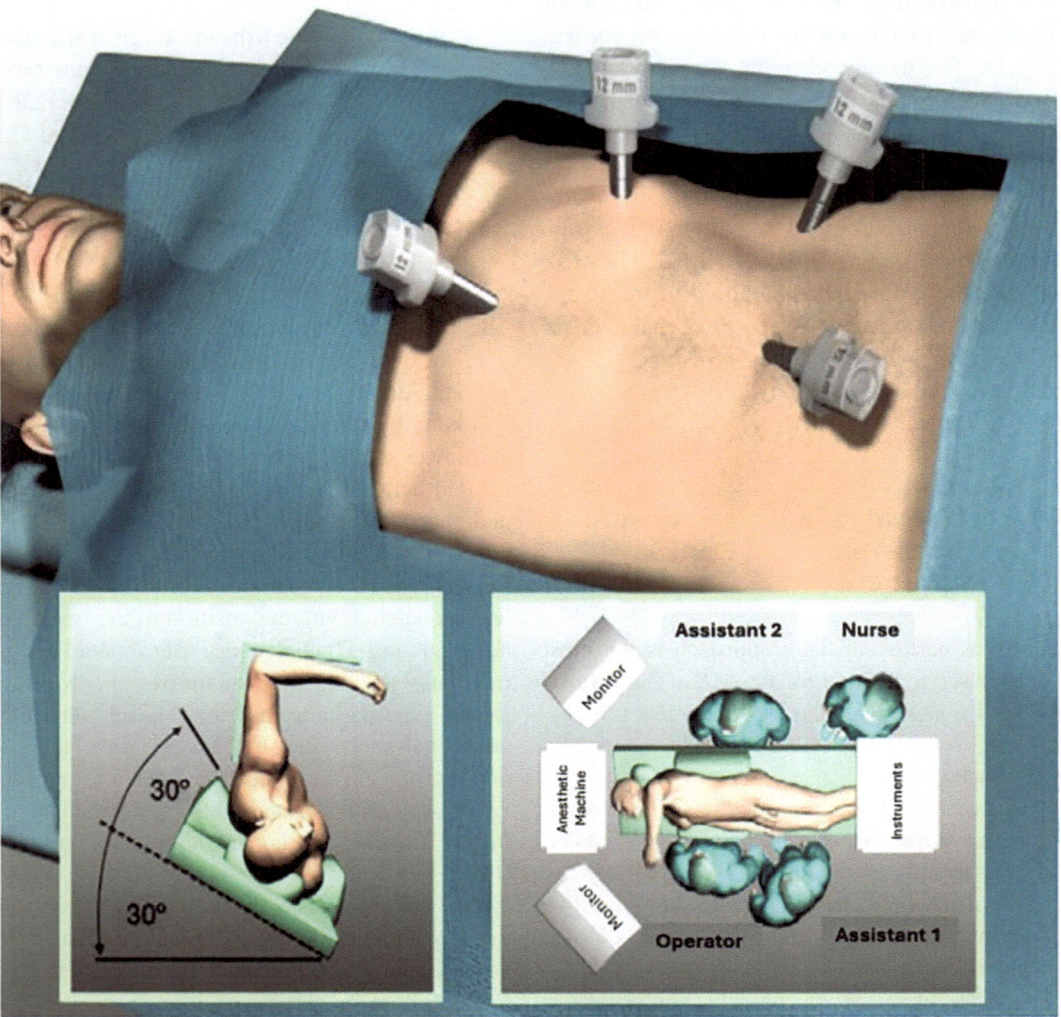

Fig. 24.2 Monitor and operator positioning

space encumbrance, the first and second operators can be placed on the opposite side to that of the first surgeon (Fig. 24.2).

24.4.2 Trocar Placement for the Right MIA (Fig. 24.3)

• The first trocar, usually a Hasson trocar, or T1, of 10 mm, is positioned 3 cm below the costal arch at the level of the right anterior axillary line and is used for the insertion of the optic at

30° and for the extraction of the surgical piece at the end of the operation.

• The second and third trocars, T2 and T3 (10–12 mm and 5 mm, respectively), are positioned approximately 4–5 cm far from T1, respectively, on the right and left, 1–5 cm from the costal arch. T2 receives the instruments of the operator's right hand (dissecting, cutting, hemostasis, and aspiration instruments) and the T3 those of the left hand (grasping and aspiration instruments). The fourth trocar, T4 (10 mm), is positioned in the

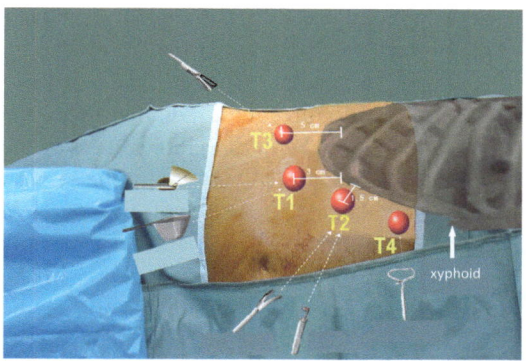

Fig. 24.3 Trocars position and function in right adrenalectomy

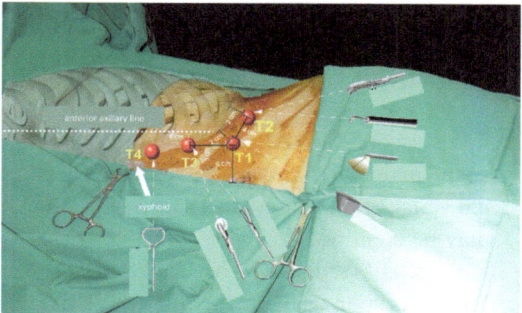

Fig. 24.4 Trocars position and function in left adrenalectomy

para-xiphoid area and receives the hepatic retractor.

- In the most difficult right adrenalectomies, a fifth trocar, T5, is sometimes necessary to create a further liver retraction or to allow the first aid to assist more intensely the action of the first operator (hemostasis, aspiration, various structures).

24.4.3 Trocar Placement for the Left MIA (Fig. 24.4)

- The first Hasson trocar, T1, is positioned 1–3 cm below the costal arch at the level of the left anterior axillary line and is used for the insertion of the 30 ° laparoscope and for the extraction of the operative piece at the end of the operation.
- The second and third trocars, T2 and T3 (10–12 mm and 5 mm, respectively), are positioned approximately 4–5 cm on the right and left of T1 1–2 cm from the costal arch. T2 receives the instruments of the operator's right hand (dissecting, cutting, and hemostasis and aspiration instruments) and the T3 those of the left hand (grasping, suction instruments).
- A fourth additional trocar, T4 (5 or 10 mm), is positioned in the para-xiphoid area and gets a retractor that can be used when the spleno-pancreatic block does not fall spontaneously medially or when an accessory working trocar is required for aspiration and continued washing of the operating field.

24.4.4 Right MIA Operative Times

- I time: Exploration. After the introduction of the optic and trocars, first the exploration of the adrenal lodge is performed, delimited at the top by the right lobe of the liver, laterally by the vena cava and inferiorly by the ipsilateral renal vein and by the superior pole of the kidney.
- II time: Exposure. The first step after the liver retraction consists in the section of the posterior parietal peritoneum at the subhepatic level, preserving a small peritoneal flap adhering to the adrenal gland, which can be used for delicate maneuvers of grasping and spreading of the gland. The section of the peritoneal sheet is continued toward the right triangular ligament of the liver. After incision of the peritoneum, the retroperitoneum is exposed, opening the vision to the adrenal mass and the inferior vena cava into the subhepatic space. The inferior vena cava must be identified and its position must be kept in mind throughout the execution of the adrenalectomy.
- III time: Lower Medial Dissection. The dissection then proceeds downward until it reaches the renal vein. The right margin of the vena cava is then gently and gradually freed from the medial aspect of the adrenal gland.
- IV time: Ligature of the Middle Vein. The latter maneuver is done up to the dihedral angle between the vena cava and the lower edge of the liver, where the outlet of the middle adrenal vein is identified. Any retraction maneuver must be done with great caution. A curved dis-

sector can be useful to completely isolate it. Then, it is clipped with two clips on the caval (medial) side and one on the lateral side of the gland. Finally, the vein is cut with unelectrified scissors. Sometimes, an abnormal outlet of the main adrenal vein or an accessory adrenal vein (20% of cases) in a supra-hepatic vein may be identified.

- V time: Dissection Of The Upper And Lower Poles. As soon as the main vein (or veins) has been dissected, the dissection and control of the upper margin is performed. Here the upper adrenal arterioles reach the gland coming from the phrenic vessels. These vessels, except for pheochromocytomas, are usually small in size and their section and hemostasis can be easily achieved. The dissection is then conducted downward, where the lower adrenal vessels, coming from the renal vessels, are demonstrated.

- VI time: Postero-Lateral Dissection. The gland is progressively elevated with atraumatic forceps, and the dissection is completed on the outer margin. The fat tissue over the pole of the kidney is removed together with the gland, thus revealing the posterior muscular plane which is constituted by the psoas-square muscle of the loin.

- VII time: Extraction, Hemostasis, Drainage, and Closure. Once detached from all the anchors, the gland is inserted into a laparoscopic pouch before being extracted through the orifice of T1, possibly enlarged by sectioning the muscle fascia. The adrenal lodge is washed to remove all the little clots and residual tissues, and the hemostasis of the operating field is carefully checked and completed. It is always preferable to leave a capillary drainage in suction at the adrenal lodge.

24.4.5 Left MIA Operative Times

- I time: Exploration. Conversely to what occurs in the right adrenalectomy, the exploration time of the adrenal area on the left is limited by the overlapping of the spleen and the ipsilateral colic angle. Therefore, the optimal vision of the adrenal region is possible only after these organs have been at least partially mobilized.

- II time: Exposure (Colic and Spleno-Pancreatic Mobilization). On this side, the operation begins with the mobilization of the left colonic flexure and then with the section of the lateral ligaments of the spleen. Complete mobilization of the spleno-pancreatic block is achieved by continuing the dissection of the posterior spleno-renal ligament up to the hilum of the spleen and posterior ligaments of the pancreatic tail. This procedure allows to have the gradual fall of the spleno-pancreatic block medially and therefore a total exposure of the retroperitoneum at the level of the left adrenal lodge.

- III time: Lower Medial Dissection. The left renal vein is then identified at the lower part of the operative field. This vena is the landmark for the identification of the left main adrenal vein.

- IV time: Ligature of Middle and Accessory Vein. Once the adrenal vein has been identified and isolated with a dissector, the section is made after clipping it as usual. The release of the gland then proceeds medially, and, during this phase, one or more accessory veins are invariably encountered and clipped.

- V time: Dissection of the Upper and Lower Poles. Thus, the gradual release of the adrenal gland from the upper pole of the kidney begins by electrocautery cutting the lower arterial vessels that come from the renal vessels. Only in cases of functioning pheochromocytomas or neo-vascularization may it be necessary to use clips. The cutting of the arterial upper venous vessels coming from the diaphragmatic arteries is instead frequently performed using high-energy instruments. As already mentioned for the right adrenalectomy, the retraction of the gland must always be very delicate in order not to cause lacerations of the glandular parenchyma.

- VI time: Postero-Lateral Dissection. The isolation of the posterior and lateral aspects of the adrenal gland is a delicate maneuver. Although the posterolateral adrenal plane is usually avascular, it is sometimes possible to encounter accessory polar vessels for the kidney which obviously must be controlled.

- VII time: Extraction, Drainage, and Closure. The operation ends, as from the right side, with the extraction of the gland, after being inserted in an endo-bag, the control of the hemostasias and the positioning of drainage in the retro-peritoneum.

24.5 Operative Technique of MIA: Trans-Peritoneal Anterior Approach

24.5.1 Advantages, Limits, and Indications

- The anterior trans-abdominal approach is currently used by a minority of authors since it presents many unfavorable anatomy-surgical conditions [6–8]. The following are a few advantages:
  - It allows a traditional view of the abdomen and therefore a good overall abdominal exploration
  - It gives the possibility of removing both glands at a single time in the the case of bilateral pathology (bilateral adrenalectomy) without the need to repositioning the patient
- Conversely, these are the defects of this kind of technique:
  - Worse exposition due to the necessity:
    On the left of the complete mobilization of the right colon by the complete section of the left parieto-colic shower and

the mobilization of the tail of the pancreas
On the right to lift the liver and move it medially, to mobilize and retract inferiorly the transverse colon and hepatic flexure and often kocherize the duodenum
  - High effort required to retract the adjacent abdominal organs
  - Need to place additional trocars
- The main indication is the rare cases in which simultaneous bilateral adrenalectomy is needed. In fact, this approach allows a significant reduction in intra-operative dead times, eliminating the need for patient repositioning

24.5.2 Patient and Trocar Position

It is performed with the patient in supine decubitus equipped with special hip supports to allow a slight inclination of the operating table to the side opposite the lesion. In most cases, the method requires the introduction of six to eight trocars 2 of which are bilateral, which are kept in place when the patient's position is changed (Fig. 24.5).

- T1, used for the insertion of the optics and as a way of removing the removed gland, is positioned at the umbilical level with the open technique.
- T2 is inserted in correspondence with the paramedian line four transverse fingers above the umbilicus.
- T3, in the xyphoid region, immediately to the right of the midline.
- T4 (two trocars) on the midclavicular line cranially with respect to the umbilicus.
- T5 (two trocars) on the side along the middle axillary line, two fingers below the costal arch.
- T6 possible additional trocar on the right or left in case of difficult adrenalectomy.

24.5.3 Operative Technique

The laparoscopic surgical technique for this type of access does not differ significantly from the

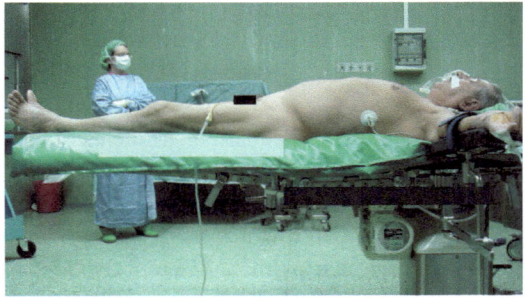

Fig. 24.5 Supine position of the patients for the anterior trans-abdominal approach

technique already described in the previous chapter.

Access to the adrenal space on the left involves the mobilization and lowering of the left colon and the mobilization of the tail of the pancreas. The first step is to medialize the descending colon and dissect the spleno-colic and colic ligaments. With the aid of a retractor inserted through the trocar in the xiphoid region, the stomach is lateralized and at the same time the splenic flexure is pulled medially and downward; in this way, the gastro-colic ligament is put in tension and can be sectioned. The descending colon is then lateralized bluntly, dissected by the Gerota's fascia which is dissected in correspondence with the adrenal lodge. With the aid of a retractor introduced through the trocar located in the xiphoid region, the tail of the pancreas and the stomach are gently retracted. In fact, the gland is located posteriorly, and the spleen is not mobilized with this technique, as occurs instead in the lateral position. Successively, the intervention is conducted for the access on the side.

The right adrenal gland is also difficult to approach with such access, especially since the main adrenal vein on the right is particularly deep and located in the posterior retro-caval position. It is therefore necessary to lift the liver and move it medially. In addition, the transverse colon and the hepatic flexure must be mobilized and retracted inferiorly, and often the duodenum must be kocherized. In any case, the complete dissection of the adrenal vein involves the displacement of the vena cava with a high risk of vascular injury. In the lateral access that places the adrenal vein anterior to the visual field, this inconvenience is greatly reduced.

24.6 Operative Technique of MIA: Retroperitoneal Approach

24.6.1 Advantage, Indications, and Contraindications

- The retroperitoneal localization of the adrenal gland makes this approach anatomically ideal; in fact, it represents direct access to the adre-

nal gland, which does not require the mobilization of the adjacent structures since this gland is one of the first structures encountered during the surgical dissection [9]. Of course, extensive experience in adrenal surgery and in-depth knowledge of the anatomy of the retroperitoneum are essential prerequisites for its success The following are the advantages:
  - Absence of intra-abdominal scar
  - Lower risk of intra-operative intestinal perforation
  - Lower incidence of post-operative ileus
  - In the case of bilateral adrenalectomy, repositioning of the patient is avoided, and therefore the operating times are significantly reduced
- The main indications are represented by:
  - Presence of intraperitoneal adhesions that contraindicate the transperitoneal laparoscopic approach
  - Small lesions (< 6 cm) due to limited dissection space for this approach. However, this group of lesions include the majority of adrenal tumors, both functioning (cortisol-secreting adenomas, cortisol-secreting macro- and micronodular hyperplasia, aldosteronomas, pheochromocytomas) and non-functioning (incidentalomas)
- On the contrary, the contraindications are the following:

  - Malignant lesions with evident infiltration of adjacent structures
  - Suspicious lesions due to lack of adequate control of intra-abdominal organs and vessels

24.6.2 Instruments and Patients/ Operators Position (Fig. 24.6)

- In addition to the standard instruments of each advanced laparoscopy procedure, a CO_2 insufflator for the creation of the retropnemoperitoneum which is connected to a blunt tip trocar with a 12 mm balloon is specific to this type of approach. The balloon is then inflated with 15 cc of saline.

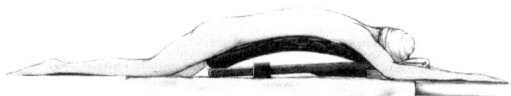

Fig. 24.6 Supine position kept by the Wilson bridge for the retroperitoneal approach

- The patient is positioned on the operating table in the prone position, using the Wilson bridge, which supports the chest and abdomen. The operators remain throughout the operation on the side of the lesion to be operated on. The laparoscopic column is positioned contralaterally to the lesion (and to the operators) at the level of the patient's head.

24.6.3 Operative Technique

- The first incision (1.5 cm) is made immediately below the end of the XII rib. The subcutaneous tissue is then incised, and the muscle plane is opened with a blunt dissection. After passing the muscular plane, the retroperitoneal space is encountered. The operator then creates with the index finger a space in the retroperitoneum, remaining in contact with the anterior face of the XII rib (superficially with respect to the Gerota fascia, which is not yet opened). This space must be large enough for the positioning of the medial and lateral trocars. The use of a dissecting balloon has also been proposed for the initial dissection of the retroperitoneum, although digital dissection is currently the preferred method.
- A 10 mm incision is then made about 2 cm inferior to the lower edge of the XII rib, 4–5 cm medial to the first incision, near the lateral margin of the sacro-spinal muscle. A 12 mm trocar is then inserted under digital guidance at this level, in a cranial direction. The index finger of the operator's left hand introduced at the level of the first skin incision, feels and guides the tip of the trocar that goes beyond the muscular plane and reaches the retroperitoneal space.
- Another incision is made 4–5 cm laterally to the first. A second trocar is then placed under digital guidance. Usually, the most lateral tro-

car is 5 mm although the placement of a 12 mm trocar may be useful in some circumstances.
- At this point, the blunt tip trocar with a 12 mm balloon is placed at the level of the first incision. The balloon is then inflated with 15 cc of saline. The CO_2 insufflator is then connected to this last trocar and the retropneumoperitoneum is induced, maintaining an insufflation pressure of about 20 mmHg.
- During this phase of the operation, the endoscope is introduced at the level of the central trocar. The Gerota fascia is then opened bluntly. The opening must be wide in order to have ample access to the retroperitoneum. After opening the fascia of the Gerota, the retroperitoneal fat must be dissected downward, so as to medially expose the paravertebral muscles, cranially the diaphragm, and laterally the peritoneum. This step is of fundamental importance, as it serves to create adequate space for subsequent dissection.
- Following the creation of an adequate dissection chamber, the upper pole of the kidney must be exposed and freed, which represents the most important landmark in this operation. The release of the upper pole of the kidney must be as complete as possible. This maneuver allows adequate lowering of the upper pole of the kidney necessary for complete exposure of the lower portion of the adrenal gland and for the identification and dissection of the main adrenal vein.
- In the right adrenalectomy, the small arterial branches that pass posteriorly to the vena cava must be dissected, using clips or high-energy instruments. At this point, the adrenal gland is raised with the instrument on the left hand in order to expose the posterior aspect of the inferior vena cava, in its cranial retroperitoneal portion. In this way, the main (middle) adrenal vein is tensioned and then identified. Its preparation and the subsequent section between clips are then realized.
- In left adrenalectomy, the release of the left adrenal gland begins from the medial and inferior aspect. At the level of the medial aspect of the adrenal, there are usually arterial vessels that must be dissected or cut, before identifying the main adrenal vein. Once prepared, the

latter is sectioned between metal clips. The inferior diaphragmatic vein is sometimes identifiable, which sometimes represents an important landmark for finding the main adrenal vein. It can be sectioned between clips although this maneuver is not usually necessary.

- After dissecting the main adrenal vein, the dissection of the adrenal gland is completed at the lateral and, ultimately, the cranial portion. All maneuvers on the adrenal gland must in any case be carried out with extreme caution and with non-traumatic instruments in order to avoid capsular breaks. Once adrenalectomy is completed, after a careful check of hemostasis, the surgical piece is extracted through the first trocar orifice using an endobag. In some cases, it may be useful to leave a suction drain in place.

24.7 Other less Usual Operative Techniques of MIA

24.7.1 Adrenal Sparing Surgery and Cryo-Surgery

- The laparoscopic technique was also used to perform partial adrenalectomy in selected series [10]. In most cases, it is possible to maintain the integrity of the main adrenal vein
- The main indications are represented by
  - Small peripheral tumors
    Aldosteronoma
    Corticosteroid adenomas
    Non-functioning adenomas
  - Bilateral lesions
    Familial pheochromocytomas
    MEN
  - Mono-adrenal patients
    E.g., pituitary adenoma Cushing's syndrome in patients with previous adrenalectomy
- Despite the apparent success of this technique, total adrenalectomy remains preferable since the potential for a "spillage" of tumor cells, resulting in tumor relapse, even in cases of benign tumors, is probably higher in subjects with partial adrenalectomy
- Recently, reports of technologies for the cryo-ablation of adrenal tumors have also appeared,

in selected series, with somewhat partial results for the moment. Of course, the correct and safe application of cryosurgery cannot be separated from a previous rather accurate radiological mapping, currently possible, thanks to new imaging technologies

24.7.2 Virtual Laparoscopic MIA

- Currently, computerized image acquisition technology has generated a series of new software capable of carrying out an accurate three-dimensional reconstruction of each organ or body region The fundamental advantage of this "virtual reality" lies in the possibility of allowing the surgeon to achieve an absolute understanding of the anatomy of the surgical field or the morphological characteristics of a lesion and, even, to interact with the image as if it existed in reality [11]
- Laparoscopy assisted by virtual reality reconstruction has multiple advantages:
  - Greater sensitivity in preoperative diagnostic procedures: 3-D reconstruction can allow us to diagnose adrenal cancer and to better evaluate incidentalomas, establishing the presence or absence of vascular infiltration or monitoring more accurately the dimensional growth of the tumor in the time (the so-called 4-D reconstruction)
  - Greater knowledge of the patient's anatomy
  - Possible preoperative establishment of the correct therapeutic plan
  - Planning the correct positioning of the trocars and instruments to optimize the "triangulation" configuration
  - Easier retrieval of the main landmarks and basically of the venous pedicles
  - Easier and faster survey of small masses (ultrasound-laparoscopy is also useful in this case)
  - Easy identification of various anatomical and in particular vascular anomalies (double venous district, abnormal outlets)
  - Possible performance of laparoscopic "training" applied to the individual patient

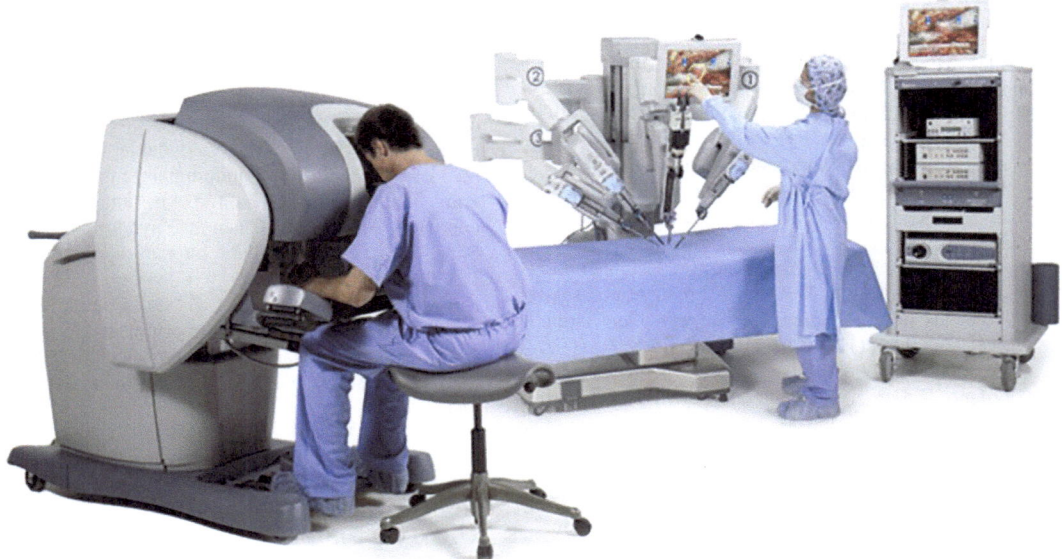

Fig. 24.7 Robotic adrenalectomy

24.7.3 Robotic MIA (Fig. 24.7)

- Another technological innovation of recent years is represented by the use of the robot. Such a device can increase the articulation capacity of intra-operative movements by the operator, overcoming the characteristic limits of laparoscopic surgery [12]
- Its advantage consists therefore in
  - Improvement of the mechanics and electronic control of the system:
    - Instruments with multiple degrees of freedom
    - Electronic control directly adjusted on the tip of the instruments
    - Elimination of physiological tremors by the electronic system, with reduction of the learning curve of complex interventions
  - Three-dimensional vision monitor
  - Possibility of having "virtual" tactile feedback
  - Ergonomics designed for the surgeon's comfort
- About adrenal surgery, several reports in the literature suggest that robot-guided laparoscopy is currently technically feasible and can

be performed effectively and safely, especially in particularly complex cases due to the size or the expansive/infiltrative tendency of the mass (see malignant pathology)

24.7.4 Single-Port MIA

- This is a little-used minimally invasive technique that involves the use of only one access in the abdominal cavity.
- Technically, a trans-abdominal single-port adrenalectomy requires a 2–3 cm incision at the umbilicus for the placement of a multiport device and the utilization of extra-long instruments able to reach the adrenal gland. The right adrenalectomy needs the help of an additional 2 mm needle-scopic port for liver retraction.
- Several authors reported the outcomes with single-incision adrenalectomy, and some studies compared the conventional laparoscopic approach with single-port adrenalectomy, demonstrating no significant differences in patient length of stay or morbidity and a small benefit in cosmesis and post-operative pain but longer operative times with single-port laparoscopy.
- Data on this approach remain limited.

References

1. Uludağ M, Aygün N, İşgör A. Surgical indications and techniques for adrenalectomy. Sisli Etfal Hastan Tip Bul. 2020;54(1):8–22. https://doi.org/10.14744/SEMB.2019.05578.

2. Bancos I, Prete A. Approach to the patient with adrenal incidentaloma. J Clin Endocrinol Metab. 2021;106(11):3331–53. https://doi.org/10.1210/clinem/dgab512.

3. Fiori C, Checcucci E, Amparore D, Cattaneo G, Manfredi M, Porpiglia F. Adrenal tumours:open surgery versus minimally invasive surgery. Curr Opin Oncol. 2020;32(1):27–34. https://doi.org/10.1097/CCO.0000000000000594.

4. Giordano A, Feroci F, Podda M, Botteri E, Ortenzi M, Montori G, Guerrieri M, Vettoretto N, Agresta F, Bergamini C. Minimally invasive versus open adrenalectomy for adrenocorticalcarcinoma: the keys surgical factors influencing the outcomes-a collective overview. Langenbeck's Arch Surg. 2023;408(1):256. https://doi.org/10.1007/s00423-023-02997-z.

5. Pedullà G, Sapienza P, Paliotta A, Giordano A, Crocetti D, Toma DE, G. Surgical considerations for removal of giant tumor of the right adrenal. Anticancer Res. 2014;34(9):5087–90.

6. Bergamini C, Martellucci J, Tozzi F, Valeri A. Complications in laparoscopic adrenalectomy:the value of experience. Surg Endosc. 2011;25(12):3845–51. https://doi.org/10.1007/s00464-011-1804-0.

7. McKinlay R, Mastrangelo MJ Jr, Park AE. Laparoscopic adrenalectomy: indications and technique. Curr Surg. 2003;60(2):145–9. https://doi.org/10.1016/S0149-7944(02)00801-2.

8. Pennestrì F, De Crea C, Voloudakis N, Raffaelli M. Laparoscopic transabdominal anterior bilateral adrenalectomy (La-TABA): an alternative approach for severe Cushing's syndrome. Updat Surg. 2023;75(8):2403–11. https://doi.org/10.1007/s13304-023-01653-x.

9. Liu Z, Li DW, Yan L, Xu ZH, Gu GL. Comparison of lateral transperitoneal and retroperitoneal approaches for homolateral laparoscopic adrenalectomy. BMC Surg. 2021;21(1):432. https://doi.org/10.1186/s12893-021-01422-w.

10. Perysinakis I, Aggeli C, Kaltsas G, Zografos GN. Adrenal-sparing surgery: current concepts on a theme from the past. Hormones (Athens). 2020;19(3):317–27. https://doi.org/10.1007/s42000-020-00202-0.

11. Shiozawa M, Sata N, Endo K, Koizumi M, Yasuda Y, Nagai H, Takakusaki H. Preoperative virtual simulation of adrenal tumors. Abdom Imaging. 2009;34(1):113–20. https://doi.org/10.1007/s00261-008-9364-z.

12. Makay O, Erol V, Ozdemir M. Robotic adrenalectomy. Gland Surg. 2019;8(Suppl 1):S10–6. https://doi.org/10.21037/gs.2019.01.09.

Minimally Invasive Bariatric/ Metabolic Surgery

Mary Giuffrè ⓘ, Niccolò Petrucciani ⓘ, Angelo Iossa ⓘ, and Gianfranco Silecchia ⓘ

25.1 Introduction

Obesity is a major public health and is defined as *"a chronic multifactorial disease related to the excess of the fat mass"* [1]. According to the 2021 National Health Statistics Reports [2], the prevalence of obesity reaches 41.9% among adults and 19.7% among children and adolescents aged 2–19 years old. Specifically, 9.2% adults in the United States have a body mass index (BMI, calculated as weight [kg]/height^2 [m] > 40 (severe obesity, class III). Obesity is considered as one of the leading preventable causes of mortality due to its relationship to cardiovascular diseases, type 2 diabetes, liver disease, chronic kidney disease, obstructive sleep apnea syndrome (OSAS), osteoarthritis, and cancer.

The management of obese patients involves several health professionals in the setting of a multidisciplinary approach. Unfortunately, diet and a healthier lifestyle alone are unable to achieve significant and sustainable weight loss with consequent remission of related comorbidities in the long term. Bariatric surgery, on the other hand, has been shown to be able to achieve long-term weight loss [EWL up to 30% at 20 years according to the data by the Swedish Obese Subjects [SOS] study [3, 4]] with remission/cure of associated comorbidities and, at present, represents the most durable and effective treatment for morbid obese patients. Today, laparoscopic surgery is considered the gold standard approach for bariatric/metabolic surgery.

Different procedures can be carried out, which are divided into two main categories:

- Pure restrictive.
- Mixed restrictive and malabsorptive/ hypo-absorbitive.

In the following chapter, we will explore the standard perioperative management and bariatric surgery techniques together with the specific operative setting and instruments needed.

M. Giuffrè · A. Iossa
Department of Medical-Surgical Sciences and Biotechnologies, Faculty of Pharmacy and Medicine, Sapienza University of Rome, Rome, Italy
e-mail: angelo.iossa@uniroma1.it

N. Petrucciani (✉) · G. Silecchia
Division of General Surgery, Department of Medical Surgical Sciences and Translational Medicine, Faculty of Medicine and Psychology, Sapienza University of Rome, Sant'Andrea Hospital, Rome, Italy
e-mail: niccolo.petrucciani@uniroma1.it;
gianfranco.silecchia@uniroma1.it

25.2 Perioperative Management

25.2.1 Prevention of Venous Thromboembolism

Death from VTE is a fearsome event after bariatric surgery. The incidence of VTE after bariatric surgery is around 0.5% [5], and the risk of mortality is 28-fold higher in patients with VTE compared to patients without VTE [6]. Furthermore, these high-risk patients may experience VTE and related complications despite using all available perioperative prophylaxis options [7]. Operative time is strictly related to the incidence of VTE, with a 3.75-fold higher incidence of VTE in patients who had operative time longer than 300 min compared to those who had operative time lower than 180 min [8]. The methods used for VTE prophylaxis are administration of subcutaneous unfractionated heparin, pneumatic compression stockings, and subcutaneous low molecular weight heparins [9].

Currently, there is no agreed-upon standard VTE prophylactic treatment in patients candidates for bariatric surgery. Types of anticoagulants to be prescribed, such as unfractionated heparin, low-molecular-weight heparin (LMWH), or warfarin, as well as their dosages and lengths of usage, are still discussed. However, guidelines for best clinical practice recommend LMWH during the perioperative period starting immediately after surgery up to 15–21 days [9, 10]. The most used treatment protocol is the administration of a dose of LMWH (3000 to 4000 anti-Xa IU 12 h^1 subcutaneously) depending on BMI for obese patients with a lower risk of VTE (Grade 2B according to the European Guidelines) and the administration of a higher dose of LMWH (4000 to 6000 anti-Xa IU 12 h^1 subcutaneously) for obese patients with a higher risk of VTE (Grade 2B) [9].

The use of intermittent pneumatic compression devices worn on the lower limbs represents a common practice (Fig. 25.1). These devices facilitate venous blood flow from the lower limbs during surgery by inflating and compressing approximately every 40 s. Evidence suggests that intermittent pneumatic compression can reduce

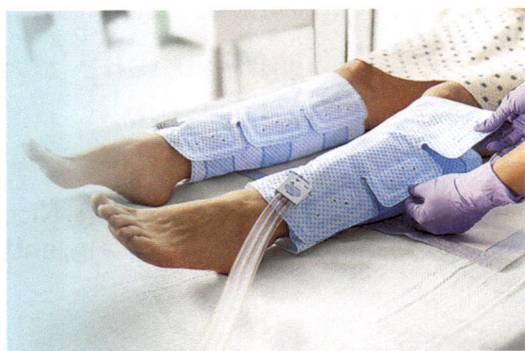

Fig. 25.1 Intermittent pneumatic compression devices for the lower limb

the VTE rate after bariatric surgery, and its use is recommended by the European Guidelines on perioperative venous thromboembolism prophylaxis [9]. After surgery, patients should stand up as quickly as possible, generally within 10–12 h wearing elastic stockings, as early ambulation is also recommended [9].

Recommendations: Minimize operating times, early postoperative ambulation, and calf-length pneumatic compression devices (intraoperative and early postoperative). LMWH for 15–21 days after discharge.

25.2.2 Venous Access in Obese Patients

Obesity is recognized as one of the main causes of venous access placement failure. Excess adiposity makes it difficult to visualize or palpate veins in the arms. According to the literature, in obese patients venous cannulation time is longer, successful cannulation on the first attempt is lower, and the need for more than 1 new venous cannula is higher compared with normal weight population [11]. Blind attempts at IV placement yield low success rates. Several methods can help improve successful cannulation. Warm compresses may be used to obtain vasodilation and better vein visualization. Displacing excess tissue by pulling the skin taut may also be useful. Real-time ultrasound is a very effective method to locate veins and guide venous cannulation.

Longer cannulas are helpful to penetrate through the excess layer of adipose tissue and go deep enough into the vessels to avoid dislodgment or infiltration. If venous access is needed for a longer time or to administer parenteral nutrition, placement of a peripherally inserted central catheter (PICC) line should be considered.

Key Points
- Obese patients are difficult-vascular-access patients.
- Intravenous site assessment should be conducted during the initial patient assessment before surgery.
- Real-time ultrasonography in conjunction with longer peripheral IV cannulas improves outcomes.

25.2.3 Operative Table Positioning

Safe transfer to the operating table, neutral positioning of the major joints and extremities, prevention of pressure injuries to skin and nerves, easy access to the operative field by the surgical team, and patient security on the table are the primary objectives in preparing an obese patient for bariatric surgery.

Patients are transported to the operation room on stretchers. The team could safely and comfortably transfer the patient from the transport stretcher or bed to the operation table using a lateral transfer device (Fig. 25.2). Automatic devices have been developed with the aim of

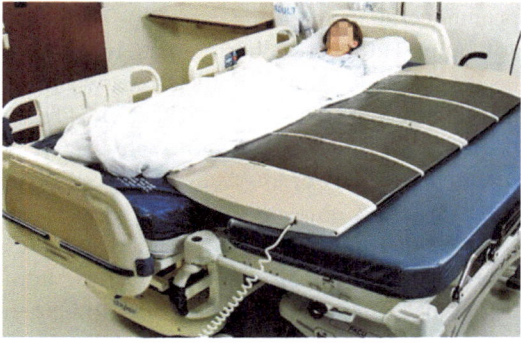

Fig. 25.2 Lateral transfer automatic device (PowerNurse© 2012 Astir Technologies)

reducing injuries to healthcare professionals due to patients' transfer, while minimizing the discomfort to the patient. In Fig. 25.2, one of these automatic tools is shown (PowerNurse© 2012 Astir Technologies). Two caregivers are needed, one for each side of the patient, and very little pushing or pulling force is required.

On the operating table, the patient is usually placed in the supine position with legs and arms abducted. The position is established after induction of anesthesia and orotracheal intubation. Ramping devices or pillows are placed under the patient's head and shoulder to facilitate intubation and airways management. When the patient is in place, the table straps are fastened around the waist. The tape is applied to the patient's legs to prevent the knees from flaring apart as the patient is positioned in reverse Trendelenburg position, facing backwards. A footboard is used to give their feet a stable location to rest on the table. The table should support all of the patient's weight, with no part of the patient's body or limbs dangling off.

The surgical team should be aware of the technical characteristics of the operating table and its maximum load. The patient's weight must be checked upon entering the operating room to verify that it does not exceed the limit imposed by the operating table. The use of heavy-weight operating tables specifically developed for severe obese patients is encouraged to guarantee patients' safety in bariatric surgical unit. For bariatric surgery, tables with at least 1000 lb. (454 kg) capacities are advised, even if, for the majority of patients, a 500 lb. (227 kg) capacity is sufficient. The table weight capacity should be checked not only in the static position but also during articulation (reverse Trendelenburg, beach chair position), as they may significantly differ. Tables with accessories, such as width extenders, leg and foot support, and arm support, are recommended. Tables with the lowest minimum height possible are advised as they facilitate patients' transfer to the table and improve nurses' and surgeons' comfort during patients' preparation and surgical procedures.

A "final check" of patient's position on the table must be performed before preparing and

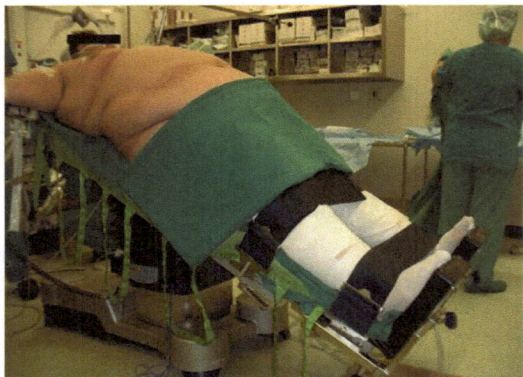

Fig. 25.3 An obese patient positioned on the operating table in reverse Trendelenburg position before

draping the patient. Nurses, anesthesiologists, and surgeons should verify that the position guarantees the correct execution of the various steps of the procedure and the safety of the patient. This check includes the verification that no excessive pressure is put on sensitive areas (such as the side, arms, hands, head, feet, and gluteal area). Attachments to the table should be adequately cushioned to prevent painful pressure sores and nerve damage. The patient's stability on the table and the neutrality of the limb joints are rechecked as well, moving the table in a "stressful" position. When working in cold conditions for an extended period, heating blankets are useful for preventing hypothermia caused by sweat and breathlessness. Figure 25.3 shows an obese patient positioned in reverse Trendelenburg position before bariatric surgery. After the verification of the patient's position, compression devices are activated and, if requested, the urinary catheter is placed (sometimes requiring two staff members, one for exposure and one for catheter insertion).

25.2.4 Surgical Team

The setting of the operating room for bariatric surgery includes the positioning of laparoscopic equipment and the placement of the surgical team. The main screen is placed at the patient's head, and it is usually part of a laparoscopic column including the source of CO_2, the light source,

and the camera and video tool with documentation systems. In our practice, the anesthesiology devices are placed to the right of the patient's head and the laparoscopic column to the left of the patient's head. It is fundamental that all the team has an optimal view of the screen. The use of large screen and of more than one screen in the operating room is advised for this purpose. The scrub nurse and the table for the instruments are placed on the patient's left. The surgeon is between the patient's legs, and the first assistant is at the surgeon's right. The second assistant is at the patient's right. The same surgical team positioning is used for all bariatric procedures.

25.3 Surgical Equipment

25.3.1 Pneumoperitoneum Creation

Due to the difficulty in performing an open cutdown procedure (Hasson) in bariatric patients, the pneumoperitoneum is usually induced with a Veress needle (length 12–15 cm) in obese patients. The Veress needle is stainless steel with a spring-loaded stylet that retracts when inserted into the abdomen. The stylet then advances to shield the needle once the needle tip enters the abdominal cavity, and it is used for induction of pneumoperitoneum. The water drop test or measuring CO_2 pressures and flow are used to confirm that the Veress needle is in the correct place once it has entered through the abdominal wall. The needle insertion at the Palmer point is the most recommended approach for inducing a safe pneumoperitoneum using a long needle of 150 mm. However, some authors recommend needle insertion in the umbilical area where the abdominal wall is less thick [12]. CO_2 infusion begins at a flow of 1–2 L/min. Schwartz et al. reported the safety of this technique in 600 obese patients [13]. Complete filling of the abdomen occurred after infusion of 4 L or more at a pressure limit of 15 mmHg in their series. Intraabdominal pressures are set at 15 mmHg to guarantee a correct working space in obese patients.

The alternative technique to insert the first trocar is the "Hasson" technique, where the abdomen is entered under direct vision. It may be very difficult in patients with a thick abdominal wall (super obese), and it is used only by a minority of surgeons in the field of bariatric surgery.

This technique can be used to enter into any quadrant of the abdomen, but it is most commonly employed at the central umbilical site.

25.3.2 Trocars

Trocars are used for laparoscopic and robotic bariatric procedures, and their size, number, and positions vary according to the different procedures performed and the type of abdomen profile and class of obesity (Fig. 25.4a and b). Trocars may be either reusable or disposable. Reusable trocars are made of stainless steel and may be cleaned, sterilized, and reused, whereas disposable trocars are made of plastic. Reusable trocars are advantageous to reduce the environmental and economic impact of laparoscopic surgery. Typically, trocars have a diameter of 5 mm (allowing passage of 5 mm diameter instruments)

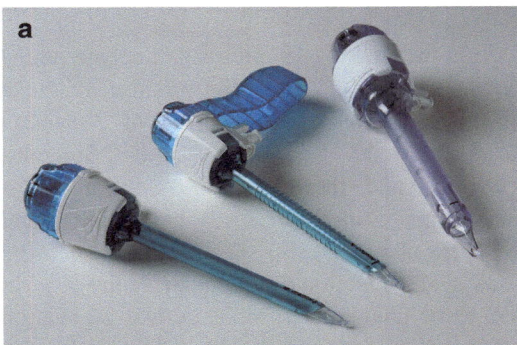
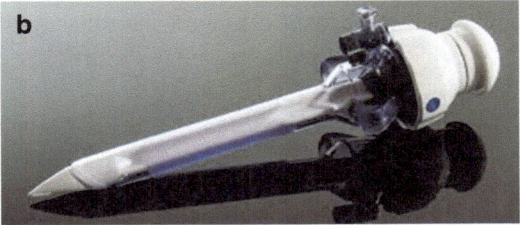

Fig. 25.4 (**a** and **b**) Trocars of various types and sizes for laparoscopic surgery

or 12 mm (to allow the introduction of staplers). For bariatric surgery, longer trocars are available, with lengths ranging from 100 to 150 mm, to facilitate good penetration and stability during the procedure. Trocars may be equipped with a retractile blade, which facilitates the penetration into the abdominal cavity. They are usually equipped with a safety lock to inform the user when the blade is exposed and have a parabolic shield designed to retract over the blade once into the peritoneal cavity. The blade is sharpened on both sides to divide tissue cleanly and precisely with control upon insertion through the abdominal wall. In our practice, after induction of the pneumoperitoneum set at a 15-mmHg pressure, we insert a first-bladed trocar. Also extra long (15 mm) optical trocars are available, which contain a see-through chuck tip that facilitates insertion into the abdomen using the laparoscope.

25.3.3 Tissue Dissection and Coagulation

Surgery is based on tissue dissection and coagulation, and several options are available in the setting of bariatric surgery to divide tissues and guarantee hemostasis. A profound knowledge of the different types of energy is mandatory for the surgical team to maximize patients' safety [14].

The energy sources available for laparoscopic bariatric surgery are:

- *Monopolar Energy*: In monopolar electrosurgery, the active electrode represents one pole, and the patient return electrode represents the other. The tissue effects available with monopolar electrosurgery include vaporization (tissue destruction and cutting), fulguration (tissue destruction and small vessel hemostasis), desiccation (cell wall rupture and cytoplasm boiling), and coaptation (vessel sealing owing to denaturation and renaturation of proteins). The major disadvantage of monopolar electrosurgery is the rare but unavoidable risk of stray current injury.
- *Bipolar Energy*: In bipolar electrosurgery (including advanced bipolar modalities), the

active and return electrodes are the two jaws of the energy source. It was introduced to eliminate the risk of stray current injury, while at the same time a means of sealing larger vessels. Bipolar electrosurgery results in tissue desiccation and vessel coaptation. A major advantage of conventional bipolar over monopolar electrosurgery is the ability to seal (coapt) vessels up to ~5 mm in diameter.

- *Advanced Bipolar Energy*: Advanced bipolar energy sources are revolutionary in several ways. Firstly, a propriety electrosurgical unit using a computer-controlled tissue feedback system controls each device. The tissue impedance is monitored with continuous adjustment of the generated voltage and current to maintain the lowest possible power setting to achieve the desired tissue effect, at which time an audio signal alerts the surgeon that the endpoint has been reached. In this way, the risk of lateral thermal spread as well as charring of the tissue and adherence of tissue to the device jaws is minimized. Second, these energy sources were the first to be approved by the US Food and Drug Administration (FDA) to seal vessels up to 7 mm in diameter.

- *Ultrasonic Energy:* Ultrasonic energy sources convert electrical energy into vibrations in the handpiece of the device at frequencies more than 20,000 cycles per second, that is, above the audible range. These vibrations oscillate the non-articulating jaw of the instrument. Tissue is compressed between an articulating jaw and the non-articulating jaw to impart the tissue effects derived from the combination of thermal and mechanical energy: desiccation and vessel sealing are achieved at lower frequencies, and tissue cutting occurs at higher frequencies. Specifically developed for larger vessel sealing and cutting, this device has been rated by the FDA to seal vessels up to 7 mm in diameter.

The diameter of monopolar, bipolar, advanced bipolar, and ultrasonic energy instruments is such that it fits into a 5 mm trocar. Also 10 mm advanced bipolar instruments with larger jaws are available.

Several instrument lengths are available for use in normal-weight and obese patients. For bariatric surgery, most surgeons use for dissection and sealing ultrasonic energy devices or advanced bipolar and choose long instruments.

Specifically, the LigaSure™ Maryland Jaw (advanced bipolar) exists in 3 lengths: 23 cm, 37 cm, and 44 cm. The first one is used in open procedures, the second in standard laparoscopic surgery, whereas the latter is conceived for obese and super-obese patients and guarantees patients' safety and surgeons' comfort. Caiman® is also based on advanced bipolar energy, and it is available in the 44 cm length. The ultrasound scalpel HARMONIC ACE® + 7 Shears with Advanced Hemostasis also exists in several lengths, including 23 cm for open surgery, 36 cm for standard laparoscopy, and 45 cm for laparoscopic surgery in obese patients. Thunderbeat® Type S has been designed for laparoscopic surgery and provides both advanced bipolar energy and ultrasonic energy. It is available in several lengths, including 45 cm for bariatric surgery.

25.3.4 Smoke Evacuation

During the COVID-19 outbreak, a debate on the potential threat of evacuation of surgical smoke and CO_2 started. The Society of American Gastrointestinal and Endoscopic Surgeons (SAGES) and the European Association for Endoscopic Surgery (EAES) have highlighted concerns about surgical smoke possibly causing COVID-19 infection during laparoscopy [15]. In the early phase, the use of smoke evacuation devices (SEDs) equipped with special filters was suggested. No evidence support the efficacy of disposable filters used at the end of the procedure to evacuate intrabdominal smoke and CO_2.

Multiple smoke alarm systems are available. Homemade devices for smoke evacuation have been developed and connected to a 10-mm trocar: this SED was built using an ordinary electrostatic filter found in ventilation systems, which is very effective at filtering loads of bacteria and viruses. Regular tubing can be used to attach this filter to the trocar's evacuation port. The endotracheal tube connector is used to connect the filter to the tubing. The homemade device was connected via standard tubing to an active suction system in order to maintain constant low-pressure wall suction during the procedure.

Another option is a framework with a filtered cardiovascular flow design (particles equal to 0.01 m), allowing for simultaneous insufflation and pressure sensing. Unlike conventional insufflators with flow systems and cyclical inflation, it provides constant smoke evacuation, which briefly stops for pressure sensing function.

25.3.5 Surgical Staplers

Surgical staplers (Fig. 25.5) are mechanical devices used to suture and cut several types of tissues, including the bowel, solid organs, and vessels. They are also used to fashion gastrointestinal anastomoses. In the field of obesity surgery, laparoscopic staplers are employed in the majority of the procedures.

The staples are made of titanium, and they have different types of chargers. Chargers are manufactured in various colors that correspond to the length of the staples, which is tailored to the tissue's characteristics and thickness. The pins in a given charger can vary in height or remain at a constant size. These chargers also have various

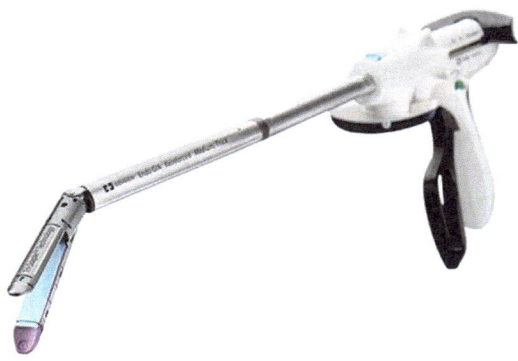

Fig. 25.5 A laparoscopic surgical stapler used to seal and cut different types of tissue and to fashion gastrointestinal anastomoses

lengths (30, 45, or 60 mm) and shapes (straight tip or curved tip for improved tissue grasping) to facilitate their use on the target tissue. The surgeon can choose between a short, regular, or long stapler shaft. Because of the increased abdominal thickness of patients undergoing obesity surgery, longer staplers (about 50 to 60 cm in length) are usually chosen in this setting.

Staplers can be either rigid or articulated (at 45°), and articulated staplers are mostly used as they allow a larger range of movements into the abdomen.

There are various suppliers of linear cutter staplers with a long shaft adapted for bariatric surgery, including:

- Medtronic's EndoGiaTMTriStaple has an XL version for obese patients.
- Medtronic Signia Stapling system also has an XL version for obese patients.
- Echelon FlexTM, by Johnson & Johnson, which is available in a long version of 44 cm.
- Panther endo linear stapler is also available with an extra long shaft (handle length = 26 cm).

25.3.6 Motorized Stapler

Motorized stapling is preferable to hand-stapling because it eliminates the micro-tremors that can occur while using a traditional stapler. Furthermore, during manual stapling, the force applied by the surgeon may not be homogeneous on the target tissue, whereas the mechanical stapler applies a constant and homogeneous force.

Motorized staplers are around 20% more expensive than their manual counterparts.

There are currently two motorized linear cutting staplers:

- Medtronic's SigniaTM stapler has three adjustable speeds. It uses a dial to provide the surgeon's feedback on how far along the abdominal stapling procedure is. A built-in chip in the grip allows it to identify individual charging devices by their unique I.D.s.

- The handle is sterilized after each use and can be used repeatedly (up to 300 times). There is a 50-use sterilization limit on shaft adapters. It is available as an XL version for bariatric procedures.
- Echelon Flex Powered PlusTM by Johnson & Johnson is a one-of-a-kind product designed for specific use. The long version of 44 cm is available.

25.3.7 Suture Reinforcements

The European Association for Endoscopic Surgery (EAES) has strongly recommended staple line reinforcement during sleeve gastrectomy as it reduces the risk of staple-line complications [16]. Buttressing material is the most preferred suture line reinforcement tool. Suture reinforcement with buttressing material has been developed to reduce the chance of leakage and bleeding on the staple lines. They are films applied on the charges of the mechanical staplers, made of biodegradable material, developed to reinforce the staple line and reduce the risk of suture bleeding. Given that the reinforcement layer causes an increase in thickness, it is customarily essential to pair it with a staple height higher than that initially given. The staple lines are fundamental to guarantee a good sealing of the suture, so the material chosen to reinforce them is crucial. In addition to being biodegradable and possessing the necessary strength, thickness, and uniformity over time, this material is also designed to reduce the risk of tissue erosion.

The three most common manufacturers of suture reinforcements are as follows:

- Polyglycolic acid (PGA) and trimethylene carbonate (TMC) copolymers make up GORE's Endoscopic SeamguardTM EBSGTM. It is a 0.5 mm thick film placed between the stapler's jaws before use. It completely dissolves in 6 months.

- Medtronic has introduced the EndogiaTM Tri-StapleTM, a customized stapler magazine with built-in reinforcement. Biotin film, a polyglycolic acid reinforcement (absorbed in 28 days), is already attached to the stapler's jaws. Only Medtronic EndoGIATM Staplers can be charged using these adapters.
- Gunze: NeoveilTM (sold by Europrisme Medical in France) is a poly-glycolic acid fabric reinforcing system that is both soft and strong. In its first appearance, it presents itself as a sleeve that can be inserted into the stapler's jaws. It is completely absorbed in 15 weeks. It is usable with EchelonTMFlex and EndoGIATM staplers.

25.3.8 Trocar Port-Site Closure

At the end of the surgical procedure, fascial opening of the 10–12 mm size trocar must be closed, to reduce the risk of incisional hernia, as recommended by the guidelines released by the European Hernia Society [17]. Closing the trocar incision during a laparoscopic procedure can be very difficult in morbid obese patients, for the thickness of the subcutaneous tissue. Complications from port-site trocars incisional hernia may have severe consequences, including the need for additional surgery or bowel resections. Herniation, bleeding, discomfort, and nerve trapping are potential complications from surgical sealing of the trocar sites. Specialized instruments and suturing techniques are studied to reduce the risk of port-site problems after laparoscopic surgery [18].

There are countless laparoscopic instruments available from over 20 companies that can be used for laparoscopic port-site closure (e.g., the Weck EFx Endo Fascial Closure, the NeatStitch laparoscopic port closure, the Vector X™ neoClose™ Closure, and the laparoscopic suture passer). The choice is up to surgeon's preference.

The Weck® EFx Shield® Fascial Closure System from Teleflex includes a shielded wing

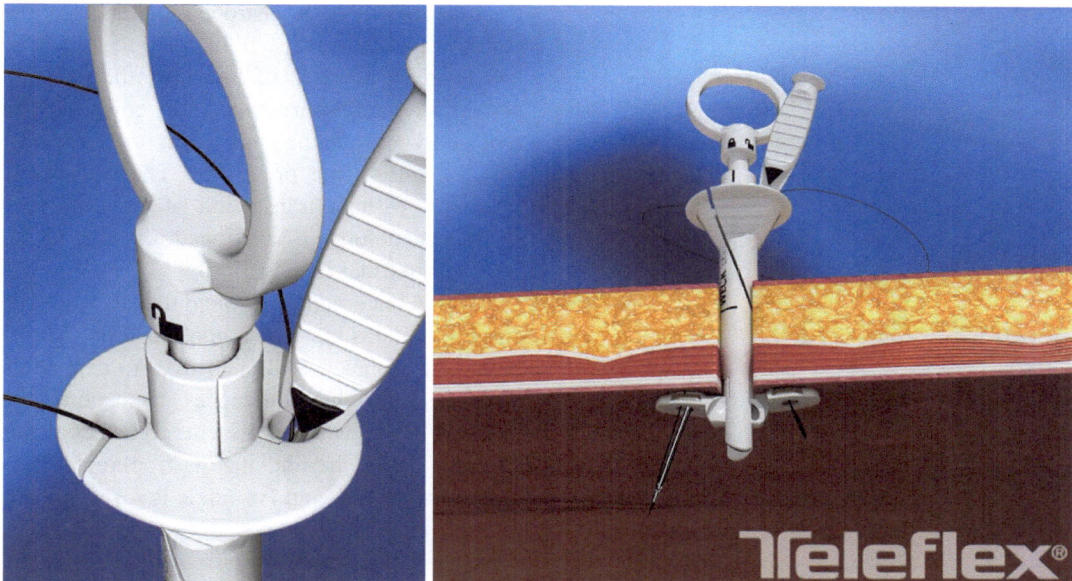

Fig. 25.6 The Weck® EFx Shield® Fascial Closure System device from Teleflex

Fig. 25.7 The Vector Neoclose device

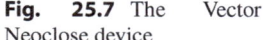

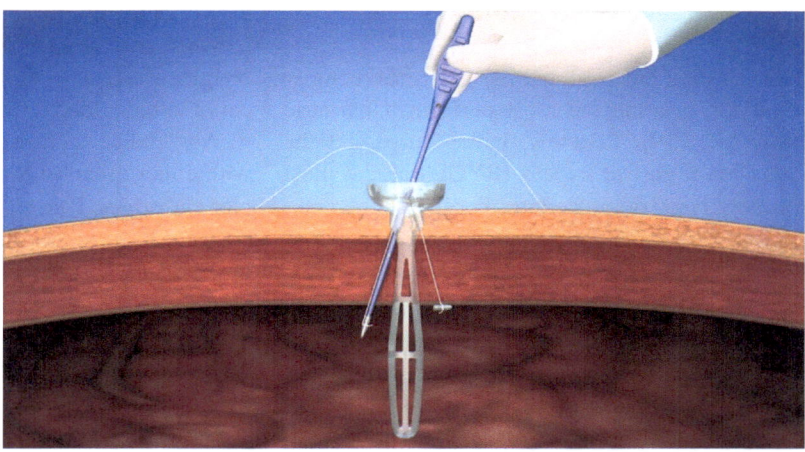

design for enhanced sharps protection, an intuitive wing deployment, and a suture retrieval system for unassisted fascial closure, as shown in Fig. 25.6. This instrument helps the surgeon pass the sutures into the aponeurosis and is used for defects of 10 mm or more. The NeatStich and the Vector Neoclose are similar port closure devices that internally suture tissues during minimally invasive laparoscopic surgical procedures (Fig. 25.7). Various types of laparoscopic suture passers (Fig. 25.8), disposable or reusable, have been designed to easily pass the sutures throughout the fascia and peritoneum.

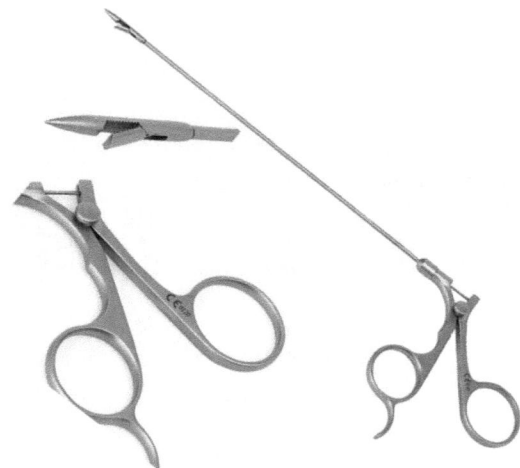

Fig. 25.8 Suture passer device

25.4 Bariatric Laparoscopic Procedures: Technical Details

25.4.1 Sleeve Gastrectomy

Worldwide, laparoscopic sleeve gastrectomy (SG) has become the most performed bariatric procedure [19]. Recently, it has surpassed the Roux-en-Y gastric bypass (RYGB) as the most frequent bariatric procedure.

25.4.2 Surgical Technique

Two 12-mm and two 5-mm ports are usually needed to perform the procedure. In challenging circumstances, additional ports may be necessary. The camera port is placed first, around 15 cm below the xiphoid process in the upper abdomen. For the best visual representation of the Angle of His and hiatus, a 30° telescope is recommended. A 12-mm port is positioned in the right midclavicular line, and a 5-mm port is set in the right anterior axillary line. The second port, measuring 5 mm in diameter, is placed in the left midclavicular line for the second surgeon.

At the outset, the lesser sac is opened, and the small branches of the gastroepiploic arcade are cut. Then, the advanced bipolar cutting device or the ultrasonic scalpel is used to dissect along the larger gastric curve, keeping close to it dividing the branches of both gastroepiploic arteries and the short gastric vessels. To increase the exposure and decrease the risk of bleeding, the assistant performs a lateral retraction of the omentum and repeatedly moves the instrument to a superior position during the procedure. The gastrocolic ligament (without transection of the gastroepiploic vasculature) is sectioned distally up to 2–6 cm proximal to the pylorus.

Cutting the omentum around the larger gastric curve facilitates the gastric mobilization. At this point, the stomach is flipped over to expose its backside, and the adherences connecting the stomach to the pancreas are cut. To detect a concomitant hiatal hernia, the gastrophrenic ligament is separated, and His angle is revealed. The left crus is also fully exposed.

After the complete mobilization of the stomach, a sufficient gastric lumen is maintained by inserting from the mouth a 34–40 Fr bougie into the stomach before stapling. Safe placement of the bougie requires constant back-and-forth between the surgeon and anesthesiologist. The bougie must be positioned toward the smaller curve to be guided to the pylorus.

Absorbable buttress material may be used with either green (4.8 mm) or black (5 mm) stapler cartridges. If no absorbent buttressing materials are utilized, the first two cartridges will be green or black, and the remaining cartridges will be yellow or blue. Usually, 60 mm cartridges are used. The stomach is stapled to create a gastric tube along the boogie, avoiding kinking or twisting.

During the stapling of the stomach, the assistant stretches the patient's stomach to the left, and the surgeon puts the stapler so that its anterior and posterior edges are at the same distance from the lesser curvature. The residual stomach's anterior wall should not be smaller than the stomach's posterior wall. As an added precaution against "dog-ears" on the stomach's edge that can lead to ischemia, a stapler should be put at a right angle to the preceding one. A wiggle test of the bougie after each firing helps the anesthesiologist ensure the sleeve is not excessively tight and that the bougie has not been stapled.

After the gastric resection, one of the 12-mm ports is used to extract the stomach. 50–100 cc of methylene blue in saline solution may be injected into the stomach to check the staple line and verify there is no leak. A drain may be placed according to the surgeon's choice. Figure 25.9 reports a graphical representation of sleeve gastrectomy.

What Instruments Should the Scrub Nurse Have on the Table?

- Laparoscopic kit including laparoscopic atraumatic forceps, liver retractor, suction/irrigation device, and a 30° laparoscope.
- Orogastric tube 36–40 Fr (for the anesthesiologist).
- Two 10–12 mm and 2–3 5 mm trocars.
- Laparoscopic monopolar hook.
- Device for laparoscopic dissection based on advanced bipolar energy or ultrasonic energy (according to the surgeons' preference).
- Laparoscopic stapler with different types of cartridge.
- Buttressing material for the laparoscopic stapler.
- Suture passer or any device for fascial closure.
- Retrieval bag (optional).
- Fascial and skin sutures.

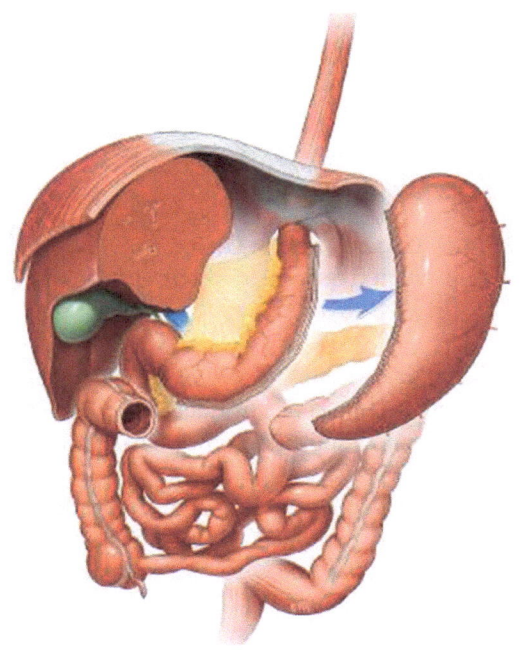

Fig. 25.9 Graphical representation of sleeve gastrectomy

Key Learning Points

- Excessive stomach narrowing can occur if no close attention is paid during the first and last stapler firings.
- The surgeon must take care to avoid including too much tissue into the stapler to prevent bunching of tissues.
- The gastric sleeve rotation may occur if different tractions are applied to the anterior and posterior stomach walls.
- Accurate hemostasis is mandatory as bleeding is a frequent complication.
- In many cases, a leakage can develop after a hematoma on the staple line.

25.4.3 Laparoscopic Roux-En-Y Gastric Bypass (LRYGB)

Laparoscopic Roux-en-Y gastric bypass (LRYGB) has been in the past the most performed bariatric procedure and still represents an effective procedure with durable results on weight loss and resolution of comorbidities.

25.4.4 Surgical Technique

Usually, four or five trocars are needed to perform the procedure, even if considerable heterogeneity in port placement exists between surgeons and patients. A liver retractor is inserted through a 5-mm incision in the epigastrium. Four additional trocars are placed for the camera port, the two hands of the surgeon, and the hand of the first assistant.

The Roux-en-Y gastric bypass involves the creation of a small gastric pouch of a volume of 15–25 mL, completely separated from the gastric remnant and anastomosed with a jejunal loop, measured 75 cm distal to the Treitz ligament, with recanalization of the bilio-pancreatic tract at a distance between 150 cm. Measures of the alimentary and biliary limbs vary according to surgeons' choice and patient's characteristics.

After exposure of the hiatal region with a hepatic retractor, the surgeon proceeds to the dissection of the angle of Hiss to obtain a good exposure of the left diaphragmatic pillar.

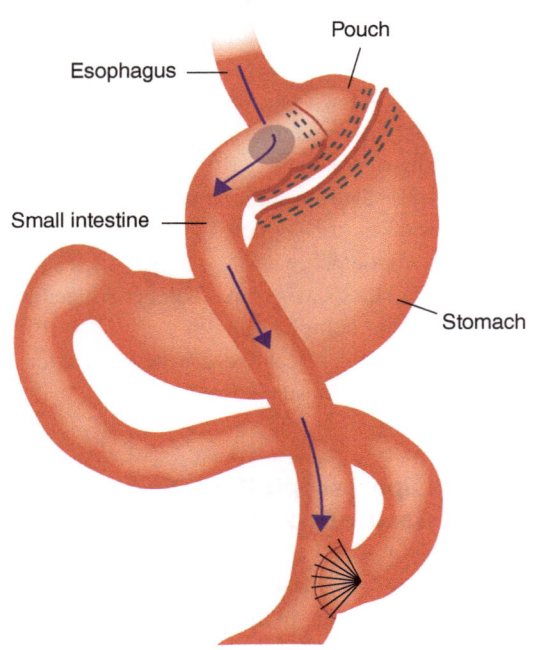

Fig. 25.10 Graphical representation of Roux en Y gastric bypass

Approximately 4 cm below the gastroesophageal junction, the omental bursa is opened, and the stomach is resected horizontally with a linear stapler for approximately 4 cm in length. After dissection of the posterior gastric wall, the stomach is completely resected vertically with a linear stapler until the Hiss angle is reached and the gastric pouch is created. By lifting the transverse colon, the Treitz ligament is identified, and 75 cm of the jejunal intestine is measured distally, which is anastomosed with the gastric pouch. 150 cm distally, the entero-enteric anastomosis is made between the bilio-pancreatic and the alimentary loop. Then, the two limbs are disconnected. The final result is shown in Fig. 25.10. The gastrojejunal anastomosis is verified with a methylene blue test through a nasogastric probe. The mesenteric defects are closed to avoid the potential development of internal hernias.

What Instruments Should the Scrub Nurse Have on the Table?

- Laparoscopic kit including laparoscopic atraumatic forceps, scissors, liver retractor, suction/irrigation device, needle-holder, and a 30° laparoscope.
- Orogastric tube 36–40 Fr (for the anesthesiologist).
- Two/three 10–12 mm and 2–3 5 mm trocars.
- Laparoscopic monopolar hook.
- Device for laparoscopic dissection based on advanced bipolar energy or ultrasonic energy (according to the surgeons' preference).
- Laparoscopic stapler with different types of cartridge.
- Sutures to close the enterotomy (usually barbed absorbable sutures, such as V-lock® or Stratafix®).
- Sutures to close the mesenteric defects (usually non-resorbable 2–0 Prolene® sutures).
- Suture passer or any device for fascial closure.
- Fascial and skin sutures.

Key Learning Points

- RYGB is a complex procedure and should be performed by a trained team:
- Laparoscopic instruments including staplers, needle holders, and cutting and sealing devices should be carefully prepared.
- The main steps of the procedure are the creation of a small gastric pouch, the fashioning of a gastrojejunal anastomosis, and a jejuno-jejunal anastomosis.

25.4.5 Laparoscopic One-Anastomosis Gastric Bypass (OAGB)

Rutledge introduced the OAGB in 1997 [20]. It has been developed as a variant of the RYGB in the effort to simplify the procedure and reduce post-operative risks.

This technique involves the creation of an end-to-lateral (or latero-lateral) anastomosis between a narrow and long gastric pouch and a jejunal loop about 150–200 cm distal to the Treitz's ligament.

Weight loss occurs not only through a restrictive effect but also through a hypo-absorptive mechanism.

25.4.6 Surgical Technique

The first 10–12 mm trocar is placed in the midline, between the xiphoid process and the navel; the second (5 mm) and third (12 mm) trocars are placed in the right and left hypochondrium. The fourth trocar (11 mm) is placed below the xiphoid process, and the fifth (12 mm) is positioned in the right quadrant on the midclavicular, 3 cm below the costal arch.

Identified the "crow's foot," where the branches of the vagus nerve divide at the level of the small gastric curve, a window is created in the small omentum to access the posterior wall of the stomach.

A 45 mm linear stapler is inserted through the created window, and the horizontal section of the stomach is performed. Then, the procedure continues with the vertical section of the stomach up to the corner of Hiss.

The short gastric vessels are not dissected, and the anterior and posterior vagus nerves are preserved.

Once the Treitz ligament has been identified, the jejunum is measured for a length of 150–200 cm, and a gastro-jejunal anastomosis is made.

A methylene blue test through the orogastric tube is suggested. Figure 25.11 shows the anatomy after OAGB.

What Instruments Should the Scrub Nurse Have on the Table?
- Laparoscopic kit including laparoscopic atraumatic forceps, scissors, liver retractor, suction/irrigation device, needle-holder, and a 30° laparoscope.
- Orogastric tube 36–40 Fr (for the anesthesiologist).
- Two/three 10–12 mm and 2–3.5 mm trocars.
- Laparoscopic monopolar hook.
- Device for laparoscopic dissection based on advanced bipolar energy or ultrasonic energy (according to the surgeons' preference).
- Laparoscopic stapler with different types of cartridge.
- Sutures to close the enterotomy (usually barbed absorbable sutures, such as V-lock® or Stratafix®).

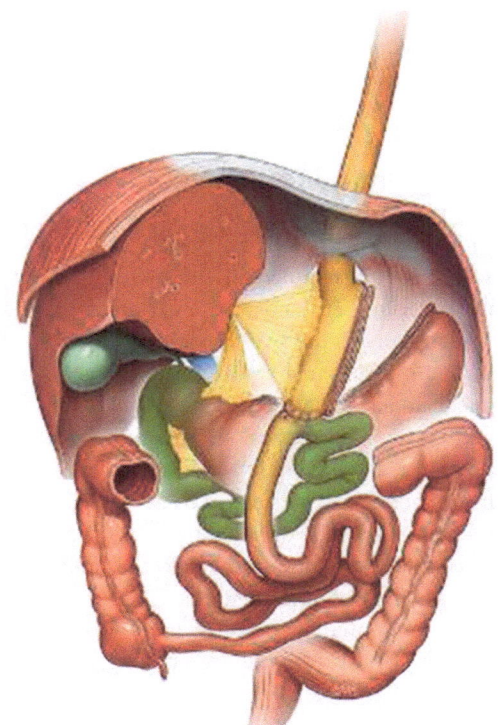

Fig. 25.11 Graphical representation of one anastomosis gastric bypass

- Suture passer or any device for fascial closure.
- Fascial and skin sutures.

Key Learning Points
- OAGB is a variant of the RYGB developed to simplify the procedure, reduce the postoperative risks, and reduce the operating time.
- The main step of the procedure is the creation of a side-to-side anastomosis between a narrow and long gastric pouch and a jejunal loop (biliary limb).

25.4.7 SADI-S (Single Anastomosis Duodenal-Ileal Bypass with Sleeve Gastrectomy)

Developed as a simplified Biliopancreatic Diversion Duodenal Switch, the SADI is described as a safe second-step operation after SG (for weight recidivism) or as a malabsorptive procedure in super obese patients (BMI >50 kg/

m²) combining the sleeve restriction with intestinal bypass consisting in a duodenal-ileal omega anastomosis.

25.4.8 Surgical Technique

Technically, the first optical trocar (10–12 mm) is inserted in the paramedian supraumbilical position. Two other 10- and 12-cm trocars are placed symmetrically in the two hypochondria. A 5-mm trocar is inserted under the xiphoid process and another under the left costal arch.

After hepatic retraction, the first operative time is the establishment of the sleeve gastrectomy as previously described. After this step, the posterior wall of the duodenum is dissected from the pancreas, paying attention to the upper border and the hepatic pedicle. The dissection should be as small as possible to avoid devascularization of the duodenum, but mobilization should be sufficient to make a tension-free anastomosis.

The right gastro-epiploic pedicle is dissected.

The section of the duodenum with a linear stapler represents the next operative time.

At 300 cm from the ileocecal valve, the ileal loop is brought up near the duodenum. A duodenotomy and an enterotomy of approximately 20–30 mm are then performed.

A manual end to lateral ileal-duodenal anastomosis is performed. The intervention ends with a test with methylene blue, and the nasogastric tube is withdrawn. In Fig. 25.12, the graphical aspect of SADI-S is shown.

What Instruments Should the Scrub Nurse Have on the Table?
- Laparoscopic kit including laparoscopic atraumatic forceps, scissors, liver retractor, suction/irrigation device, needle-holder, and a 30° laparoscope.
- Orogastric tube 36–40 Fr (for the anesthesiologist).
- Two/three 10–12 mm and 2–3.5 mm trocars.
- Laparoscopic monopolar hook.
- Device for laparoscopic dissection based on advanced bipolar energy or ultrasonic energy (according to the surgeons' preference).

- Laparoscopic stapler with different types of cartridge.
- Sutures to perform an intestinal anastomosis (usually barbed absorbable sutures, such as V-lock® or Stratafix®).
- Sutures to close the mesenteric defects (usually non-resorbable 2–0 Prolene® sutures).
- Suture passer or any device for fascial closure.
- Fascial and skin sutures.

Key Learning Points
- The SADI-S is a mixed surgical technique (restrictive and malabsorptive) born as a simplification of the duodenal switch.
- The first step involves the creation of a Sleeve Gastrectomy with the removal of 80% of the stomach.
- The second step involves the creation of a duodenal-ileal anastomosis using an ileal limb 300 cm distant from the ileocecal valve.

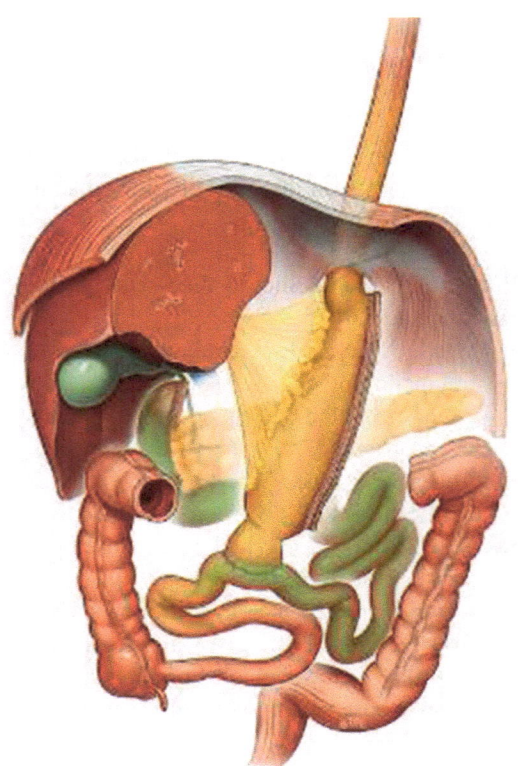

Fig. 25.12 Graphical representation of sleeve-single anastomosis duodenal ileal bypass

- SADI is more effective for weight control and diabetes control than SG but has a major impact on the nutrient absorption and higher risk of malnutrition.

25.4.9 Robotic Approach

Over the past decade, the intraoperative and post-operative complications rate has decreased significantly in high-volume bariatric surgery centers, thanks to a minimally invasive approach. The use of laparoscopic surgery has allowed not only the decrease of postoperative complications but also faster recovery and better patient acceptance. Consequently, laparoscopic bariatric surgery has boomed in the last 30 years. More refined instruments have been developed over time to improve the safety of laparoscopic bariatric procedures. In Fig. 25.5, a modern stapler is shown. The search for new techniques, instruments, and tools that offer risk reduction, better postoperative results, and faster recovery is still ongoing. Laparoscopy does not entirely satisfy surgical teams as it is limited by a two-dimensional (2D) perspective and its challenging ergonomics (particularly in super obese patients). Recent advances in robotic surgery have overcome some drawbacks of laparoscopy by providing high-definition 3D imaging and much more comfortable and flexible tools that better respond to precise surgical movements. In Fig. 25.13, the Da Vinci Xi robot and its console are shown.

The surgical robot consists of a control console with a display in front of which the surgeon, by placing his eyes in front of a binocular optical system, will then direct the robotic arms using two joysticks and several pedals, and a bed-side robot with four articulated arms in which the surgical instruments are connected. The dual console option includes a second screen for training; a technological column supports the tower housing the main computer, the CO_2 insufflator, and the numerous generators; and the screen retransmits the image of the operative field.

In comparison to human hands, robotic arms can twist and bend in seven directions instead of three, allowing for the creation of complex angles that facilitate the reaching of deep planes and the increased precision afforded by the use of miniaturized, articulated pliers that contribute to the arms' minimally invasive nature. Many consumable tools are stored on the robot's robotic arm, including staplers, section coagulation devices, needle holders, clip applicator forceps, scissors, pliers, and so on. Their multi-planar technology makes the ability to spin in a full 360°. A chip built into each consumable keeps track of how many times it has been sterilized.

During robotic procedures, the assistant at the table may use laparoscopic staplers from its port, and when robotic staplers were not still available, it was a common practice. In the last years, robotic staplers controlled by the main surgeon at the console have been introduced.

As teams conducting robotic surgery have gained experience and technical skills, they have been able to treat complex operations, such as bariatric procedures. Robotic surgery can increase precision and provide greater comfort for the surgeon, especially during technically challenging procedures, as it is more ergonomic and offers hand tremor filtration, which allows the robot's mechanical arm to remain stable at all times. The actual value of robotic bariatric surgery to the patient has yet to be defined; nevertheless, advantages like reduced surgical process times, greater visualization clarity because of high-definition 3D imaging, and the simplicity of suturing exist.

The exact advantages of robotics in bariatric surgery may become clearer as the direct and ancillary expenses of using a robot decrease, and surgical experience increases with longer patient follow-up periods [21].

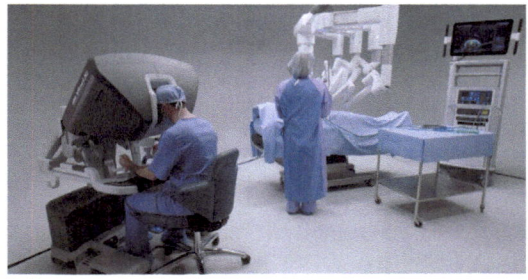

Fig. 25.13 The Da Vinci console and surgical robot

Regarding bariatric surgery, there is currently no evidence in the literature that demonstrates the superiority of the robotic technique over laparoscopy, although it appears to be more comfortable for the surgeon. The robotic approach may be useful in the future to perform revisional bariatric surgery, where the alteration of anatomical structures and the presence of adhesions require high laparoscopic skills [22]. Certainly, more studies are needed to define the role of the robot in this field.

References

1. The World Health Organization. Obesity and overweight. 2020. http://www.who.int/fr/news-room/fact-sheets/detail/obesity-and-overweight/.
2. Centers for Disease Control and Prevention. Obesity and Overweight. 2022. https://www.cdc.gov/nchs/fastats/obesity-overweight.htm.
3. Sjöström L. Review of the key results from the Swedish obese subjects (SOS) trial - a prospective controlled intervention study of bariatric surgery. J Intern Med. 2013;273(3):219–34.
4. Sjöholm K, Sjöström E, Carlsson LMS, Peltonen M. Weight change-adjusted effects of gastric bypass surgery on glucose metabolism: 2- and 10-year results from the Swedish obese subjects (SOS) study. Diabetes Care. 2016;39(4):625–31.
5. Becattini C, Agnelli G, Manina G, Noya G, Rondelli F. Venous thromboembolism after laparoscopic bariatric surgery for morbid obesity: clinical burden and prevention. Surg Obes Relat Dis. 2012;8(1):108–15.
6. Aminian A, Andalib A, Khorgami Z, Cetin D, Burguera B, Bartholomew J, et al. Who should get extended Thromboprophylaxis after bariatric surgery?: a risk assessment tool to guide indications for post-discharge Pharmacoprophylaxis. Ann Surg. 2017;265(1):143–50.
7. Jogiat U, Mocanu V, Verhoeff K, Dang J, Birch DW, Switzer NJ, et al. Method of venous thromboembolism prophylaxis is not a predictor of pulmonary embolus following elective bariatric surgery: a retrospective cohort study of 135,409 patients. Surg Obes Relat Dis. 2022;S1550-7289(22):00643–8.
8. Dang JT, Switzer N, Delisle M, Laffin M, Gill R, Birch DW, et al. Predicting venous thromboembolism following laparoscopic bariatric surgery: development of the BariClot tool using the MBSAQIP database. Surg Endosc. 2019;33(3):821–31.
9. Venclauskas L, Maleckas A, Arcelus JI. ESA VTE guidelines task force. European guidelines on perioperative venous thromboembolism prophylaxis: surgery in the obese patient. Eur J Anaesthesiol. 2018;35(2):147–53.
10. American Society for Metabolic and Bariatric Surgery Clinical Issues Committee. ASMBS updated position statement on prophylactic measures to reduce the risk of venous thromboembolism in bariatric surgery patients. Surg Obes Relat Dis. 2013;9(4):493–7.
11. Nafiu OO, Burke C, Cowan A, Tutuo N, Maclean S, Tremper KK. Comparing peripheral venous access between obese and normal weight children. Paediatr Anaesth. 2010;20(2):172–6.
12. Pantoja Garrido M, Frías Sánchez Z, Zapardiel Gutiérrez I, Torrejón R, Jiménez Sánchez C, Polo Velasco A, et al. Direct trocar insertion without previous pneumoperitoneum versus insertion after insufflation with Veress needle in laparoscopic gynecological surgery: a prospective cohort study. J Obstet Gynaecol. 2019;39(7):1000–5.
13. Schwartz ML, Drew RL, Andersen JN. Induction of pneumoperitoneum in morbidly obese patients. Obes Surg. 2003;13(4):601–4; discussion 604.
14. Olasehinde O, Owojuyigbe A, Adeyemo A, Mosanya A, Aaron O, Wuraola F, et al. Use of energy device in general surgical operations: impact on peri-operative outcomes. BMC Surg. 2022;22(1):90.
15. Bracale U, Silvestri V, Pontecorvi E, Russo I, Triassi M, Cassinotti E, et al. Smoke evacuation during laparoscopic surgery: a problem beyond the COVID-19 period. A quantitative analysis of CO_2 environmental dispersion using different devices. Surg Innov. 2022;29(2):154–9.
16. Di Lorenzo N, Antoniou SA, Batterham RL, Busetto L, Godoroja D, Iossa A, et al. Clinical practice guidelines of the European Association for Endoscopic Surgery (EAES) on bariatric surgery: update 2020 endorsed by IFSO-EC, EASO and ESPCOP. Surg Endosc. 2020;34(6):2332–58.
17. Muysoms FE, Antoniou SA, Bury K, Campanelli G, Conze J, Cuccurullo D, et al. European hernia society guidelines on the closure of abdominal wall incisions. Hernia. 2015;19(1):1–24.
18. Andraos Y. Safety and efficacy of trocar port-site closure using a biological plug closure in laparoscopic bariatric surgery: a prospective study. Obes Surg. 2022;32(11):3796–806.
19. Angrisani L, Santonicola A, Iovino P, Ramos A, Shikora S, Kow L. Bariatric surgery survey 2018: similarities and disparities among the 5 IFSO chapters. Obes Surg. 2021;31(5):1937–48.
20. Rutledge R. The mini-gastric bypass: experience with the first 1,274 cases. Obes Surg. 2001;11(3):276–80.
21. Fantola G, Moroni E, Runfola M, Lai E, Pintus S, Gallucci P, et al. Controversial role of robot in primary and Revisional bariatric surgery procedures: review of the literature and personal experience. Front Surg. 2022;9:916652.
22. Vanetta C, Dreifuss NH, Schlottmann F, Mangano A, Cubisino A, Valle V, et al. Current status of robot-assisted Revisional bariatric surgery. J Clin Med. 2022;11(7):1820.

Laparoscopic Treatment of Gallbladder Diseases

26

Fabio Cesare Campanile and Tiziana Placidi

26.1 Introduction

Laparoscopic cholecystectomy has been the first largely practiced minimally invasive procedure. Since its introduction in the late 1980s, it has rapidly become the gold standard for treating gallstone-related disease, and now, it is one of the most common general surgical procedures all over the world. It is performed, as an elective or urgent procedure, by expert operators, but it is also one of the first supervised surgical operations assigned to residents and in-training surgeons. Surgery can be straightforward, but the team can face exceedingly challenging and risky situations because the clinical and anatomical scenarios are extremely assorted.

Several diagnostic modalities may be part of the surgical procedure (intraoperative cholangiography with iodinated contrast media, intraoperative ultrasound, cholangioscopy, and indocyanine green fluorescence cholangiography); their need can be planned before surgery or arise in the middle of it.

Therefore, the surgical team (surgeons, anesthesiologists, scrub, and circulating nurses) must keep a versatile disposition and be prepared to deal with all those possibilities.

After a first description by the German surgeon Erich Mühe in 1986, the introduction of laparoscopic cholecystectomy is generally ascribed to the French surgeon Phillipe Mouret during the following year. Soon, two other French surgeons (François Dubois and Jacques Perissat) introduced the procedure in their practice. Shortly thereafter, some American surgeons (Barry McKernan, William Saye, Eddie Reddick, Douglas Olsen) started their laparoscopic cholecystectomy practice and the first educational program about it, training several US surgeons.

The French and American techniques are still commonly adopted in our operating rooms today, the first more common in Europe (mainly France and Germany), the second elsewhere.

In our chapter, we will take into account both varieties.

26.2 Operating Room Setup and Patient Positioning

The patient's position on the operating table and the surgical team's disposition vary between the French [1] and the American [2] techniques. In both cases, the laparoscopic cart with video monitor, insufflator, light source, camera system, and recording devices is placed at the right of the patient's head. Recently, in most operating rooms, video monitors are mounted on articulated arms either on the laparoscopic cart or on

F. C. Campanile (✉) · T. Placidi
Division of General Surgery, ASL Viterbo, Hospital
San Giovanni Decollato Andosilla,
Civita Castellana VT, Italy
e-mail: campanile@surgical.net

ceiling-mounted trolleys; they can be easily positioned at the head of the patient, right in front of the surgical team. Multiple monitors are often available.

Before starting surgery, the operating room staff will ensure that all the necessary equipment is available and correctly functioning. A standardized checklist generally accomplishes this.

26.2.1 French Technique

The French technique's patient positioning is shown in Fig. 26.1:

- The patient is supine with the legs astride.
- The surgeon between the patient's thighs.
- The assistant on either side of the patient.
- The scrub nurse and the instrument table either between the surgeon and the assistant or on the opposite side of the assistant.
- The anesthesiologist at the patient's head.

26.2.2 American Technique

The American technique's patient positioning is shown in Fig. 26.2:

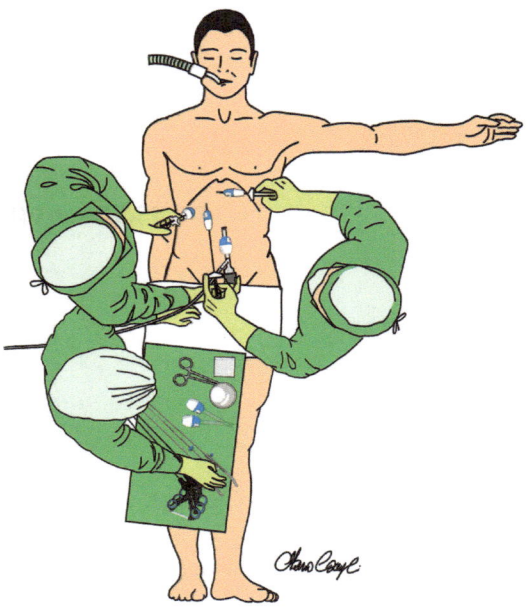

Fig. 26.2 American technique's patient positioning

- The patient is supine with the legs closed.
- The surgeon on the patient's left.
- The assistant on the opposite side, if available, a second assistant (camera operator) at the left of the surgeon.
- The scrub nurse and the instrument table on the right side of the first assistant (or at the left of the surgeon if there is no second assistant).
- The anesthesiologist at the patient's head.

26.3 Port Placement

The first trocar is at the umbilicus; it accommodates the laparoscope. The rest of the trocars are placed under direct laparoscopic view. The American and French techniques differ in the typical port placement, although several variations have been described.

In the American technique, a 10–12 mm trocar is positioned at the epigastrium, below the xiphoid process, just to the right of the falciform ligament. Two additional 5-mm ports are placed on the right anterior axillary line at the level of the umbilicus and on the midclavicular line, 2 cm below the right costal margin [2]. In the original description, the surgeon operated one-handed

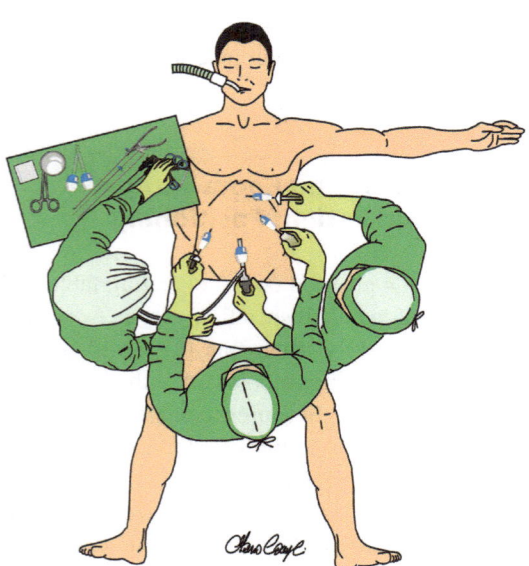

Fig. 26.1 French technique's patient positioning

using the epigastric port, while the assistant exposed the gallbladder using both 5 mm ports; nowadays, most surgeons prefer a two-handed dissection using the epigastric and the midclavicular ports; the assistant retracts the fundus of the gallbladder cephalad through the axillary line trocar.

In the French technique, two 5-mm trocars are inserted in the epigastrium and on the right anterior axillary line, similar to the American technique; a 10-mm trocar is placed in the left hypochondrium [1]. The operator, standing between the patient's legs, uses the dissecting instruments through the 10 mm port and holds the Hartmann's pouch with holding forceps in the axillary line port. The assistant retracts the gallbladder cephalad through the epigastric port.

26.4 Surgical Steps and Related Instruments

A laparoscopic cholecystectomy may be completed with a variety of laparoscopic instruments and energy sources. It is usually performed in a retrograde fashion (*bottom-up*; dissecting the structures within the Calot's triangle first, then detaching the gallbladder from the liver bed), but sometimes an antegrade dissection (*top-down*; separating the gallbladder from the liver bed first, leaving the section of cystic duct and artery as the last step)[1] is preferable and safer, especially if the dissection at the infundibulum is difficult for adhesions, fibrosis, or inflammation [3]. If a challenging situation is found, the team must be ready to change the operative plan and keep a flexible but rigorous attitude.

Blunt or sharp dissection is appropriate in different phases of the procedure. The most commonly utilized laparoscopic instruments are listed in Table 26.1.

Monopolar current is generally employed for dissection and bleeding control. It can be applied on a variety of laparoscopic instruments accord-

Table 26.1 Open surgery instruments

n.	Instrument	Length
1	Scalpel with a stainless steel blade (size #11 or 15)	
1	Narrow tip forceps (for coagulation)	18 cm
2	Forester ring clamps	24 cm
2	Toothed tissue forceps	18 cm
2	Smooth tissue forceps	18 cm
2	Toothed Adson forceps	12 cm
2	Farabeuf retractors	12 cm
2	Stainless steel bowl	12 cm
2	Backhaus clamp	13 cm
6	Curved Crile (or Kelly, Rochester, Pean) hemostatic forceps	16 cm
4	Straight Kocher clamp	16.5 cm
1	Needle holder	16 cm
1	Needle holder	18 cm
2	Curved Mayo scissors	17 cm
1	Curved Metzenbaum scissors	18 cm

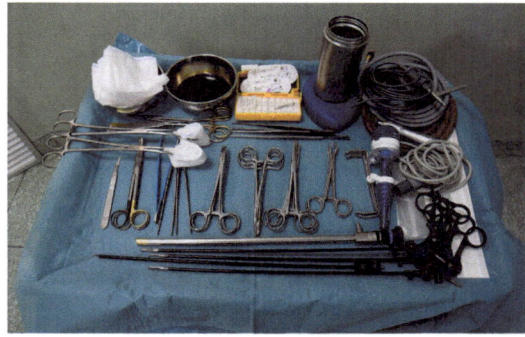

Fig. 26.3 First Mayo stand with instruments

ing to the surgeon's preference, most commonly a curved dissector, scissors, or a hook (also known as crochet in French, particularly common in Europe). Using the ultrasonic dissector as the preferred energy source is also possible [4, 5]. Lasers have been employed in the past, but they are no longer used for cholecystectomy [6].

A typical instrument table setup is shown in Table 26.1. The reusable instruments will be prepared on one or two Mayo stands (Figs. 26.3 and 26.4), while the circulating nurse may open the disposable tools when needed.

---

[1] Several terms are used to define antegrade cholecystectomy: anterograde, top-down, fundus-first, fundus-down, and dome-down.

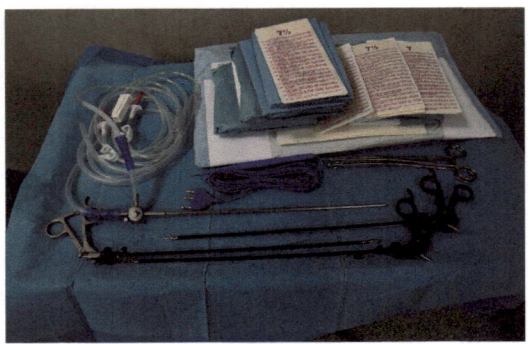

Fig. 26.4 Second Mayo stand with instruments

26.4.1 Preparation, Access, and Exposure

The patient is prepped and draped. The abdomen is completely exposed; the xiphoid process, costal margin, umbilicus, and pubis are accessible as anatomical landmarks. Before starting surgery, the scrub and circulating nurses set up the laparoscopic equipment. They jointly cover the camera and its connecting cable with a sterile plastic sleeve and connect it to the imaging system processor; the scrub nurse handles the proper extremity of the light cord, monopolar cable, and, eventually, harmonic ultrasonic cable to the circulating nurse who connects them to the appropriate equipment. The irrigation and suction tubing are also set up at this moment.

The first (umbilical) port can be placed with an open technique (a Hasson cannula is generally used for this purpose), an optical trocar, or blindly, with a penetrating trocar, after having induced the pneumoperitoneum through a Veres needle (commonly misspelled as Veress or Verres [7]). The first approach's clear superiority over the others has never been demonstrated [8, 9].

The blind or optical trocar access only requires a #11 blade, the Veres needle, a syringe with a few milliliters of normal saline solution for the drop test, and the chosen trocar. If a Hasson technique is selected, open surgery instruments will be used according to the surgeon's preferences. In our habitual practice, we use a #11 (or #15) scalpel blade, tissue forceps, and Metzenbaum dissection scissors for blunt dissection to visualize the umbilical ring and the abdominal fascia, one Backhaus clamp to circle the umbilical ring at its base and lift it; a small Farabeuf retractor on the opposite skin border. Once the fascia is well visualized, two traction stitches are placed (they will also serve to hold the Hasson cannula in place), the aponeurosis is divided between them; and the peritoneum is pinched with two curved Kelly clamps (three or four of them may be used in sequence to obtain the proper hold) and divided between them. More details about the access techniques can be found in Chap. 6 and 7.

Once all the ports are placed (as described above) and the abdominal cavity explored, the dissection generally starts at the infundibulum of the gallbladder (Hartmann's pouch). The assistant's upward and backward retraction of the fundus rotates the liver and exposes its inferior surface, the hepato-duodenal ligament, and the Calot's triangle. The operator's left hand alternatively retracts the infundibulum laterally to expose the Calot's triangle and medially to release the lateral peritoneal layer on the gallbladder. These maneuvers usually require a firm grip with a grasper on the fundus but a gentler hold with atraumatic laparoscopic holding forceps (e.g., Johann or Croce-Olmi forceps) on the infundibulum.

Often, in particular for acute cholecystitis, the gallbladder is distended, tense, and has a very thick wall, making it impossible to obtain a proper grasper bite on its fundus. In this situation, it may be necessary to decompress the organ, suctioning part of its content with a needle introduced through the abdominal wall. A large bore venous access cannula can be used for this purpose, but a Veres needle is an excellent choice.

26.4.2 Cystic Pedicle Dissection

The cystic duct and artery can be exposed and isolated in several manners after having sectioned the lateral and medial peritoneal layers at the level of the infundibulum (and above it). The complete dissection of the cystic duct until its junction with the common bile duct was strongly suggested in the early infundibular technique description [10], but it is no longer considered necessary and, in fact, is discouraged with the broadly adopted critical-view-of-safety technique [11, 12]. The latter is considered safer and recommended by several guidelines [4, 13]. The critical-view-of-safety mandates that a large window between the gallbladder and the liver surface, at the Calot's triangle, be bluntly dissected until the cystic duct and artery are circumferentially isolated. The dissection is easily done with a curved Maryland dissector or another instrument, but the blunt tip of a suction-irrigation device is an excellent tool for this maneuver as long as the tissues are soft enough.

Once the two structures are safely identified, they can be divided among titanium or non-absorbable polymer clips with scissors, but the harmonic-shear is sufficient to seal them clipless if correctly applied [14]. The use of monopolar, endoloops, ligatures, or even stapling devices has also been described, but they are seldom used [4, 15].

Clips are available in several sizes and types: titanium or non-absorbable polymer, disposable multiple clip or reusable single clip applier, and 10- or 5-mm diameter devices. More than one alternative is usually present in any operating room; the scrub nurse and the operating room staff are generally aware of the surgeon's preferences, but a different choice is possible for local conditions.

26.4.3 Gallbladder Separation from the Liver Bed

Unless a top-down dissection is done, the gallbladder is separated from the inferior surface of the liver after securing the pedicle structures.

The instruments are the same used in the preceding step: grasper for the fundus of the gallbladder, atraumatic holding forceps, and the energy-delivering device (hook, scissors, spatula, or harmonic shears) in the left and right hand of the surgeon.

Bleeding from the liver bed is easily controlled; occasionally, hemostatic agents may be used and should be handy. If the bleeding is both-

ersome, the surgeon may ask for a small gauze to insert in the sub-hepatic space. It may temporarily control the bleeding and increase the luminosity in the surgical field. The scrub nurse will use a radio-opaque marked gauze for this purpose and accurately verify the gauze count at the end of the procedure, even when sure that the gauze was removed.

Although generally not necessary, a soft suction drain (Jackson Pratt, Blake, or similar) may be placed, at this time, in the sub-hepatic space under direct vision and immediately secured to the skin with a suture.

26.4.4 Specimen Extraction

The dissected gallbladder is extracted through the umbilical or epigastric port at the end of the procedure. The specimen can be placed in a retrieval bag or directly extracted unprotected [13]. In the latter case, it will be held by a grasper or passed to claw forceps for a firmer grip.

The trocar will be removed from the chosen site, and the incision enlarged to allow the passage of the largest gallstone. It is also possible to open the gallbladder at the incision site and extract or break up the stones to facilitate the retrieval. The retrieval bag can be used as a wound protector during this phase.

In this step, open surgery instruments will be necessary to enlarge the incision (tissue forceps, scalpel, Metzenbaum or Mayo scissors, curved Kelly or similar clamps, electrocautery, and Farabeuf or Mathieu retractors), extract the stones (Kocher clamps, ring clamps, straight or slightly curved Randall stone extraction forceps, Yankauer suction cannula), and close the incisions (needle-holder, tissue forceps, and sutures).

26.5 Tools Required in Selected Cases

26.5.1 Subtotal Cholecystectomy

Subtotal cholecystectomy is a bailout procedure when the surgeon judges that the local conditions are unsafe to pursue secure identification of cystic duct and artery. If severe adhesions, intense fibrosis, or inflammation at the infundibulum and the pedicle area prevent obtaining a critical-view-of-safety, it is possible to proceed with a top-down cholecystectomy; it usually allows the secure identification of cystic structures. In particularly difficult situations, it may be too dangerous to move toward the pedicle in this way too. At this point, the surgeon may decide not to carry on a total cholecystectomy and proceed with a partial cholecystectomy, leaving the infundibulum (or part of it) in place [4].

The fundus and the body of the gallbladder are removed. It is necessary to meticulously collect all the stones. They can be placed, with the gallbladder wall, in a retrieval bag (sometimes more than one is required to facilitate this tedious part of the procedure).

The gallbladder remnant can be left open (to reduce the incidence of biliary fistula; eventually, a suture can be placed on the internal orifice of the cystic duct, if visible) or sutured to reconstitute a small gallbladder. Laparoscopic needleholders and sutures (usually cut at 13 cm length by the scrub nurse before their introduction in the operating field) become necessary at this point. Each of the two alternatives has its advantages and disadvantages, but their discussion is outside the purpose of this chapter [16, 17].

26.5.2 Intraoperative Cholangiogram

The adjunct of an intraoperative X-ray cholangiography is sometimes required for cholecystectomy. In this chapter, we will not get into its indications and controversies but will examine only some technical aspects related to the necessary tools.

The procedure requires a C-arm fluoroscopy device and enough space to fit it into the operating room and on the operating table. All the involved personnel will have to wear protective aprons and neck shields. The scrub nurse will cover the upper part of the C-arm with a sterile

Table 26.2 Laparoscopic instruments

n.	Instrument	Size
1	30° laparoscope	10 mm
1	Hasson cannula	12 mm
1	10–12 mm trocar	12 mm
2	5 mm trocar	5 mm
1	Specimen retrieval bag	10 mm
1	Croce-Olmi forceps	5 mm
2	Johann forceps	5 mm
1	Maryland dissector	5 mm
2	Grasper (with or without ratchet)	5 mm
1	Laparoscopic scissors	5 mm
1	Hook electrode	5 mm
1	Unipolar high-frequency cord	
1	Light cable	
1	Suction/irrigation cannula with tubing	
1	CO2 tube	
1	Thermos-type laparoscope warmer	
2	Clip appliers (according to the available clip models)	

plastic cover before it is pushed above the operative field and prepare the devices necessary for the procedure (Table 26.2).

Scissors are necessary to create a cystic duct opening to insert the 6-Fr cholangiography catheter. Depending on the catheter type, an Olsen cholangiogram clamp or a plastic guide can facilitate its introduction. If the catheter has a retention balloon, a small syringe will be necessary to inflate it. The scrub nurse will prepare one syringe with diluted radio-opaque cholangiography contrast dye and one with plain normal saline solution (to flush the contrast out of the common bile duct after the procedure and avoid undue irritation), marking them accordingly. It is essential to prevent air bubbles in the solutions: although harmless, they can be mistaken for stones on X-ray imaging. Ten-milliliter syringes are an excellent choice because they make injecting the dense contrast into the small caliber catheter easier. Also, a 3-way stopcock valve may be placed on the catheter extremity to accommodate the two syringes (contrast and saline), avoiding excessive manipulation and reducing the risk of injecting air bubbles in the duct.

26.5.3 Indocyanine Green Fluorescence Cholangiography

Intraoperative indocyanine green (ICG) fluorescent cholangiography is increasingly used to identify the extrahepatic biliary anatomy. Unlike X-ray cholangiography, it allows real-time visualization of the biliary tree during cholecystectomy. The patient receives an intravenous injection of indocyanine green about 45–60 min before surgery (but various dosage and timing protocols have been suggested); a near-infrared light source and camera (see Chap. 10) are necessary to manifest the fluorescence of the dye excreted in the bile and enhance the visualization of the bile ducts [18].

With the near-infrared imaging system, it is possible to switch between near-infrared and xenon light during the procedure, therefore continuing the dissection with an improved understanding of the biliary anatomy.

Besides the intravenous administration of the ICG, the possibility of obtaining a fluorescence cholangiography by direct injection of the dye in the gallbladder has been described, although not standardized. In this case, a 27-gauge needle punctures the gallbladder through the abdominal wall [19].

26.5.4 Conversion to Open Surgery

Conversion to open surgery must not be considered a complication, although a complication may suggest a conversion. When a surgeon thinks that laparoscopic surgery is no longer safe, the procedure continues with a laparotomy incision. Therefore, we will address the topic here and not in the section dedicated to complications.

When the need for conversion arises, a large number of additive instruments becomes necessary in a short time if bleeding is the cause of it. In addition, it may be convenient to withdraw all the laparoscopic equipment from the field. Therefore, it may be an intense moment for the operating room nurses, and extra help, if available, could be useful.

According to the local organization, the operating room nurses may have prepared the instrument for conversion on an additional stand or have a complete kit readily accessible in case of need.

The laparotomy can be started with the instruments already on the laparoscopic setup (scalpel, Kelly clamps, Metzenbaum scissors), but full instrumentation for open cholecystectomy will be necessary (see Table 26.1).

26.6 Intraoperative Complications

26.6.1 Management and Tools

When a conversion is not required, the most frequent intraoperative complications during a laparoscopic cholecystectomy can usually be managed with the same equipment already available for the procedure,

If bleeding is an issue, it is imperative to have a well-functioning suction/irrigation device to keep clean the operative field and allow the best visibility. Monopolar or bipolar current is usually the best choice for parenchymal or small vessel bleeding; occasionally, clips may be needed. Topical hemostatic agents are also used, mainly oxidized regenerated cellulose and Floseal® (Baxter International, Inc., Deerfield, IL, USA) hemostatic matrix.

Acknowledgments We are very grateful to Mario Campli, MD, for his excellent drawings.

References

1. Dubois F, Icard P, Berthelot G, Levard H. Coelioscopic cholecystectomy. Preliminary report of 36 cases. Ann Surg. 1990;211:60–2. https://doi.org/10.1097/00000658-199001000-00010.
2. Reddick EJ, Olsen DO. Outpatient laparoscopic laser cholecystectomy. Am J Surg. 1990;160:485–7. https://doi.org/10.1016/S0002-9610(05)81009-8.
3. Garzali IU, Aburumman A, Alsardia Y, Alabdallat B, Wraikat S, Aloun A. Is fundus first laparoscopic cholecystectomy a better option than conventional laparoscopic cholecystectomy for difficult cholecystec-

tomy? A systematic review and meta-analysis. Updat Surg. 2022;74:1797–803. https://doi.org/10.1007/s13304-022-01403-5.

4. Agresta F, Campanile FC, Vettoretto N, Silecchia G, Bergamini C, Maida P, Lombari P, Narilli P, Marchi D, Carrara A, Esposito MG, Fiume S, Miranda G, Barlera S, Davoli M, Italian Surgical Societies Working Group. Laparoscopic cholecystectomy: consensus conference-based guidelines. Langenbecks Arch Surg Dtsch Ges Für Chir. 2015;400:429–53. https://doi.org/10.1007/s00423-015-1300-4.

5. Jiang H-P, Liu Y-D, Li Y-S, Shen Z-L, Ye Y-J. Ultrasonic versus electrosurgical device for laparoscopic cholecystectomy: a systematic review with meta-analysis and trial sequential analysis. Int J Surg. 2017;40:24–32. https://doi.org/10.1016/j.ijsu.2017.02.020.

6. Southern Surgeons Club. A prospective analysis of 1518 laparoscopic cholecystectomies: the southern surgeons club. N Engl J Med. 1991;324:1073–8. https://doi.org/10.1056/NEJM199104183241601.

7. Szabó I, László A. Veres needle: in memoriam of the 100th birthday anniversary of Dr János Veres, the inventor. Am J Obstet Gynecol. 2004;191:352–3. https://doi.org/10.1016/j.ajog.2004.01.030.

8. Ahmad G, Baker J, Finnerty J, Phillips K, Watson A. Laparoscopic entry techniques. Cochrane Database Syst Rev. 2019;1:CD006583. https://doi.org/10.1002/14651858.CD006583.pub5.

9. Sultan AI, Ali SH, Ghareeb OA. Port site consequences after laparoscopic cholecystectomy using an open versus closed approach of Pneumoperitoneum. Cureus. 2022;14:e26499. https://doi.org/10.7759/cureus.26499.

10. Peters JH, Ellison EC, Innes JT, Liss JL, Nichols KE, Lomano JM, Roby SR, Front ME, Carey LC. Safety and efficacy of laparoscopic cholecystectomy. A prospective analysis of 100 initial patients. Ann Surg. 1991;213:3–12.

11. Strasberg SM, Hertl M, Soper NJ. An analysis of the problem of biliary injury during laparoscopic cholecystectomy. J Am Coll Surg. 1995;180:101–25.

12. Vettoretto N, Saronni C, Harbi A, Balestra L, Taglietti L, Giovanetti M. Critical view of safety during laparoscopic cholecystectomy. JSLS J Soc Laparoendosc Surg Soc Laparoendosc Surg. 2011;15:322–5. https://doi.org/10.4293/108680811X13071180407474.

13. Fisher AT, Bessoff KE, Khan RI, Touponse GC, Yu MMK, Patil AA, Choi J, Stave CD, Forrester JD. Evidence-based surgery for laparoscopic cholecystectomy. Surg Open Sci. 2022;10:116–34. https://doi.org/10.1016/j.sopen.2022.08.003.

14. Abounozha S, Alshahri T, Alammari S, Ibrahim R. Clipless laparoscopic cholecystectomy is a better technique in reducing intraoperative bleeding. Ann Med Surg. 2021;62:431–4. https://doi.org/10.1016/j.amsu.2021.01.039.

15. Arkle T, Lam S, Toogood G, Kumar B. How should we secure the cystic duct during laparoscopic cholecystectomy? A UK-wide survey of clinical practice and systematic review of the literature with meta-analysis. Ann R Coll Surg Engl. 2022;104:650–4. https://doi.org/10.1308/rcsann.2021.0264.

16. Strasberg SM, Pucci MJ, Brunt LM, Deziel DJ. Subtotal cholecystectomy-"Fenestrating" vs "reconstituting" subtypes and the prevention of bile duct injury: definition of the optimal procedure in difficult operative conditions. J Am Coll Surg. 2016;222:89–96. https://doi.org/10.1016/j.jamcollsurg.2015.09.019.

17. Yildirim AC, Zeren S, Ekici MF, Yaylak F, Algin MC, Arik O. Comparison of Fenestrating and reconstituting subtotal cholecystectomy techniques in difficult cholecystectomy. Cureus. 2022;14:e22441. https://doi.org/10.7759/cureus.22441.

18. Lie H, Irawan A, Sudirman T, Budiono BP, Prabowo E, Jeo WS, Rudiman R, Sitepu RK, Hanafi RV, Hariyanto TI. Efficacy and safety of near-infrared florescence cholangiography using Indocyanine green in laparoscopic cholecystectomy: a systematic review and meta-analysis. J Laparoendosc Adv Surg Tech A. 2022;33(5):434–46. https://doi.org/10.1089/lap.2022.0495.

19. Castagneto-Gissey L, Russo MF, Iodice A, Casella-Mariolo J, Serao A, Picchetto A, D'Ambrosio G, Urciuoli I, De Luca A, Salvati B, Casella G. Intracholecystic versus intravenous Indocyanine green (ICG) injection for biliary anatomy evaluation by fluorescent cholangiography during laparoscopic cholecystectomy: a case-control study. J Clin Med. 2022;11:3508. https://doi.org/10.3390/jcm11123508.

Robotic Treatment of Gallbladder Diseases

27

Dario Ribero [iD], Diana Baldassarri,
Sellitri Domenico, and Giuseppe Spinoglio

27.1 Introduction

Gallbladder disorders encompass a wide breadth of diseases that vary in clinical presentation and severity. Among the various nosological entities, including acute acalculous cholecystitis, gallbladder dyskinesia, gallbladder polyps, gallbladder hydrops, porcelain gallbladder, and gallbladder cancer, gallstones disease represents the most frequent one. In most of the developed countries, gallstones disease is common with a significant economic and health impact due to its high frequency and related morbidity. Although accurate epidemiological data are not available for every European country, in Europe the reported median prevalence ranges from 4.4% to 21.9%, with the highest rates seen in Norway (21.9%) and former East Germany (19.7%) and the lowest rates in Italy (4.4%) [1, 2]. Prospective ultrasound-based surveys have also assessed the gallstone incidence in Europe, showing rates of <1/100 persons per year (0.67% in Italy, 0.93% in Denmark) [2, 3].

Of the newly diagnosed patients with gallstone disease, up to 70% are asymptomatic at diagnosis with the large majority remaining asymptomatic during a lifetime. The GREPCO group studied the natural history of gallstones over a 10-year period in an Italian population sample of 118 asymptomatic patients [4]. The authors reported a cumulative probability of developing biliary colic of 11.9% at 2 years, 16.5% at 4 years, and 25.8% at 10 years. Interestingly, none of the variables considered as possible modifiers of natural history were found to increase the risk of developing biliary colic. These data are similar to that observed in other longitudinal studies reporting no more than 18% of patients becoming symptomatic over a 20-year period [5, 6]. Among the third of patients with gallstones who develop symptoms, different clinical scenarios are possible, from a mild biliary colic to an acute or chronic cholecystitis, a choledocholithiasis with or without cholangitis, a Mirizzi syndrome, and a Bouveret syndrome. The most frequent symptom is biliary colic: it is estimated that 70–80% of patients experience biliary colic [7] with more than 90% having recurrent pain in 10 years [8, 9]. Overall, symptomatic gallstones disease is the most common abdominal conditions for which patients in

D. Ribero (✉)
The Division of General and Oncologic Surgery, AO Santa Croce e Carle, Cuneo, Italy
e-mail: ribero.d@ospedale.cuneo.it

D. Baldassarri
The Division of General Surgery, Ospedale San Gaudenzio, Novara, Italy

S. Domenico
Ospedale Civile Lorenzo Bonomo Andria (BA)l, Andria, Italy

G. Spinoglio
Department of Colorectal Robotic Surgery, IRCAD, Strasbourg, France

© The Author(s), under exclusive license to Springer Nature Switzerland AG 2024
M. Milone et al. (eds.), *Scrub Nurse in Minimally Invasive and Robotic General Surgery*,
https://doi.org/10.1007/978-3-031-42257-7_27

Western countries are admitted to hospitals [9], and this frequency has increased since the 1950s [10].

Gallstone disease is "a surgical disease": in fact, only a cholecystectomy permits to definitively treat symptomatic gallstones. It took 103 years since the first cholecystectomy performed by Carl Langenbuch in 1882 to enter into a new surgical era. On September 12, 1985, Erich Mühe of Böblingen, Germany, performed the first laparoscopic cholecystectomy [11] followed, 2 years later, by Phillipe Mouret of Lyon, France [12]. These experiences paved the way for a revolution in the surgical approach to gallbladder diseases. Within a few years, multiport laparoscopic cholecystectomy has become the gold standard technique in both acute and elective settings. During the late 1990s, a further evolution was introduced: in an attempt to achieve even more enhanced cosmesis and to decrease postoperative pain, the single-site technique was developed. However, technical difficulties of the procedure and concerns about increased complications such as hernias, wound infection, and pain [13] have been deterrents in its wide diffusion.

In 2000, the introduction of the da Vinci® robotic platform (Intuitive Surgical Inc., Sunnyvale, CA) into clinical practice expanded the possibilities of a minimally invasive approach to gallbladder diseases [14]. The advantages offered by the robotic platform, such as three-dimensional optics, stable view of the operative field, tremors' filtration with motion scaling, and improved dexterity with superior dissection capabilities, led to its rapid adoption. Using the largest US national database, Aguayio et al. [15] observed a dramatic increase in the use of robotic-assisted cholecystectomy from 0.02% in 2008 to 3.2% in 2017. However, despite a rapid expansion, questions remain about its benefits and utility. A recent systematic review of four RCTs, four propensity-matched studies, and 36 observational studies showed that robotic cholecystectomy is not inferior to laparoscopic cholecystectomy with no evidence of differences in major clinical outcome (conversion rates, intraoperative complications, estimated blood loss, length of stay, surgical site infection, and readmission rates) with longer operative time associated with the use of the robot [16]. However, due to the nuanced nature of the factors contributing to OR time, this difference may represent a variety of modifiable factors such as surgeon learning curve, OR staff efficiency, and case selection. Interestingly, when analyzing single studies, it emerged a reduced conversion rate in subgroups of patients at high risk [17–20] and, overall, a reduced incidence of bile duct injuries (BDI) [18, 21] when the robotic approach is used.

The development of dedicated robotic instruments for single-port surgery has also partially revitalized the interest in this technique since most of the traditional challenges and limitations of a single-entry site are overcome. While no significant differences in clinical outcome were noted when comparing single-port robot-assisted to single-port laparoscopic cholecystectomy [16], in a randomized controlled trial [22] the large 95% confidence interval includes a more than 30% reduction in complications for the robotic arm. In addition, Spinoglio et al. [23] showed a significantly reduced operative time for the robotic approach (62.7 min vs. 83.2 min; $p < 0.001$) with a shorter learning curve. Table 27.1 summarizes the key advantages of robotic cholecystectomy.

The purpose of this chapter is to briefly review the indication for surgery and to present the technique of robotic cholecystectomy, providing details for OR setup, patients' positioning, port placement, and surgical instruments needed using the robot da Vinci® Xi.

Table 27.1 Clinical benefit of robotic cholecystectomy in subgroups of patients

Reported benefits	Clinical settings	Reference and level of evidence
Reduction in the risk of open conversion[a]	Patients who have at baseline a higher risk of conversion: • Patients with one or more of the following risk factors: Age > 40 years, intraoperative diagnosis of acute or gangrenous cholecystitis and/or male gender • Obese Male (mean BMI 31.2 kg/m²), chronic cholecystitis • Patients with advanced liver disease (MELD score 21–30)	Huang et al. (2017) [17] meta-analysis Gangemi et al. (2017) [18] retrospective review Strosberg et al. (2017) [19] retrospective review Aziz et al. (2020) [20] retrospective review
Successful completion of surgery for complex gallbladder disease	Patients who present with: • Mirizzi syndrome • Gangrenous cholecystitis • Cholelithiasis with choledocholithiasis not treatable with ERCP • ERCP refractory choledocholithiasis	Magge et al. (2017) [24] review Ji et al. (2011) [25] case series
Reduced rates of bile duct injuries	Any patients (in particular, reduce risk with the use of ICG cholangiography)	Dip et al. (2021) [21] systematic review Gangemi et al. (2017) [18] retrospective
Improved postoperative outcomes (length of hospital stay, estimated blood loss, 30-day readmission rates, postoperative complications)	Patients at higher risk: • Obese male (mean BMI 31.2 kg/m²), chronic cholecystitis • Patients with advanced liver disease (MELD score 21–30) Patients undergoing single-site procedures (more than 30% reduction in complications for the robotic arm in a RTC)	Tao et al. (2021) [26] retrospective review Aziz et al. (2020) [20] retrospective review Grochola et al. (2019) [22] randomized controlled trial
Avanced training for surgical residents	Improved surgical performance, reduced complications, reduced learning curve, higher competence	Willuth et al. (2021) [27] randomized cross-over study

BMI body mass index, *MELD* model for end-stage liver disease, *ERCP* endoscopic retrograde cholangiopancreatography
[a]Overall, based on randomized controlled trial data, the certainty of evidence for no difference in conversion rates is high, albeit a meta-analysis by Huang et al. [2017] showed a trend in reduced open conversion for the robotic approach

27.2 Indications

In 2015, an Italian consensus conference, held under the auspices of the EAES, updated the clinical guidelines on laparoscopic cholecystectomy [28]. Although robotic assistance has not been proven to have significant advantages over the conventional laparoscopic approach, at present, there is no documented clinical contraindication that would warrant laparoscopic cholecystectomy to be chosen over robotic cholecystectomy assuming that the operating surgeon is adequately trained in the robotic approach. Therefore, the two techniques share the same indications.

Cholecystectomy is indicated in the presence of symptoms in patients who can tolerate general anesthesia. In asymptomatic patients, the annual risk for severe and nonsevere events decreases with time, with an annual complication rate of 0.3–3% [4, 29]. The majority of patients rarely develop gallstone-related complications without first having at least one episode of biliary pain [30]. Thus, prophylactic cholecystectomy is not recommended with most authors adopting a "watch and wait" policy. The only exceptions might be (1) the presence of microcalculi or sludge. In fact, an association between acute pancreatitis and small gallbladder stones or sludge has been described, especially if gallbladder motility is preserved. Therefore, in these patients a prophylactic cholecystectomy might be indicated [31, 32]; (2) patients with asymptomatic porcelain gallbladder and selective mucosal calcifications since this feature seems to be at a higher risk of association with gallbladder cancer; (3) risk of malignancy based on ethnicity, geographic area, and gallbladder imaging; and (4) post-cardiac transplant recipients due to increased mortality and morbidity. Conversely, an expectant management is to be preferred in kidney, pancreas, and/or pulmonary transplant recipients. Cholecystectomy might also be indicated in patients with gallbladder polyps, although the treatment algorithm of this disease is complex [33]: Cholecystectomy is recommended in patients with polypoid lesions measuring 10 mm or more; cholecystectomy is also recommended in patients fit for, and who accept surgery, in the presence of a 6–9 mm polypoid lesion and one or more risk factors for malignancy (age > 60 years, history of primary sclerosing cholangitis, Asian ethnicity, sessile polypoid lesion—including focal gallbladder wall thickening >4 mm). If the patient has either no risk factors for malignancy and a 6–9 mm polypoid lesion, or risk factors for malignancy and a polypoid lesion of ≤ 5 mm, a follow-up with ultrasound is recommended at 6 months, 1 year, and 2 years. If during follow-up the polypoid lesion grows to 10 mm, then cholecystectomy is advised. If the polypoid lesion grows by 2 mm or more within the 2-year follow-up period, then the current size of the polypoid lesion should be considered along with patient risk factors.

27.3 Robotic Cholecystectomy with the da Vinci® Xi

In the following sections, we will present relevant aspects of robotic cholecystectomy.

27.3.1 Operating Room Setup

The setup of the operating room is shown in Fig. 27.1. The patient cart is positioned at 90° to the right of the operating table; however, the angle of the patient cart base is not critical. The vision cart is placed to the left of the patient, at

Fig. 27.1 Schematic operating theater setting for robotic cholecystectomy

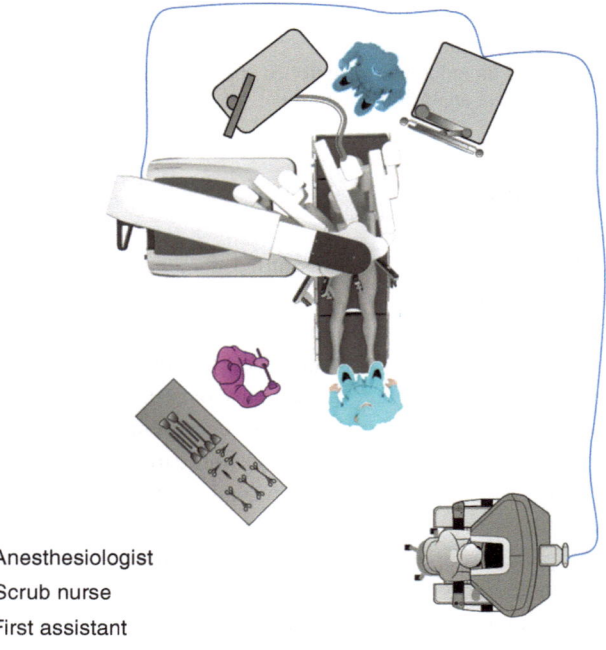

■ Anesthesiologist
■ Scrub nurse
■ First assistant

the level of the left shoulder. The surgical console is positioned in one of the operating room corners, ideally permitting the operating surgeon, in case of arms' conflicts, to observe the position of the robotic arms while sitting at the console. The first assistant sits at the operating table positioned between the patient's legs. The scrub nurse stands to the right or left of the first assistant based on the operating room spaces with the serving cart closed to him/her.

Of note, the position of the patient cart and vision cart might be switched based on the OR spaces.

27.3.2 Patient Positioning

The patient is positioned supine with a slight reverse Trendelenburg (inclination of ~10°) and a left lateral rotation of 5–10°. The arms are tucked in at the body side, albeit the left arm might be kept open based on anesthesiologist's preferences. Legs are spread apart.

27.3.3 Port Placement, Robotic Docking, and Instruments' Insertion

A 12-mmHg pneumoperitoneum is established through a Veress needle inserted in the Palmer point. Then, with a sterile marker, a line is drawn from the anterior superior iliac spine to the umbilicus. Port 3 is placed in the umbilicus. Ports 1, 2, and 4 are inserted at a distance of 6–8 cm from other ports on this line. Port 1 might be shifted 2 cm upwards based on the patient's habitus. In difficult cases, a 4-arm procedure might be planned adding an assistant port on the left flank. In easy cases, a 3-arm procedure might be a safe option: Robotic camera and instruments are positioned in ports 2 and 1 and 3, respectively, while an assistant port might be inserted where usually port 4 is placed (Fig. 27.2a, b). In very obese patients, in whom the umbilicus can be displaced lower than normal, the surgeon should consider to draw the ports line more cranially considering

that the distance between the passing line for ports and target anatomy should not exceed 20 cm. After docking the camera port (port 3 with arm 3 in the 4-arm procedure; port 2 with arm 3 in the 3-arm procedure since in this case arm 1 remains stowed), the targeting is carried out pointing to the hepatic pedicle. Then, all remaining arms are docked to the corresponding ports and the instruments are inserted under vision.

When a single-port robotic procedure is planned, a midline incision of approximately 2 to 2.5 cm is created within the umbilicus. After entering the abdomen, the single-site port is grabbed using an atraumatic forceps that clamps the port above both the lower rim and the insufflation adapter barb. Then, the leading edge of the clamped port is inserted into the incision with a downward motion until the entire lower rim of the port is inside the abdomen. The arrow depicted on the port is pointed toward the target anatomy and the abdomen is insufflated. In some patients, an additional port for the assistant might be necessary: This is placed in the right flank (Fig. 27.2c). Similarly to multiport procedures, in obese individuals the entering midline incision should be more cranial. Then, the cannula for the endoscope is inserted aligning the top line on the cannula with the top of the port: This ensures that the cannula is fully inserted and the remote center is correctly positioned. The cannula is docked on arm 3 (arm 1 is stowed), and the targeting is performed in the same way as for multiport. Then, the endoscope is positioned perpendicular to the port and retracted just within the tip of the cannula: This provides the correct angle for visualizing insertion of the curved cannulae. While holding the port to prevent its displacement, the first curved cannula is inserted into the first curved cannula lumen using a diagonal path until the "V" mark on the cannula reaches the top of the port. Then, the curved cannula bowl is lifted up and the cannula fin is rotated to face in the direction of the port arrow until the tip comes into view. The second cannula is inserted in the same way. When insertion is complete, both curved cannulae should be angled toward the target anatomy and docked to arms 2 and 4. Of note, the Xi

Fig. 27.2 Robotic and assistant port position in the (**a**) four-arm, (**b**) 3-arm, and (**c**) single-port robotic cholecystectomy

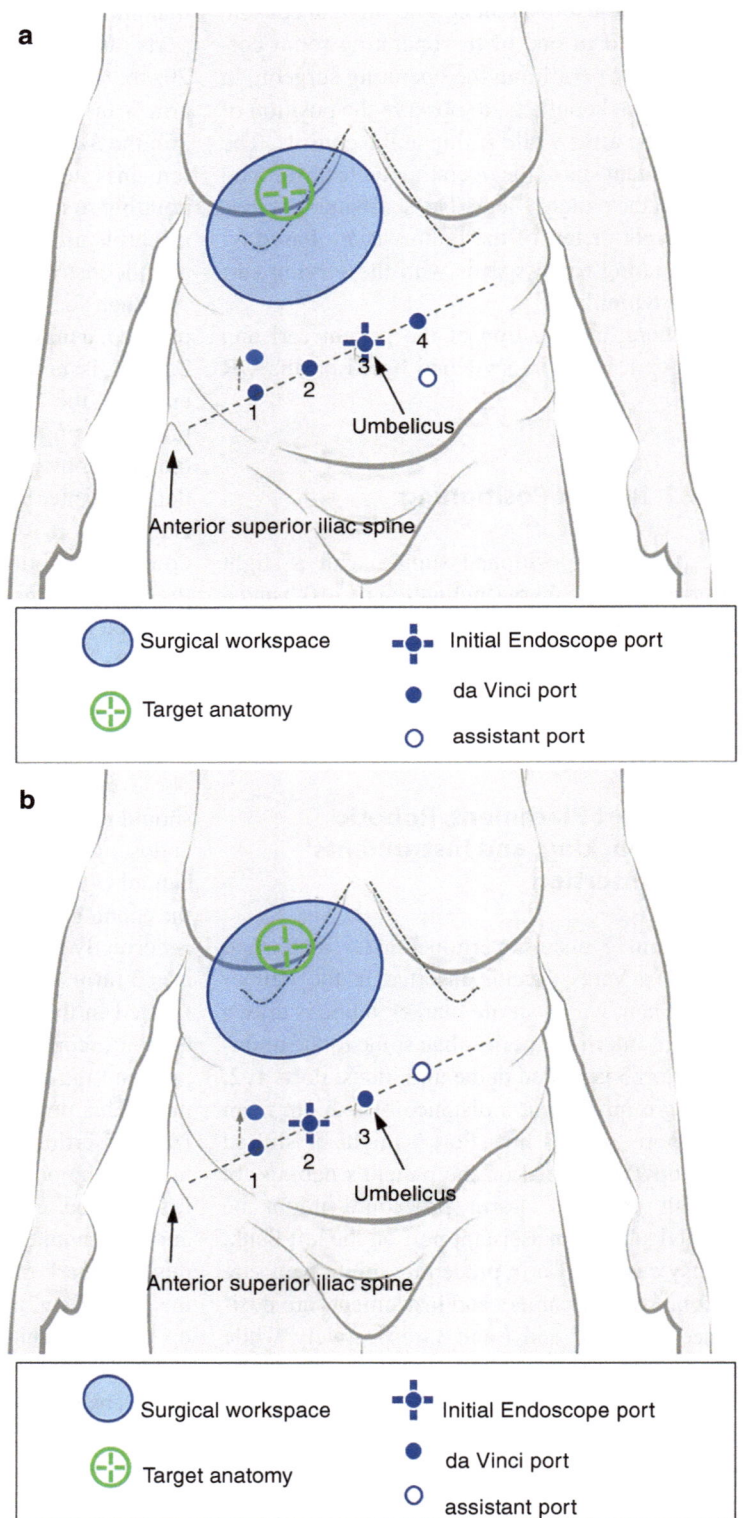

Fig. 27.2 (continued)

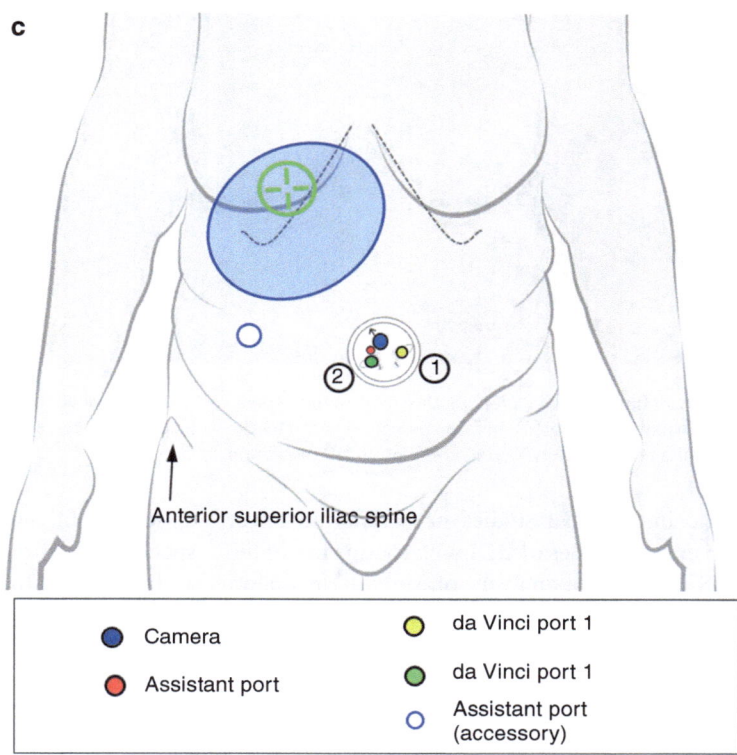

single site requires a second neutral grounding pad as a patient dispersive electrode: this pad is connected through a grounding cable plugged into the endoscope cannula.

27.3.4 Surgical Technique of Cholecystectomy

Regardless of the adopted technique, either multiport or single port, surgical steps of robotic cholecystectomy are identical. First, the gallbladder is identified and the fundus is retracted cephalad toward the right shoulder to expose the infundibulum. Adhesions with the omentum, transverse colon, or duodenum, if present, are dissected. Then, the infundibulum is retracted inferolaterally to expose the hepatocystic triangle formed by the cystic duct, the common hepatic duct, and the lower border of the liver. This anatomical area contains the cystic artery that forms with the cystic duct and the main bile duct an isosceles trian-

gle, known as the "Triangle of Calot." The next step is complete dissection of the hepatocystic triangle. Dissection, usually performed with an electrocautery, begins from the junction of the infundibulum with the cystic duct, keeping the dissection plane always close to the gallbladder or the cystic duct. The lower third of the gallbladder is separated from the liver by incising both the ventral and dorsal sierosa: This permits to widen the hepatocystic triangle and to facilitate clearance of all fatty and fibrous tissue. Of note, the common bile duct and the common hepatic duct are searched for but not completely exposed. At the end of dissection, full exposure of the Calot's triangle is achieved: two, and only two structures entering the gallbladder (i.e., the cystic duct and artery), should be seen in the anterior and posterior views of the triangle of Calot (Fig. 27.3). This is the "Critical View of Safety" (CVS) [34], which is emerging as the preferred method for preventing BDI. Two lines of indirect evidence support its use. First, a number of large

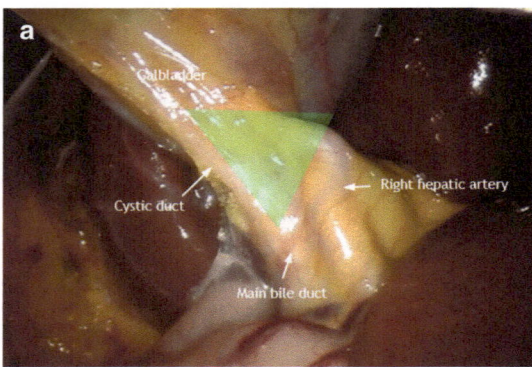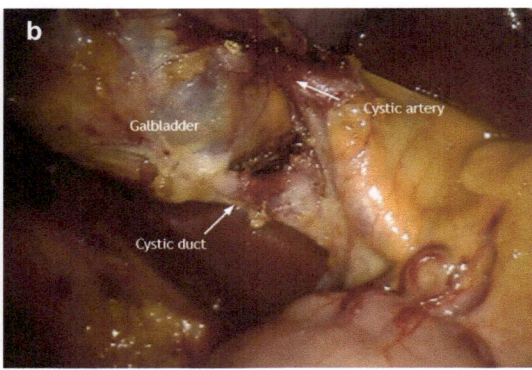

Fig. 27.3 Intraoperative pictures showing (**a**) the hepatocystic triangle (in green) before dissection and (**b**) the "critical view of safety" after completion of dissection

with identification of only two structures entering the gallbladder: the cystic duct and the cystic artery

single institutional studies have reported lower than expected rates of BDI with routine use of the CVS. In a meta-analysis of single-arm cohort studies of sample size ≥400 cases, the pooled incidence of BDI was 2 in one million cases when CVS was used [35]. Second, case series of BDIs that have analyzed the circumstances of the injury, either on the operative reports or the videos of laparoscopic cholecystectomy, have shown that BDIs usually occurred in patients when the CVS was not attained [36–38]. Overall, the ability to achieve the CVS is reported to be 85–95% of attempted cases with no substantial evidence that reasonable efforts to achieve the CVS have been harmful. Consequently, practice guidelines, elaborated during a recent multi-society consensus conference on the prevention of BDI during cholecystectomy, suggested the routine use of CVS for anatomic identification of the cystic duct and artery [35].

After the cystic duct and cystic artery are clearly identified, they are both clipped three times, with space to allow two clips to remain on the proximal end of both the artery and duct. Then, the artery is sectioned first followed by the cystic duct. The gallbladder is dissected from the liver bed using a monopolar instrument. If a posterior branch of the cystic artery is encountered, this can also be clipped or cauterized. Before completion of the gallbladder detachment, the liver bed is inspected for hemostasis. After the

dissection of the gallbladder is completed, the specimen is extracted in an endobag.

In the next lines, details on the instruments used are provided. Monopolar dissection can be done with the use of either the cautery hook or the monopolar curved scissor positioned in port on the right of the camera while a Cadiere forceps or a bipolar forceps is inserted in port on the left. When a 3-arm procedure is adopted, the assistant uses its port to retract the fundus with a Johann grasper or to insert a clip applier or a suction-irrigator instrument if needed. In the 4-arm procedure, a Cadiere forceps is used in arm 1; when the cystic duct and artery are to be secured, the right-hand instrument (arm 4) is exchanged for a Hem-o-lok® robotic clip applier. When the single-site technique is used, a bipolar forceps is inserted into robotic arm 1 and the monopolar cautery hook is inserted into robotic arm 2. After the assistant has grasped the fundus of the gallbladder, the endoscope is retracted, repositioned under the grasper, and reinserted, a maneuver that lifts the grasper and the fundus of the gallbladder upwards. At the end of the hepatocystic triangle dissection, the skeletonized cystic duct and cystic artery are clipped with a Hem-o-lock® ML clip applier (positioned in arm 2) which is then exchanged with a curved scissors used to transect the cyst duct and artery transected above the first two clips.

27.3.5 ICG Cholangiography

Although careful hepatocystic dissection with the achievement of the CVL mitigates significantly the risk of BDI, in some circumstances, an accurate evaluation of the biliary anatomy is essential. While intraoperative cholangiography has some disadvantages, such as a longer operative time, the need for a multidisciplinary team and dedicated equipment (i.e., the C-bow), and exposure of the patient and the surgical staff to radiation, use of the indocyanine-green (ICG) fluorescent cholangiography represents a valid option. In fact, it has been demonstrated that there exists a significant correlation between intraoperative near-infrared (NIR) biliary imaging with ICG and MRCP in the proper delineation of the common bile duct. Recently, the results of a single-blind multicenter, randomized controlled trial of NIR and white light versus white light alone have been published [39]. The trial showed that the detection rates for each biliary structure (cystic duct, right hepatic duct, common hepatic duct, common bile duct, cystic-common bile duct junction, cystic-gallbladder junction, and accessory ducts) were significantly higher for the NIR group before dissection with odd ratios ranging from 2.3 (95% CI 1.6–3.2) for the cystic-gallbladder junction to 3.6 (95% CI 1.6–9.3) for the right hepatic duct. After dissection, similar differences were observed for all structures except the cystic duct and cystic-gallbladder junction. Interestingly, the authors found that body mass index (BMI), level of inflammation, patient age, and surgeon experience significantly affected detection rates. Overall, BMI reduced visualization by 6% per BMI unit increase albeit visualization remained better with NIR compared to white light. Similarly, a reduction of 40–70% of the detection rate was registered among patients with moderate-to-severe inflammation as compared to those with minimal inflammation. Surgeon experience in years was also directly proportional to detection rates. In the study, there were two "mild" BDIs out of 639 patients, both in the white light-only group. In a separate randomized trial comparing laparoscopic or robotic cholecystectomy with versus without ICG cholangiography, the use of ICG fluorescent cholangiography sizably decreased duct injury and conversion to open surgery rates relative to cholecystectomy under white light alone; the effect on conversion was particularly marked in the robotic group (12 vs 322/10,000) [21]. Therefore, expert consensus suggests that the use of NIR imaging may be an adjunct to white light alone for identification of biliary anatomy during cholecystectomy albeit it cannot substitute a proper dissection and identification technique [35].

The technique of ICG cholangiography is as follows [40]: A dose of 2.5 mg of ICG, at a dilution of 0.5 mg/dl, is administered intravenously approximately 30–45 min before surgery. If fluorescence is not detected in the liver after 60 min, an additional dose of 2.5 mg of ICG is again injected intravenously. Of note, IGC is presented in vials of 25 or 50 mg of lyophilized powder for solution for injection. It should be diluted with sterile distilled water and not sodium chloride (NaCl) as the latter could cause aggregation; in addition, after preparation, the solution must be stored in a dark and cool place to avoid rapid deterioration of the whitening fluorescence.

27.4 Conclusions

Robotic cholecystectomy is a safe and valuable option in the treatment of gallbladder diseases. Future studies are needed to better define its role in the daily routine maximizing cost benefits. Continued development of new robotic technologies will probably expand its use and curb economic concerns.

References

1. Aerts R, Penninckx F. The burden of gallstone disease in Europe. Aliment Pharmacol Ther. 2003;18(Suppl. 3):49–53.
2. Festi D, Dormi A, Capodicasa S, et al. Incidence of gallstone disease in Italy: results from a multicenter, population-based Italian study (the MICOL project). World J Gastroenterol. 2008;14(34):5282–9.
3. Jorgenson T, et al. Eleven-year cumulated incidence of gallstone formation in unselected Danish popula-

tion. Gastroenterology. 1996;110(Suppl. 4):A21. (Abstract)

4. Attili AF, et al. The natural history of gallstones; the GREPCO experience. The GREPCO Group. Hepatology. 1995;21:655–60.

5. Zubler J, Markowski G, Yale S, Graham R, Rosenthal TC. Natural history of asymptomatic gallstones in family practice office practices. Arch Fam Med. 1998;7(3):230–3.

6. Gracie WA, Ransohoff DF. The natural history of silent gallstones: the innocent gallstone is not a myth. N Engl J Med. 1982;307(13):798–800.

7. Abraham S, Rivero HG, Erlikh IV, Griffith LF, Kondamudi VK. Surgical and nonsurgical management of gallstones. Am Fam Physician. 2014;89(10):795–802.

8. Donovan JM. Physical and metabolic factors in gallstone pathogenesis. Gastroenterol Clin N Am 1999;28(1):75–97.

9. Russo MW, Wei JT, Thiny MT, et al. Digestive and liver diseases statistics, 2004. Gastroenterology. 2004;126:1448–53.

10. Bateson MC. Gallstones and cholecystectomy in modern Britain. Postgrad Med J. 2000;76:700–3.

11. Walker R. The first laparoscopic cholecystectomy. JSLS. 2001;5(1):89–94.

12. Mouret P. Interview by GS Litynski. In: Litynski GS. Highlights in the history of laparoscopy. Frankfurt/Main, Germany: B. Bernert Verlag; 1996.

13. Marks JM, Phillips MS, Tacchino R, et al. Single-incision laparoscopic cholecystectomy is associated with improved cosmesis scoring at the cost of significantly higher hernia rates: 1-year results of a prospective randomized, multicenter, single-blinded trial of traditional multiport laparoscopic cholecystectomy vs single-incision laparoscopic cholecystectomy. J Am Coll Surg. 2013;216(6):1037–47. discussion 1047-8

14. Maeso S, Reza M, Mayol JA, et al. Efficacy of the da Vinci surgical system in abdominal surgery compared with that of laparoscopy: a systematic review and meta-analysis. Ann Surg. 2010;252(2):254–62.

15. Aguayo E, Dobaria V, Nakhla M, et al. National trends and outcomes of inpatient robotic-assisted versus laparoscopic cholecystectomy. Surgery. 2020;165:625–30.

16. Shenoy R, Mederos MA, Ye L, et al. Intraoperative and postoperative outcomes of robot-assisted cholecystectomy: a systematic review. Syst Rev. 2021;10:124.

17. Huang Y, Chua TC, Maddern GJ, et al. Robotic cholecystectomy versus conventional laparoscopic cholecystectomy: a meta-analysis. Surgery 2017;161(3):628–36.

18. Gangemi A, Danilkowicz R, Bianco F, et al. Risk factors for open conversion in minimally invasive cholecystectomy. J Soc Laparoendosc Surg. 2017;21(4):e2017.00062.

19. Strosberg DS, Nguyen MC, Muscarella P 2nd, et al. A retrospective comparison of robotic chole-cystectomy versus laparoscopic cholecystectomy: operative outcomes and cost analysis. Surg Endosc. 2017;31(3):1436–41.

20. Aziz H, Zeeshan M, Kaur N, et al. A potential role for robotic cholecystectomy in patients with advanced liver disease: analysis of the NSQIP database. Am Surg. 2020;86(4):341–5.

21. Dip F, Lo Menzo E, White KP, Rosenthal RJ. Does near-infrared fluorescent cholangiography with indocyanine green reduce bile duct injuries and conversions to open surgery during laparoscopic or robotic cholecystectomy? - a meta-analysis. Surgery. 2021;169(4):859–67.

22. Grochola LF, Soll C, Zehnder A, Wyss R, Herzog P, Breitenstein S. Robot-assisted versus laparoscopic single-incision cholecystectomy: results of a randomized controlled trial. Surg Endosc. 2019;33(5):1482–90.

23. Spinoglio G, Lenti LM, Maglione V, et al. Single-site robotic cholecystectomy (SSRC) versus single-incision laparoscopic cholecystectomy (SILC): comparison of learning curves. First European experience. Surg Endosc. 2012;26(6):1648–55.

24. Magge D, Steve J, Novak S, et al. Performing the difficult cholecystectomy using combined endoscopic and robotic techniques: how I do it. J Gastrointest Surg. 2017;21(3):583–9.

25. Ji WB, Zhao ZM, Dong JH, Wang HG, Lu F, Lu HW. One-stage robotic-assisted laparoscopic cholecystectomy and common bile duct exploration with primary closure in 5 patients. Surg Laparosc Endosc Percutaneous Tech. 2011;21(2):123–6.

26. Tao Z, Emuakhagbon VS, Pham T, Augustine MM, Guzzetta A, Huerta S. Outcomes of robotic and laparoscopic cholecystectomy for benign gallbladder disease in veteran patients. J Robot Surg. 2021;15(6):849–57.

27. Willuth E, Hardon SF, Lang F, et al. Robotic-assisted cholecystectomy is superior to laparoscopic cholecystectomy in the initial training for surgical novices in an ex vivo porcine model: a randomized crossover study. Surg Endosc. 2022;36(2):1064–79.

28. Agresta F, Campanile FC, Vettoretto N, et al. Laparoscopic cholecystectomy: consensus conference-based guidelines. Langenbeck's Arch Surg. 2015;400(4):429–53.

29. Gurusamy KS, Davidson BR. Surgical treatment of gallstones. Gastroenterol Clin N Am. 2010;39(2):229–44.

30. Festi D, Reggiani ML, Attili AF, et al. Natural history of gallstone disease: expectant management or active treatment? Results from a population-based cohort study. J Gastroenterol Hepatol. 2010;25:719–24.

31. Venneman NG, Renooij W, Rehfeld JF, et al. Small gallstones, preserved gallbladder motility, and fast crystallization are associated with pancreatitis. Hepatology. 2005;41:738–46.

32. Colecchia A, Sandri L, Bacchi-Reggiani ML, et al. Is it possible to predict the clinical course of gallstone disease? Usefulness of gallbladder motility evaluation in a clinical setting. Am J Gastroenterol. 2006;101:2576–81.

33. Foley KG, Lahaye MJ, Thoeni RF, et al. Management and follow-up of gallbladder polyps: updated joint guidelines between the ESGAR, EAES, EFISDS and ESGE. Eur Radiol. 2022;32(5):3358–68.

34. Strasberg SM, Hertl M, Soper NJ. An analysis of the problem of biliary injury during laparoscopic cholecystectomy. J Am Coll Surg. 1995;180(1):101–25.

35. Brunt M, Deziel DJ, Telem DA, et al. Safe cholecystectomy multi-society practice guideline and state-of-the-art consensus conference on prevention of bile duct injury during cholecystectomy. Ann Surg. 2020;272(1):3–23.

36. Booij KA, de Reuver PR, Nijsse B, et al. Insufficient safety measures reported in operation notes of complicated laparo- scopic cholecystectomies. Surgery. 2014;155:384–9.

37. Strasberg SM, Eagon CJ, Drebin JA. The "hidden cystic duct" syndrome and the infundibular technique of laparoscopic cholecystectomy–the danger of the false infundibulum. J Am Coll Surg. 2000;191(6):661–7.

38. Nijssen MA, Schreinemakers JM, Meyer Z, et al. Complications after laparoscopic cholecystectomy: a video evaluation study of whether the critical view of safety was reached. World J Surg. 2015;39(7):1798–803.

39. Dip F, LoMenzo E, Sarotto L, et al. Randomized trial of near-infrared incisionless fluorescent cholangiography. Ann Surg. 2019;270:990–9.

40. Spinoglio G, Priora F, Bianchi PP, et al. Real-time near- infrared (NIR) fluorescent cholangiography in single- site robotic cholecystectomy (SSRC): a single-institutional prospective study. Surg Endosc. 2013;27(6):2156–62.

Laparoscopic Treatment of Hepatic Diseases

28

Andrea P. Fontana, Monica Fiorentini, Nadia Russolillo, Ilaria Cesari, and Alessandro Ferrero

28.1 Terminology of Liver Anatomy and Resections

Liver surgery, in contrast to the other surgical interventions in abdominal surgery, includes an almost limitless number of different resections with a different degree of complexity and extension. Therefore, definition of liver resection is rather difficult.

According to the Brisbane Classification [1] (Fig. 28.1), the liver is subdivided, by the portal pedicles, into three successive orders of division: liver or hemilivers (*right* and *left liver* or *hemiliver*), sections (*right posterior section*, *right anterior section*, *left medial section*, and *left lateral section*), and segments (from *Sg1* to *Sg8*). Every liver segment is further subdivided into subsegmental units, each fed by a third- or fourth-order portal branch named "cone units" [2–4].

Therefore, several anatomical resections are defined by adding the suffix *-ectomy* to the name of the excised portion of the liver. For example, resection of the right liver is defined as *right hepatectomy* or *right hemihepatectomy*, resection of the right posterior section as a *right posterior sectionectomy*, and resection of segment 7 as *segmentectomy 7*. Anatomical liver resections are further classified as "minor" or "major" based on the number of segments removed (less or more than 3, respectively).

In contrast with anatomical liver resections, non-anatomical resections (also defined as wedge, atypical, or limited resections) are characterized by the removal of the tumor with a free resection margin without regarding the segmental anatomy of the liver.

The spread of laparoscopic liver surgery has been slower than in other fields of oncological surgery. However, the three consensus conferences held in Louisville (2008) [5], Morioka (2014) [6], and Southampton (2018) [7] have certified the advantages of laparoscopic liver resections compared to the traditional open technique: less intraoperative bleeding, less morbidity, and shorter length of hospital stay with comparable long-term outcomes.

One peculiarity of laparoscopic surgery is the extensive use of technology in almost all the phases of resection. Therefore, it is essential for the scrub nurse to know the fundamental principles and the main criticisms of this type of approach.

A. P. Fontana · M. Fiorentini · N. Russolillo
I. Cesari · A. Ferrero (✉)
Department of General and Oncological Surgery,
Ordine Mauriziano Hospital, Turin, Italy
e-mail: aferrero@mauriziano.it

Fig. 28.1 First (**a**), second (**b**), and third (**c**) order liver division with the correspondent anatomical term, liver segment referred to the term for the surgical resection, and schematic diagram of the surgical resection. (From Strasberg SM et al. The Brisbane 2000 Terminology of Liver Anatomy and Resections. HPB 2000; 2:333–339; with permission)

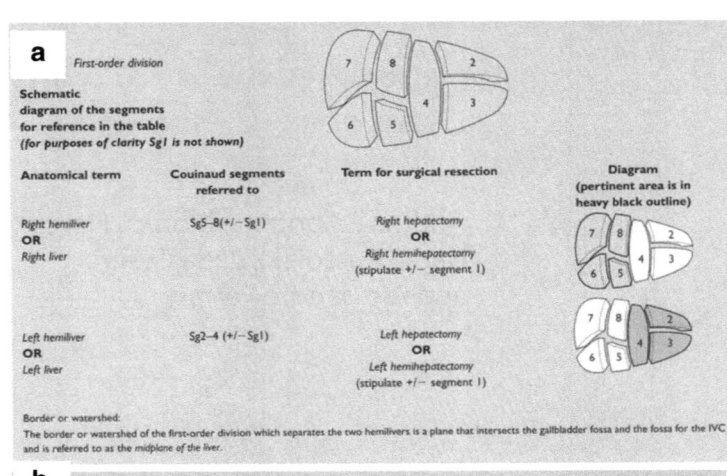

28.2 Description of the Surgical Technique

A laparoscopic liver resection surgery consists of several phases, which can be summarized as follows.

28.2.1 Exploratory Laparoscopy

- To rule out peritoneal carcinomatosis.
- To assess the macroscopic liver aspect and detect superficial liver lesions not visible at the preoperative imaging.

28.2.2 Laparoscopic Ultrasound (LUS)

- To confirm the presence and location of known liver nodules and search for any new liver lesions. It should always be performed before any mobilization maneuver to avoid artifacts.
- To study the patient's liver anatomy.
- To guide the surgeon during the liver parenchymal dissection [8].

28.2.3 Preparation of the Pringle Maneuver

- Partial division of the lesser omentum.
- Encircle the hepatic hilum through the foramen of Winslow with a nylon tape fixed with a clip and a 5-cm rubber tube.
- The nylon tape ends can be cut and remain within the abdomen, clamping the hepatic hilum through the placement of a Hem-o-lok (intracorporeal Pringle maneuver) [9] or brought out through the temporary placement of a 5-mm trocar and using a Mayo clamp to tighten the tourniquet around the hepatic hilum (extracorporeal Pringle maneuver) [10].

28.2.4 Hepatic Hilum Dissection and in-Flow Control

- This phase is needed in some anatomical liver resections (e.g., major hepatectomies) in order to reduce the risk of bleeding and to obtain ischemic demarcation on the liver surface.
- The ischemic demarcation can be further improved by infusion of indocyanine green fluorescent dye (ICG), using a specific near-infrared light range (NIR) camera. The perfused liver will be green, unlike the parenchyma excluded by the ligation of the portal pedicles (negative staining technique).
- If required by the histotype of the liver tumor (intrahepatic cholangiocellular carcinoma or perihilar cholangiocellular carcinoma), regional lymphadenectomy is performed during this phase removing the retropancreatic, the hepatic hilum, and the common hepatic artery lymph nodes.

28.2.5 Liver Mobilization

- Section of the round and falciform ligament.
- Section of the coronary ligament and dissection of the bare area exposing the hepatocaval confluence.
- Section of the right (in case of right liver mobilization) or the left (in case of left liver mobilization) triangular ligament.
- Section of the hepatocaval ligament (Makuuchi ligament) to have complete right liver mobilization and access to the right hepatic vein.
- Section of the Arantius' ligament if common trunk isolation is needed.
- Ligation and section of the accessory hepatic veins if Sg1 mobilization is needed.
- In some cases, it can be useful to control hepatic veins by encircling with a tape in order to clamp or tie them during the parenchymal transection phase (e.g., liver resection with extensive exposition of hepatic veins or major hepatectomy).

28.2.6 Parenchymal Transection

- Usually, it starts without any Pringle maneuver in order to "test" the consistency of the liver parenchyma. However, laparoscopic liver resections often require intermittent clamping of the hepatic hilum (15′ of inflow occlusion alternating to 5′ of reperfusion).
- The transection of the liver parenchyma can be performed with different techniques according to the type of instruments used.
- For selective techniques, devices (e.g., ultrasonic dissector) capable of fragmenting and selectively dividing parenchyma while preserving vascular and biliary structures are used.
- For non-selective techniques, devices (e.g., radiofrequency-ablation dissector) which cannot discriminate between vascular structures and parenchyma are used.

28.2.7 Division of Vascular and Biliary Structures

- Vessel coagulations can be achieved by placing clips, using sealer-divider devices like LigaSure™, Harmonic®, or Thunderbeat® or with sutures. The choice of the technique mainly depends on the vessel size.
- Staplers are particularly useful in dividing the major trunk of hepatic veins, main portal branches, and right or left bile duct during major hepatectomies.

28.2.8 Specimen Extraction Phase

- After inserting the specimen into an endobag.
- Through a mini-laparotomy (usually a Pfannenstiel incision).
- For small specimens, through a 1- or 2-cm enlargement of a 12-mm trocar incision.
- Other site in case of previous midline, subcostal, or other abdominal incision.

28.2.9 Hemostasis and Biliostasis

- The cut surface of the liver is double-checked and any blood or bile leaks are sutured or coagulated at the end of parenchymal transection.

28.2.10 Falciform Ligament Reconstruction

- In case of right hepatectomy or extended hepatectomy of the right liver, it is mandatory to reconstruct the falciform ligament to avoid the rotation of the left liver which would obstruct proper outflow through the residual hepatic vein(s).

As already mentioned, given the variety of possible liver resections, not all of these phases are always necessary in every laparoscopic liver resection.

28.3 Operating Theater Setting

The operating theater setting is schematized in Fig. 28.2:

- The surgeon stands between the patient's legs.
- The first assistant stands on the right side of the patient.
- The second assistant stands on the left side of the patient.
- The scrub nurse stands on the left side of the patient, next to the second assistant. The nurse is positioned sideways so that she/he can serve the surgeon frontally but also be able to see the screen.
- Back table is placed next to the scrub nurse.
- The main screen (a 55-inch 4 K monitor) is placed behind the patient's head, right in front of the main surgeon. The upper surgical drape is placed directly in contact with the patient's face without any support to avoid interfering with the surgeon's view of the screen.

Fig. 28.2 Scheme of the operative theater setting. (Lap, laparoscopic; Surg, surgeon; Ass, assistant)

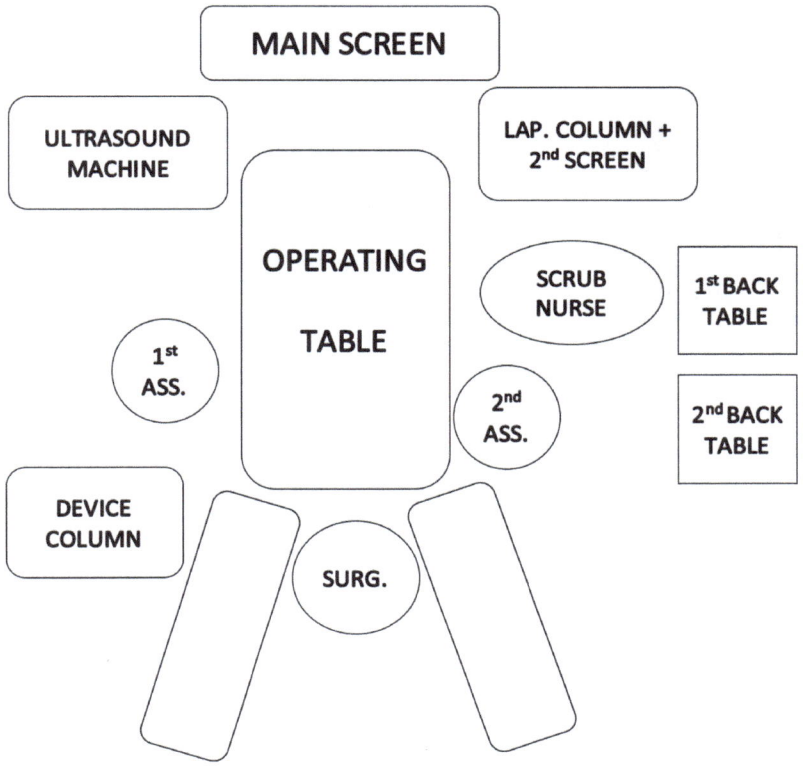

- The laparoscopic column along with the second screen (sometimes used for intraoperative visualization of 3D reconstructions) is on the left side of the patient's head.
- The ultrasound machine is on the right side of the patient's head.
- The energy devices column (monopolar, bipolar, radiofrequency, and ultrasonic dissector) next to the patient's right leg.

28.4 Patient Positioning

The patient is positioned as shown in Fig. 28.3:

- Supine.
- 20° reverse Trendelenburg position.
- Split legs, secured on surgical boot stirrups.
- Right arm adducted along the body; left arm open.
- Only in the case of right posterior segment resection (Sg6; Sg7; Sg8d), an atraumatic gel positioner pad is placed behind the back in

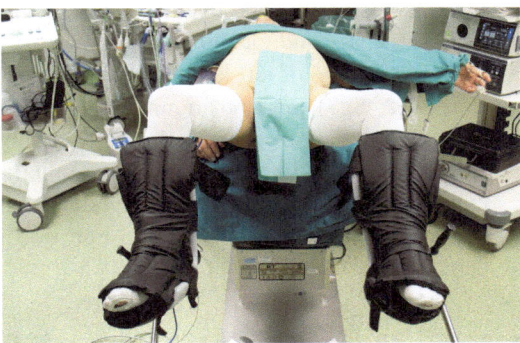

Fig. 28.3 Patient position

order to obtain a partial left rotation (hybrid position).

28.5 Port Placement

After an open or closed laparoscopy entry and pneumoperitoneum creation, the laparoscopic trocars are placed as schematized in Fig. 28.4a:

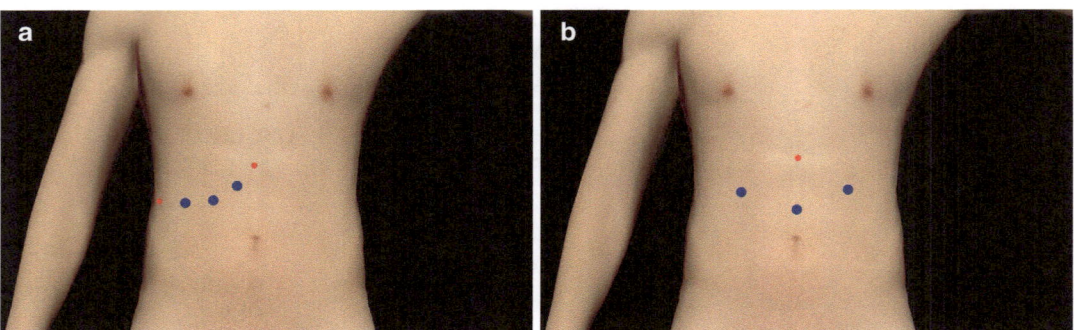

Fig. 28.4 (**a**) Typical port placement; (**b**) port placement for left lateral segments (Sg2 and Sg3) resections. (Blue dot: 12-mm port; red dot: 5-mm port)

- The laparoscopic trocars are positioned along an "ideal right subcostal J-shaped line," which is also used in the case of laparotomic conversion.
- 3 "central" subcostal 12-mm trocars. The first one along the midclavicular line.
- 2 "lateral" subcostal 5-mm trocars. The "right lateral" along the anterior axillary line. The "left lateral" subxiphoid.
- The "ideal right subcostal J-shaped line" may be slightly higher or lower depending on the patient's abdominal and liver conformation as well as the size and location of the lesions.
- Only in the case of left lateral segment resection (Sg2; Sg3), port positioning is different (Fig. 28.4b). Four trocars are placed. A 12-mm trocar on the midline 4 cm above the umbilicus. Two 12-mm trocars on the right and left hypochondrium, respectively. A 5-mm trocar subxiphoid.

28.6 Surgical Instruments Required

Figure 28.5 shows the scrub nurse's two back tables.

All laparoscopic instruments as well as those for performing open laparoscopy are arranged on the first back table (Fig. 28.5a). The instruments for the minilaparotomy for specimen extraction (usually a Pfannenstiel incision) or the eventual laparotomic conversion are arranged on the second back table (Fig. 28.5b). Furthermore, two large sterile plastic adhesive bags, containing the instruments equipped with a cable, are placed on the patient's sides.

Monopolar hook, bipolar forceps, and ultrasonic dissector are placed in the right plastic bag, whereas suction/irrigation system, laparoscopic ultrasound probe, and radiofrequency sealer-divider device are on the left.

Laparoscopic Instruments (Figs. 28.5a and 28.6):

- 5 disposable ports (three 12-mm ports and two 5-mm ports).
- 30° laparoscopic endoscope with 4 K NIR/ICG camera.
- Scope warmer.
- 3 reusable Johann forceps.
- 2 reusable right-angle dissectors (10 mm and 5 mm, respectively).
- 1 reusable Kelly forceps.

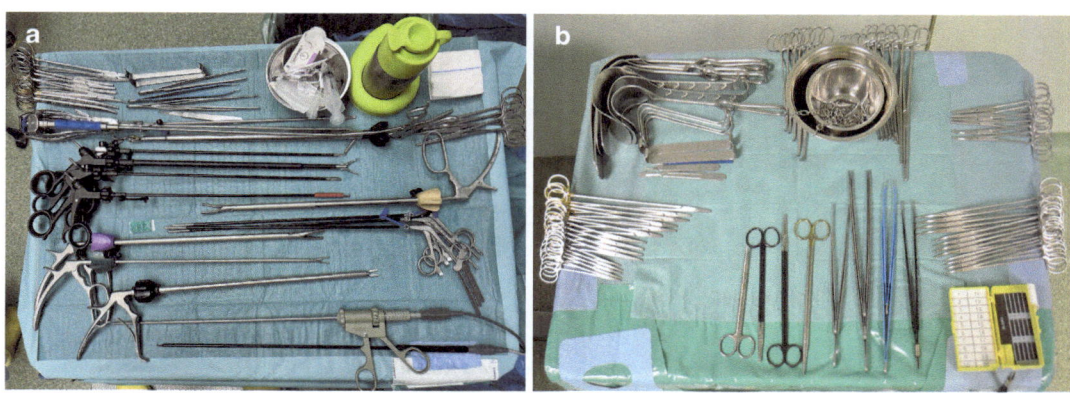

Fig. 28.5 (**a**) Scrub nurse first back table for laparoscopic instruments; (**b**) scrub nurse second back table for minilaparotomy and conversion instruments

- 2 reusable needle holders (1 curved and 1 straight).
- 2 reusable scissors (1 curved and 1 straight).
- 10-mm titanium clip applier.
- 3 Hem-o-lok clip appliers (small/medium/large).
- 1 rubber tourniquet and 1 nylon tape.
- 1 bulldog clip applied and removing forceps.
- Rubber vessel loops.
- 1 "Gold finger" liver retractor.
- 1 atraumatic "snake" liver retractor.

- 1 monopolar hook.
- 1 bipolar forceps.
- 1 sealer-divider instrument (radiofrequency or ultrasonic device).
- 1 ultrasonic surgical aspirator.
- 1 laparoscopic 4-way ultrasound probe.
- 1 suction/irrigation system.
- 5 × 5 cm gauze swabs.
- Peanut swabs.
- Endo GIA.
- Endobag.

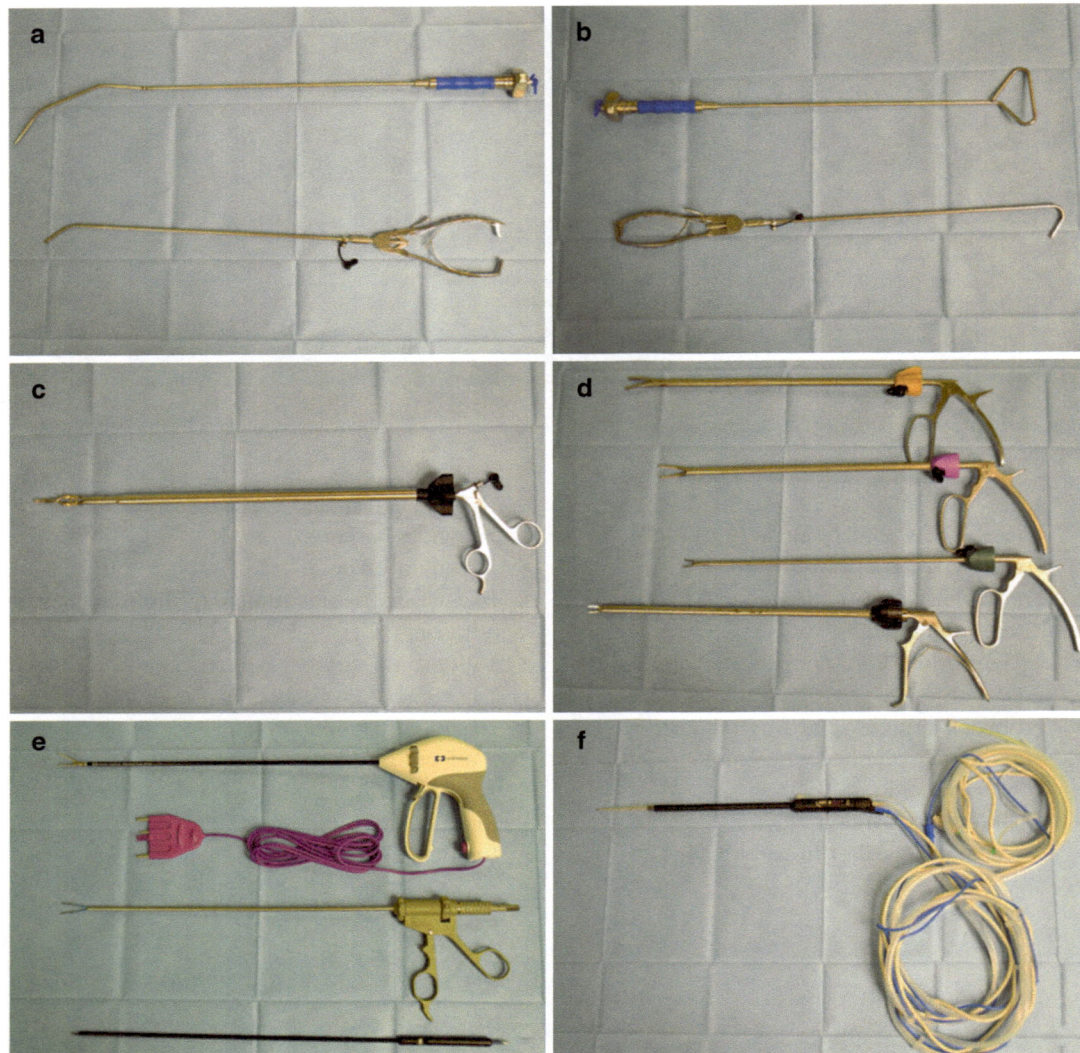

Fig. 28.6 Detail of some instruments. (**a** and **b**). Atraumatic "snake" retractor and "Goldfinger" retractor, open (**a**) and closed (**b**); (**c**) bulldog clip applied forceps; (**d**) Hem-o-lok clip appliers (small/medium/large) and a 10-mm titanium clip applier; (**e**) LigaSure™, bipolar forceps and monopolar hook; (**f**) ultrasonic surgical aspirator

28.7 Surgical Steps and Related Instruments

Below is a detailed description of the surgical instruments used in the various phases of the operation already described above.

28.7.1 Exploratory Laparoscopy

- 2 Johann forceps
- Scissors, if a peritoneum biopsy is necessary.
- Monopolar hook, bipolar forceps, and vessel sealer, in case of peritoneal adhesion.

28.7.2 Laparoscopic Ultrasound (Fig. 28.7)

28.7.3 Preparation of the Pringle Maneuver (Fig. 28.8)

- Laparoscopic 4-way or 2-way ultrasound probe.

- 2 Johann forceps.

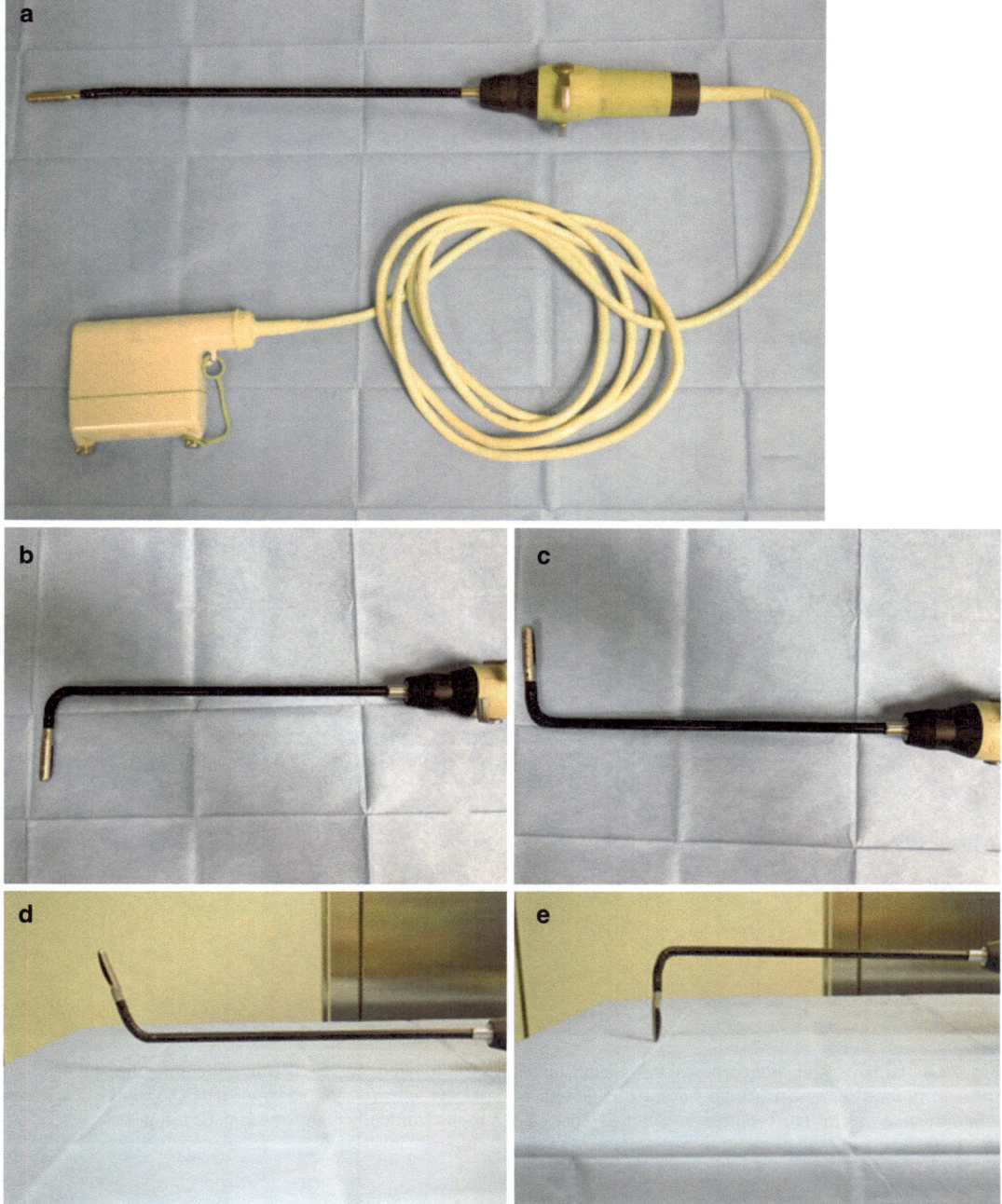

Fig. 28.7 (**a**) Laparoscopic 4-way ultrasound probe; (**b**–**e**) four possible directions (right, left, down, up) in which to move the probe; (**f**) intraoperative laparoscopic ultrasound

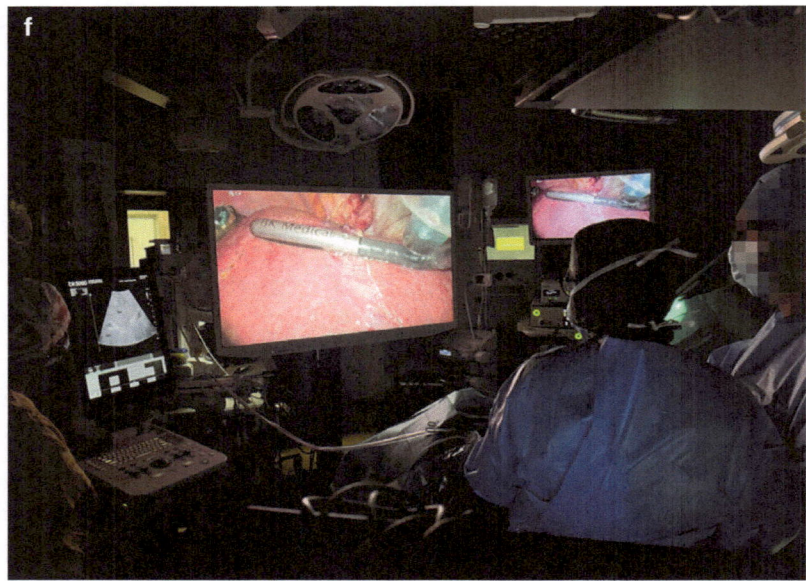

Fig. 28.7 (continued)

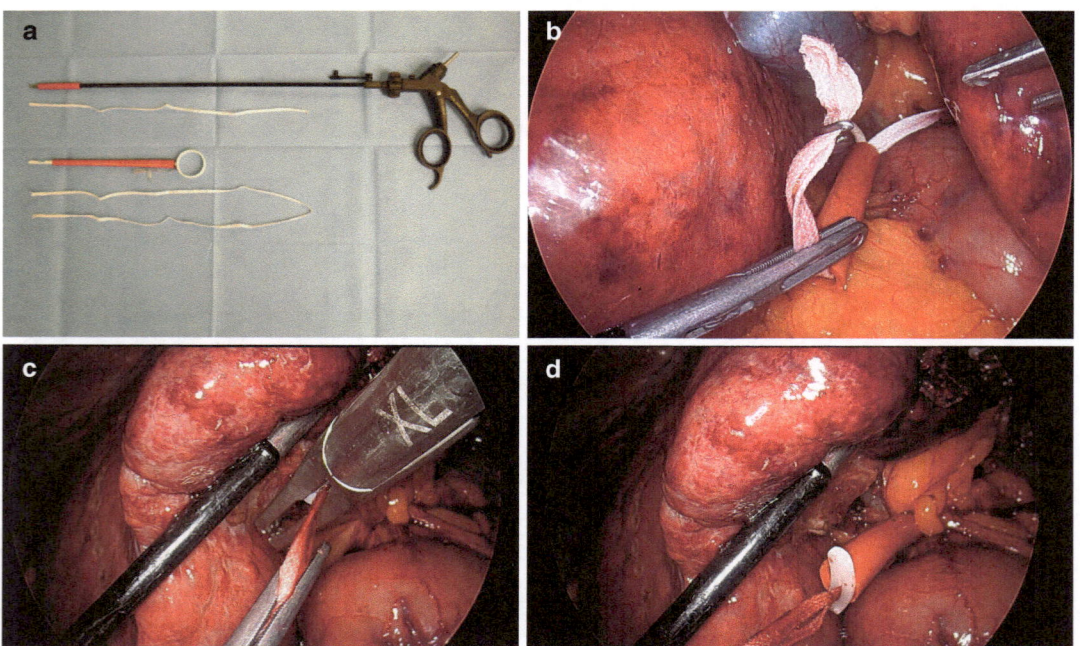

Fig. 28.8 Laparoscopic intracorporeal Pringle maneuver. (**a**) The rubber tourniquet should be cut to a length of approximately 5 cm; (**b**) the hepatic hilum is encircled with a nylon tape fixed with a titanium clip and the 5-cm rubber tube; (**c** and **d**) a large size (XL) Hem-o-lok is used to intermittently clamp the hepatic hilum

- Sealing instrument, to cut the lesser omentum.
- "Gold finger" liver retractor or Johann forceps to encircle the hepatic hilum.
- 12F (intracorporeal Pringle) or 20 F (extracorporeal Pringle) rubber tourniquet and 1 nylon tape.
- 1 titanium clip.
- 1 large size Hem-o-lok/Mayo clamp.
- Scissors, to cut the nylon tape.

28.7.4 Hepatic Hilum Dissection and in-Flow Control

- 2 Johann forceps.
- Atraumatic "snake" liver retractor.
- Monopolar hook, bipolar forceps, and sealing instrument, to dissect the hepatic hilum.
- Curved scissors, to dissect the hepatic hilum.
- Rubber vessel loops to encircle the pedicle to be clamped and sectioned.
- Bulldog clips, to temporarily clamp the pedicle.
- Laparoscopic 4-way ultrasound probe, to check, using the color Doppler, the correct clamping of the pedicle, and the patency of the remnant pedicles.
- Hem-o-lok clips and straight scissors or Endo GIA (vascular load) to section the pedicle.

- ICG, to enhance the ischemic demarcation and facilitate the execution of the parenchymal transection.

28.7.5 Liver Mobilization

- 2 Johann forceps.
- Atraumatic "snake" liver retractor.
- "Gold finger" liver retractor.
- Monopolar hook, bipolar forceps, sealing instrument.
- Curved scissors.
- 2 right angle dissectors (10 mm and 5 mm, respectively).
- Titanium and Hem-o-lok clips and scissors, to section the accessory hepatic vein and the hepatocaval ligament.
- Nylon tape or vessel loop for the possible encircling of a major hepatic vein.

28.7.6 Parenchymal Transection (Fig. 28.9)

- Laparoscopic 4-way ultrasound probe, to plan the resection and to draw with the monopolar hook the sketch of the principal vessels involved in the resection.

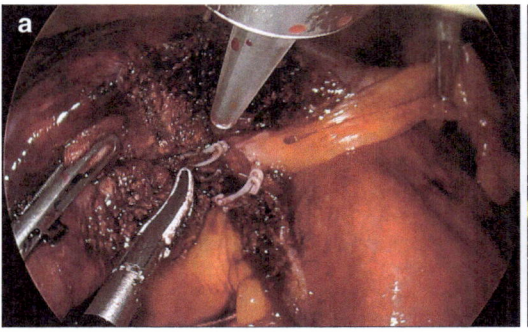 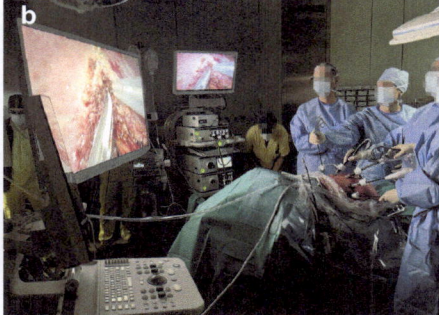

Fig. 28.9 Parenchymal transection. (**a** and **b**) The liver parenchyma is selectively divided with an ultrasonic dissector (surgeon's right hand), and vascular and biliary structures are clipped or sealed by a radiofrequency sealer-divider (surgeon's left hand) depending on their diameter. First assistant, standing on the right side of the patient, holds the scope with the right hand, and Johann forceps with a peanut swab on the tip for an atraumatic retraction of the cut surface with the left hand. Second assistant, standing on the left side of the patient, retracts the liver through the round ligament stump with a Johann forceps

- 2 Johann forceps, one to retract the liver (sometimes from the round ligament previously sectioned), one with a peanut swab on the tip, used as a retractor on the cut surface.
- "Gold finger" liver retractor.
- Atraumatic "snake" liver retractor.
- Ultrasonic dissector for liver parenchyma transection.
- Sealing instrument (radiofrequency or ultrasonic device), to seal and cut the smaller vessels.
- Suction/irrigation system.
- 2 right angle dissectors (10 mm and 5 mm, respectively).
- Titanium clips, Hem-o-lok clips, and scissors, to section the vessels not amenable to be sectioned by the sealing instrument.
- Rubber vessel loops, to encircle a bigger pedicle or a major hepatic vein.
- Bulldog clips, to temporarily clamp a pedicle.
- Curved needle holder with 4/0, 5/0, 6/0 Prolene or Nylon suture, for hemostasis or biliostasis.
- Bipolar forceps, for hemostasis.
- Endo GIA (vascular load), in case of major hepatic vein resection or first−/second-order bile duct resection.

28.8 Specimen Extraction Phase

- Endobag.
- Scalpel (blade 24).
- Diathermy.
- 2 anatomical forceps.
- 2 Farabeuf retractors.
- 3 straight Klemmers to grasp the fascia and the peritoneum.
- 1–2 absorbable suture for closing the peritoneum (based on the surgeon request).
- 1–2 absorbable suture for closing the fascia (based on the surgeon request)
- Skin stapler/suture for closing the skin.

28.8.1 Hemostasis and Biliostasis

- Suction/irrigation system.

- 5 × 5 cm gauze swabs.
- Titanium and Hem-o-lok clips.
- Curved needle holder with 4/0, 5/0, 6/0 Prolene or Nylon suture.

28.8.2 Falciform Ligament Reconstruction

- Curved needle holder with 3/0 PDS barbed suture.

References

1. Strasberg SM, Belghiti J, Clavien P-A, Gadzijev E, Garden JO, Lau W-Y, Makuuchi M, Strong RW. The Brisbane 2000 terminology of liver anatomy and resections. HPB. 2000;2:333–9.
2. Takasaki K. Glissonean pedicle transection method for hepatic resection: a new concept of liver segmentation. J Hepato-Biliary-Pancreat Surg. 1998;5:286–91.
3. Majno P, Mentha G, Toso C, Morel P, Peitgen HO, Fasel JHD. Anatomy of the liver: an outline with three levels of complexity--a further step towards tailored territorial liver resections. J Hepatol. 2014;60:654–62.
4. Wakabayashi G, Cherqui D, Geller DA, et al. The Tokyo 2020 terminology of liver anatomy and resections: updates of the Brisbane 2000 system. J Hepatobiliary Pancreat Sci. 2022;29:6–15.
5. Buell JF, Cherqui D, Geller DA, et al. The international position on laparoscopic liver surgery: the Louisville statement, 2008. Ann Surg. 2009;250:825–30.
6. Wakabayashi G, Cherqui D, Geller DA, et al. Recommendations for laparoscopic liver resection: a report from the second international consensus conference held in Morioka. Ann Surg. 2015;261:619–29.
7. Abu Hilal M, Aldrighetti L, Dagher I, et al. The Southampton consensus guidelines for laparoscopic liver surgery: from indication to implementation. Ann Surg. 2018;268:11–8.
8. Russolillo N, Langella S, Lo Tesoriere R, Zingaretti CC, Fontana AP, Ferrero A. Ultrasound liver map technique for laparoscopic liver resections: tips and tricks. Mini-invasive Surg. 2023;7:3. https://doi.org/10.20517/2574-1225.2022.74.
9. Laurenzi A, Cherqui D, Figueroa R, Adam R, Vibert E, Cunha AS. Totally intra-corporeal Pringle maneuver during laparoscopic liver resection. HPB. 2018;20:128–31.
10. Rotellar F, Pardo F, Bueno A, Martí-Cruchaga P, Zozaya G. Extracorporeal tourniquet method for intermittent hepatic pedicle clamping during laparoscopic liver surgery: an easy, cheap, and effective technique. Langenbeck's Arch Surg. 2012;397:481–48.

Robotic Surgical Treatment of Hepatic Diseases

29

Gianluca Cassese, Mariano Cesare Giglio, and Roberto Ivan Troisi

29.1 Introduction

Despite the introduction of minimally invasive liver surgery (MILS) dates back to 1991, this approach had a slower diffusion when compared with other surgical subspecialties because of both technical difficulties and patients' characteristics [1]. Nonetheless, laparoscopic liver resection (LLR) has clearly shown several benefits, such as reduced postoperative pain, lower adhesions, lower surgical site infections, lower rates of incisional hernia, and shorter hospital stay, while having affordable costs [2]. Thus, after the first two consensus conferences held in Louisville in 2008 and in Morioka in 2014 recommending a safe implementation of the laparoscopic approach, MILS is currently recommended for most surgical liver pathologies by the latest international guidelines [3–5].

The first robotic liver resection (RLR) was reported in 2003; however, a significant increase in case numbers was recorded only after a period of 10 years, whereas the safety and reproducibility were first confirmed at the first international consensus statement on RLR in 2018 [6, 7]. The robotic approach has several advantages when compared to LLR, such as 360° of freedom of the wrist (simulating open liver resections), tremor filtration, and steady high-definition camera [8]. Despite such advantages, there remain some controversies around robotic surgery when compared with laparoscopic surgery, such as the higher cost without strong evidences about its clinical superiority. Similarly, there is also a lack of agreement on whether they should be compared against each other or directly compared to open surgery. However, in the latest series RLR accounts for 16–22% of all major resections at referral high volume centers, confirming the importance of this technique [9].

In this chapter, we describe the key aspects of robotic hepatobiliary surgery, with a focus on technical descriptions and the optimal settings of the robotic platform.

G. Cassese · M. C. Giglio · R. I. Troisi (✉)
Division of HPB, Minimally Invasive and Robotic Surgery, Renal Transplantation Service, Department of Clinical Medicine and Surgery, Federico II University Hospital, Naples, Italy

29.2 Technique

Robotic liver surgery has evolved from laparoscopy, with some similarities that can be easily found. However, the robotic platform with its instruments, the equipment and setting of the operation room, and the economy of movements are very different from the laparoscopic approach and should be mastered by the whole surgical and paramedic teams. Local expertise, surgeon's preferences, and patient's specific conditions may modify the standard approach, but there are some common principles. Actually, there is only one robotic platform available, and therefore, the development of alternative robotic systems in the future may bring some different technical concepts.

Furthermore, the robotic platform has the advantage, compared to laparoscopic surgery, of having a second workstation (double console). This eases the proctorship of surgeons in training, with continuous education and training to improve their ability under the guidance of an expert robotic surgeon. In addition, the second workstation provides young surgeons and residents with a more immersive and immediate learning experience [10].

29.2.1 Setup and Docking

Patient positioning is similar to laparoscopic approach. The supine position with open legs and one extended arm is the most common, but several variations can be found according to surgeon's experience and preferences. Left prone or semi-prone position can be preferred in case of surgeries involving the right posterior segments. Four robotic operating trocars are placed (one camera, three robotic arms), and one or two assistant trocars. It is essential to prevent instrument clashing when deciding port placement. Furthermore, port positioning in laparoscopic surgery is more versatile, while robotic surgery demands wider space between trocars without any port caudal or cephalic to another one (com-monly they must be positioned in a rectilinear-shaped line). The assisting surgeon is commonly placed between the legs.

Robotic ports are inserted under laparoscope vision guidance; then, the robotic cart is positioned within the surgical field and the arms docked. The distances and positions of the arms are calibrated by the robotic system itself, based on the target organ and the position of the camera itself. Bedside units are placed cephalic to the surgical field for most hepatobiliary and upper gastro-intestinal procedures. Newer versions allow the cart to be docked sideways to the patient. This adds the benefit of better access to the patient's airway for the anesthetic team.

Irrespective of the system, close collaboration with the nurses and the anesthetist is essential at the time of docking.

29.2.2 Robotic Instrumentation

Some instruments routinely used for laparoscopic liver surgery are not available for the robotic platform. Actually, the cavitron ultrasonic surgical aspirator (CUSA) is one of the most effective and widely used devices for liver parenchymal transection, but it is still not available for robotic platform. It can be used only through the assistant port, but its movements can be restricted by the presence of the robotic arms [11] (Fig. 29.1). The combination of robotic and laparoscopic approaches could solve such criticisms, maximizing human performance while keeping all the advantages of minimal invasiveness (hybrid approach) [12–14]. This robotic-laparoscopic technique also offers the possibility of improving the expertise and to shorten the learning curve of the side-table surgeon, allowing them to face the challenges of the parenchymal transection phase in an "assisted" fashion. Furthermore, the use of laparoscopic devices by the table assistant surgeon may sensibly reduce the costs related to robotic surgery, since they are cheaper than the corresponding robotic devices (such as laparoscopic harmonic, scissors, clip-appliers, staplers, CUSA).

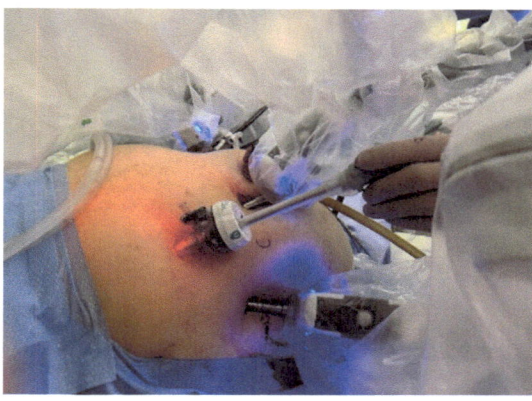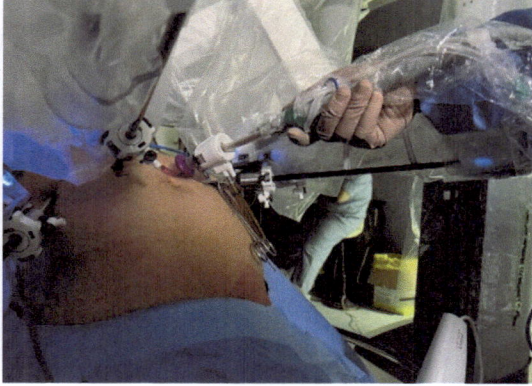

Fig. 29.1 "Hybrid" robotic approach for parenchymal transection, with the use of CUSA by the side-table surgeon

The Harmonic Scalpel is available for RLR, but while being effective for parenchymal transection, it shows some limitations about the control of moderate bleedings when transecting portal vessels, or a difficult recovery of bile ducts after their section. A new Endowrist Vessel Sealer® is now available, but more studies about its outcomes are still needed. There are other techniques for parenchymal transection that can be used as an alternative to CUSA dissection, widely depending on the surgeon's experience. However, parenchymal transection is a crucial part of the operation and is still considered as one of the limiting factors in the diffusion of RLR. In the authors' opinion, in light of the published results of RLR, these aspects should not hinder the diffusion of this approach.

Robotic surgery could improve the suturing capacity of the surgeon when compared to laparoscopy, thanks to the mobility of the operator's hands and wrists. This could help the bleeding control in difficult circumstances, together with the possibility to use the traditional laparoscopic instruments and stapling devices (i.e., stapling hepatic veins or hilar structures) and in all cases of tissue reconstruction.

29.2.3 Hepatic Inflow Control

Both surgeons and anesthesiologists must contribute to decreasing intraoperative blood loss.

Surgeons can use vascular clamps intraoperatively. A Pringle maneuver (selective or not) should be prepared when performing major resections, as recently shown in a propensity-matched analysis on 209 patients [15]. However, in some small resections on a normal liver it can be avoided, in order to prevent any ischemic injury to the remaining liver and intestinal congestion. Montalti et al. in a setting of hepatic resections on postero-superior segments, found that the average clamping time was significantly longer in RLR than in LLR (76.7 vs. 24.6 min, $p < 0.001$) [16]. However, some other authors tend to use the Pringle maneuver less frequently when operating robotically than in an open fashion (8.3% vs. 90.9%, $p < 0.001$ in a recent series) when considering non-difficult positions [17].

Similarly, Glissonean approach for selective inflow control has been reported as safe and effective, by using the same technique as in laparoscopy (Fig. 29.2) [18]. This term was first used by Takasaki in 1986, referring to a right sectionectomy when dealing with the so-called extrafascial technique for inflow control (even if already described by Couinaud, together with the classical intrafascial, the extrafascial, and the extrafascial-transfissural approaches) [19]. Recently, the study group of precision anatomy for minimally invasive hepato-biliary-pancreatic surgery (PAM-HBP), composed of the major worldwide experts in MILS, concluded several advantages of the Glissonean approach compared

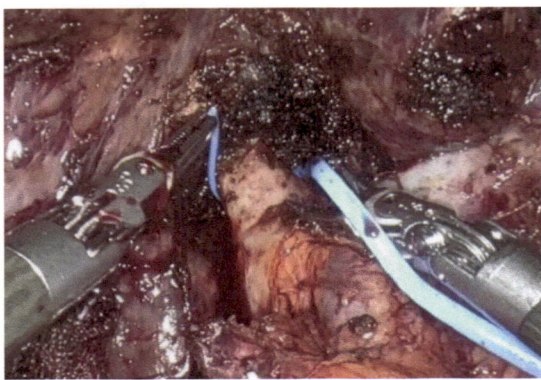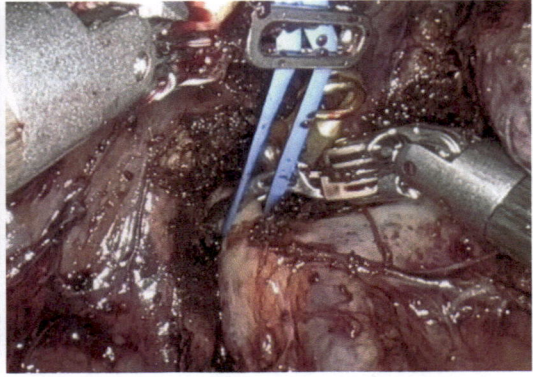

Fig. 29.2 Robotic Glissonean approach for the inflow control of the right anterior pedicle

to the conventional hilar approach for performing minimally invasive anatomic liver resections [20, 21].

29.2.4 Augmented Reality in Robotic Liver Surgery

The robotic platform delivers an immersive surgical experience. Highly magnified 3DHD vision gives a true depth perception. Furthermore, in liver surgery, the use of 3D reconstruction is very helpful for both correct preoperative planning and intraoperative guidance [22]. Also in this case, the intuitive robotic platform provides the surgeon with the *TilePro* system that is able to visualize the 3D models directly into the robotic console (Fig. 29.3a).

Intraoperative ultrasound (IOUS) is a key point in liver surgery, in both conventional and minimally invasive approaches. It is fundamental to identify the lesion and its relationship with liver and vascular elements, as well as to guide the transection line and to confirm the preoperative diagnosis [23]. The authors recommend a standard routine four-step protocol: exploration, verification, guidance, and confirmation [24]. There are some differences regarding the use of IOUS

between RLR and LLR. Only one type of ultrasound probe is currently compatible with robotic trocars (Robotic Drop-In Ultrasound Transducer-BK-Medical) while any other type of ultrasound probe can only be used by the assistant surgeon [24]. The number of assistant trocars (1 or 2 in robot-assisted procedures, 4 or 5 in laparoscopy) and their different positions could need initial training.

Indocyanine green (ICG) has many applications in hepatobiliary surgery, enhancing a better visualization of liver lesions (with different doses and timing of infusion, as described elsewhere [25]), of vascular and biliary structures, hepatic segmental limits, lymph nodes, and peritoneal metastases, with many clinical potential advantages [25]. The green light fluorescence needs specific equipment, with a camera able to filter the green wavelengths and a high-definition monitor. Such equipment is integrated into the last version of Da Vinci Xi® (Firefly® fluorescence imaging) (Fig. 29.3b). ICG seems to be a promising technology applied to RLR for malignancies, as two-dimensional laparoscopy lacks depth perception: The additional visual information guides the transection, making up for the technical difficulties given by a minimally invasive approach [8, 26].

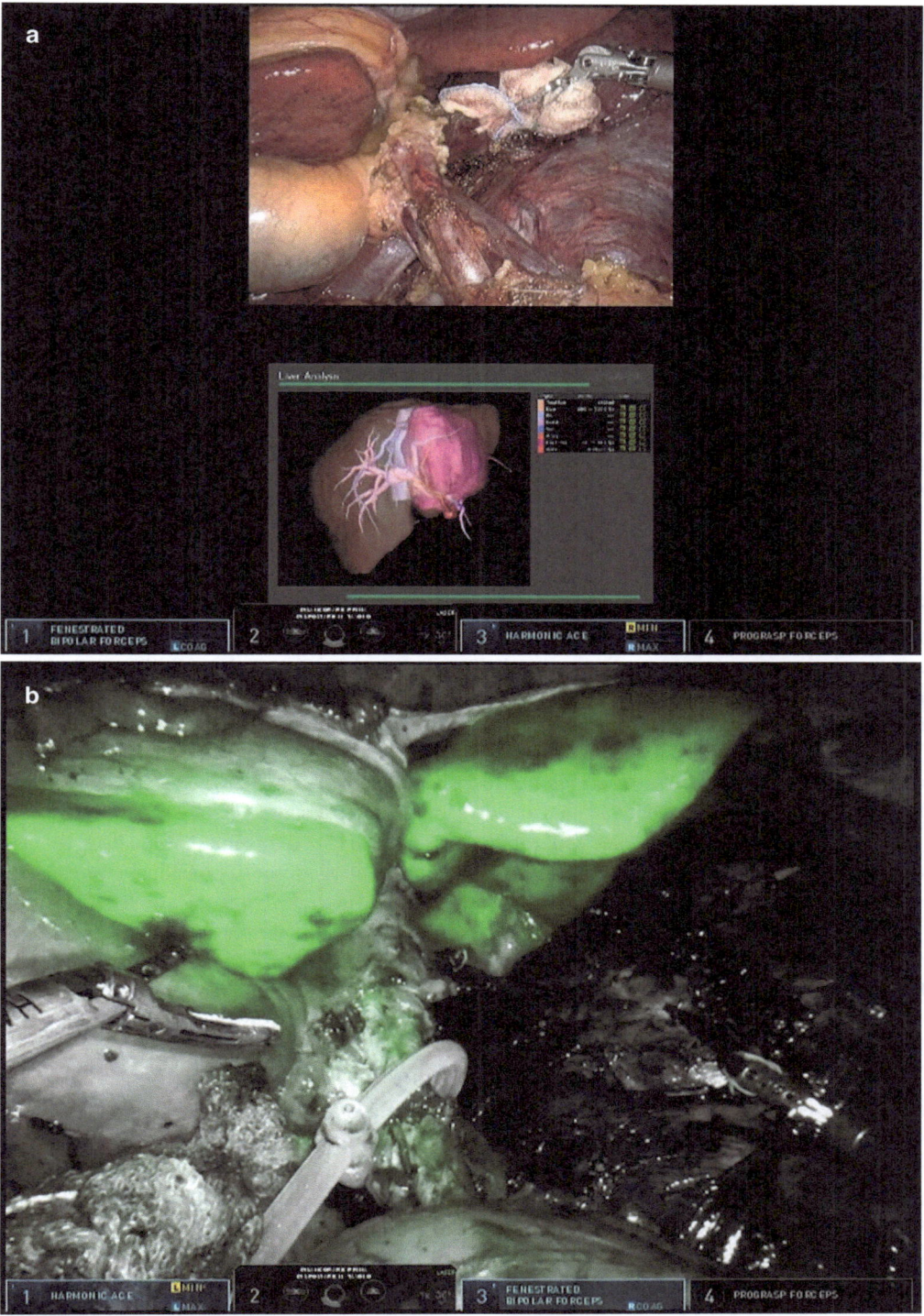

Fig. 29.3 Augmented reality in robotic surgery. (**a**) Intraoperative visualization of a 3D rendering through the TilePro system; (**b**) ICG-guided negative counterstaining during robotic liver resection through the firefly system

29.2.5 Biliary and Vascular Reconstructions

There are few studies about both robotic or laparoscopic biliary reconstructions, mainly performed for Klatskin tumors or during pancreatic or bariatric surgery. The robotic approach could indeed be a valid option for the reconstruction of biliary tract, as the augmented degrees of freedom, the increased steadiness of the camera, the tremor filtration, and the better suturing process could provide some advantages [8, 27]. The few results of robot-assisted operations on the biliary tract are generally encouraging, such as for the first comparison between robotic and open techniques for choledochotomies that reported a lower complication rate in the robotic group [28, 29].

Currently, only a few studies described minimally invasive vascular reconstructions, mainly during pancreatic resections or living hepatectomy for liver transplantation [30, 31]. Vascular reconstructions during liver resection are a challenge for minimally invasive techniques and are currently considered as relative contraindications to the minimally invasive approach. There are few data about vascular reconstructions carried out using a robotic platform, but vascular reconstructions could be technically easier with robotic assistance thanks to endowristed robotic instruments [32].

29.2.6 Specimen Extraction

There is no difference in specimen extraction technique between robotic and laparoscopic surgery at this point. The specimen is extracted through a retrieval bag, following the undocking of the robotic arms. Options for specimen extraction include extension of an existing port site, a previous midline, or transverse incision or a new incision. There is little evidence comparing all available options, but there seems to be a preference toward the Pfannenstiel incision, thanks to lower postoperative pain and rate of incisional hernia [33].

29.2.7 Conversions

A conversion to open laparotomy is always possible during a liver resection; therefore, the operation room must always have the laparotomic vascular and abdominal instrumental equipment for open surgery. The most common event that requires a conversion is uncontrollable bleeding, but long operative time has also been found as associated with open conversions, as well as morbid obesity and the intraoperative finding of a more extensive disease burden [34–36].

The conversion rate has been proposed as a method to assess the quality of a minimally invasive procedure, as it usually decreases with experience [37]. Recently, a meta-analysis including 11 studies showed no significant difference between the RLR group and LLR group in conversion rate (6.1% vs. 8.8%, p 0.27), while a subgroup analysis of studies published after 2010 showed a lower incidence of conversions in the robotic group (4.6% vs. 13%, p 0.02) [38].

A multicentric study on 3880 conventional and minimally invasive major liver resections (including also right sectoriectomies) showed that male gender, laparoscopic approach, liver cirrhosis, previous abdominal surgery, concomitant other surgery, ASA score 3/4, larger tumor size, conventional MH, and Institute Mutualiste Montsouris classification group III procedures were associated with an increased risk of conversion. Although RMH showed a decreased risk of conversion than LMH (OR 0.39, $p < 0.001$), converted RMH showed increased blood loss, blood transfusion rate, postoperative major morbidity, and 30- and 90-day mortality compared to converted LMH [39].

A need to carry out an emergency conversion to open surgery and the relatively longer timing needed for the de-docking should not "destabilize" the surgical team. A key role is played by the surgeon and his side-table attendee: coordinating work in giving the right instructions to the team while providing temporarily a bleeding control should attempt in preparing the de-docking. Like in laparoscopic approach, the use of a long vascular clamp available "just in case" could help for this.

29.3 Indications

MILS is performed for almost every liver disease that can benefit from surgical treatment; LRR and RLR have similar indications [40, 41]. However, there are some challenging situations, such as surgeries requiring biliary or vascular reconstructions, in which still there is not enough evidence supporting the minimally invasive technique, even if the robotic approach could represent useful support.

29.3.1 Hepatocellular Carcinoma

Hepatocellular carcinoma (HCC) represents the main indications for MILS worldwide [42]. In the past, the specific surgical and anesthesiologic risks linked to HCC surgery represented one of the main obstacles for the spread of the laparoscopic approach [43]. Indeed, HCC arises from an underlying liver cirrhosis in 90% of cases [44]. Liver cirrhosis carries a high risk of bleeding because of impaired coagulation or low platelets, as well as a high risk of post-hepatectomy liver failure (PHLF) and other postoperative complications [45]. Differently from CRLM, there is still no RCT comparing LLR and OLR. However, propensity score-matched studies showed the aforementioned encouraging results [46]. Additional studies reported similar results in cirrhotic patients. Recently, Kabir et al. published a meta-analysis on eleven studies including 1618 HCC patients: The results showed a 16–26% reduction in the hazard ratio of death for patients with HCC and cirrhosis undergoing LLR when compared to OLR, as well as reduced blood loss, reduced major complications, and shorter length of hospital stay [47]. Furthermore, when dealing with cirrhotic patients, it is important to consider not only the oncological and perioperative outcomes but also the surgical stress. Indeed, minimally invasive liver surgery in cirrhotic patients is reported to be associated with lower incidence of PHLF and ascites, probably thanks to reduced interruption of portosystemic shunts, preservation of abdom-inal musculature with subcutaneous vessels, together with lower electrolyte imbalances due to minimal exposure of the abdominal content to the air [48]. Furthermore, the advantages of LLR have also been reported in Child-B cirrhotic patients, with reduced blood loss, morbidity, and major complications after laparoscopic approach in this setting of patients [49].

The first studies about RLR for HCC confirmed similar advantages to LLR. The first 42 cases showed similar oncological and survival outcomes than LLR although the operative time was longer for the robotic group [13]. Recently, a wider series of 140 consecutive robot-assisted liver resections confirmed the safety and feasibility of RLR for HCC, showing a learning curve of about 30 consecutive cases at a CUSUM analysis [50]. Furthermore, recent studies are reporting very encouraging results from long-term follow-up of RLS. A recent propensity score-matched study on 3049 patients from a national American database showed improved 5-year overall survival (OS) compared with laparoscopic surgery (HR = 0.64, 95% CI: 0.43–0.96 for intent to treat, and HR = 0.59, 95% CI: 0.39–0.90 for end treatment).

29.3.2 Colorectal Liver Metastases (CRLM)

CRLM is the second worldwide indication for MILS, recently validated by the first-ever randomized controlled trial (RCT) of LLR, the OSLO-COMET [51]. Additional propensity score-matched studies confirmed the feasibility and eligibility of LLR for CRLM, suggesting up to 70% of patients with indication for laparoscopic approach at referral centers, with lower severe complications and shorter length of hospital stay when compared to OLR [52]. MILS has shown to be a viable option also for parenchymal-sparing hepatectomies that are currently considered the standard of care surgical therapy, thanks to decreased postoperative complications without affecting oncological outcomes, while improving subsequent resections [53]. Although the laparoscopic approach can be applied for selected cases of parenchymal-sparing resections, there are several biases which should be taken into account, firstly, the number of resected lesions in the case of CRLM. Looking to the literature and current practice, multiple nodules are still more often associated with open approach, even if LLR associated with thermal ablation can be proposed with this intent [54].

RLR for CRLM has been reported to be able to carry out parenchymal-sparing hepatectomies, with some authors proposing some advantages for difficult positions and postero-superior segments when compared to LLR [55]. However, such a hypothesis must be confirmed in more appropriate studies.

A recent propensity score-matched studies confirmed similar perioperative outcomes of RLR than LLR [56]. Similarly, regarding the long-term outcomes of RLR for CRLM, 5-year OS and DFS were 61% vs. 60%, $p = 0.78$, and 38% vs. 44% DFS, $p = 0.62$, respectively [56]. Appropriate oncological results have also been reported in an Italian multicentric analysis from the IgoMILS registry, whereas 1030 points, 953 LLR (92.5%), and 77 (7.5%) RLR, have been compared confirming similar outcomes but with an R1 rate with wider margins significantly lower in the RLR group ($p = 0.025$ and $p < 0.001$, respectively) [57].

Another interesting scenario is the surgical treatment of synchronous CRLM since there is still not enough evidence about the superiority of a liver-first approach over a simultaneous resection. Herein the possibility of a simultaneous minimally invasive surgical approach of both primary tumors and CRLM could be a valid option in selected cases. LLR could be more manageable than RLR as there is no need for patient's repositioning and robot's re-docking. To date, only one case series of six patients reported the safety and feasibility of the robotic approach [58].

29.3.3 Cholangiocarcinoma (CCC)

Surgical treatment of biliary tract malignancies is traditionally considered a "non-laparoscopic approach" because of the need for extensive and technically challenging liver resection, together with systematic lymphadenectomy. Recently, laparoscopic approach for intrahepatic CCC (iCCC) and hilar CCC (hCCC) has shown in several propensity score-matched studies similar survival outcomes than open approach, with a reduction in blood loss, even if the need for further studies with an appropriate design has been stressed [59, 60]. Other experiences reported the feasibility and effectiveness of an accurate lymphadenectomy [61]. For gallbladder cancer (GBC), several retrospective comparisons have shown that the laparoscopic approach can provide similar oncological results and the laparoscopic extended cholecystectomy has comparable outcomes compared to open surgery in expert centers [62]. The laparoscopic approach is also a viable option in case of re-operation after incidental GBC [63]. For T3/T4 stages, we still have low evidence that surgery and LLR can significantly modify the prognosis [64]. In 2019, the first expert consensus meeting on laparoscopic surgery for GBC treatment was held in Seoul, Korea, and the first expert consensus statement was established [65, 66]. The consensus meeting concluded that laparoscopic surgery does not worsen the prognosis of patients with resectable GBC, with accurate lymphadenectomy, acceptable morbidity, and survival outcomes also after bile duct resection.

Of course, there are even fewer studies in literature about RLR for CCC, with small case series, reaching a low level of evidence [67]. Even if the robotic approach could be more feasible than pure laparoscopy, thanks to the tridimensional movements of its wristed instruments, a recent series by Xu et al. comparing 10 RLR with 32 open resections for hCCC, the robotic group showed a significantly longer surgical time and an increased morbidity rate (90% vs. 50%; p 0.031), with a third of robotic patients experiencing a complication ≥3a according to Clavien-Dindo. For GBC, several reports have been published [68]. Goel et al. showed their results on 27 patients undergoing robotic surgery, with lower intraoperative bleeding and length of hospital stay when compared with open approach, confirming its safety and feasibility [69].

We can conclude that the robotic approach for iCCC and hCCC is technically challenging and still limited to expert centers, as it can require single or multiple biliodigestive reconstructions, complete regional lymphadenectomy (stations 12, 5, 8, 9, 7, and 16), vascular reconstructions in some cases, and fine dissection of the liver parenchyma.

29.3.4 Benign Lesions

Up to 35% of all LLR and RLR are performed for benign indications [40, 41]. Although fewer literature studies are available, all the papers report excellent results for liver hemangiomas and hepatocellular adenomas, even in young or pregnant patients [70–72]. Similarly, robotic approach could be particularly beneficial for the treatment of hepatolithiasis, as it allows for easier exploration of the proximal biliary system and, when needed, an easier biliodigestive reconstruction than laparoscopy [73, 74]. However, more appropriate studies are needed to confirm it.

29.4 Contraindications

In parallel with a wide spread of MILS, its absolute contraindications have constantly decreased. Actually, difficult positions, tumor size, tumor numbers, and underlying liver disease are not considered contraindications anymore, similarly for patients' age and BMI.

The invasion of major vessels (a main division of the portal vein, hepatic veins confluence, and inferior vena cava), the need for vascular reconstruction, and the resection of main bile ducts generally represent relative contraindications for minimally invasive surgery, waiting for more consistent results from literature; however, this could be easier by the robotic approach [28, 75].

The appropriate management should be decided following a multidisciplinary team discussion, giving each patient tailored indications.

References

1. Reich H, McGlynn F, DeCaprio J, Budin R. Laparoscopic excision of benign liver lesions. Obstet Gynecol. 1991;78(5 Pt 2):956–8.
2. Cassese G, Han HS. Minimally invasive surgery for HCC. Hepatoma Res. 2022;8:24. https://doi.org/10.20517/2394-5079.2022.15.
3. Buell JF, Cherqui D, Geller DA, et al. The international position on laparoscopic liver surgery: the Louisville statement, 2008. Ann Surg. 2009;250(5):825–30. https://doi.org/10.1097/sla.0b013e3181b3b2d8.
4. Wakabayashi G, Cherqui D, Geller DA, et al. Recommendations for laparoscopic liver resection: a report from the second international consensus conference held in Morioka. Ann Surg. 2015;261(4):619–29. https://doi.org/10.1097/SLA.0000000000001184.
5. Abu Hilal M, Aldrighetti L, Dagher I, et al. The Southampton consensus guidelines for laparoscopic liver surgery: from indication to implementation. Ann Surg. 2018;268(1):11–8. https://doi.org/10.1097/SLA.0000000000002524.
6. Giulianotti PC, Coratti A, Angelini M, et al. Robotics in general surgery: personal experience in a large community hospital. Arch Surg Chic Ill 1960. 2003;138(7):777–84. https://doi.org/10.1001/archsurg.138.7.777.
7. Liu R, Wakabayashi G, Kim HJ, et al. International consensus statement on robotic hepatectomy surgery in 2018. World J Gastroenterol. 2019;25(12):1432–44. https://doi.org/10.3748/wjg.v25.i12.1432.
8. Giannone F, Felli E, Cherkaoui Z, Mascagni P, Pessaux P. Augmented reality and image-guided robotic liver surgery. Cancer. 2021;13(24):6268. https://doi.org/10.3390/cancers13246268.
9. Dagher I, Gayet B, Tzanis D, et al. International experience for laparoscopic major liver resection. J Hepato-Biliary-Pancreat Sci. 2014;21(10):732–6. https://doi.org/10.1002/jhbp.140.
10. Broering DC, Elsheikh Y, Alnemary Y, et al. Robotic versus open right lobe donor hepatectomy for adult living donor liver transplantation: a propensity score–matched analysis. Liver Transpl. 2020;26(11):1455–64. https://doi.org/10.1002/lt.25820.
11. Choi GH, Chong JU, Han DH, Choi JS, Lee WJ. Robotic hepatectomy: the Korean experience and perspective. Hepatobiliary Surg Nutr. 2017;6(4):230–8. https://doi.org/10.21037/hbsn.2017.01.14.
12. Lai ECH, Tang CN, Li MKW. Robot-assisted laparoscopic hemi-hepatectomy: technique and surgical outcomes. Int J Surg Lond Engl. 2012;10(1):11–5. https://doi.org/10.1016/j.ijsu.2011.10.005.
13. Lai ECH, Yang GPC, Tang CN. Robot-assisted laparoscopic liver resection for hepatocellular carcinoma: short-term outcome. Am J Surg. 2013;205(6):697–702. https://doi.org/10.1016/j.amjsurg.2012.08.015.
14. Hawksworth J, Radkani P, Nguyen B, et al. Improving safety of robotic major hepatectomy with extrahepatic

inflow control and laparoscopic CUSA parenchymal transection: technical description and initial experience. Surg Endosc. 2022;36(5):3270–6. https://doi.org/10.1007/s00464-021-08639-z.

15. Al-Saeedi M, Ghamarnejad O, Khajeh E, et al. Pringle maneuver in extended liver resection: a propensity score analysis. Sci Rep. 2020;10:8847. https://doi.org/10.1038/s41598-020-64596-y.

16. Montalti R, Scuderi V, Patriti A, Vivarelli M, Troisi RI. Robotic versus laparoscopic resections of posterosuperior segments of the liver: a propensity score-matched comparison. Surg Endosc. 2016;30(3):1004–13. https://doi.org/10.1007/s00464-015-4284-9.

17. Lee SJ, Lee JH, Lee YJ, et al. The feasibility of robotic left-side hepatectomy with comparison of laparoscopic and open approach: consecutive series of single surgeon. Int J Med Robot Comput Assist Surg MRCAS. 2019;15(2):e1982. https://doi.org/10.1002/rcs.1982.

18. Lee JH, Han DH, Jang DS, Choi GH, Choi JS. Robotic extrahepatic Glissonean pedicle approach for anatomic liver resection in the right liver: techniques and perioperative outcomes. Surg Endosc. 2016;30(9):3882–8. https://doi.org/10.1007/s00464-015-4693-9.

19. Couinaud C. Surgical anatomy of the liver revisited. C. Couinaud; 1989.

20. Morimoto M, Tomassini F, Berardi G, et al. Glissonean approach for hepatic inflow control in minimally invasive anatomic liver resection: a systematic review. J Hepato-Biliary-Pancreat Sci. 2022;29(1):51–65. https://doi.org/10.1002/jhbp.908.

21. Nakamura M, Wakabayashi G, Tsuchida A, Nagakawa Y. Study group of precision anatomy for minimally invasive Hepato-biliary-pancreatic surgery (PAM-HBP surgery). Precision anatomy for minimally invasive hepatobiliary pancreatic surgery: PAM-HBP surgery project. J Hepato-Biliary-Pancreat Sci. 2022;29(1):1–3. https://doi.org/10.1002/jhbp.885.

22. Liu JP, Lerut J, Yang Z, Li ZK, Zheng SS. Three-dimensional modeling in complex liver surgery and liver transplantation. Hepatobiliary Pancreat Dis Int. 2022;21(4):318–24. https://doi.org/10.1016/j.hbpd.2022.05.012.

23. Schneider CM, Peng PD, Taylor RH, et al. Robot-assisted laparoscopic ultrasonography for hepatic surgery. Surgery. 2012;151(5):756–62. https://doi.org/10.1016/j.surg.2011.07.040.

24. Zhu P, Liao W, Ding ZY, et al. Intraoperative ultrasonography of robot-assisted laparoscopic hepatectomy: initial experiences from 110 consecutive cases. Surg Endosc. 2018;32(10):4071–7. https://doi.org/10.1007/s00464-017-5854-9.

25. Cassese G, Troisi RI. Indocyanine green applications in hepato-biliary surgery. Minerva Surg. 2021;76(3):199–201. https://doi.org/10.23736/S2724-5691.21.08809-2.

26. Marino MV, Di Saverio S, Podda M, Gomez Ruiz M, Gomez FM. The application of Indocyanine green fluorescence imaging during robotic liver resection: a case-matched study. World J Surg. 2019;43(10):2595–606. https://doi.org/10.1007/s00268-019-05055-2.

27. Guerra F, Amore Bonapasta S, Di Marino M, Coratti F, Annecchiarico M, Coratti A. Surgical revision of benign hepaticojejunostomy stricture using a robotic system (with video). J Visc Surg. 2016;153(5):389–90. https://doi.org/10.1016/j.jviscsurg.2016.05.006.

28. Giulianotti PC, Quadri P, Durgam S, Bianco FM. Reconstruction/repair of iatrogenic biliary injuries: is the robot offering a new option? Short clinical report. Ann Surg. 2018;267(1):e7–9. https://doi.org/10.1097/SLA.0000000000002343.

29. Almamar A, Alkhamesi NA, Davies WT, Schlachta CM. Cost analysis of robot-assisted choledochotomy and common bile duct exploration as an option for complex choledocholithiasis. Surg Endosc. 2018;32(3):1223–7. https://doi.org/10.1007/s00464-017-5795-3.

30. Chen KH, Huang CC, Siow TF, et al. Totally laparoscopic living donor right hepatectomy in a donor with trifurcation of bile duct. Asian J Surg. 2016;39(1):51–5. https://doi.org/10.1016/j.asjsur.2015.01.012.

31. Dokmak S, Chérif R, Duquesne I, et al. Laparoscopic Pancreaticoduodenectomy with reconstruction of the portal vein with the parietal peritoneum. Ann Surg Oncol. 2016;23(8):2664. https://doi.org/10.1245/s10434-016-5207-2.

32. Wang J, Jin Z, Xu B, et al. First robotic hepatectomy with middle hepatic vein reconstruction using ePTFE graft for hepatic adenoma: a case report. Front Surg. 2022;9:904253. https://doi.org/10.3389/fsurg.2022.904253.

33. Luijendijk RW, Jeekel J, Storm RK, et al. The low transverse Pfannenstiel incision and the prevalence of incisional hernia and nerve entrapment. Ann Surg. 1997;225(4):365–9. https://doi.org/10.1097/00000658-199704000-00004.

34. Troisi RI, Montalti R, Van Limmen JGM, et al. Risk factors and management of conversions to an open approach in laparoscopic liver resection: analysis of 265 consecutive cases. HPB. 2014;16(1):75–82. https://doi.org/10.1111/hpb.12077.

35. Khan S, Beard RE, Kingham PT, et al. Long-term oncologic outcomes following robotic liver resections for primary hepatobiliary malignancies: a multicenter study. Ann Surg Oncol. 2018;25(9):2652–60. https://doi.org/10.1245/s10434-018-6629-9.

36. Becker F, Morgül H, Katou S, et al. Robotic liver surgery - current standards and future perspectives. Z Gastroenterol. 2021;59(1):56–62. https://doi.org/10.1055/a-1329-3067.

37. Vigano L, Laurent A, Tayar C, Tomatis M, Ponti A, Cherqui D. The learning curve in laparoscopic liver resection: improved feasibility and reproducibility. Ann Surg. 2009;250(5):772–82. https://doi.org/10.1097/SLA.0b013e3181bd93b2.

38. Guan R, Chen Y, Yang K, et al. Clinical efficacy of robot-assisted versus laparoscopic liver resection: a meta analysis. Asian J Surg. 2019;42(1):19–31. https://doi.org/10.1016/j.asjsur.2018.05.008.

39. Montalti R, Giglio MC, Troisi R, Han H-S, Goh BK, The International robotic and laparoscopic liver resection study group investigators. Risk factors and outcomes of open conversion during minimally-invasive major hepatectomies and impact of robotic assistance: an international multicentre study on 3880 procedures. Ann Surg Oncol. 30(8):4783–96.

40. Ciria R, Cherqui D, Geller DA, Briceno J, Wakabayashi G. Comparative short-term benefits of laparoscopic liver resection: 9000 cases and climbing. Ann Surg. 2016;263(4):761–77. https://doi.org/10.1097/SLA.0000000000001413.

41. Ciria R, Berardi G, Alconchel F, et al. The impact of robotics in liver surgery: a worldwide systematic review and short-term outcomes meta-analysis on 2,728 cases. J Hepato-Biliary-Pancreat Sci. 2022;29(2):181–97. https://doi.org/10.1002/jhbp.869.

42. Guro H, Cho JY, Han HS, Yoon YS, Choi Y, Periyasamy M. Current status of laparoscopic liver resection for hepatocellular carcinoma. Clin Mol Hepatol. 2016;22(2):212–8. https://doi.org/10.3350/cmh.2016.0026.

43. Cassese G, Han HS, Lee B, Lee HW, Cho JY, Troisi R. Leaping the boundaries in laparoscopic liver surgery for hepatocellular carcinoma. Cancer. 2022;14(8):2012. https://doi.org/10.3390/cancers14082012.

44. El-Serag HB, Rudolph KL. Hepatocellular carcinoma: epidemiology and molecular carcinogenesis. Gastroenterology. 2007;132(7):2557–76. https://doi.org/10.1053/j.gastro.2007.04.061.

45. Cassese G, Han HS, Lee B, Lee HW, Cho JY, Troisi RI. The role of minimally invasive surgery in the treatment of HCC. Hepatoma Res. 2022;8:26. https://doi.org/10.20517/2394-5079.2022.14.

46. Han HS, Shehta A, Ahn S, Yoon YS, Cho JY, Choi Y. Laparoscopic versus open liver resection for hepatocellular carcinoma: case-matched study with propensity score matching. J Hepatol. 2015;63(3):643–50. https://doi.org/10.1016/j.jhep.2015.04.005.

47. Kabir T, Tan ZZ, Syn NL, et al. Laparoscopic versus open resection of hepatocellular carcinoma in patients with cirrhosis: a meta-analysis. Br J Surg. 2021;109(1):21–9. https://doi.org/10.1093/bjs/znab376.

48. Morise Z. Laparoscopic liver resection for the patients with hepatocellular carcinoma and chronic liver disease. Transl Gastroenterol Hepatol. 2018;3:41. https://doi.org/10.21037/tgh.2018.07.01.

49. Troisi RI, Berardi G, Morise Z, et al. Laparoscopic and open liver resection for hepatocellular carcinoma with child-Pugh B cirrhosis: multicentre propensity score-matched study. Br J Surg. 2021;108(2):196–204. https://doi.org/10.1093/bjs/znaa041.

50. Zhu P, Liao W, Ding ZY, et al. Learning curve in robot-assisted laparoscopic liver resection. J Gastrointest Surg Off J Soc Surg Aliment Tract. 2019;23(9):1778–87. https://doi.org/10.1007/s11605-018-3689-x.

51. Fretland ÅA, Dagenborg VJ, Bjørnelv GMW, et al. Laparoscopic versus open resection for colorectal liver metastases: the OSLO-COMET randomized controlled trial. Ann Surg. 2018;267(2):199–207. https://doi.org/10.1097/SLA.0000000000002353.

52. Ratti F, Fiorentini G, Cipriani F, Catena M, Paganelli M, Aldrighetti L. Laparoscopic vs. open surgery for colorectal liver metastases. JAMA Surg. 2018;153(11):1028–35. https://doi.org/10.1001/jamasurg.2018.2107.

53. Alvarez FA, Sanchez Claria R, Oggero S, de Santibañes E. Parenchymal-sparing liver surgery in patients with colorectal carcinoma liver metastases. World J Gastrointest Surg. 2016;8(6):407–23. https://doi.org/10.4240/wjgs.v8.i6.407.

54. Cipriani F, Rawashdeh M, Stanton L, et al. Propensity score-based analysis of outcomes of laparoscopic versus open liver resection for colorectal metastases. Br J Surg. 2016;103(11):1504–12. https://doi.org/10.1002/bjs.10211.

55. Troisi RI, Patriti A, Montalti R, Casciola L. Robot assistance in liver surgery: a real advantage over a fully laparoscopic approach? Results of a comparative bi-institutional analysis. Int J Med Robot Comput Assist Surg MRCAS. 2013;9(2):160–6. https://doi.org/10.1002/rcs.1495.

56. Beard RE, Khan S, Troisi RI, et al. Long-term and oncologic outcomes of robotic versus laparoscopic liver resection for metastatic colorectal cancer: a multicenter, propensity score matching analysis. World J Surg. 2020;44(3):887–95. https://doi.org/10.1007/s00268-019-05270-x.

57. Masetti M, Fallani G, Ratti F, et al. Minimally invasive treatment of colorectal liver metastases: does robotic surgery provide any technical advantages over laparoscopy? A multicenter analysis from the IGoMILS (Italian Group of Minimally Invasive Liver Surgery) registry. Updat Surg. 2022;74(2):535–45. https://doi.org/10.1007/s13304-022-01245-1.

58. Dwyer RH, Scheidt MJ, Marshall JS, Tsoraides SS. Safety and efficacy of synchronous robotic surgery for colorectal cancer with liver metastases. J Robot Surg. 2018;12(4):603–6. https://doi.org/10.1007/s11701-018-0813-6.

59. Brustia R, Laurent A, Goumard C, et al. Laparoscopic versus open liver resection for intrahepatic cholangiocarcinoma: report of an international multicenter cohort study with propensity score matching. Surgery. 2022;171(5):1290–302. https://doi.org/10.1016/j.surg.2021.08.015.

60. Jinhuan Y, Yi W, Yuanwen Z, et al. Laparoscopic versus open surgery for early-stage intrahepatic Cholangiocarcinoma after mastering the learning curve: a multicenter data-based matched study. Front Oncol. 2022;11. https://www.frontiersin.org/articles/10.3389/fonc.2021.742544. Accessed 8 Sep 2022

61. Ratti F, Cipriani F, Ariotti R, et al. Safety and feasibility of laparoscopic liver resection with associated lymphadenectomy for intrahepatic cholangiocarcinoma: a propensity score-based case-matched analysis from a single institution. Surg Endosc. 2016;30(5):1999–2010. https://doi.org/10.1007/s00464-015-4430-4.

62. Cassese G, Han HS, Yoon YS, et al. Preoperative assessment and perioperative Management of Resectable Gallbladder Cancer in the era of precision medicine and novel technologies: state of the art and future perspectives. Diagn Basel Switz. 2022;12(7):1630. https://doi.org/10.3390/diagnostics12071630.

63. Han S, Yoon YS, Han HS, Lee JS. Laparoscopic bile duct resection with lymph node dissection for gallbladder cancer diagnosed after laparoscopic cholecystectomy. Surg Oncol. 2020;35:475. https://doi.org/10.1016/j.suronc.2020.10.006.

64. Kim S, Yoon YS, Han HS, Cho JY, Choi Y. Laparoscopic extended cholecystectomy for T3 gallbladder cancer. Surg Endosc. 2018;32(6):2984–5. https://doi.org/10.1007/s00464-017-5952-8.

65. Yoon YS, Han HS, Agarwal A, et al. Survey results of the expert meeting on laparoscopic surgery for gallbladder cancer and a review of relevant literature. Dig Surg. 2019;36(1):7–12. https://doi.org/10.1159/000486208.

66. Han HS, Yoon YS, Agarwal AK, et al. Laparoscopic surgery for gallbladder cancer: an expert consensus statement. Dig Surg. 2019;36(1):1–6. https://doi.org/10.1159/000486207.

67. Goja S, Singh MK, Chaudhary RJ, Soin AS. Robotic-assisted right hepatectomy via anterior approach for intrahepatic cholangiocarcinoma. Ann Hepato-Biliary-Pancreat Surg. 2017;21(2):80–3. https://doi.org/10.14701/ahbps.2017.21.2.80.

68. Belli A, Patrone R, Albino V, et al. Robotic surgery of gallbladder cancer. Mini-Invasive Surg. 2020;4:77. https://doi.org/10.20517/2574-1225.2020.70.

69. Goel M, Khobragade K, Patkar S, Kanetkar A, Kurunkar S. Robotic surgery for gallbladder cancer: operative technique and early outcomes. J Surg Oncol. 2019;119(7):958–63. https://doi.org/10.1002/jso.25422.

70. Gryspeerdt F, Aerts R. Laparoscopic liver resection for hemorrhagic hepatocellular adenoma in a pregnant patient. Acta Chir Belg. 2018;118(5):322–5. https://doi.org/10.1080/00015458.2017.1379790.

71. Giulianotti PC, Addeo P, Bianco FM. Robotic right hepatectomy for giant hemangioma in a Jehovah's witness. J Hepato-Biliary-Pancreat Sci. 2011;18(1):112–8. https://doi.org/10.1007/s00534-010-0297-x.

72. Pietrabissa A, Giulianotti P, Campatelli A, et al. Management and follow-up of 78 giant haemangiomas of the liver. Br J Surg. 1996;83(7):915–8. https://doi.org/10.1002/bjs.1800830710.

73. Lee KF, Fong AKW, Chong CCN, Cheung SYS, Wong J, Lai PBS. Robotic liver resection for primary Hepatolithiasis: is it beneficial? World J Surg. 2016;40(10):2490–6. https://doi.org/10.1007/s00268-016-3528-8.

74. Shu J, Wang XJ, Li JW, Bie P, Chen J, Zheng SG. Robotic-assisted laparoscopic surgery for complex hepatolithiasis: a propensity score matching analysis. Surg Endosc. 2019;33(8):2539–47. https://doi.org/10.1007/s00464-018-6547-8.

75. Giulianotti PC, Bianco FM, Daskalaki D, Gonzalez-Ciccarelli LF, Kim J, Benedetti E. Robotic liver surgery: technical aspects and review of the literature. Hepatobiliary Surg Nutr. 2016;5(4):311–21. https://doi.org/10.21037/hbsn.2015.10.05.

Laparoscopic Treatment of the Extrahepatic Biliary Duct Disease and Biliodigestive Anastomosis

30

Carlo Bergamini

30.1 Definition

The extrahepatic bile ducts (EHBD) are part of the biliary system (Fig. 30.1). They are tubes that go outside the liver and carry bile from the liver and gallbladder to the small intestine. Such ducts are made up of the peri-hilar region (the area that is closest to the liver and includes the common hepatic duct) and the distal region (the area that is farthest from the liver and includes the common bile duct).

30.2 Etiologic Classification

The etiology of EHBD diseases can be broadly classified as benign or malignant. Since the first ones usually cause obstruction, they are usually defined as benign biliary strictures (BBSs) [1]. Many possible origins have been described, each with a different natural history and each demonstrating a different response to treatment (Table 30.1). They can be divided into lithogenic and non-lithogenic, the first being largely more frequent. Among the latter, iatrogenic causes, such as post-cholecystectomy and orthotopic liver transplantation, are the most common causes of BBSs. Postoperative biliary strictures can be further classified as anastomotic or non-anastomotic. Other causes include inflammatory, autoimmune, or immunoglobulin G4-related cholangiopathy, radiation-induced sclerosing cholangitis, ischemia, and infections.

On the other hand, malignant BSs (MBSs) usually result from local malignancy, most commonly cholangiocarcinoma, pancreatic adenocarcinoma, liver metastases, hepatocellular carcinoma, ampullary carcinoma, or gallbladder adenocarcinoma. Other causes can finally include lymphoma and metastasis to the regional lymph nodes.

30.3 Laparoscopic Treatment of Common Bile Duct Lithiasis

Gallstones are a very common condition among the general population. Generally, this situation does not cause symptoms, but 10–25% of affected people may have specific symptoms, such as biliary pain and acute cholecystitis and 1–2% of these may have major complications. In most cases, symptoms and major complications occur due to the migration of stones into the common bile duct (CBD), and this circumstance can cause obstruction of the bile flow in the small intestine, resulting in pain, jaundice, and sometimes cholangitis. Primary choledocholithiasis refers to stones formed directly within the biliary tree,

C. Bergamini (✉)
Department of Emergency Surgery, University Hospital of Careggi, Florence, Italy

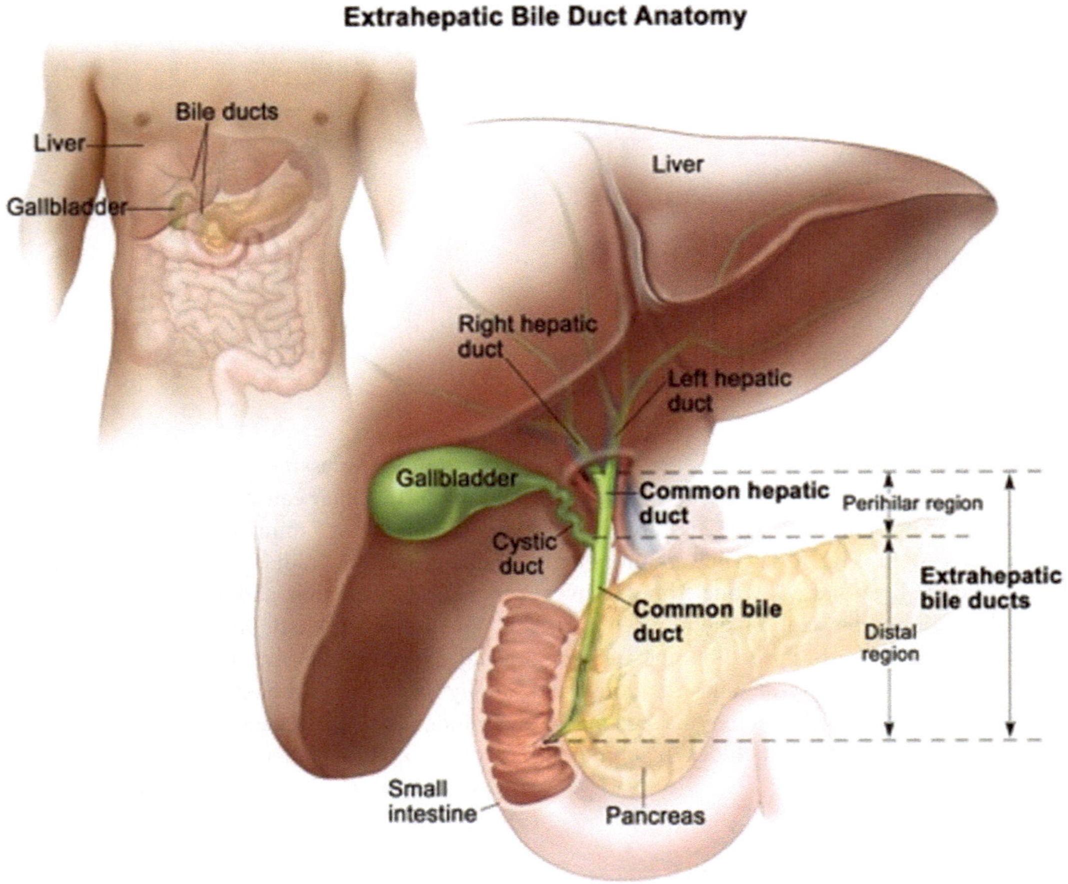

Extrahepatic Bile Duct Anatomy

Fig. 30.1 Extrahepatic bile duct anatomy

Table 30.1 Most common extrahepatic bile duct diseases

Type of Disease	Description
	Benign
Iatrogenic	Postendoscopic sphincterotomy, posthepatobiliary surgery
Inflammatory	Primary and secondary sclerosing cholangitis, acute or chronic pancreatitis
Ischemic	Hepatic artery stenosis or thrombosis
Infectious	Recurrent pyogenic cholangitis, human immunodeficiency virus cholangiopathy, tuberculosis, sarcoidosis, parasitic, choledocholithiasis
Autoimmune	Immunoglobulin G4 cholangitis
Miscellaneous	Portal biliopathy, trauma, papillary stenosis
	Malignant
Cholangiocarcinoma	Involving intra- and extrahepatic bile ducts
Carcinoma in the head of the pancreas, ampullary or duodenal malignancies	Distal common bile duct stricture
Carcinoma in the gallbladder	Invading the biliary ducts
Lymphoma and metastatic lymphadenopathy	Compressing biliary ducts
Intrahepatic metastases	Invading or compressing biliary ducts

while secondary choledocholithiasis refers to stones migrated from the gallbladder. Of the total of cholecystectomies performed every year for cholelithiasis, the presence of CBD stones (CBDSs) is 5–15%; another small percentage of these will develop CBDS after intervention.

The management of CBDSs represents an important clinical problem. In symptomatic patients, the primary goal is to obtain complete clearance of the CBD and cholecystectomy; on the contrary, in asymptomatic patients, there is still no shared diagnostic and therapeutic path. In the last 20 years, the development of new technologies has allowed new diagnostic and therapeutic scenarios, with a consequent critical evaluation of management options. All these have led to a more cautious and patient-tailored preoperative workup based on the patient's risk and ultimately to a multidisciplinary approach. However, if on the one hand multidisciplinarity has improved the management of patients with symptomatic cholelithiasis, on the other hand it has shown non-unanimous consent in the choice of treatment for choledocholithiasis: endoscopic or surgical?

To date, many therapeutic options are available, including laparoscopic, endoscopic, percutaneous, and traditional open techniques, applied both as a combination in a simultaneous way or as a gradual sequence. The most followed therapeutic options are preoperative endoscopic retrograde cholecystopancreatectomy (ERCP) followed by laparoscopic cholecystectomy (LC); LC plus intraoperative laparoscopic CBD exploration (LCBDE); LC plus intraoperative ERCP (*rendez-vous* technique); and, finally, LC plus postoperative ERCP. The preference between one technique and the other is, most of the time, guided by the presence of professional resources and local skills rather than by its verified effectiveness.

30.3.1 Two-Round Approach [2]

Preoperative ERCP followed by LC is the most frequently used treatment worldwide. Various studies have shown that this two-session approach is safe and effective. Its limits are represented by a percentage between 40% and 70% of negative

results that expose patients to unnecessary and risky endoscopic maneuvers. The development of diagnostic techniques such as magnetic resonance cholangiography (MRC) and endoscopic ultrasonography (EUS) has increased the anatomical visualization of the biliary tract and has shown a high sensitivity and specificity for preoperative diagnosis of CBDS. However, preoperative ERCP followed by LC often requires two rounds of anesthesia and two hospitalizations, and in the time between the two procedures, some patients may escape LC, being satisfied by the results of the preoperative ERCP. Therefore, for this treatment modality, it is a good rule not to delay the LC too much and to avoid the occurrence of recurrent events.

Another option is LC followed later by postoperative ERCP. This technique is rarely performed as the first choice for the treatment of cholelithiasis with choledocholithiasis because in a low percentage of cases it fails the intended purpose. The failure may be due to the operator's lack of experience, the absence of a guide wire, and a site altered by the previous surgery for inflammatory phenomena. The postoperative ERCP retains a role when the intraoperative laparoscopic exploration fails or during an LC, the presence of CBDS is found with the impossibility of performing it intraoperatively.

30.3.2 One Round Approach [3]

One-session procedures have confirmed benefits, both in suspected cases and in proven cases of CBDS. These procedures are believed to be efficient, safe, convenient, and well-accepted by patients, as the two different pathological conditions are resolved in a single surgery with single anesthesia. Regarding laparoscopic exploration of the CBD (Fig. 30.2), some authors have described stone removal rates ranging from 94% to 98%, low morbidity, and a mortality rate of 0%. Through laparoscopic exploration, negative events that can occur during endoscopic sphincterotomy, such as pancreatitis, perforation, bleeding, cholangitis, and malignancies of the CBD, are avoided.

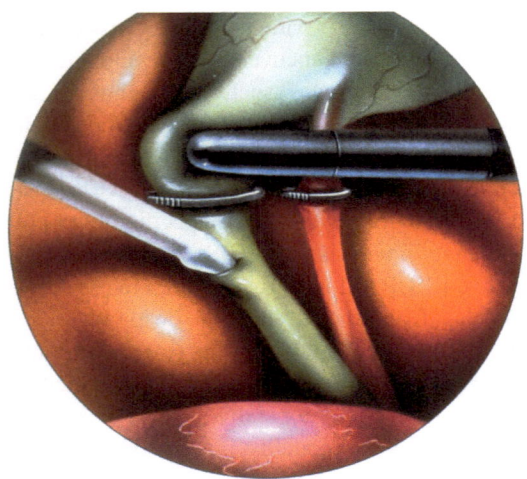

Fig. 30.2 Laparoscopic exploration of CBD

However, this technique has some drawbacks. First, the procedure requires high-level skills in laparoscopic surgery with long learning curves and there is a need for dedicated instruments; it is understandable that these qualities may not be present in all treatment centers. Many surgeons prefer the trans-cystic approach, which is considered less invasive and less complicated; however, choledochotomy is recommended in cases of dilated CBD, large diameter, or multiple stones, impacted stones, and stones with intrahepatic localization. The trans-cystic exploration route is often more challenging due to a small diameter and tortuous and low-base implant duct.

During laparoscopic exploration, stone removal can be guided fluoroscopically or by choledochoscopy. The use of a flexible choledochoscope is the most preferred because it increases precision and is under direct visual control. The choledochoscope also presents some criticalities; first, it is a fragile instrument that can break during the procedure, thereafter needing a double monitor for laparoscopic and choledochoscopic viewing and causing an increase in costs. Fluoroscopic guidance exposes the patient to radiation, increases the length of the procedure, and requires instrumentation that can hinder the operator's movements.

After the choledochotomy, the closure of the CBD can be performed directly or with the positioning of the T-tube endoprosthesis. The T-tube provides easy percutaneous access for cholangiography and extraction of preserved stones. However, the T-tube can accidentally detach, promoting CBD obstruction, bile loss, persistent biliary fistulas and skin abrasions, cholangitis from exogenous sources through the T-tube, and dehydration and salt depletion. The T-tube also requires long and continuous management, limiting the patient's quality of life. Some authors have concluded that primary closure is preferred over T-tube placement, as the latter increases operative time and hospital stay. The most common complications of this technique are CBD tearing, leakage of bile, stitched T-tubes, and the formation of strictures.

Another single-session minimally invasive procedure for the treatment of cholecystocholedocholithiasis is ERCP during the LC, also called the *rendezvous* technique. This approach was found by many experts to be safe and effective and to require single hospitalization and single anesthesia. For the exploration and extraction of the stones, the CBD is not opened, postoperative ERCP is avoided, and in case of extraction failure, surgical exploration is carried out during the same operation, with cost reduction. Despite these benefits, the procedure is not widespread, probably because operative endoscopy is not present in all treatment centers, and often when this exists, there is no expert operator.

The appropriate management of patients with CBD stones should be determined according to the condition of the patient, expertise of operators, and local resources. With advancing technology and minimally invasive surgery, laparoscopic CBD exploration has the potential to become more efficient and cost-effective.

30.4 Laparoscopic Treatment of Other Benign Causes of Common Bile Duct Disease

30.4.1 Iatrogenic Lesions [4]

We will be treating the other most common cause of benign CBD disease that is represented by iatrogenic lesions. To systemize the various possible anatomic configuration and, consequently, to establish the best treatment, many classifications have been described. However, the most followed is the Strasberg classification (Table 30.2) that was originally described for the CBD injured laparoscopic injuries of the biliary ducts.

Intraoperatively during any cholecystectomy, active effort should be made to avoid a CBD injury. The "critical view of safety" should be established before clips are deployed in the Calot triangle (Fig. 30.3). Failure to identify the anat-

Table 30.2 Strasberg classification of CBD iatrogenic injury

Type	Description
A	Leak from the cystic duet or a small duct in the liver bed
B	Occlusion of an aberrant right hepatic duct
C	Transection of an aberrant right hepatic duct without ligation
D	Lateral injury to a major bile duct
E1	Distal CHD stricture with a CHD stump ≥ 2 cm long
E2	Proximal CHD stricture with a CHD stump < 2 cm long
E3	Hilar stricture with no CHD stump but with preservation of the hilar confluence
E4	Hilar stricture with loss of communication between the right and left hepatic ducts
E5	Aberrant right hepatic duct stricture with or without concomitant CHD stricture

omy or achieve the critical view may be an indication for conversion to open surgery; however, subtotal cholecystectomy with removal of all stones from the gallbladder is another method for definitively managing gallbladder inflammation and preventing an injury. The presence of a short cystic duct can be particularly challenging.

If a CBD injury is suspected intraoperatively, intraoperative cholangiography should be used to confirm the diagnosis. In cases of limited injury, we advocate leaving a drain in place with a view to treating the injury conservatively with a biliary stent. In all other cases, definitive repair is achieved with hepaticojejunostomy or hepaticoduodenostomy, discussed below. The hepatic arteries should be carefully visualized to ensure that there is no vasculo-biliary injury in every case.

When a patient presents in the postoperative period with evidence of bile leak or peritonitis, laparoscopy can be a useful diagnostic and therapeutic tool. The first step at relaparoscopy is to perform an extensive washout of the abdominal cavity to help control and treat the sepsis and to allow for identification of the source of the bile leak. Although the most likely source is somewhere in the biliary tree, the small bowel and, in particular, the duodenum should be inspected to rule out inadvertent injury there, which could give rise to a similar presentation.

Fig. 30.3 "Critical view of safety" during laparoscopic cholecystectomy

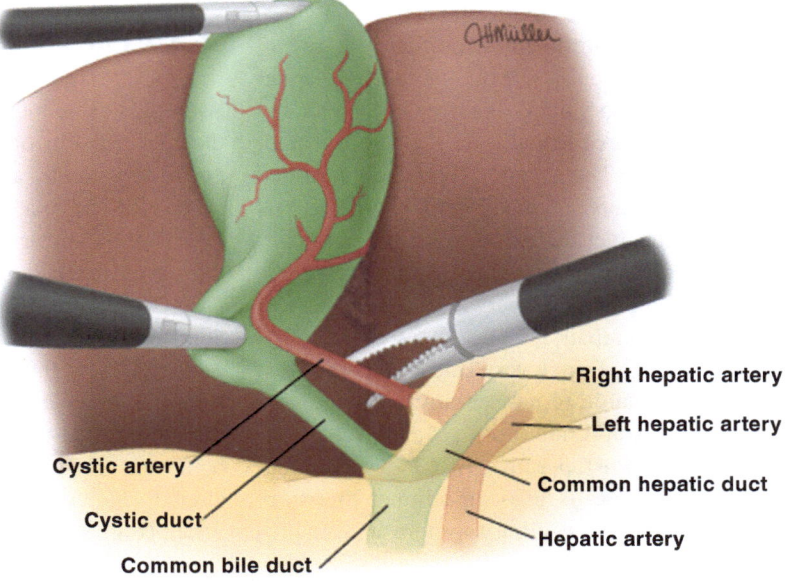

Right hepatic artery

Left hepatic artery

Common hepatic duct

Cystic artery

Hepatic artery

Cystic duct

Common bile duct

In situations where bile is leaking from a small defect in the cystic duct, common hepatic duct, or CBD, laparoscopic peritoneal lavage is often the only surgical intervention needed to control the spillage and prevent severe sepsis. Endoscopic retrograde cholangiopancreatography and sphincterotomy, with or without biliary stenting, can help to ensure low pressure in the biliary tract, which will allow the defect to seal itself with time. There are several reports of leaks from small ducts in the gallbladder bed, the duct of Luschka, or small accessory hepatic ducts being successfully controlled with laparoscopic suturing.

An option during this procedure is to place a drain, which can help to control or prevent the progression of sepsis. This method can be used to treat the injury conservatively or to stabilize the patient while definitive repair is planned.

At this point of the procedure, the surgeon must make a judgment call on whether to proceed with immediate repair or to delay repair of the injury, depending on the location and extent of injury, the patient's overall stability, and local expertise.

Bilio-enteric anastomosis in the form of hepaticojejunostomy or hepaticoduodenostomy is the definitive treatment for a severe CBD injury and has shown good long-term results (see next paragraph).

In the index operation, if a bile leak is found intraoperatively, the source should first be elucidated through careful inspection and the use of suction and irrigation to examine the gallbladder fossa for accessory ducts, the liver surface for any tears, and the extrahepatic biliary tree for inadvertent injury. The diagnosis can be confirmed with intraoperative cholangiography. The arterial supply to the duct should be examined; an injury there often requires open reconstruction if there has been minimal delay between identification of the injury and repair.

If the leak is from a very small CBD lesion, it may be amenable to conservative management with a Jackson–Pratt drain to achieve a controlled leak. Postoperative ERCP with sphincterotomy can be used as an adjunct to ensure low pressure in the biliary system and to pro-

mote healing. In selected cases of an aberrant or liver bed bile duct leak where the duct orifice is very small ($\leq$ 2–3 mm) and cholangiography shows it to be draining only a small section of the liver, that duct orifice may be simply ligated. The criteria for laparoscopic repair are the same as those used for open repair. If the injury is fresh ($\leq$ 72 h), an early repair with laparoscopic bilio-enteric anastomosis is preferable. If the duct is small (< 3 mm), if anatomy or injury complexity precludes straightforward repair, or if port positioning is awkward for laparoscopic repair, an open approach is demanding. Any free bile should be suctioned and the abdomen irrigated to control sepsis. A surgical drain is routinely left.

In situations where the operating surgeon does not feel comfortable performing the repair, the CBD can be stented or cannulated and an abdominal drain placed to stabilize the patient and control sepsis while they are transferred to a tertiary care center for delayed repair. In this setting, laparoscopic repair is feasible if inflammation in the porta hepatis is not too extensive.

If there is a healthy duct with good arterial blood supply, an end-to-side bilio-enteric anastomosis is performed. If there is any concern regarding the blood supply, a side-to-side repair incorporating the anterior wall of the bile duct near the biliary bifurcation is favored.

30.4.2 Choledochal Cyst [5]

Although choledochal cysts are a rare disease, they occur more commonly in young women and pediatric patients, and the advantage of the cosmetic effect in laparoscopic surgery is maximized in these patient groups. Several centers have attempted laparoscopic excision of choledochal cysts and have reported surgical outcomes in adult patients. Therefore, most studies have recommended the feasibility and safety of the laparoscopic procedure for choledochal cysts and have suggested that laparoscopic surgery would be advantageous and the treatment of choice for choledochal cysts, replacing open surgery in the future (Fig. 30.4).

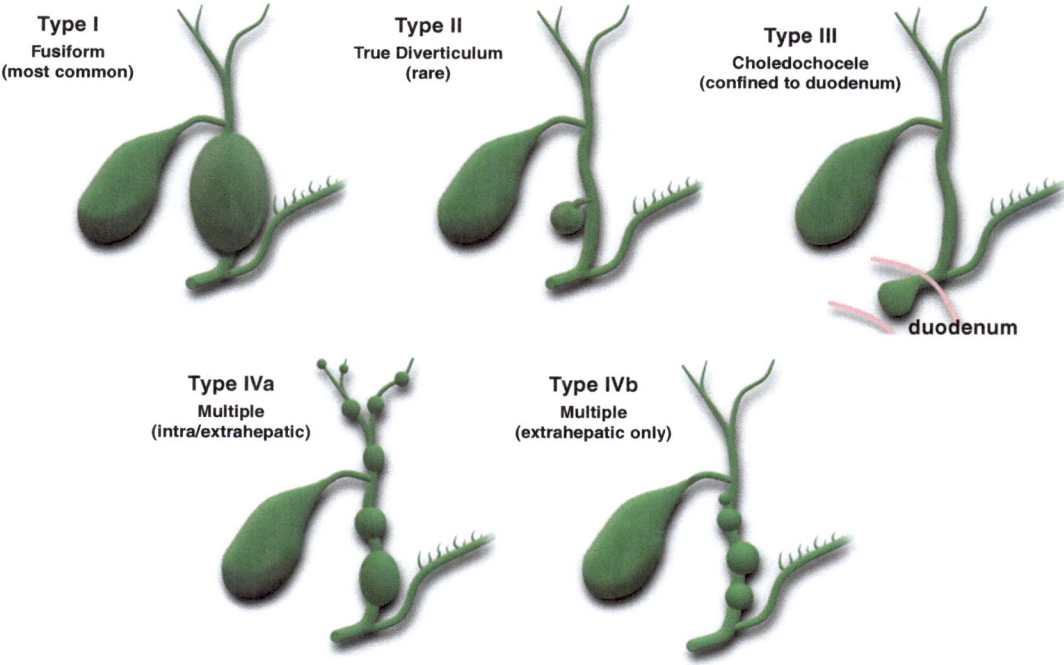

Fig. 30.4 Different anatomical variants of choledochal cysts

Several difficulties are associated with hepaticojejunostomy and jejunojejunostomy, which are time-consuming procedures. A particular advantage of robotic surgery is that hepaticojejunostomy anastomosis is far easier and more precise with robotic techniques than with conventional laparoscopic techniques. Choledochal cysts can be dissected easily, precisely, and safely using a three-dimensional operative field, and the surgeon could reproduce the same procedures of hepaticojejunostomy as are performed in open surgery. However, despite the advantages of robotic surgery including a three-dimensional view, tremor filtering, and an ergonomically designed console, the disadvantages include a prolonged operative time, high cost, and need for specially trained tableside assistants. In the future, most of the problems will be solved by accumulation of surgical experiences and the development of robotic technology including more convenient and cheaper instruments.

30.5 Laparoscopic Treatment of Malignant Causes of Common Bile Duct Disease

Obstruction of the extrahepatic bile ducts from a malignant process presents both a diagnostic and therapeutic challenge [6]. It is a common problem, with as many as 70% of pancreatic cancer patients presenting with obstruction upon diagnosis. Obstruction may serve as the initial sign of disease—such as in the classic presentation of painless jaundice in pancreatic ductal adenocarcinoma—or may occur during the progression of malignancy once the diagnosis is established.

The two most common malignant neoplasms known to occlude the bile ducts are pancreatic ductal adenocarcinoma and primary bile duct cancer (cholangiocarcinoma). Other causes of malignant biliary obstruction can include ampullary carcinoma, primary duodenal adenocarcinoma, pancreatic neuroendocrine tumors, or occlusion of the hepatic hilum due to lymphadenopathy at the porta hepatis (as seen in metastatic colon cancer or lymphoma). Of note, some premalignant lesions such as biliary papillomatosis may cause an obstructive picture like malignancy. Benign conditions such as autoimmune cholangiopathy must also be ruled out, so obtaining tissue via endoscopic retrograde cholangiography (ERCP) with brush biopsy or core biopsy or endoscopic ultrasound with fine-needle aspiration (FNA) is paramount.

Only once a firm diagnosis of malignancy is secured can the final choice of treatment be made. Occlusion of the bile ducts may cause debilitating symptoms such as pruritus and malaise, and thus treatment is often recommended on that basis alone. This may come in the form of surgical resection if the patient presents with resectable disease. However, both pancreatic cancer and cholangiocarcinoma are notorious for presenting at an advanced stage in which immediate surgery is contraindicated.

Treatment goals for these patients include downstaging of the tumor with chemoradiotherapy or strictly palliative measures. Relief of biliary obstruction is recommended in either setting. Treatment of distal malignant biliary obstruction from pancreatic cancer is typically managed by an endoscopically placed single biliary prosthesis, whereas hilar strictures can be more challenging to manage due to the need to access the left and right systems of the biliary tree. Malignant obstruction of the extrahepatic bile ducts at the liver hilum can be much more difficult to treat, given the possible involvement of the left and right hepatic ducts and the need to decompress the left and right lobes individually.

The decision whether to decompress obstructed bile ducts in a patient with resectable disease has traditionally been quite controversial. Jaundice has long been recognized as an important preoperative risk factor in the setting of malignancy. Several mechanisms have been described through which jaundice exerts its negative effects.

Complete resection is the only curative treatment for cholangiocarcinoma. Unfortunately,

most patients will present with obstructive symptoms or frank jaundice later in the disease course. Resection modalities vary depending on the location of the malignancy: Intrahepatic tumors are treated with hepatic resection while extrahepatic tumors can be classified as hilar cholangiocarcinoma (Klatskin tumor) or distal cholangiocarcinoma. The level of the cystic duct demarcates hilar vs distal tumors. Hilar cholangiocarcinoma may still require partial hepatic resection as part of definitive management.

Drainage is recommended in special situations such as cholangitis and patients with symptomatic jaundice (e.g., pruritus) or renal failure. In the absence of these factors, preoperative drainage has been previously discouraged on the basis that it confers no mortality benefit but may surgical treatment modalities.

30.5.1 Surgical Treatment

While most biliary cancer patients present when the disease is unresectable, the treatment of choice for early biliary cancers is surgical resection, even though the risk of recurrence is high. Localized diseases are generally considered resectable, whereas locally advanced or distant metastatic diseases are beyond the scope of surgery, and resection of nodal metastatic disease is still controversial. Patients with biliary cancer should be offered surgical resection as the only treatment associated with long-term survival and potential cure since there has been little progress in the development of locoregional treatments. Surgical treatment, including hemihepatectomy or extended hepatectomy, extrahepatic bile duct resection, and regional lymphadenectomy, has been performed due to a better understanding of tumor pathology. In addition, distal cholangiocarcinomas of the distal bile duct are treated with pancreaticoduodenectomy.

The surgical approaches, from completely open to laparoscopic or robotic approaches, demonstrated some changing trends. There was a noticeable increase in the minimally invasive approach in biliary cancer procedures. However, the rate of increase varied between the laparoscopic and the robotic-assisted approaches. The robotic approach increased fivefold from 2010 to 2016. The absolute number is still small compared to the number of total procedures; however, if it continues at the same rate and direction, the trajectory of increase will be noticeable. Robotic surgery as a minimally invasive approach has been gaining increasing favor due to its many advantages. Its range of applications in various procedures has been quickly expanding, as it has the potential to overcome some of the limits of laparoscopy. Even though the number of procedures performed laparoscopically was more than those performed robotically over the years, the laparoscopic approach did not show the same rate of increase. However, given the complexity of biliary procedures, the advanced disease stage at diagnosis, and the rarity of the disease, the prevalence of the minimally invasive approach in biliary cancer may not progress as in other abdominal or GI procedures.

30.6 Laparoscopic Techniques for Extrahepatic Duct Diseases and Biliodigestive Anastomosis

30.6.1 Positions of Patients, Surgeons, and Trocars

Patients are placed in the supine position or in the reverse Trendelenburg position, or they are tilted slightly to the left. Two monitors are placed on either side of the patient's head. General anesthesia is administered, and endotracheal intubation performed. A 10-mm incision is made at the right margin of the umbilicus to place a 10-mm trocar. A pneumoperitoneum is then constructed, and the laparoscope is placed through this trocar. Under the laparoscope, four more trocars are placed below the xiphoid process (12 mm) at the right subcostal margin (5 mm), at the right lumbar (10 mm), and at the left lumbar (5 mm), respectively, to place the surgical instruments. Monitors were placed on each side of the patient's head (Fig. 30.5).

30.6.2 Laparoscopic Treatment of the Common Bile Duct (CBD) According to Type of Biliary Tract Disease

First, we deal with the biliary tract disease. At the same time, we prepare the end of the residual bile duct. During this procedure, the laparoscope is put through the paraumbilical trocar. The assistant holding the laparoscope stays on the left side of the patient and watches the right monitor and the surgeon. The surgeon operates on the hepatic portal area through the right subcostal and subxiphoid trocar. The other assistant stays on the right side and operates the intestinal clamp through the right lumbar trocar.

1. For *recurrent bile duct stones*, the CBD is incised longitudinally, and all intrahepatic and extrahepatic bile duct stones are removed with a choledochoscope. The CBD is transected 2 cm distally to the bifurcation of the left and right hepatic ducts. To enlarge the diameter of the anastomosis, the CBD should be cut obliquely or longitudinally (Fig. 30.2).
2. For *congenital cystic dilatation* of the CBD, the hepatoduodenal ligament is incised longitudinally before isolating the dilated CBD (Fig. 30.6). Bleeding tends to occur near the pylorus, and electric coagulation, ultrasonographic scalpel, or the responsible vascular suture is used to stop it. Then the left and posterior wall of the CBD is isolated from the left side wall. Careful attention should be given to protecting the portal vein. Then the dilated CBD is transected from the level of maximum diameter, and the choledochoscope is inserted to confirm that no stones remained. The distal end of the CBD above the superior margin of the pancreas is closed with a double-loop ligation, and the extra CBD is resected. The proximal CBD end is trimmed, and at least 1.5 cm of CBD is left for cholangiojejunostomy. Resected lesions are removed through the subxiphoid port.
3. *For injury of the CBD*, the hepatic portal area is explored and the proximal end of the bile duct that is injured is confirmed. The CBD is trimmed obliquely, and the anterior wall is

Fig. 30.5 General and
monitor disposition

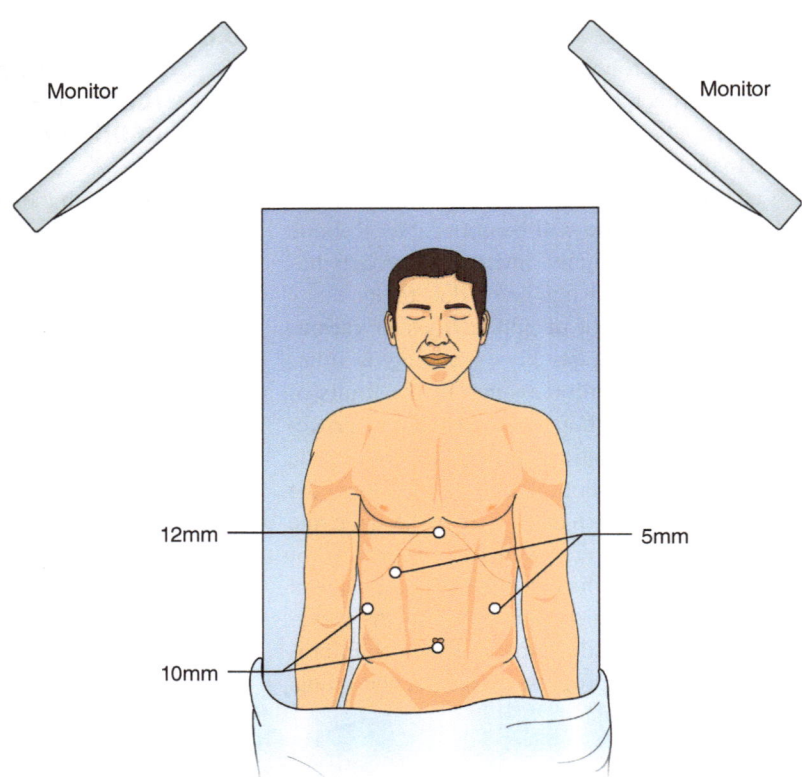

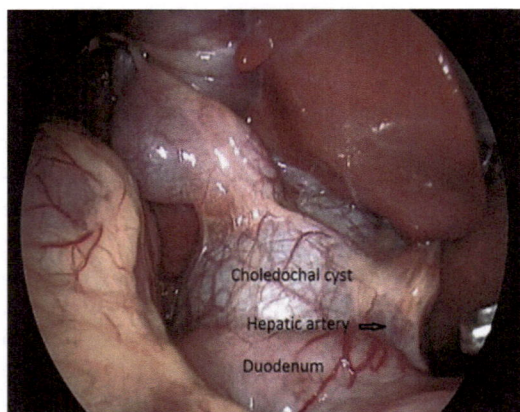

Fig. 30.6 Role of laparoscopic surgery in the treatment
of choledochal cyst

incised to enlarge the anastomotic diameter. If
the injured position of the bile duct is at a
higher level, 0.3 to 0.5 cm of the anterior wall
of each hepatic duct is longitudinally incised
to enlarge the diameter of the anastomosis.

4. For *upper cholangiocarcinoma*, the hepatoduodenal ligament, as well as internal fibro-
   fatty tissue and lymph nodes, is resected using
   the ultrasonographic scalpel. After isolating
   the duodenal segment of the CBD, two Hem-
   o-lok clips are placed on the unaffected bile
   duct distal to the tumor. The bile duct is transected between two Hem-o-lok clips. The surgeon then lifts the proximal bile duct with his
   left hand and dissects it with the ultrasonographic scalpel in his right hand. The common
   hepatic duct or the left and right hepatic ducts
   are cut, and resected tumor tissue is taken out
   through the subxiphoid port. The caudate lobe
   of the liver is resected. Bipolar electrocoagulation is used to stop bleeding on the liver
   surface.

If the transaction is around the bifurcation of
the left and right hepatic ducts or a higher level,
"basin-like bile duct plasty" is needed to enlarge
the diameter of the hepatic bile duct to facilitate

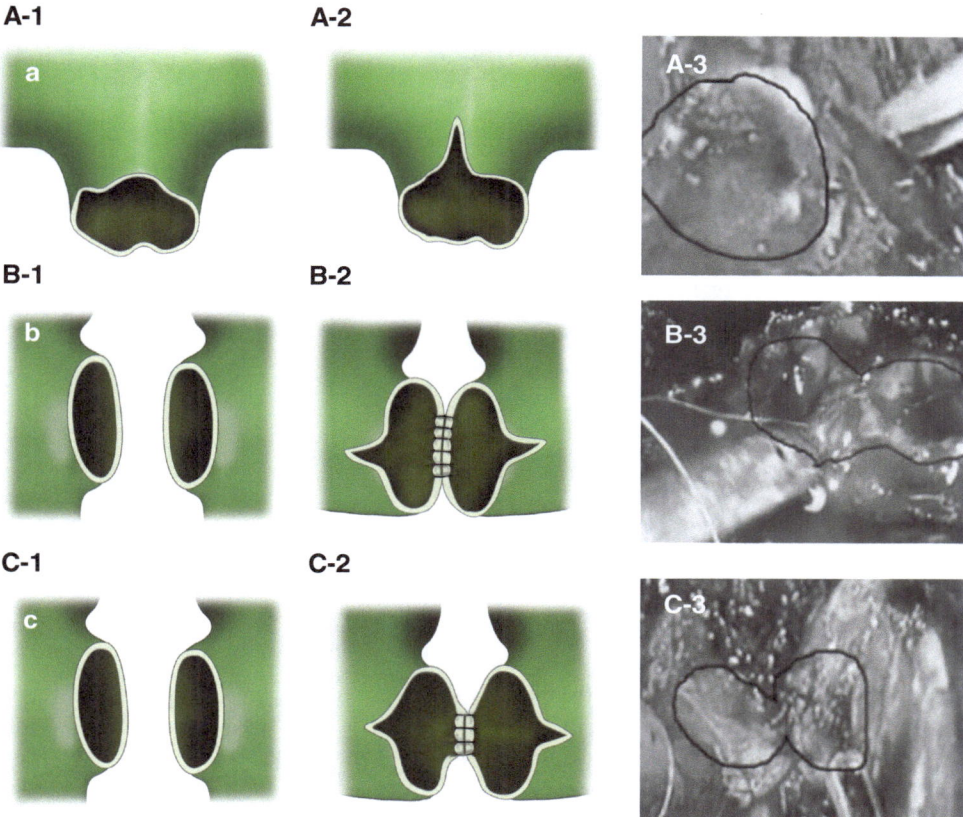

Fig. 30.7 Basin-like bile duct angioplasty. a), b), and c) correspond to the three possible ways to perform a bile duct plasty (see text)

the hepaticocholangiojejunostomy (Fig. 30.7). There are three ways to perform basin-like bile duct plasty. (A) For residual bile duct distal to the confluence of the hepatic duct, a 3-mm incision is made in the side wall of the bile duct to enlarge the diameter of the anastomosis. (B) If the residual ducts are closely located left and right hepatic ducts, the inside wall of each hepatic duct was cut, respectively. Then 5–0 absorbable sutures are used to suture the upper and lower margins of the incision. Finally, each outside wall of the bile duct is cut properly to form a basin shape. (C) If the left and right hepatic ducts are far apart and difficult to bring close together, the hepatic tissue between the ducts is resected. We then sutured the inside wall of each hepatic duct.

30.6.3 Totally Laparoscopic Roux-En-Y Jejunojejunostomy

The laparoscope is inserted into the right lumbar trocar for JJS. The assistant holding the laparoscope is on the right side of the patient. The surgeon stays on the left side of the patient and operates via the subcostal trocar with his left hand and the trans-umbilical trocar with his right hand. The first assistant is at the left side of the patient using the left trocar to lift the greater omentum and the transverse colon with the intestinal clamp. The Treitz ligament and the upper jejunum are then exposed. The mesentery of the jejunum is isolated and cut along the line of the mesenteric artery 15 to

Fig. 30.8 Totally
laparoscopic Roux-en-Y
jejunojejunostomy

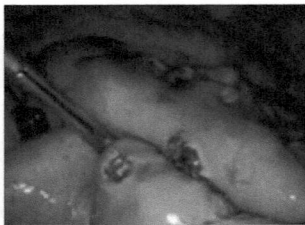

Before JJS

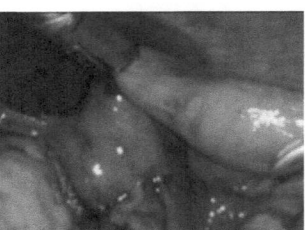

Performing JJS

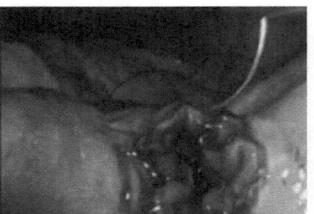

Suture the incisions used to put Endo-GIA

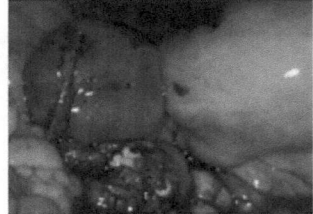

After JJS

20 cm distal to the Treitz ligament. Then the jejunum is transected with Endo-GIA. A hiatus 45 cm away from the end of the distal limb (the biliary limb) and another hiatus 5 cm away from the end of the proximal limb (jejunum limb) at the antimesenteric border were made. With a subxiphoid trocar, the Endo-GIA is put through the two hiatuses and is fired to complete the jejunojejunal anastomosis. The stapler is then taken out, and the residual incision is sutured using a double-layer suture (Fig. 30.8).

References

1. Kapoor BS, Mauri G, Lorenz JM. Management of Biliary Strictures: state-of-the-art review. Radiology. 2018;289(3):590–603. https://doi.org/10.1148/radiol.2018172424.

2. Zepeda-Gómez S, Baron TH. Benign biliary strictures: current endoscopic management. Nat Rev Gastroenterol Hepatol. 2011;8(10):573–81.

3. Cianci P, Restini E. Management of cholelithiasis with choledocholithiasis: endoscopic and surgical approaches. World J Gastroenterol. 2021;27(28):4536–54.

4. Strasberg SM, Hertl M, Soper NJ. An analysis of the problem of biliary injury during laparoscopic cholecystectomy. J Am Coll Surg. 1995;180(1):101–25.

5. El Mouhadi S, Arrivé L. Choledochal cyst. Gastroenterol Clin Biol. 2010;34(6-7):347.

6. Tuma F, Abbaszadeh-Kasbi A, Munene G, Shebrain S, Durchholz WC. Trends of the extra-hepatic biliary cancer and its surgical management: a cross-sectional study from the national cancer database. Cureus. 2022;14(8):e27584.

G. Ceccarelli, F. Rondelli, A. Palazzini, A. Santarelli, M. Silvestrini, S. Capezzali, M. I. Ceccarelli, and M. De Rosa

31.1 Introduction

Bile duct exploration is the surgical procedure to remove gallstones blocked in the common bile duct (CBD) (Fig. 31.1). This condition, defined as choledocholithiasis, may be characterized by jaundice or infections (cholangitis) and usually requires emergency surgery. Surgical exploration of CBD is rarely indicated, as endoscopic retrograde cholangiopancreatography (ERCP) with endoscopic sphincterotomy is generally the first choice, but in some circumstances it is not possible or contraindicated.

The procedure may be associated with gallbladder removal and is performed under general anesthesia.

CBD resection and the consequent hepaticojejunostomy are two technical steps common to surgical operations for different diseases such as biliary, pancreatic, or ampullary cancer, biliary duct injuries, benign biliary disease (choledochal cyst, choledocholithiasis, etc.), and other biliopancreatic diseases [1–4].

A Roux-en-Y hepaticojejunostomy is generally performed to establish biliary-enteric continuity after resection.

The non-dilated proximal biliary duct, with an orifice diameter of 5–6 mm, represents a technically challenging aspect of this surgery. In selected cases, in order to achieve a sufficient bile duct caliber, the left hepatic duct is opened keeping the posterior wall of the bifurcation, according to the "Hepp-Couinaud technique" [5, 6].

G. Ceccarelli (✉) · A. Palazzini · A. Santarelli · M. Silvestrini · S. Capezzali · M. I. Ceccarelli
General and Robotic Surgery Unit, "San Giovanni Battista" Hospital, Foligno (PG), Italy

San Matteo" Hospital, Spoleto (PG), Italy
e-mail: graziano.ceccarelli@uslumbria2.it; annalisa.sanatrelli@uslumbria2.it; marco.silvestrini@uslumbria2.it; Stefano.capezzali@uslumbria2.it

F. Rondelli
Department of General Surgery, University of Perugia, "Santa Maria" Hospital, Terni, Italy

M. De Rosa
General and Robotic Surgery Unit, "San Giovanni Battista" Hospital, Foligno (PG), Italy
e-mail: michele.derosa@uslumbria2.it

Fig. 31.1 (**a**) Anatomy of liver pedicle. (**b–d**) Most frequent bile duct diseases requiring hepaticojejunostomy, (**b**) bile duct stones, (**c**) bile duct tumors, and (**d**) iatrogenic injury of bile duct

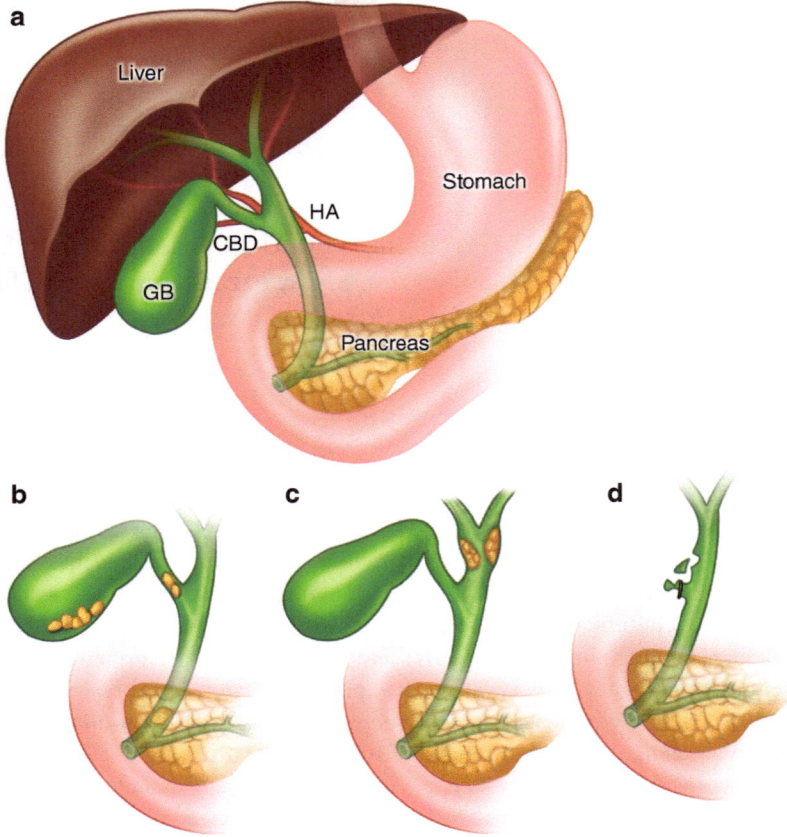

31.2 Operating Theater Setup

The operating theater (possibly a shielded room) for robotic CBD exploration or hepaticojejunostomy is set as follows (Fig. 31.2):

- Operating table in the center of the theater.
- Vision cart to the right of the patient, at the level of the right patient flank.
- Patient cart to the patient's head (according to Si or Xi device).
- Surgeon at the surgical console.
- First assistant at the operating table between the patient's legs.
- Instrument nurse to the right of the first assistant.
- Serving cart to the left of instrument nurse.
- Anesthesiologist at patient's head.

31.3 Patient Positioning

Patient positioning is performed as shown in Figs. 31.2 and 31.3:

- Supine position in reverse Trendelenburg with an inclination of about 15°–20°.
- Spread legs.
- Arms adducted along the body (in case an X-ray cholangiography is necessary).

The operating table is therefore prepared with a sliding prevent mat (Pink Pad®) or, in its absence, fixing the legs with bandages to prevent the patient falling from the operating table.

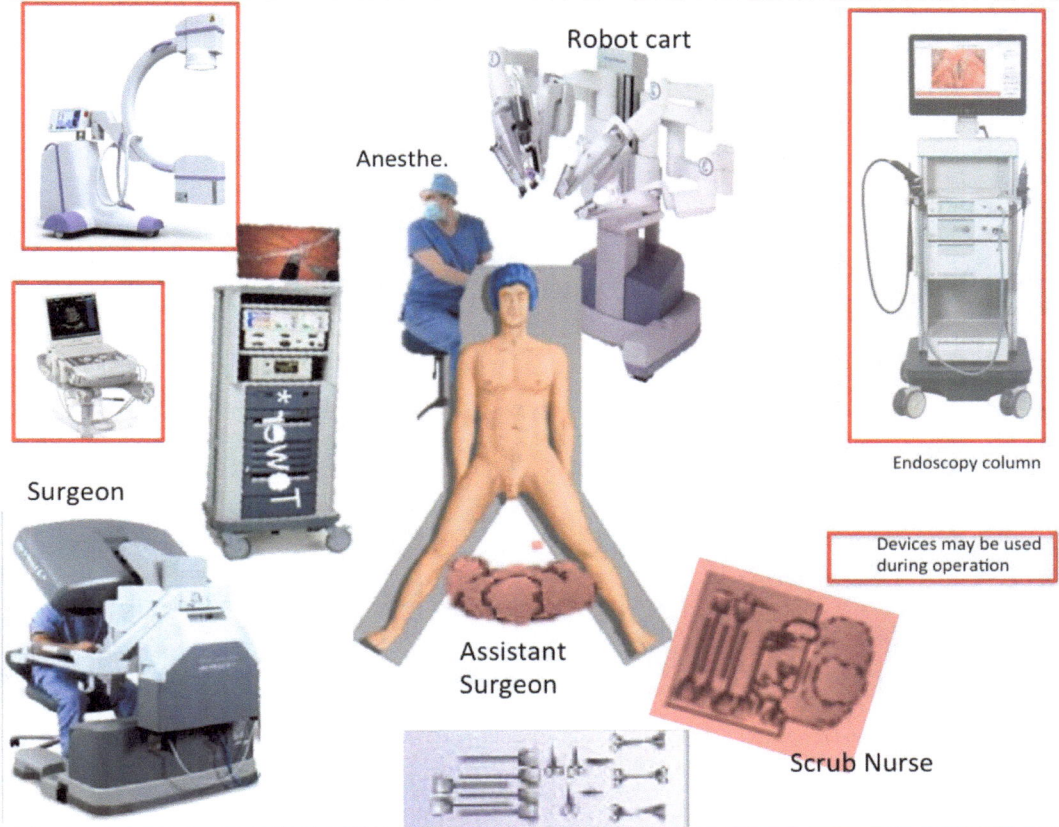

Fig. 31.2 Schematic operating theater setting (any devices are optional)

31.4 Port Placement and Robot Docking

In robotic surgery, ports are placed 8 cm from each other along a straight transverse line located approximately at the transverse umbilical line (Fig. 31.3a).

A 12-mm additional port for the assistant surgeon (generally the AirSeal trocar) is placed 3 cm below the umbilical line, between umbilicus scar (port 3) and the left robotic port (port 4).

One additional 5-mm port may be useful in challenging cases and is usually placed at the level of 12-mm port between robotic trocars 1 and 2.

Different trocar dispositions in terms of height and distance may be necessary, according to patient's characteristics (obesity, brachytype morphology, adhesions, etc.).

The "targeting" (centering of target anatomy for working) is carried out on the liver pedicle (Fig. 31.3b).

Once the ports have been positioned and the patient cart is approximated at the operating table, the instrument nurse connects the arm that accommodates the endoscope and the first assistant at the table performs the targeting. Once it is complete, the other arms are docked and the robotic instruments are inserted by the instrument nurse, after positioning the reducers on the 12-mm ports to avoid loss of pneumoperitoneum.

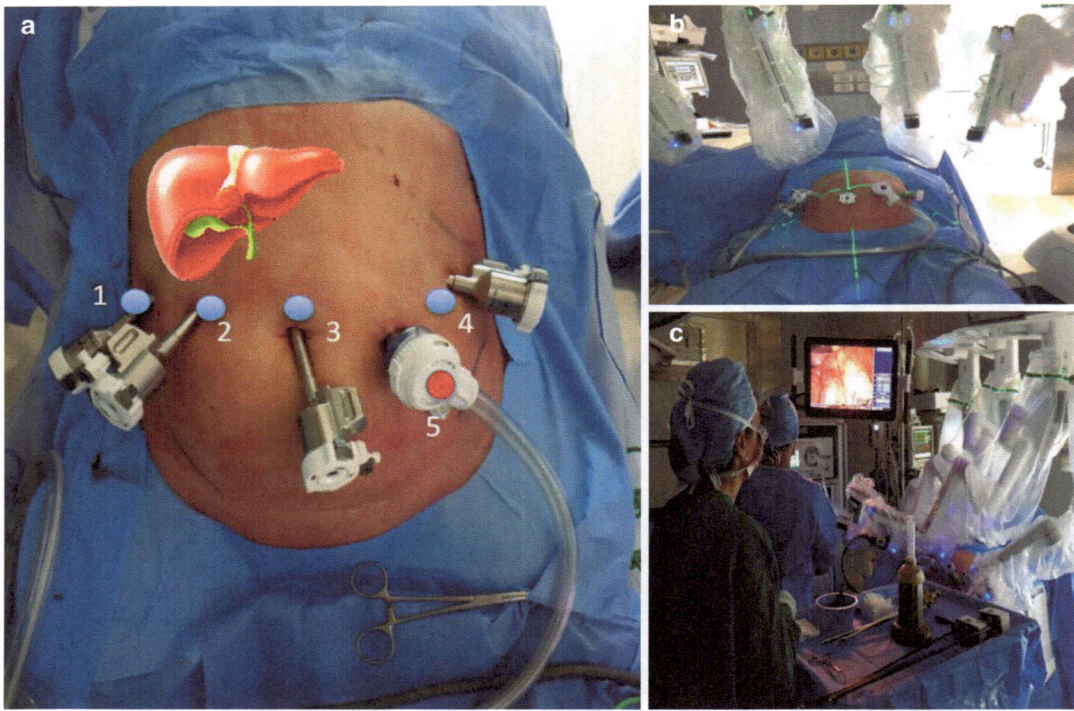

Fig. 31.3 Trocar site and robot docking. (**a**) 1, 2, 3, and 4 robotic ports – 5 auxiliary ports (AirSeal), (**b**) robot targeting and docking, and (**c**) nurse placement in the operating theater

31.5 Surgical Instruments Required

The preparation of the robotic and laparoscopic instruments table and the serving cart is carried out as shown in Figs. 31.4 and 31.5.

31.5.1 Robotic Instruments: "Robotic Table" (Fig. 31.4)

- 4 robotic ports (8 mm).
- 1 port with tubing set for the stabilization of pneumoperitoneum (AirSeal System).
- 30° robotic endoscope (the Xi last device is equipped for ICG view).
- 1 grasping forceps (ProGrasp Forceps® or Cadiere Forceps®).
- 1 bipolar forceps (Fenestrated or Maryland Bipolar Forceps®).

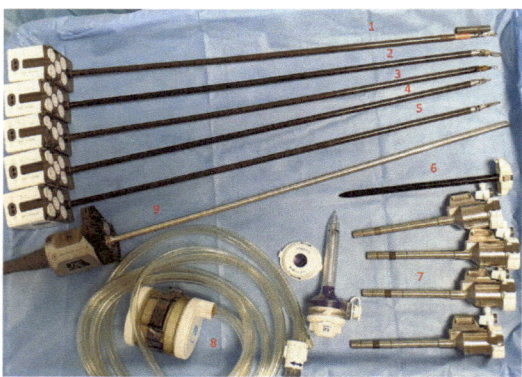

Fig. 31.4 Robotic instruments (more frequently used): (1) Scissors, (2) Maryland bipolar forceps, (3) Hook, (4) Needle driver, (5) Cadiere forceps, (6, 7) Robotic ports and trocar, (8) AirSeal system, (9) Robotic camera

- 1 monopolar instrument (Permanent Cautery Hook® or Hot Shears®).
- 1 needle holder (Large Needle Driver® or Black Diamond®).

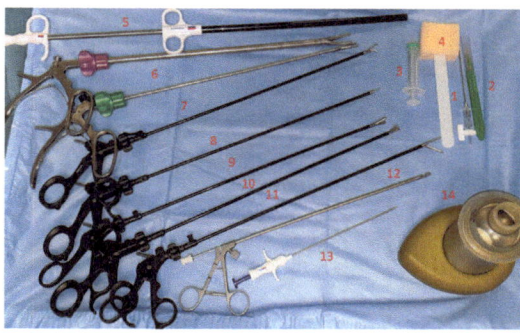

Fig. 31.5 Laparoscopic instruments (more frequently used): (1) Veress needle, (2) scalpel, (3) syringe, (4) sponge, (5) endoscopic bag, (6) Hem-o-lock applier, (7) laparoscopic scissors, (8–11) laparoscopic forceps, (12) laparoscopic device for cholangiography, (13) device for trocar site closure, (14) scope warmer

31.5.2 Laparoscopic Instruments: "Laparoscopic Table" (Fig. 31.5)

- 1 Veress needle.
- 1 20-mL syringe (for drop test).
- 1 scope warmer.
- 1 or 2 laparoscopic grasping forceps (Croce-Olmi forceps, Grasper or Johann forceps).
- 1 laparoscopic suction/irrigation system.
- Hem-o-lok or other laparoscopic clips applier of various sizes (small/medium/large).
- 1 laparoscopic scissors.
- 1 laparoscopic cholangiogram forceps.
- 1 laparoscopic bulldog applier (with different bulldogs).
- 1 Endo close suture device.
- 1 endobag (small size).

31.5.3 Open Instruments

- 2 scalpels with stainless steel blade (sizes 11 and 24).
- 1 or 2 kidney basins/Janach (steel bowls).
- 2 anatomical tissue forceps.
- 2 toothed forceps.
- 4 curved Klemmer clamps.
- 4 curved Kocher clamps.
- 1 sponge holder.

- 1 Mayo scissors and Nelson-Metzenbaum dissection scissors.
- Gauze of different sizes.
- 4 Backhaus clamps.
- 1 Mixter right angle forceps.
- 1 curved Bengolea forceps.
- 1 set of Randall forceps (for CBD exploration).
- 2 Mathieu retractors.
- 2 Langenbeck retractors.
- 1 monopolar electric scalpel.
- 1 needle holder.
- Fogarty balloon set.
- Drains.
- T-tube set.
- Set for intraoperative cholangiography.
- Different sutures PDS/Vicryl 3/0,4/0, 5/0, Prolene 5/0.
- Contrast dye for cholangiography.
- 1 abdominal wall retractor.

31.5.4 Indocyanine Green (ICG)

The indocyanine green fluorescent dye (IGC) is presented in vials of 25 mg of powder for solution for injection (Fig. 31.6):

- Use in concentrations of 0.1–0.5 mg/mL.
- Dilute with sterile distilled water (10–20 mL) and not sodium chloride as the latter could cause aggregation.
- After preparation, the solution must be stored in a dark and cool place to avoid rapid deterioration of the whitening fluorescence.
- For the dosage to be administered, follow the instructions of the anesthetist present in the theater.

31.6 Surgical Steps and Related Instruments

31.6.1 Hasson Technique for Laparoscopic Access

- 1 scalpel (blade 11).
- 2 anatomical tissue forceps.

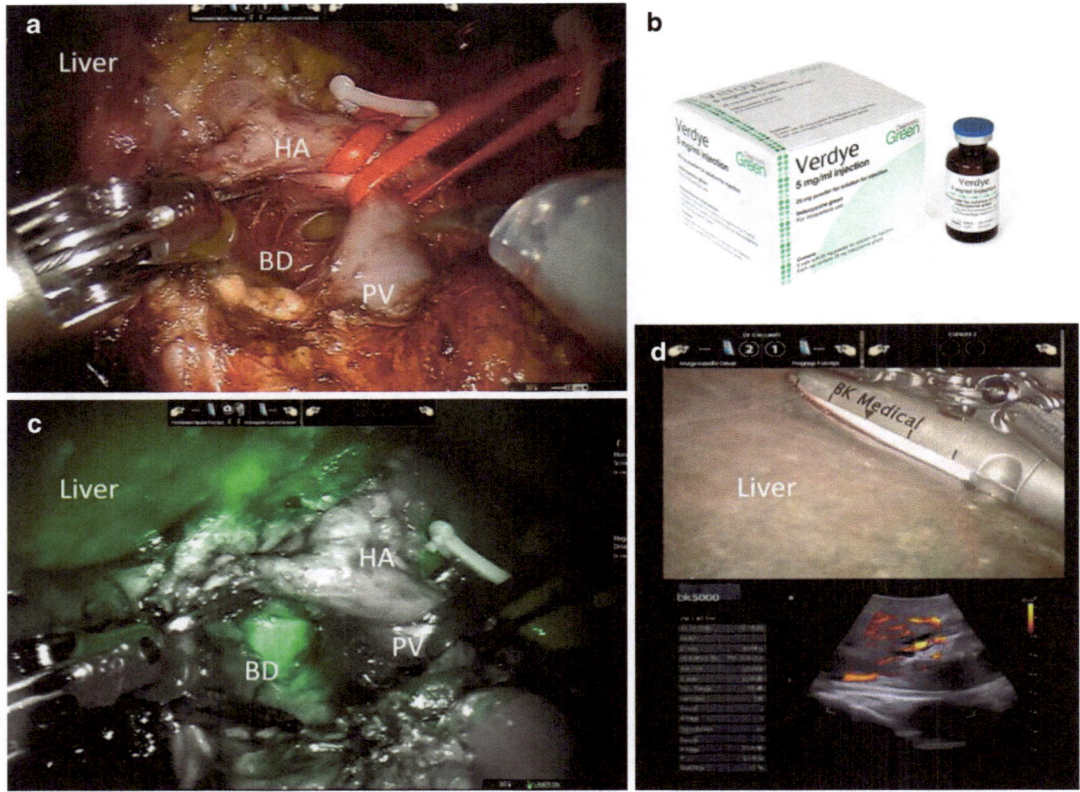

Fig. 31.6 (**a**) Normal view, (**b**) indocyanine green (ICG) dye, (**c**) view using scope for indocyanine green fluorescence, (**d**) endoscopic US probe for robotic surgery

- 2 Mathieu retractors.
- 1 Nelson-Metzenbaum dissection scissors.
- 2 curved Kocher clamps to grasp fascia.
- 2 curved Klemmer clamps to grasp parietal peritoneum.

31.6.2 Veress Technique for Laparoscopic Access

- Scalpel (blade 11).
- Veress needle.
- Syringe for saline drop test.

The specimen is extracted enlarging the periumbilical incision or the 12-mm port incision. For larger specimens, a Pfannenstiel minilaparotomy is performed using a wound protector/retractor.

During the specimen extraction phase, the required instruments are as follows:

- 1 scalpel (blade 24).
- 1 monopolar electric scalpel.
- 2 anatomical/toothed tissue forceps (based on the surgeon's requests).
- 3 Mathieu retractors.
- 1 Nelson-Metzenbaum dissection scissors.
- 2 curved Kocher clamps to grasp fascia.
- 2 curved Klemmer clamps to grasp parietal peritoneum.
- 1 wound protector/retractor to extract specimen safely.
- 1 adsorbable suture for peritoneum.
- 1 looped/monofilament/braided suture (based on the surgeon's request) to perform closure of fascia.

- 1 monofilament/braided suture (based on the surgeon's request) to perform a suture of the subcutaneous plane.
- Titanium skin clips/suture to perform closure of skin.

31.7 Tools Required in Selected Cases

- Intraoperative ultrasound examination (Figs. 31.2, 31.6).
- X-ray cholangiography (Fig. 31.2).
- Jejunostomy Kit (when a postoperative enteral nutrition may be indicated).

31.7.1 Robotic Common Bile Duct Exploration: Step-by-Step Surgical Phases

- Operating theater setup (Fig. 31.2).
- Trocar is positioned and robot is docked (Fig. 31.3).
- Robotic instruments are generally scissors on the right and a bipolar forceps on the left (Fig. 31.4).
- Liver is retracted upward, using the auxiliary robotic arm with a Cadiere forceps, thus exposing the hepatic pedicle.
- If gallbladder is still in place, it is dissected from the fundus (anterograde technique or fundus-down cholecystectomy) to cystic duct insertion. A previous cholecystectomy makes the dissection of the area challenging for the presence of adhesions.
- A minimal duodenal mobilization (Kocher maneuver) may be performed.
- The common bile duct is identified (the presence of stones makes its diameter larger than usual), and the duct may be isolated with a vessel loop.
- An intraoperative ultrasound evaluation may be used (Fig. 31.6).
- The use of ICG-fluorescence may ease the dissection (Fig. 31.6).
- 1–2 cm choledochotomy (according to stone size) is generally performed longitudinally, in

the supraduodenal CBD (under the cystic insertion) using robotic scissors and bipolar forceps.
- Two 3/0 stitches of polyglactin 910 (Vicryl) or polydioxanone (PDS) may be used to lift and keep the edges open (Fig. 31.7).
- A Fogarty balloon catheter may be introduced into the CDS and passed into the duodenum, the balloon is inflated, and the catheter is withdrawn. Stones can be felt against the shaft of the catheter, which is gradually and gently pulled up to the choledochotomy site, taking care to prevent stones slipping into the proximal biliary tree. The catheter is easily addressed using the articulated tips of robotic bipolar forceps. The procedure may be repeated several times.
- The CBD irrigation may help to complete the procedure since small stones floating into the water are easily removed through the opening.
- If available, together with an endoscopic column, a choledochoscope can be used through the opening for a final check or to remove residual fragments using the operative channel (Fig. 31.7).
- T-tube of adequate size is inserted and choledochotomy closed with 4/0 PDS or Vicryl interrupted stitches (Fig. 31.7).
- An X-ray cholangiography is useful to evaluate the final result of surgery or possible biliary tree anatomical variations. It requires an X-ray-screened operating room and enough space to fit the C-arm device (Fig. 31.2).
- Gallbladder, if present, is finally removed into a plastic bag.
- A perihepatic drain is left in place.

31.7.2 Hepaticojejunostomy: Step-by-Step Surgical Phases

- Operating room setup and trocar positioning are the same as described above.
- If gallbladder is still in place, we start with its dissection from the fundus (anterograde technique or fundus-down cholecystectomy) to cystic duct insertion.

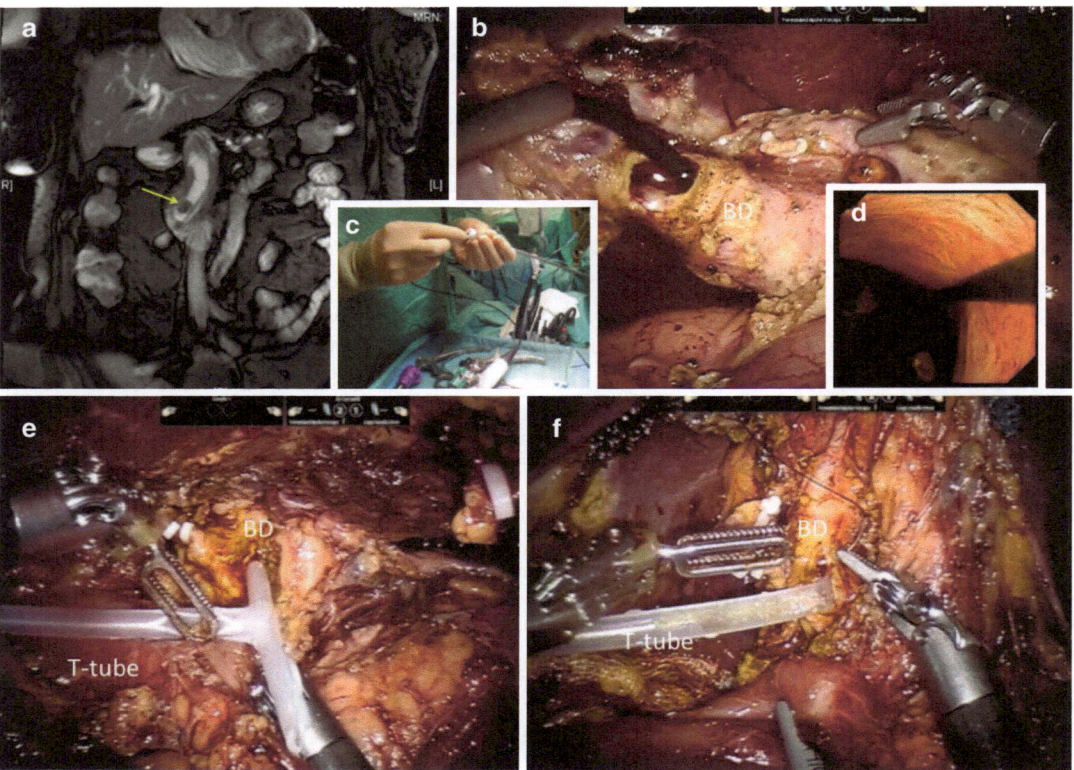

Fig. 31.7 (**a**) Cholangio-RMI with stones inside the common bile duct, (**b**) common BD exploration using choledocoscopy, (**c**) External view, (**d**) view inside the CBD, (**e**) T-tube placement, (**f**) Robotic CBD suture

- ICG-fluorescence is generally used (Fig. 31.6).
- The common bile duct is identified and isolated using a vessel loop.
- The jejunal limb for the Roux-en-Y technique is prepared by transecting the jejunum about 20–30 cm distal from the Treitz ligament, then brought in a retrocolic (antroduodenal, if present) fashion, right to the middle colic vessels, up to the hilar plate. Attention must be taken to ensure a tension-free limb.
- A small orifice (about 5 mm according to duct diameter) at the anti-mesenteric side of the Roux limb, 2–3 cm distal to the stapled jejunal stump, is created. The diameter of the jejunal orifice should always be smaller than the width of the hepatic duct. The mucosa of the intestinal orifice is slightly inverted and sometimes partially resected. Two 4–0 or 5–0 PDS running sutures for bilioenteric anastomosis is performed, one on the posterior side and the

other on the anterior one (Figs. 31.8, 31.9). The two sutures are secured together at the corners that are kept in traction to facilitate the maneuver.
- When a simultaneous pancreatoduodenectomy is performed, if the same ileal loop is used for reconstruction, a distance of 10–15 cm between the pancreaticojejunostomy and the hepaticojejunostomy should be left.
- On the anterior side of the anastomosis, additional 5/0 interrupted stitches are placed mainly to reduce the traction on the anastomosis.
- During anastomotic construction, the needle is passed so as to have the knot tied outside of the anastomotic channel. The passing of all stitches should take a good amount of tissue (at least 4–5 mm) of small bowel seromuscular in order to hold the mucosa inside the bile duct and to avoid tearing and ischemia.

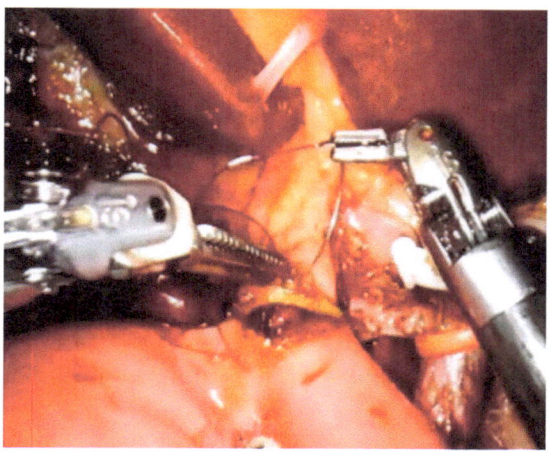
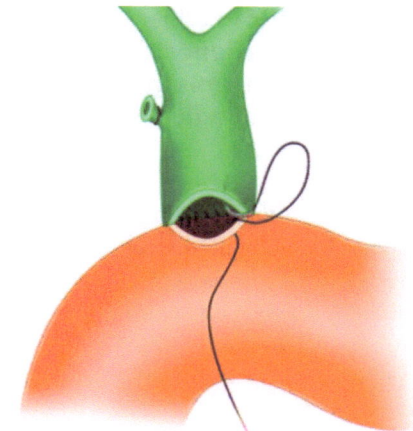

Fig. 31.8 Robotic suture during hepaticojejunostomy

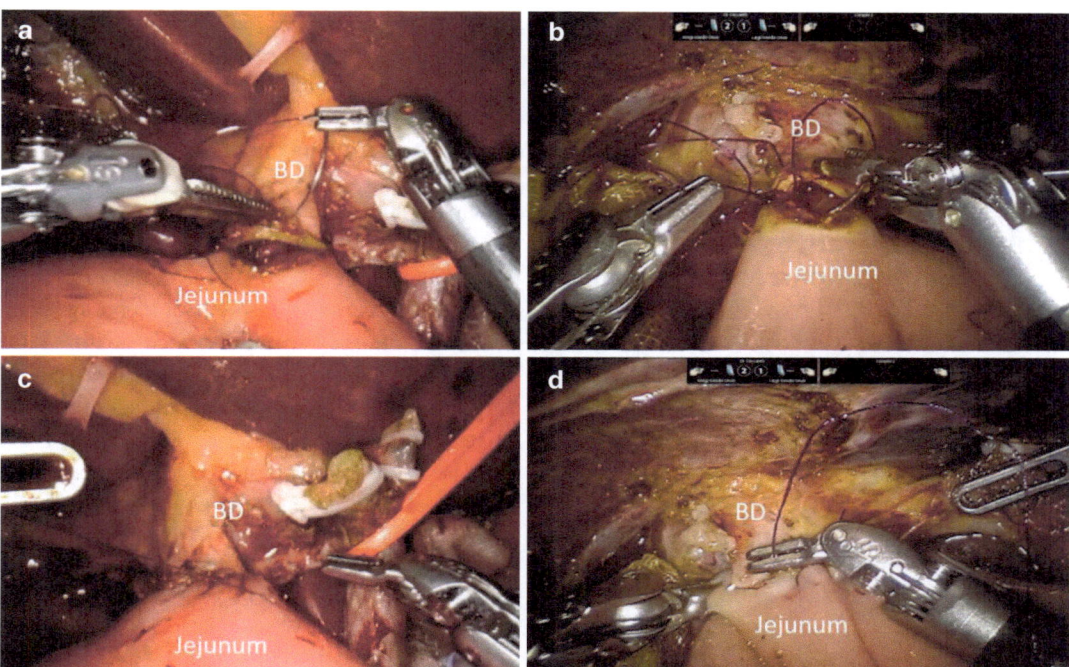

Fig. 31.9 Different frames of hepaticojejunostomy robot-assisted sutures. (**a-b**) Hand-sewn 2-layer hepaticojejunstomy; (**c**) completion of the first layer; (**d**) second layer

- If we use the technique of interrupted stitches, the number of stitches to use is related to the caliber of the bile duct and the surgeon's experience. In this case, the posterior wall is generally performed from the left to the right side. All the knots of the posterior wall remain outside of the anastomosis.

- A trans-anastomotic stent (a piece 8–10 French Nelaton catheter) may be left in place in order to protect and improve the patency of the anastomosis in the early postoperative period, especially if the bile duct diameter is small. The stent is fixed using a 5–0 Vicryl-rapid suture.

31.7.3 Hepatic Pedicle Lymphadenectomy or Lymph Node Sampling for Oncological Diseases

Hepatic lymph node metastases have a strong impact on the prognosis for oncological diseases. Systemic lymph node dissection or simple sampling may be requested in selected cases. Minimally invasive dissection may be facilitated by robotic device.

Robotic lymphadenectomy can be performed in different ways:

- En bloc: All lymph node stations are extracted together with the surgical specimen and sent to the pathology laboratory for analysis.
- For each station: Each lymph node station is removed by the surgeon separately and therefore as different samples.
- A node sampling: The lymph node is close to the lesion or only enlarged nodes are removed.

31.8 Intraoperative Complications: Management and Tools

The most frequent intraoperative complications to manage during a robotic hepaticojejunostomy are basically hemorrhage and injuries of parenchymatous organs (pancreas, liver), often requiring conversion to open surgery.

In these circumstances, the following instruments should be readily available:

- Laparoscopic suction/irrigation system.
- Laparoscopic bulldog clamps (to manage the problem using the minimally invasive setting), a set of open vascular clamps/bulldogs.
- 10 cm × 10 cm gauze to be passed to the assistant at the request of the surgeon.
- 5- or 10-mm endoscopic clip applier (titanium clips or others).
- Laparoscopic Hem-o-lok applier (remember that once these clips are positioned, their removal is very difficult!).
- Robotic needle holder (the best for microsuture is the so-called black diamond) and

monofilament suture with small gauge needle to attempt a repair of the bleeding vessel or, in case of injury of parenchymatous organ, needle holder, and monofilament/barbed suture to repair it.
- 5/0 Prolene vascular suture for vascular repair or 4/0 or 5/0 PDS for bile duct suture. Intestinal sutures may be treated by absorbable 3/0 PDS or Vicryl sutures.

31.8.1 Conversion to Open Surgery

The majority of intraoperative complications may be adequately resolved using the robotic device. Anyway open conversion may be the consequence of a situation impossible to manage in a minimally invasive setting. The surgical table for conversion to open surgery needs to include the tools for laparotomy. The conversion may be an emergent decision or the result of a planned decision. The instruments necessary to continue the procedure with open approach are listed in the previous chapter. Unmanageable hemorrhage as a consequence of vascular injury requires an immediate conversion: Bulldog clamps for artery or portal vein are used to control bleeding, while vascular sutures are performed with 5–6/0 Prolene stitches. Ample abdominal incision and self-retaining retractors are essential for an adequate exposure, and vascular forceps or grafts may be used according to the injury type, while the use of magnifying glasses may improve the vision of the surgeon.

In these circumstances, the following instruments should always be available:

- Scalpel and electrocautery.
- Open suction system.
- Self-retaining retractor (Rochard model preferable).
- 10 cm x 10 cm gauze.
- Mikulicz spatulas.
- Stitches for hemostasis (Prolene 4–5/0) PDS or Vicryl.
- Open Hem-o-lok applier, or clips applier.
- Vascular clamps and other vascular scissors.
- Other instruments are related to the cause of conversion.

References

1. Robinson J, Tschuor C, McKillop IH, Baker EH, Iannitti DA, Vrochides D, Martinie JB. Robotic revision of Hepaticojejunostomy for benign biliary stricture. Am Surg. 2022;89(6):2455–9. https://doi.org/10.1177/00031348221096834.
2. Morikawa T, Ohtsuka H, Takadate T, Ishida M, Miura T, Mizuma M, Nakagawa K, Kamei T, Naitoh T, Unno M. Laparoscopic and robot-assisted surgery for adult congenital biliary dilatation achieves favorable short-term outcomes without increasing the risk of late complications. Surg Today. 2022;52(7):1039–47. https://doi.org/10.1007/s00595-021-02438-8.
3. Varshney VK, Swami A. Total robotic choledochal cyst excision with Roux-en-Y hepaticojejunostomy in adults. Langenbecks Arch Surg. 2022;407(4):1727–32. https://doi.org/10.1007/s00423-021-02395-3. Epub.
4. Sucandy I, Ross SB, Crespo KL, Rosemurgy AS. Robotic extrahepatic biliary resection with roux-en-Y Hepaticojejunostomy for type 2 Klatskin tumor. Ann Surg Oncol. 2022;29(1):339–40. https://doi.org/10.1245/s10434-021-10562-5.
5. Robinson J, Watson M, Baimas-George M, Iannitti D, Martinie J, Vrochides D. Objective evaluation of technical dexterity in robotic hepaticojejunostomy: assessment of hepatopancreatobiliary fellows using cumulative sum analytics. Int J Med Robot. 2021;17(5):e2294. https://doi.org/10.1002/rcs.2294. Epub 2021 Jun 7
6. Sucandy I, Giovannetti A, Spence J, Ross S, Rosemurgy A. Robotic roux-en-Y Hepaticojejunostomy for right hepatic duct transection. Application of minimally invasive technique for high bile duct injury. Am Surg. 2021:3134820956358. https://doi.org/10.1177/0003134820956358.

Laparoscopic Treatment of Splenic Disease

32

Diego Cuccurullo, Stefano Reggio, Luigi Mauriello, and Salvatore Errico

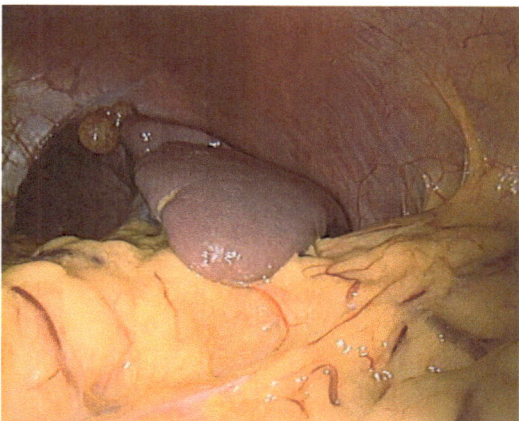

Table 32.1 Indications of splenectomy [1]

Idiopathic thrombocytopenic purpura
Hereditary spherocytosis
Splenomegaly in cirrhosis patients
Splenic cysts
Thalassemia
Myeloproliferative disorders
Lymphomas
Autoimmune hemolytic anemia
Sarcoma
Splenic abscess
Splenic aneurysm
Metastatic disorders
Hematologic hypersplenism
Subcapsular splenic hematoma

32.1 Indications (Table 32.1)

Contradictions: These are relative and not absolute, uncorrected coagulopathy and severe portal hypertension, as significant venous collaterals may be very difficult to control laparoscopically; however, splenectomy in the context of liver cirrhosis has been performed with good results in patients with Child's class A and class B [1]. Very massive splenomegaly (25 cm craniocaudal length) remains a relative contraindication to a laparoscopic approach as the technical difficulties in exposure and manipulation of these organs become increasingly difficult, and the advantages of the laparoscopic approach become less clear.

32.1.1 Preoperative Preparation

- Xipho sub-umbilical trichotomy.
- Antibiotic prophylaxis: Cephalosporin.
- Urinary catheter and nasogastric tube (placed when patient is in supine position).

D. Cuccurullo (✉) · S. Reggio · L. Mauriello
S. Errico
General, Laparoscopic and Robotic Surgery Unit, A.O.R.N. dei Colli, Monaldi Hospital, Naples, Italy
e-mail: diego.cuccurullo@ospedalideicolli.it;
stefano.reggio@ospedalideicolli.it;
salvatore.errico@ospedalideicolli.it

32.1.2 Description of the Patient Positioning

32.1.2.1 Right Lateral Decubitus

Left arm is adducted and suspended on an armrest (a thigh support in this case also can be useful for arm's positioning) or fixed on an arch while right arm is adducted and positioned on another armrest (placed perpendicular to surgical bed). A lateral support is tangentially positioned on the patient's left side at buttocks height to keep him in a 45° position, and a second support is transversely positioned between shoulder and waist. The lower leg (right leg) is flexed, while the upper leg (left leg) is extended. A memory foam pillow is positioned between two legs to prevent decubitus injury. Another pillow is positioned on the right patient side to expose the spleen (Fig. 32.1).

The table is then tilted in a slight reverse Trendelenburg, putting the iliac crest patient at the level of table's fulcrum, and flexed 30° in order to open the space between the iliac crest and the costal margin.

At last, we control shoulders, and it is important that they are on the axis, especially the right one in order to avoid nerve injuries caused by body weight. The left arm suspended on the armrest needs to keep a curved position to not stretch the brachial nerve.

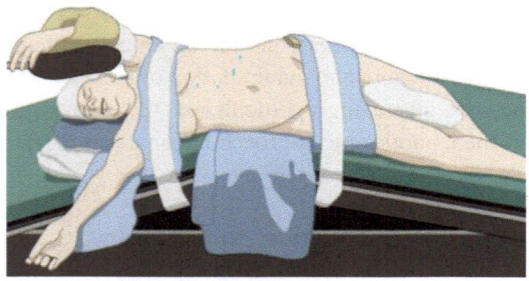

Fig. 32.1 Patient positioning [1]

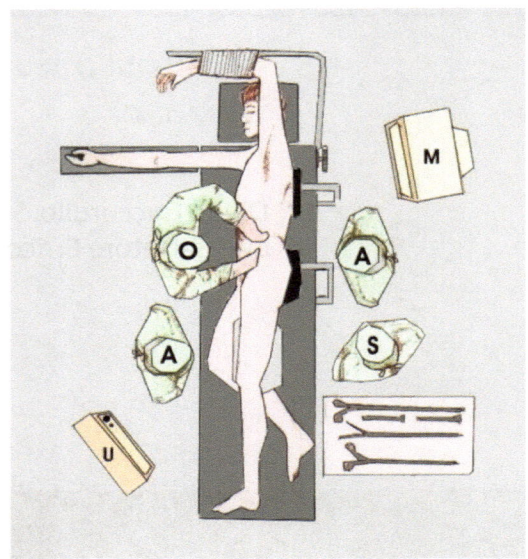

Fig. 32.2 Splenectomy. *Patient, operators and monitor positioning* [3]

32.1.3 Description of the Operating Theater Setting

The surgeon and the cameraman stand on the patient's ventral side and the second assistant with the scrub nurse are positioned on the dorsal side. The video monitor is placed in front of the surgeon at the level of the patient's shoulder (Fig. 32.2).

32.1.4 Trocars Position

We routinely use four trocars with a 30° HD 3D scope and atraumatic grasper. The first 10–12 mm trocar for the camera is placed 2 cm above the costal margin at the anterior axillary line, a 10–12 mm trocar and a 5 mm trocar, respectively, on the right and left, below the costal edge (for the right and left hand of the surgeon), and finally a fourth 5 mm more lateral trocar on the posterior axillary line (second assistant) (Fig. 32.3).

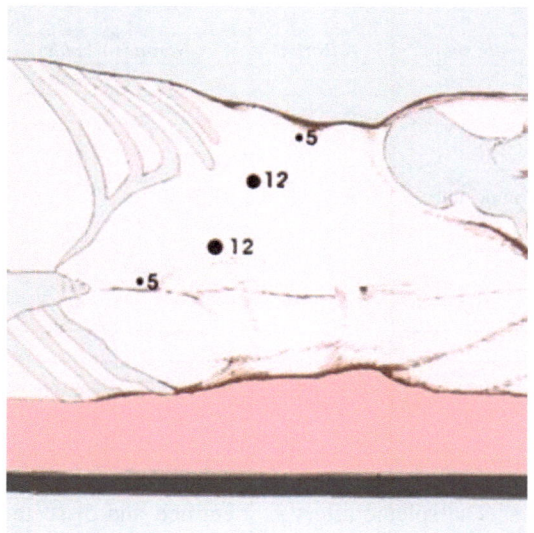

Fig. 32.3 Splenectomy. *Trocars positioning* [3]

32.1.5 Surgical Instruments

For a laparoscopic splenectomy, the following are required [2, 3]:

Laparoscopic instruments		
Syringe with 2 cc saline solution [for drop test]		1
Veress needle		1
Trocar	10–12 mm	2
Trocar	5 mm	2
Johann forceps	5 mm	4
Grasper forceps	5 mm	1
Delaitre forceps	10 mm	1
Videoendoscope 3D 30°	10 mm	1
Ultrasound instrument (Thunderbeat® or Ultracision®)	5 mm	1
Laparoscopic needle holder	5 mm	1
Suction and irrigation cannula	5 mm	1

Instruments for laparoscopic approach	
Dressing forceps	2
Disposable scalpel	1
Medium curved Metzenbaum scissor	1
Mayo scissor	1
Needle holder	2
Curved Klemmer forceps	2
Curved Kocher forceps	4
Langenbeck retractors	2
Tampon forceps Collin	1
Foerster forceps	1
Backhaus forceps	4
Round dish bowl	1
Mathieu retractors	2

Medical and surgical device	No.
Monopolar electric scalpel	1
Insufflation tube	1
Suction and irrigation tube	1
Endo-bag 15 mm	1
Scope warmer	1
Drainage tube 18 French	1
Gauze (size 10 × 60; 15 × 2,5; 30 × 45)	–

Suture				
	Suture USP	Needle shape	Adsorbable	Non-adsorbable
Polyglactin 910 (Vicryl®)	0	5/8	×	
Polyglactin 910 (Vicryl Rapide®)	3/0	3/8	×	
Silk	1	1/2		×
In case of necessity				
Polyglactin 910 (Vicryl®)	2/0	Composite	×	

Metallic suture		
	Diameter	Size
Endoclip	10 mm	ML
In case of necessity		
Endoclip	12 mm	L
Linear stapler	12 mm	35 mm (vascular)

32.1.6 In Case of Emergency, you Must Have an Instrument Stable for a Laparotomic Conversion

32.2 Splenectomy: Operative Technique

32.2.1 Step-by-Step Procedure [4, 5]

- Pneumoperitoneum is created using open Veress-assisted technique (Veress needle in Palmer point).
- The presence of an accessory spleen is always evacuated.
- Mobilization of the splenic flexure of the colon.
- Spleen meso is dissected starting from the caudal pole, and then exposure of the medial aspect of the spleen is achieved by dissection of the lateral gastrocolic and splenorenal ligaments, thus opening the lesser sac.
- All short gastric vessels are divided, and the dissection of the spleno-gastric ligament is achieved.
- The gastro-phrenic ligament is divided allowing the entire stomach to be rotated to the right. Complete opening of the lesser sac allows visualization of the pancreatic tail and the splenic vessels overlaid by the posterior peritoneum.

- The splenic artery is identified and dissected from the upper border of the pancreatic body tail and clipped 2 cm from splenic hilum (to decrease blood supply to the spleen and reduce the volume and the vein turgor).
- Mobilization of the spleen by division of the splenorenal ligament and splenopancreatic ligament.
- The splenic vein is isolated at the hilum: At this moment, its swelling is reduced and it can be easily clipped (Fig. 32.4).
- The splenic vessels are now divided, and the mobilization is completed.
- Spleen is removed using a retrieval bag (Fig. 32.5).
- Drain is inserted through the port incision on the middle axillary line.

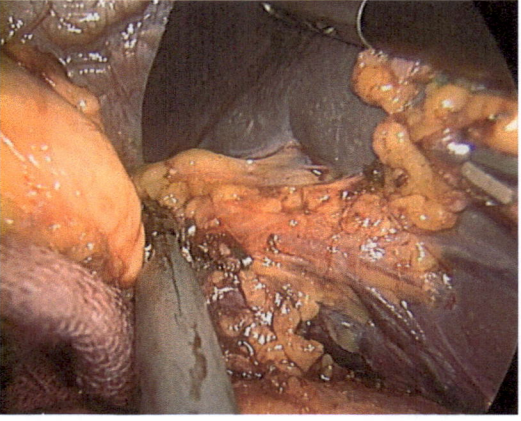

Fig. 32.4 The splenic vessels are clipped and then cutted by energy device

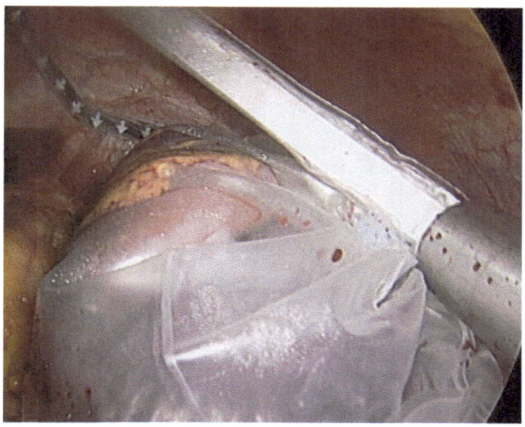

Fig. 32.5 The specimen was placed in a retrieval bag and extracted through suprapubic incision

- The spleen is morcellated in case of benign neoplasia, and the specimen is removed intact through a sovrapubic incision in case of malignancy.

32.3 Near Total Splenectomy

Indications: Indications for the procedure were a cyst of superior pole of the spleen and moderate-to-severe hereditary spherocytosis according to hematologist.

32.4 Operative Technique

32.4.1 Step-by-Step Procedure [6]

- The first step of the operation is the identification of the autonomous inferior polar artery coming from the left gastro-omental artery or coming from an early division of the splenic artery.
- The splenic artery is isolated in its course along the upper border of the pancreas at 1–2 cm from the splenic hilus and then divided in between clips.

- The splenorenal and splenodiaphragmatic ligaments are divided, freeing the lower or the upper pole of the spleen to leave the spleen completely free to rotate on its vascular axis.
- It is mandatory to look for and to preserve the most caudal vessels coming from the left gastro-epiploic vessels that supply the splenic inferior pole.
- The area to be resected is now clearly visible by the ischemia of the splenic parenchyma that is divided by using bipolar scissors and the ultrasonic device about 1 cm in the devascularized spleen.
- To reduce bleeding, in this phase, we first leave previous the splenic vein in order to allow the flow from the splenic remnant. To avoid parenchymal or vascular injuries of the residual spleen we use a "no-touch" technique.
- The splenic vein is then divided. Fibrin sealant and hemostatic sponge are applied over the residual parenchyma for further hemostatic control and also to fix the remnant to the posterior abdominal wall, in order to prevent its torsion.

References

1. Liane S. Feldman laparoscopic splenectomy: standardized approach. World J Surg. 2011;35:1487–95. https://doi.org/10.1007/s00268-011-1059-x.
2. Errico S. Protocols in laparoscopic surgery; 2002. p. 93–5.
3. Corcione F, Miranda L, Ruotolo F. Laparoscopic surgery. 3rd ed; 2019. p. 228–9.
4. Corcione F, Esposito C, Cuccurullo D, et al. Technical standardization of laparoscopic splenectomy: experience with 105 cases. Surg Endosc. 2002;16(6):972–4.
5. Corcione F, Pirozzi F, Aragiusto G, et al. Laparoscopic splenectomy: experience of a single center in a series of 300 cases. Surg Endosc. 2012;26:2870–6.
6. Tartaglia E, Reggio S, Cuccurullo D, et al. Laparoscopic near-total splenectomy: a single center experience of a standardized procedure. Minim Invasive Ther Allied Technol. 2019;28(5):298–303.

Robotic Treatment of Splenic Diseases

33

Mario Annecchiarico and Antonio Varricchio

33.1 Introduction

Minimally invasive splenectomy (laparoscopic and robotic) improved patient morbidity, reduced lenght of stay in hospital, perioperative pain and provided enhanced cosmesis.

The improvements of laparoscopic tools for ligation over time have popularized the approach [3]. However, laparoscopic splenectomy (LS) does have its limitations, such as a steep learning curve [4], unstable two-dimensional vision, and rigid instrumentation. Multiple studies have reported that in difficult operational circumstances such as splenomegaly, obesity, hematological malignancies, and previous laparotomies, LS is associated with increased morbidity and conversion rates to open surgery [5–8]. With the introduction and increasing availability of the robot in the operative arena [9, 10], general surgeons are adopting the robotic platform to benefit from its stable 3D view with 4x zoom and its markedly advanced endowristed instruments [11]. These features lead to a more meticulous hilar dissection.

33.1.1 Indications for Splenectomy

The most common indications for splenectomy include [2]:

- Blood and reticuloendothelial disorders.
  - Hemolytic (hemolytic anemia, thalassemia).
  - Hematological malignancy (acute leukemia, chronic myeloid or lymphocytic leukemia, lymphoma).
  - Myeloproliferative disorders (polycythemia vera, myelofibrosis).
  - Thrombocytopenic disorders (immune thrombocytopenic purpura).
- Infective complications (hydatid, malaria).
- Inflammatory disorders (Felty syndrome).
- Neoplastic.
- Cryptogenic disorders.
- Congestive disorders (portal hypertension).
- Metabolic storage disorders (amyloidosis, Gaucher disease).
- Splenic trauma (selected cases).

33.1.2 Contraindications for Splenectomy

Contraindications to performing minimally invasive splenectomy include uncorrected coagulopathies and severe portal hypertension from liver cirrhosis. According to Giulianotti et al. [1],

M. Annecchiarico (✉) · A. Varricchio
Surgical Oncology Unit, "San Pio" Hospital, Benevento, Italy
e-mail: mario.annecchiarico@aornsanpio.it; antonio.varricchio@aornsanpio.it

whether Robotic Splenectomy (RS) is technically challenging or not can be ascribed to four factors. Anatomy of the pancreatic tail can make complex splenic vessel dissection when a bulky or "intrasplenic" pancreatic tail is present. The anatomy of the splenic vessels is another factor. Splenic artery and vein branching off in multiple, short vessels can hamper their identification and ligation. Spleen volume and consistency are the most common factors determining the conversion of LS and the only one can be detected in the preoperative setting by CT and ultrasound exploration. The last factor impairing the good outcome of LS is related to iatrogenic conditions, such as previous radiotherapy (Fig. 33.3) [7]. With the exception of splenomegaly, it is not easy to predict preoperatively the difficulties encountered during LS. Therefore, indications for RS should be accurately evaluated during the preoperative work-up and eventual laparoscopic exploration, restricting the robot use to cases not suitable for LS.

33.1.3 Advantages of Robotic Surgery in Splenectomy and Hemisplenectomy

Robotic splenectomy gives advantages in the cases listed below:

- Multiple and short arterial and venous branches of the splenic vessels.
- Bulky or intrasplenic pancreatic tail.
- Fragile parenchyma.
- High spleen volume.
- Previous radiotherapy with extensive fibrosis and adhesions.
- Hemisplenectomy: selective small vessel isolation and ligation.

33.2 Anatomy

The spleen is placed in the splenic lodge (diaphragm on the top, left colic flexure on the bottom, the internal aspect of diaphragm laterally, posterior surface of the stomach anteriorly, the anterior side of kidney, and adrenal gland posteriorly).

The spleen's two ends are the anterior and posterior ends. The anterior end of the spleen is expanded and is more like a border; it is directed forward and downward to reach the midaxillary line. The posterior end is rounded and is directed upward and backward; it rests on the upper pole of the left kidney.

The spleen's three borders are the superior, inferior, and intermediate. The superior border of the spleen is notched by the anterior end. The inferior border is rounded. The intermediate border directs toward the right.

The two surfaces of the spleen are the diaphragmatic and visceral. The diaphragmatic surface is smooth and convex, and the visceral surface is irregular and concave and has impressions. The gastric impression is for the fundus of the stomach, which is the largest and most concave impression on the spleen. The renal impression is for the left kidney and lies between the inferior and intermediate borders. The colic impression is for the splenic flexure of the colon; its lower part is related to the phrenicocolic ligament. The pancreatic impression for the tail of the pancreas lies between the hilum and colic impression.

The spleen consists of segments or "parenchymatous units"[12], each one with its own hilar arterial blood supply and venous drainage, separated, one from the other, by paucivascular planes. The segments were named superior, mid-superior, middle, mid-inferior, and inferior (Christo 1963). The intersegmental divisional planes are transversally superposed, at higher and higher angles, in a supero-inferior direction. The division of the spleen into superior and inferior hemispleens occurs at a 90° dihedral angle.

33.3 Hilum

The hilum can be found on the inferomedial part of the gastric impression. The hilum transmits the splenic vessels and nerves and provides attachment to the gastrosplenic and splenorenal (lienorenal) ligaments.

33.4 Splenic Ligaments (See Fig. 33.1)

1. The *gastrosplenic* ligament extends from the hilum of the spleen to the greater curvature of the stomach; it contains short gastric vessels and associated lymphatics and sympathetic nerves and left gastroepiploic arteries and veins.

2. The *splenorenal* ligament extends from the hilum of the spleen to the anterior surface of the left kidney; it contains the tail of the pancreas and splenic vessels.

3. The *phrenicocolic* ligament is a horizontal fold of peritoneum that extends from the splenic flexure of the colon to the diaphragm along the midaxillary line; it forms the upper end of the left paracolic gutter.

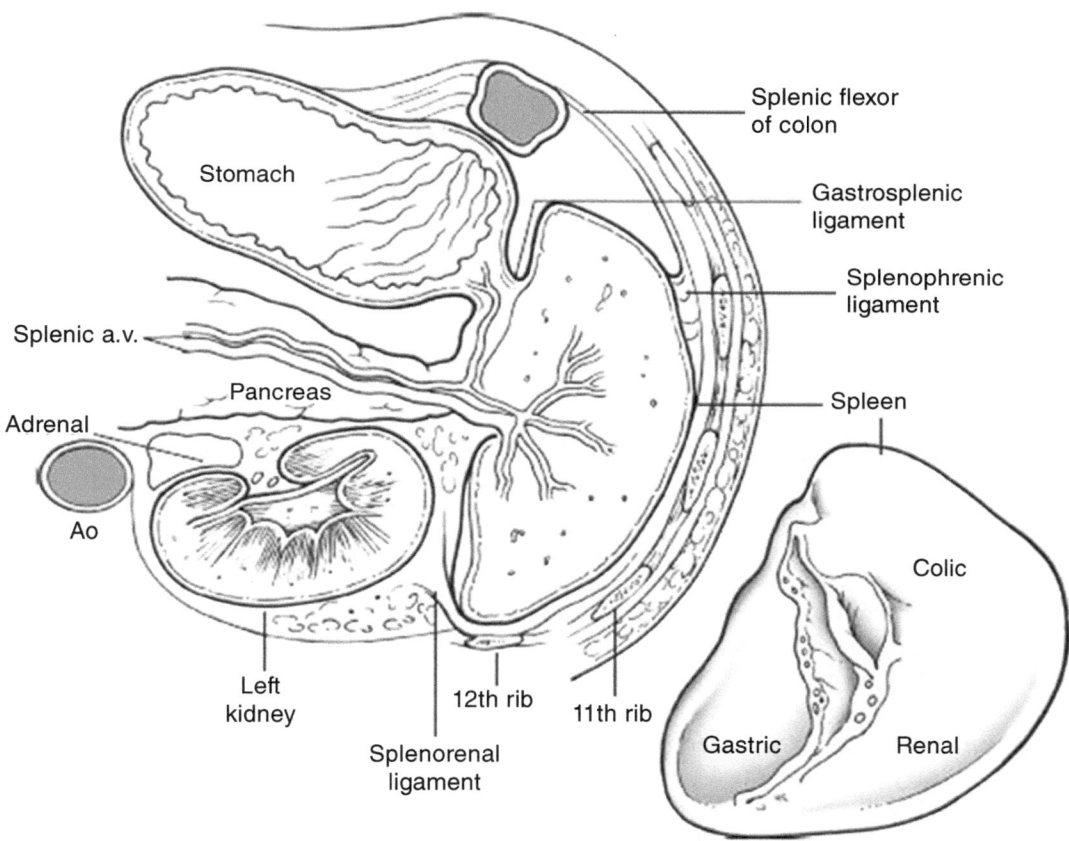

Fig. 33.1 Splenic attachments

33.5 Vascular Supply

The splenic artery supplies blood to the spleen. This artery is the largest branch of the celiac trunk and reaches the spleen's hilum by passing through the splenorenal ligament on the superior border of the pancreas till to its tail where it divides into two branches. The tortuous course of the splenic artery is considered so variable that no two arteries are alike, but the tortuosity of the artery is absent in infants and children. The splenic artery may course through the pancreas to reach the spleen. In congenital absence of the spleen (very rare), the splenic artery terminates in the pancreas.

When the splenic artery divides terminally near the spleen (~1–2 cm from the hilus), it is called a magistral splenic. This occurs in about 30% of individuals. When the division of the splenic occurs earlier, as in about 70% of individuals, in the prepancreatic segment, it is called a distributing splenic. In distributing splenic, artery dissection is easier: After division, the branches give origin to 2–4 branches where sprout 5–8 arterioles penetrating in the parenchyma.

In the magistral splenic artery, the branches are perpendicular to its axis (bifurcation or more rarely trifurcation). Venous drainage follows the arterial setting. The splenic vein is not invested in a common sheath with the artery—it is retropancreatic and never tortuous. Splenic arteries are end arteries in the strictest sense, and interference with the blood supply to the spleen will result in necrotic areas in the organ.

The variations of the splenic artery are numerous [13]. It may divide into two branches that reunite; the splenic vein passing through the loop thus formed. It may give rise to branches normally derived from other vessels, such as the left gastric, middle colic, and left hepatic.

The splenic artery supplies four to six (more or less) gastric vasa brevia arteries. These are terminal or end arteries. It can arise from the gastroepiploic artery, the splenic artery proper, the splenic branches of the splenic artery, or any combination thereof. The left gastroepiploic artery may originate from one of the splenic branches rather than from the splenic artery proper.

33.6 Surgical Instruments Required

33.6.1 Robotic Instruments

- 4 robotic ports (8 mm)
- 1 robotic port 12-mm whether stapler is required
- 1 port with tubing set for the stabilization of pneumoperitoneum
- 30° robotic endoscope
- 1 grasping forceps (Tip-up® or Cadiere Forceps®)
- 1 bipolar forceps (Maryland or Fenestrated Bipolar Forceps®)
- 1 monopolar instrument (Hot Shears®)
- 1 sealing instrument (SynchroSeal® or Harmonic Ace® 8 mm) for hemisplenectomy
- 1 stapler (SureForm EndoWrist Stapler® with vascular cartridge) if the splenic vein has large diameter
- 1 needle holder (Large Needle Driver®)
- 1 robotic clip applier with Hem-o-lok or titanium clips.

33.6.2 Laparoscopic Instruments

- Laparoscopic grasping forceps (Croce-Olmi forceps, Grasper or Johann forceps).
- Laparoscopic suction/irrigation system.
- 1 assistant port (10 mm)
- Hem-o-lok clips with laparoscopic applier of various sizes.
- Laparoscopic scissors.
- Scope warmer.

33.6.3 Open Instruments

- 2 scalpels with stainless steel blade (sizes 11 and 24)
- 1 kidney basin
- 2 Janach (steel bowls)
- 2 anatomical tissue forceps
- 2 toothed forceps
- 4 curved Klemmer clamps

- 4 curved Kocher clamps
- 1 Mayo scissors
- 1 Nelson-Metzenbaum dissection scissors
- 1 curved Bengolea forceps
- 3 Mathieu retractors
- 2 Langenbeck retractors
- 1 monopolar electric scalpel
- 1 wound protector/retractor
- Morcellator (in case of voluminous benign diseases).
- Endobag.

33.7 Patient Position (See Fig. 33.2)

Patient is placed in the dorsal supine position with arms tucked and widened legs. The operating table was jackknifed 15° and rotated 30° in the right lateral tilt, with 20° of reverse Trendelenburg in order to help expose the spleen and widen the space between the left costal margin and the anterior superior iliac spine. This procedure allows a better introduction of the trocars.

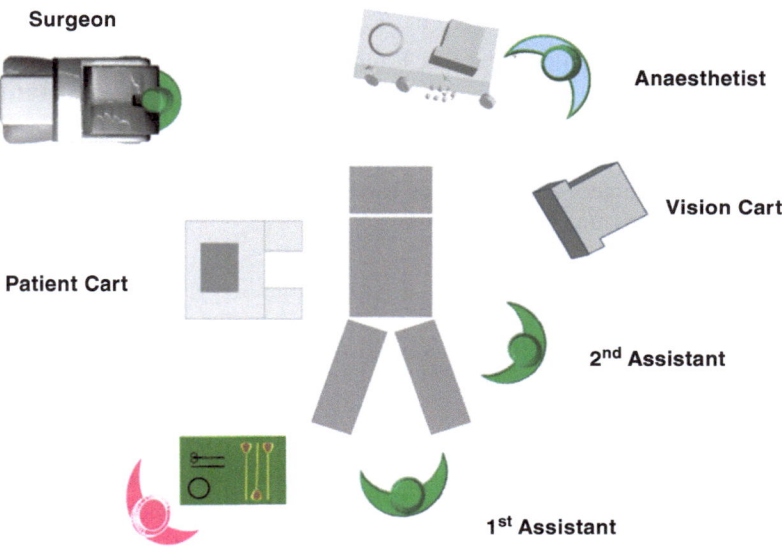

Fig. 33.2 Operating room setup

Surgeon

Anaesthetist

Vision Cart

Patient Cart

2nd Assistant

1st Assistant

Scrub Nurse

33.8 Patient Cart and Trocar Placement (See Fig. 33.3)

The patient cart is docked from the patient's right side, with the boom rotated to target the left upper quadrant. Pneumoperitoneum is induced with trans-umbilical Veress needle (in order to prevent splenic injury in case of splenomegaly) or open Hasson technique. After positioning the assistant port above the umbilicus near the midline, R2 8-mm port was placed on the midline 8–10 cm cephalad to the umbilicus with the other ports spaced 8–9 cm apart. The 8-mm robotic trocar for the camera is placed on the transverse umbilical line 5–6 cm left paraumbilical. The 8-mm robotic trocar R3 is placed in the right lateral epigastric area. The 8-mm robotic trocar R1 is in the left flank. The assistant 12-mm port is midway between the camera and R2 and is used to traction, apply clips, and provide suction.

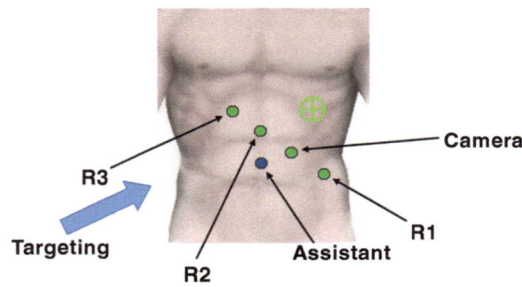

Fig. 33.3 Port placement and targeting

33.9 Splenectomy

33.9.1 Step-by-Step Description of the Procedure (Anterior Approach)

33.9.1.1 Critical Advice

The dissection of ligaments is of paramount importance for the correct approach to splenic hilum.

Do not traction directly spleen parenchyma.

33.9.2 Splenic Flexure Mobilization, Access to Lesser Sac, and Splenic Hilum Exposure

In the anterior approach, there is a vessel division without a posterior mobilization of the spleen.

At first, there is the splenic flexure mobilization. Grasper in R3 is protected by folded laparoscopic gauze tractions upward the spleen while the assistant grasps gently the colon to the opposite site. The monopolar scissor in R1 was helped by bipolar forceps in R2 sections of the phrenicocolic ligament. Patient's position helps the removal of the splenic flexure from the operative field. A complete splenic flexure mobilization with complete separation of Toldt's fascia from Gerota's fascia is rarely required.

Grasper in R3 retracts gently the posterior wall of the stomach upward and medially. A section of the gastrocolic ligament is necessary to access the lesser sac. Successively, there is the exposure of the gastrosplenic ligament where short gastric vessels run. After a section of the gastrosplenic ligament, short gastric vessels have to be sectioned. This maneuver can be performed with bipolar forceps in R2 and monopolar scissors in R1; clips or Hem-o-lok can be applied if needed.

33.9.3 Vascular Dissection

After the exposure of the pancreatic tail, the main trunk of the splenic artery is identified on its superior border. The artery is then dissected circumferentially with a monopolar scissor in R1 and bipolar forceps in R2. Sometimes, the needle holder in R1 may be helpful. After dissection, the artery is underpassed with a loop to control the inflow and clipped or ligated and divided with scissors. If the artery shows the distributing pattern, the lobar or segmental branches may be dissected, clipped, and sectioned separately. Non-adsorbable self-locking clips are usually advised for that maneuver. It is mandatory to avoid the dissection of the arteries too close to the hilum and consequently bleeding. Distal hilar bleeding is demanding to manage in mini-invasive surgery and can lead to open conversion.

After the division of the splenic artery, the splenic vein is dissected, ligated or clipped, and divided. The splenic vein can be sectioned with EndoWrist Stapler with vascular load if it has a large diameter. The risk of splenic vein thrombosis is related to the length and diameter of the splenic vein stump [14]. The splenic vein should be clipped and sectioned proximally.

33.9.4 Spleen Mobilization and Extraction

The spleen is not hanged only by the peritoneal lateral and posterior ligaments (the posterior sheet of the splenopancreatic and splenorenal ligament). The spleen is pulled cranially by tip-up in R3, and the assistant tractions, caudally, the Gerota's fascia. A suction/irrigator may be used to keep the operative field and obtain gentle tractions. The posterior peritoneal attachments of the spleen are sectioned in caudal to cephalad direction with scissors in R1 and bipolar forceps in R2.

An endobag is inserted through the assistant port for specimen extraction. The specimen is extracted after Da Vinci Xi's undocking with a Pfannenstiel laparotomy or after morcellation enlarging a trocar site.

Successively, a laparoscopic check should be performed, and a suction drain is left in the splenic lodge. Trocars are removed under vision.

33.9.5 Single-Port Robotic Splenectomy

SP surgery was reported in a few reports [16].

SP surgery can be performed with a single incision (usually Pfannenstiel incision) for removal of the intact spleen, eliminating the concern for splenosis. The SP consists of a flexible 3D camera and three flexible, interchangeable instruments, all of which pass through a 2.5-cm cannula. The instruments have mid-instrument flexion and can be manipulated immediately beyond the end of the cannula. Once deployed, the telescope and instruments are functional within a 7-cm-diameter space. This technology provides narrow, deep access, making it highly applicable to pediatric surgery.

A full array of interchangeable instruments is available for tissue manipulation, suturing, and cauterization. Notably, the SP allows the telescope to move in a full 180° arc without moving instruments relative to the tissue field, improving visualization in areas that previously were difficult to access. Finally, the robot can rotate in a complete 360° circle without changing ports, allowing the surgeon to access the complete abdomen.

33.9.6 Bench Surgery and Autotransplant

Robotic surgery allows safe and precise vascular anastomoses. Giulianotti et al. [17] reported a case of robotic splenectomy with ex vivo bench surgery and hemi-spleen autotransplant for a benign splenic cist not suitable for partial splenectomy. Mini-invasive partial splenectomy is considered technically challenging or impossible for very large cysts or cysts involving the splenic hilum. The proximal splenic artery and vein were dissected, clamped with bulldogs, and divided with a long proximal stump. A splenectomy was performed, and the specimen was extracted with a GelPort® (Applied Medical) installed through a small midline incision below the umbilicus.

The spleen was cooled with infusions at 4 °C and flushed with approximately 1.5 L of custodiol solution through the splenic artery until there was a clear flow from the splenic vein. The bench procedure started with the preparation of the hilum. Segmental arteries from the main splenic artery to the upper splenic pole containing most of the cyst were divided. The parenchymal transection was gradually performed until complete resection of the cyst. Hemostasis of the parenchymal transection plane was obtained with multiple Prolene 4-0 and 5-0 sutures. Finally, a row of 3/0 interrupted U-stitches with pledgets was placed on the transected capsule. A leak test with cooled custodiol solution through the splenic artery was performed before re-implantation to ensure good hemostasis after reperfusion. After the reintroduction in the abdominal cavity of the hemi-spleen through the midline GelPort®, arterial and venous reconstructions were performed robotically, using running 6-0 Gore-Tex suturing. Finally, indocyanine green fluorescence was used to assess splenic perfusion.

33.10 Hemisplenectomy

33.10.1 Indications

Selected benign diseases limited to a part of splenic parenchyma are suitable for robotic hemisplenectomy. Partial robotic splenectomy

seems to offer safety and all the benefits of minimally invasive surgery; it preserves the immune function of the spleen and allows the surgeon to conserve as much of the splenic parenchyma as possible [15]. The most important indications are:

- Non-parasitic cysts
- Benign tumors
- Splenic infarction
- Metastases.

33.10.2 Instruments, Patient Position, Patient's Cart, and Trocar Placement

Vessel sealer or harmonic scalpel in R2 may be used to section the spleen parenchyma after clipping and sectioning segmental vessels. Patient position, column, and trocar placement are the same as described above for splenectomy.

33.10.2.1 Critical Advice

It is important to mobilize just the part of spleen which should be removed. Ligaments tractioning the remaining part of the spleen should be preserved. This avoids splenic torsion and may ease section maneuvers.

33.10.2.2 Vessels' Dissection/ Devascularization

Two attitudes were mainly reported:

1. Division of splenic artery and vein, with the perfusion of the splenic remnant provided by collateral vessels (gastric vasa brevia/phrenic collateral vessels or left gastro-epiploic artery) [20–26], similar to Warshaw procedure when associated with distal pancreatectomy [27].

2. Division of branches from splenic vessels at the hilum of the spleen, those feeding the segment to resect [20, 26].

33.10.3 Description of the Step-by-Step Procedure

Gastrocolic ligament must be sectioned to access the lesser sac. Splenic flexure should be mobilized.

Splenic ligament mobilization should be arranged as follows based on the splenic pole to remove:

33.10.3.1 Inferior Pole Splenectomy

Section of splenocolic and phrenicocolic ligaments with R1 scissors.

33.10.3.2 Superior Pole Splenectomy

Section of lateral peritoneal adhesions and splenophrenic and posterior ligaments with R1 scissors.

33.10.3.3 Splenic Hilum Approach

Ligation of segmental vessels at the hilum is nowadays the most diffused approach. It implies the careful dissection of the splenic hilum in order to identify and severe the vessel tributary of the segment to be resected. The main technical point of regular partial splenectomy is the fine dissection and ligation of the second and third splenic pedicle vessels close to the spleen hilum, where each bundle is as small as possible while observing the spleen blood circulation. The splenic artery is dissected first with R1 scissors and R2 bipolar forceps and passed under with a loop as distally as possible for bleeding control. At this time, hilar dissection begins. All arterial branches based on anatomy and/or on intraoperative ICG test are identified and gently dissected with R1 scissors, R2 bipolar, and R1 needle holder. The same is performed for the venous branches. After the exposure of the arterial branches, vessels to preserve are identified and spared, while the other tributary vessels are ligated or clipped and sectioned.

33.11 Section of Parenchyma and Specimen Extraction

After the interruption of the vascular supply, splenic parenchyma usually shows a demarcation line.

This line may be identified with white light or fluorescence imaging system after the intravenous administration of 0,1 mg/kg on indocyanine green (ICG). The spleen is divided using the vessel sealer or the harmonic scalpel or bipolar forceps on R2. The section begins on the splenic capsule 1 cm below the demarcation line. Subsegmental arteries and veins may be skeletonized and clipped or sealed by vessel sealer. Hemostasis is carefully performed by bipolar forceps or hemostatic materials. Also, an omental flap could help the hemostasis of the remnant. The specimen is extracted with endobag enlarging a trocar site. A suction drain is left in place. The robot is undocked, and trocars are removed under laparoscopic vision.

33.12 Treatment of Splenic Artery Aneurisms (SAA)

33.12.1 Introduction

Splenic artery aneurysm (SAA) is the most frequently observed visceral artery aneurysm, with an incidence of 50–70% of all visceral aneurysms [18]. Usually, the indications for the treatment of SAA include symptomatic aneurysms and asymptomatic aneurysms >2 cm or detected in women who are pregnant or of childbearing age, in regard to the higher incidence of rupture observed in this group of patients [19]. The minimally invasive surgical technique has recently become a potential alternative to endovascular treatment when not feasible for technical or anatomical reasons. The intraoperative strategy depends on the following:

1. The specific vascular anatomy of the splenic hilum can be either magistral or distributive (see above in anatomy). In the first case, there is a higher probability that vascular anastomosis is needed to guarantee adequate spleen perfusion after the aneurysmectomy, whereas in the latter case, the arterial network provides valid collateral branches that ensure adequate spleen perfusion.
2. The localization of the aneurism when the SAA is proximal, close to the celiac trunk, or in the middle third of the artery, the flow is usually supplied by valid collateral branches, whereas when it is located at its distal third,

vascularization is usually supplied by branches from the splenic artery, short gastric vessels, or pancreatic branches, and it results in an insufficient spleen perfusion.

3. The modifications of the intrasplenic arterial flow recorded before and after the aneurysm resection.

33.12.2 Instruments

The instruments are the same as splenectomy with the addition of:

- -PTFE 0-5 sutures
- -Bulldog endoscopic clamps
- -Black Diamond needle holder
- -Microscissors
- -Hemostatic sealant patch
- -Endoscopic ecodoppler US.

33.12.3 Patient Position, Column, and Trocar Placement

Patient's position, column, and trocar placement are the same as splenectomy.

The surgical technique shares the same steps of splenectomy (see above) till the exposure of the splenic artery. After the identification and dissection of the splenic artery proximally and distally to the aneurysmatic sac, the small peripancreatic vessels arising from the splenic artery were isolated and coagulated, respecting the pancreatic parenchyma. Aneurysm is isolated, and proximal and distal vessel loops were placed to safely complete the vessel and aneurysm dissection and isolation. After intravenous administration of 5000 IU of heparin, vessel loops are temporarily replaced with two endoscopic bulldog clamps. The aneurysm is resected with robotic scissors, and the splenic artery is reconstructed by a double-running suture using PTFE 5-0 sutures using Black Diamond or a standard robotic needle holder in R1. After completing the anastomosis, an endoscopic ecodoppler US is performed to check the vessel patency flow. The hemostatic sealant patch is used to protect all

around the external suture rime. A suction drain is left in the perianastomotic area.

Robotic surgery has been widely demonstrated to represent an advantageous tool in complex vascular procedures as a result of the increased dexterity of movements due to a greater freedom of movements and elimination of the surgeon's tremor effect.

References

1. Giulianotti PC, Buchs NC, Addeo P, Ayloo S, Bianco FM. Robot-assisted partial and total splenectomy. Int J Med Robot. 2011;7:482–8.
2. Weledji EP. Benefits and risks of splenectomy. Int J Surg. 2014;12(2):113–9.
3. Misiakos EP, Bagias G, Liakakos T, Machairas A. Laparoscopic splenectomy: current concepts. World J Gastrointest Endosc. 2017;9(9):428–37.
4. Bagdasarian RW, Bolton JS, Bowden JC, Fuhrman GM, Richardson WS. Steep learning curve of laparoscopic splenectomy. J Laparoendosc Adv Surg Tech. 2009;10(6):319–23.
5. Corcione F, Pirozzi F, Aragiusto G, Galante F, Sciuto A. Laparoscopic splenectomy: experience of a single center in a series of 300 cases. Surg Endosc. 2012;26(10):2870–6.
6. Moris D, Dimitriou N, Griniatsos J. Laparoscopic splenectomy for benign hematological disorders in adults: a systematic review. In Vivo. 2017;31(3):291–302.
7. Patel AG, Parker JE, Wallwork B, Kau KB, Donaldson N, Rhodes MR, et al. Massive splenomegaly is associated with significant morbidity after laparoscopic splenectomy. Ann Surg. 2003;238(2):235–40.
8. Wysocki M, Radkowiak D, Zychowicz A, Rubinkiewicz M, Kulawik J, Major P, et al. Prediction of technical difficulties in laparoscopic splenectomy and analysis of risk factors for postoperative complications in 468 cases. J Clin Med. 2018;7(547):1–11.
9. Lane T. A short history of robotic surgery. Ann R Coll Surg Engl. 2018;100(6):5–7.
10. Sheetz KH, Claflin J, Dimick JB. Trends in the adoption of robotic surgery for common surgical procedures. JAMA Netw Open. 2020;3(1):1–9.
11. Szold A, Bergamaschi R, Broeders I, Dankelman J, Forgione A, Lango T, et al. European association of endoscopic surgeons (EAES) consensus statement on the use of robotics in general surgery. Surg Endosc. 2015;29:253–88.
12. Christo MC, Liberato JA. Di Dio, anatomical and surgical aspects of splenic segmentectomies, annals of anatomy. Anat Anz. 1997;179(5):461–74.
13. Bergman RA, Afifi AK, Miyauchi R. Splenic artery. Anatomy atlases: an anatomy digital library; 1995.
14. de Angelis N, Abdalla S, Lizzi V, Esposito F, Genova P, Roy L, Galacteros F, Luciani A, Brunetti F. Incidence

and predictors of portal and splenic vein thrombosis after pure laparoscopic splenectomy. Surgery. 2017;162(6):1219–30. https://doi.org/10.1016/j.surg.2017.07.016.

15. Vasilescu C, Tudor S, Popa M, Tiron A, Lupescu I. Robotic partial splenectomy for hydatid cyst of the spleen. Langenbeck's Arch Surg. 2010;395(8):1169–74.

16. Klazura G, Sims T, Rojnica M, Koo N. Thom lobe Single port robotic splenectomy for pyruvate kinase deficiency in a five–year-old patient, a case report of a surgical first. Int J Surg Case Rep. 2021;84:106122. https://doi.org/10.1016/j.ijscr.2021.106122.

17. Giulianotti PC, Daskalaki D, Gonzalez-Ciccarelli LF, Bianco FM, et al. J Robot Surg. 2017;11(2):243–6. https://doi.org/10.1007/s11701-016-0635-3.

18. Akbulut S, Otan E. Management of giant splenic artery aneurysm: comprehensive literature review. Medicine (Baltimore). 2015;94:e1016.

19. Yagmur Y, Akbulut S, Gumus S, et al. Giant splenic artery pseudoaneurysm: a case report and literature review. Int Surg. 2015;100:1244–8.

20. Rice HE, Oldham KT, Hillery CA, Skinner MA, O'Hara SM, Ware RE, et al. Ann Surg. 2003;237(2):281–8.

21. Sheikha AK, Salih ZT, Kasnazan KH, Khoshnaw MK, Al-Maliki T, Al-Azraqi TA, et al. Prevention of overwhelming postsplenectomy infection in thalassemia patients by partial rather than total splenectomy. Can J Surg. 2007;50(5):382–6.

22. Rosman CWK, Broens PMA, Trzpis M, Tamminga RYJ. A long-term follow-up study of subtotal splenectomy in children with hereditary spherocytosis. Pediatr Blood Cancer 2017;64(10).

23. Moorman DW, Evans DM, Wright DJ. Segmental splenectomy using the ultrasonic surgical aspirator. Am J Surg. 1988;155(2):266–7.

24. Sagar PM, McMahon MJ. Partial splenectomy for splenic cysts. Br J Surg. 1988;75(5):488.

25. Hall JG, Kurtzberg J, Szabolcs P, Skinner MA, Rice HE. Partial splenectomy before a hematopoietic stem cell transplantation in children. J Pediatr Surg. 2005;40(1):221–7.

26. Vasilescu C, Stanciulea O, Tudor S. Laparoscopic versus robotic subtotal splenectomy in hereditary spherocytosis. Potential advantages and limits of an expensive approach. Surg Endosc. 2012;26(10):2802–9.

27. Warshaw AL. Conservation of the spleen with distal pancreatectomy. Arch Surg. 1988;123(5):550–3.

Laparoscopic Treatment of Duodenal Cephalic Pancreatic Tumors

34

Giuseppe Boccia, Pasquale Ruberto, and Francesco Corcione

34.1 Introduction of Pancreas Cancer

Worldwide pancreatic cancer is considered the twelfth most common cancer and the seventh leading cause of death, and its 5-year survival rate is about 12% [1]. To date, it remains a critical global burden of disease due to its aggressive nature and poor survival rate; unfortunately, both incidence and mortality rates are stable or slightly increasing in the last few years [2]. Unfortunately, patients with pancreatic head cancer have subtle symptoms, which do not always allow early identification of the tumor; therefore, surgery remains a cornerstone in the treatment of pancreatic cancer. Moreover, the number of patients at the resectable stage is minimal. Although computed tomography (CT) and magnetic resonance imaging (MRI) remain the best modality to stage the tumor for resectability [3], laparoscopic exploration and laparoscopic ultrasonography can be considered the last step for the stadiation of this disease. Resection of the pancreatic head, also known as the Whipple procedure, is one of the most difficult surgical procedures in gastrointestinal surgery, requiring not only an excellent knowledge of upper abdominal cavity abnormalities but also the ability to preoperatively assess the severity of the disease [4]. Due to its complex nature, the use of this procedure has historically been associated with a high rate of perioperative morbidity and mortality [5]. However, recent studies regarding feasibility and postoperative outcomes have suggested that the laparoscopic approach to pancreatoduodenectomy is associated with shorter hospital stays, better lymph node dissection, and less blood loss when compared with the results of an open approach [6]. Despite this, the possibility of a laparotomic conversion must always be considered due to the onset of intraoperative complications or unknown anatomical variables. For these reasons, laparoscopic duodenopancreatectomy is the prerogative of highly experienced surgeons and is reserved for reference centers in particular with experience in the hepato-biliary-pancreatic field.

34.2 Anatomy and Physiology

The pancreas is a retroperitoneal organ and lies within the C-shaped loop of the duodenum. It is divided into the head, uncinate process, neck, body, and tail. The head and uncinate process of the pancreas receives blood from the superior and inferior pancreaticoduodenal arteries and by branches of the gastroduodenal artery and middle

G. Boccia · P. Ruberto
Department of Public Health, University of Naples Federico II, Naples, Italy

F. Corcione (✉)
Chief of General Minimally Invasive Oncology Surgery, Clinica Mediterranea, Naples, Italy
e-mail: francesco.corcione@clinicamediterranea.it

© The Author(s), under exclusive license to Springer Nature Switzerland AG 2024
M. Milone et al. (eds.), *Scrub Nurse in Minimally Invasive and Robotic General Surgery*,
https://doi.org/10.1007/978-3-031-42257-7_34

colic artery. Instead, the neck, body, and tail are supplied by the splenic artery via the dorsal pancreatic artery, transverse, and greater pancreatic arteries. The pancreatic head is primarily drained by the four pancreaticoduodenal veins, which drain into the superior mesenteric vein (SMV) or portal vein (PV). The neck, body, and tail have venous drainage into the splenic vein. The main pancreatic duct (Wirsung) begins in the tail, runs lengthwise through the pancreas, and opens into the second part of the duodenum together with the bile duct at the major duodenal papilla.

There are different critical anatomical points in pancreatic surgery to take into account. The same blood supply to the pancreas is shared with the duodenal C-loop, necessitating the removal of the duodenal C-loop along with the pancreas. The neck of the pancreas lies behind the confluence of the portal vein and is also the origin of the superior mesenteric artery (SMA). SMV is located to the right of SMA; thus, SMV is the first vascular structure encountered in the duodenal curvature. The splenic artery runs along the superior border of the pancreas. On the other hand, the splenic vein runs posteriorly through the body of the pancreas.

34.3 Indication and Contraindication for Duodenopancreatectomy

To perform duodenopancreatectomy, there are some indications to consider:

- Cancers located at the head of the pancreas.
- The pancreatic neuroendocrine tumors (PNETs).
- The gastrointestinal stromal tumor (GIST).
- The intraductal papillary mucinous neoplasms (IPMN).
- Periampullary cancer which includes distal bile duct cholangiocarcinoma (DBDC).
- The adenocarcinoma of the ampulla of Vater.
- The duodenal adenocarcinoma.
- Chronic pancreatitis with the inflammatory mass in the head of the pancreas.
- Severe pancreatic trauma [7].

As far as contraindications are concerned, it must be considered that the procedure depends on a variable number of factors. The most important is the patient's performance status since it is a very demolitive operation and above all the tumor resectability criteria. National Comprehensive Cancer Network (NCCN) defines three grades of resectability for pancreatic ductal adenocarcinoma: resectable, borderline resectable, and unresectable [8].

34.3.1 Resectable

Absence of distant metastases. Absence of infiltration of celiac axis (CA), superior mesenteric artery (SMA), or common hepatic artery (CHA). There is no contact of the tumor with the superior mesenteric vein or portal vein or contact $\leq 180°$ without vein contour irregularity.

34.3.2 Borderline Resectable

Solid tumor contact with CHA without extension to celiac axis or hepatic artery bifurcation allowing for safe and complete resection and reconstruction. Solid tumor contact with the SMA of $\leq 180°$. Solid tumor contact with variant arterial anatomy (e.g., accessory right hepatic artery, replaced right hepatic artery, replaced CHA, and the origin of replaced or accessory artery), and the presence and degree of tumor contact should be noted if present as it may affect surgical planning. Solid tumor contact with the SMV or PV of $>180°$ and contact of $\leq 180°$ with contour irregularity of the vein or thrombosis of the vein but with suitable vessel proximal and distal to the site of involvement allowing for safe and complete resection and vein reconstruction. Solid tumor contact with the inferior vena cava (IVC).

34.3.3 Unresectable for Head Tumor

Distant metastasis (including nonregional lymph node metastasis). Solid tumor contact with SMA $>180°$. Solid tumor contact with the CA $>180°$ IVC involvement. Aortic involvement. Irreparable occlusion of SMV or PV.

34.4 Perioperative Management

The role of the anesthesiologist is of fundamental importance given the duration of the procedure, to ensure good anesthesia, timely monitoring of all physiological parameters, and a prompt response in the event of unexpected blood loss. Intravenous antibiotics are given before the skin incision. The administration of octreotide depends on the preference of the surgeon.

Postoperatively, the presence of an experienced nutritionist for glucose management and a diabetes endocrinologist is important because adequate insulin therapy is required after pancreatic resection.

34.5 Positioning and Operating Room Information

34.5.1 Laparoscopic Instruments

Table 34.1 describes the tools needed for the laparoscopic procedure. It is good practice to have an open surgery instrumentation already for a possible conversion.

34.5.2 Patient Positioning and Operating Room Setup

The patient is placed supine on the operating table, with the legs spread apart and the arms along the body. Care is taken to adequately secure the patient with a thigh belt to the operating table. It is essential to guarantee the stability of the patient since the table must allow Trendelenburg and anti-Trendelenburg positions up to 35 degrees, the same as right or left laterality, in different phases of the procedure to favor the exposure of the organs during the dissection and the tissue reconstruction. It is advisable to use two monitors, positioned on both sides of the patient's head. Furthermore, the ultrasound with laparoscopic probe is essential to carry out perioperative abdominal exploration and to intraoperatively evaluate any infiltration of the vascular axis.

Table 34.1 Necessary instruments for the laparoscopic surgery

Instruments	No.
Veress needle	1
Hasson trocar 10–12 mm	1
Trocar 10–12 mm	2
Trocar 5 mm	1
10 mm 30° laparoscopes	1
Johann fenestrated grasper 5 mm	3
Laparoscopic energy device 5 mm	1
Laparoscopic bipolar forceps 5 mm	1
Laparoscopic scissors 5 mm	1
Laparoscopic dissecting forceps 10 mm	1
Laparoscopic need holder 10 mm	1
Laparoscopic suction irrigator 5 mm	1
Laparoscopic bulldog clamp	1
Vessel loops 1.2–2.5 mm	3
Endoscopic clip 5–10-12 mm clip applier 1	1
Laparoscopic endobag	1
Endoscopic stapler 60 mm	1
Stent 4–8 Fr	2
Surgical drains 19 Fr	2
Prolene 5-0 blue 36" C-1 needle	NA
Surgipro II 4-0 36" CV-23 needle	NA
Suture PDS 4-0 RB-1	NA
Suture V LOC 3–0 P-14 18" 180	NA

NA not applicable

34.5.3 Position of Surgeons

The surgeon is positioned between the patient's legs, the first assistant, who operates the camera, is on the right side of the patient, and in relation to the different steps of the operation, he will be placed on the right or left of the operating surgeon. The second assistant is to the patient's left. The scrub nurse positions himself to the patient's left (Fig. 34.1).

34.5.4 Positioning of the Trocars

Access is performed with an open Veress-assisted technique. Usually, four to six trocars are used, and this depends on the intraoperative needs. The first 10–12 mm trocar is inserted at a supraumbilical level in the midline and will be the optical trocar. The right-hand 10–12 mm trocar is placed in the left hypochondrium just above the optic

Fig. 34.1 Position of surgeons. The present figure represents the position of the surgeon (dark blue circle), the assistant (blue circle), and the scrub nurse (orange circle)

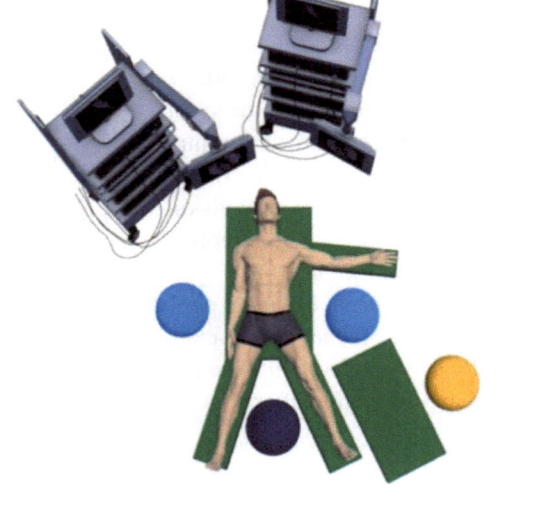

SURGEON   ASSISTANT   SCRUB NURSE

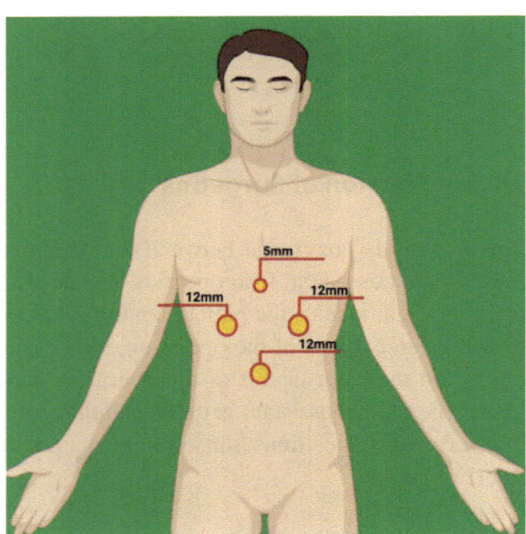
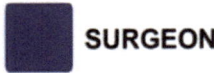
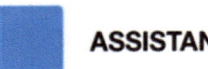

Fig. 34.2 Trocars position

trocar, on the left mammary line. The 10–12 mm left-hand trocar is placed on the right breast line a few cm higher than the right-hand trocar. Finally, the 5-mm assistant's trocar is placed in the subxiphoid position (Fig. 34.2).

34.6 Technique

34.6.1 Exploration of the Abdominal Cavity

The first phase involves exploration of the abdominal cavity to evaluate the resectability of the tumor and identify any distant metastases. Occult metastases have been identified in up to 30% of patients undergoing diagnostic laparoscopy [9]. The peritoneum, the main lymph node stations, the liver, the gastro-colic ligament, and the lesser omentum are explored. In this phase, intraoperative echolaparoscopy may be useful. Then, we move on to the section of the gastro-colic ligament. The table is tilted in reverse Trendelenburg by about 25 degrees; the assistant pulls the greater omentum upward to expose the greater gastric curvature. Thanks to an ultrasound dissector, the gastro-colic ligament is sectioned in the cranial direction and lateral to medial directions. In this way, the posterior gastric wall is freed which will allow a complete exposure of the pancreas (Fig. 34.3). The next step is the cre-

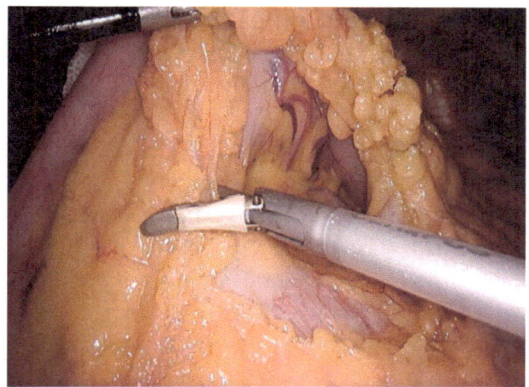

Fig. 34.3 Opening of the gastro-colic ligament

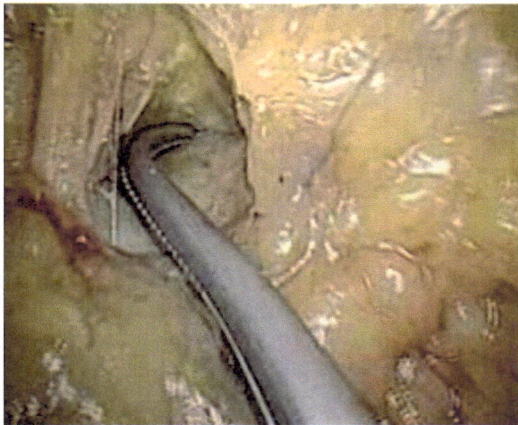

Fig. 34.4 Identification of the superior mesenteric vein

ation of the retro-pancreatic tunnel. We proceed to the identification of the superior mesenteric vein (SMV). Blunt dissection is performed by progressively separating the posterior aspect of the pancreatic neck from the SMV until the confluence between the SMV vein and the splenic vein is identified. This dissection takes place in an avascular plane and in this phase, laparoscopy offers a magnified view which is a huge advantage over a traditional approach (Fig. 34.4). At the end of the creation of the tunnel, the pancreas is passed under with a tape which will be used for the exposure maneuvers for its subsequent transection. In this way, it is possible to understand whether the superior mesenteric vessels are involved in the neoplasm. At this point, complete staging can be achieved.

34.6.2 Stomach Transection

If the operation is considered feasible, it is possible to proceed with the section of the stomach. To do this, the lesser gastric curve is prepared by opening the hepatogastric ligament. Once the stomach has been skeletonized, it is sectioned using a linear stapler, introduced by the 10-mm trocar. To improve hemostasis on the gastric suture line, a bioabsorbable reinforcement device can be used which is applied to the stapler (Fig. 34.5).

34.6.3 Preparation of the Hepatic Peduncle and Section of the Gastroduodenal Artery

By suspending the gallbladder upward, the assistant exposes the hepatic stalk, allowing the surgeon to perform lymphadenectomy of it. This maneuver can be performed with the ultrasound dissector or with the monopolar hook. To have good exposure of the structures that are isolated (right and left hepatic artery, main bile duct), it is possible to highlight them with vessel loops (Fig. 34.6). This dissection allows us to identify the gastroduodenal artery (GDA) which is isolated and dissected between metal clips. At this point, retrograde cholecystectomy is performed, after having opened the

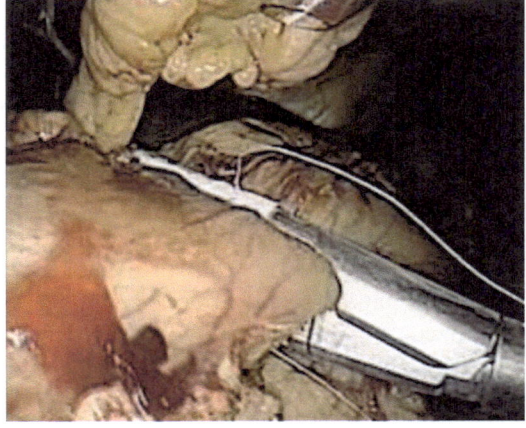

Fig. 34.5 Transection of stomach

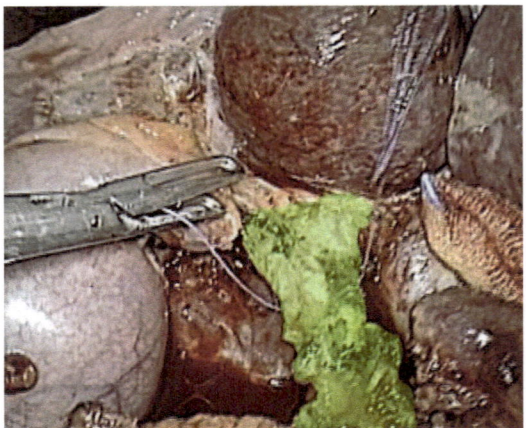

Fig. 34.6 Preparation of the common bile duct

triangle of Calot and sectioning the cystic duct and cystic artery between metal clips. The gallbladder is then placed in a bag on the right side of the abdomen to be removed at the end of the procedure. The common bile duct is then clamped, which can be performed using a bulldog clamp and its section with a cold blade immediately above the emergence of the cystic duct.

34.6.4 Mobilization of the Duodenum (Kocher's Maneuver)

The hepatic flexure and the proximal transverse colon are mobilized medially and downwards, after dissecting the hepatocolic ligament. This allows complete exposure of II and III duodenal portions. An extended Kocher maneuver is performed to allow medialization of the duodenum and pancreas from the posterior avascular plane usually using blunt dissection (e.g., using the aspirator) to allow identification of the inferior vena cava, aorta, and mesenteric superior artery. This maneuver continues until the lower duodenal knee is mobilized. At this time, it is necessary to dissect the right gastroepiploic vein and the inferior anterior pancreaticoduodenal vein.

34.6.5 Preparation of the Treitz and Section of the First Jejunal Loop

At this point, the ligament of Treitz is identified, thanks to the assistant who pulls the transverse mesocolon upward, and its complete dissection is performed. The transection of the first jejunal loop is performed about 5–7 cm from the Treitz, with a laparoscopic linear stapler, after having created a window in its meso with the ultrasound dissector.

A crucial maneuver of this procedure is then carried out, namely the passage of the dissected jejunal loop from left to right, in a retroperitoneal plane, passing under the mesenteric vessels (Fig. 34.7).

34.6.6 Preparation and Section of the Pancreas

The transection of the pancreas is then performed with the use of the ultrasound scalpel and bipolar forceps especially for the control of the pancreaticoduodenal arteries. The cut line usually falls to the left of the confluence of the superior mesenteric vein with the splenic vein.

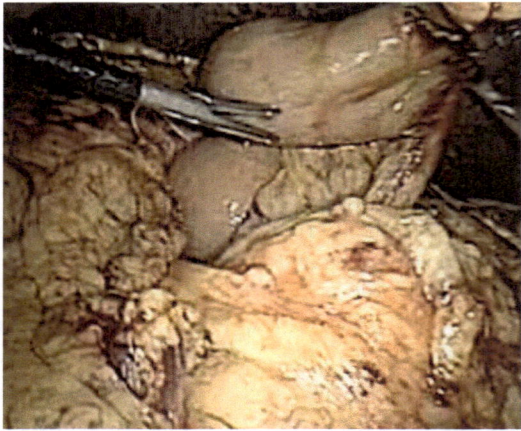

Fig. 34.7 Passage of the first jejunal loop from left to right, in a retroperitoneal plane

34.6.7 Complete Mobilization of the Duodeno-Pancreatic Bloc and Lymphadenectomy

To complete the release of the duodeno-pancreatic bloc, attention is paid to the dissection of the uncinate process from the superior mesenteric vessels. In this phase, the section of the retroportal lamina is carried out, with an ultrasound dissector and bipolar forceps. The assistant can use the aspirator to keep the field bloodless. Upon completion of the demolition phase, lymphadenectomy of stations 16 and 16b is performed, removing the paracaval, interaortocaval, and paraaortic lymph nodes. Previously, together with the removal of the distal part of the stomach, the lymph nodes of the right gastroepiploic vessels (station 4d), the lymph nodes of the right gastric artery (station 5), and those sub-pyloric (station 6) were removed. Instead, with the dissection of the hepatoduodenal ligament and the hepatic peduncle, the lymph nodes of the common hepatic artery (stations 8a and 8p), the proper hepatic artery (station 12a), the bile duct (12b), and the portal vein were removed (12p).

The reconstructive phase in surgery is a real challenge for the surgeon. Gastrointestinal and biliary transit is re-established by making four anastomoses.

34.6.8 Wirsung-Jejunal or Pancreatic-Jejunal Anastomosis

The first anastomosis is the one between the pancreas and the jejunum. It is possible to perform a Wirsung-jejunal anastomosis if there is a dilation of the Wirsung duct which allows the insertion of a guide stent inside it. In this case, an end-to-side, duct-to-mucosa pancreatic-jejunal anastomosis is then performed by bringing the free jejunal loop close to the pancreatic remnant. This begins with the construction of the posterior anastomotic row, which is contoured using a single layer 5–0 barbed suture. Then, a 2–3 mm jejunostomy is performed to allow for a duct-to-mucosa anastomosis, after inserting a stent (usually between 4

and 8 French) into the main pancreatic duct, which will serve as a temporary guide for reconstruction. Once the pancreatic duct is secured to the jejunal mucosa with a synthetic non-absorbable 5-0 Prolene suture, the pancreatic duct stent is passed through the jejunal defect and an anastomosis between the duct and the mucosa is completed using five or six additional 5-0 synthetic non-absorbable sutures in an interrupted manner. Finally, the anterior wall of the anastomosis is completed with a 5-0 Prolene suture (Fig. 34.8). The alternative is pancreatic-jejunal anastomosis, which can be considered when the Wirsung is of a small caliber. In this case, an end-to-side anastomosis between the jejunum and the pancreatic stump is then performed.

34.6.9 Choledochojejunostomy

The second anastomosis is a common bile duct-jejunum anastomosis performed approximately 40–50 cm from the first anastomosis. Also, in this case it is customary to insert a stent into the biliary tract to be used as a guide. An end-to-side ductus-to-mucosal choledochojejunostomy anastomosis is then performed using 4–0 interrupted slow-resorbing synthetic sutures, passing through the main bile duct to its full thickness and completing the posterior wall first and then the anterior wall.

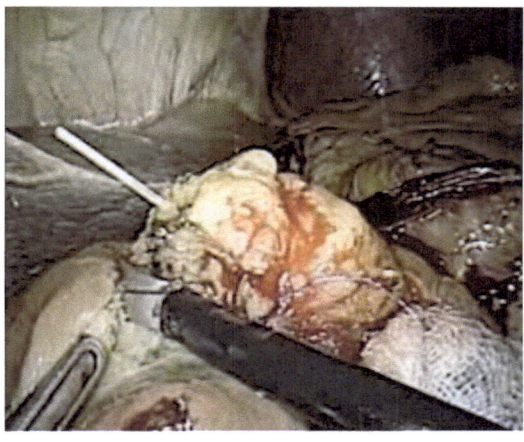

Fig. 34.8 Wirsung-Jejunal anastomosis

34.6.10 Gastro-Jejunal and Jejuno-Jejunal Anastomosis

So, a gastro-jejunal and jejuno-jejunal anastomosis are made, thus creating a Roux-en-Y reconstruction. The gastro-jejunal anastomosis is performed by cutting a jejunal loop about 60 cm from the bile duct-jejunal anastomosis and bringing it to the supramesocolic region via the antecolic route. After bringing the loop to the posterior wall of the gastric stump, anastomosis can be performed with a linear stapler, closing the enterotomy with slow resorption of 3–0 stitches. A nasogastric tube is usually placed through the anastomosis to perform a methylene air-blue test.

Finally, a jejunum-jejunum anastomosis is made in the sub-mesocolic region, with a linear stapler and closing the enterotomy with 3–0 slow-resorbing stitches (Fig. 34.9).

At the end of the reconstructive phase, the abdominal cavity is carefully washed, and hemostasis is performed if necessary. A drain is placed near the pancreatic-jejunum and gastric-jejunal anastomosis, and a second drain is placed near the common bile duct-jejunum anastomosis. Both drains can be placed through the 10–12 mm trocar holes. The resected part and the removed gallbladder are brought out via a suprapubic mini laparotomy, after being placed in a laparoscopic endobag.

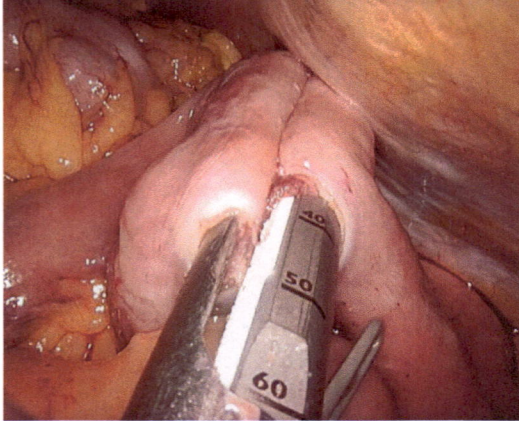

Fig. 34.9 Jejunojejunal anastomosis

34.6.11 Postoperative Management

Once the procedure is complete, the patient usually is transferred directly to the intensive care unit for about 24 h. During the initial phase of recovery, it is important to focus primarily on obtaining appropriate resuscitation with infusion therapy, pain control, and close blood glucose monitoring (i.e., <180 mg/dL). On postoperative day (POD) 1, the patient is transferred to the surgical department, continuous telemetry monitoring is performed, and early mobilization is encouraged. In addition, a diet of small, frequent, low-fat, high-carb, high-protein meals should be placed after channeling and can usually be initiated with POD 4. In the absence of serious complications, the patient can be discharged from the hospital in POD 6.

References

1. Huang J, Lok V, Ngai CH, Zhang L, Yuan J, Lao XQ, Ng K, Chong C, Zheng ZJ, Wong MCS. Worldwide burden of, risk factors for, and trends in pancreatic cancer. Gastroenterology. 2021;160:744–54.
2. Arnold M, Abnet CC, Neale RE, Vignat J, Giovannucci EL, McGlynn KA, Bray F. Global burden of 5 major types of gastrointestinal cancer. Gastroenterology. 2020;159:335–349.e15.
3. Muniraj T, Barve P. Laparoscopic staging and surgical treatment of pancreatic cancer. N Am J Med Sci. 2013;5:1–9.
4. Masiak-Segit W, Rawicz-Pruszyński K, Skórzewska MPW. Surgical treatment of pancreatic cancer. Pol Przegl Chir. 2018;90:45–53.
5. Jiang YL, Zhang RC, Zhou YC. Comparison of overall survival and perioperative outcomes of laparoscopic pancreaticoduodenectomy and open pancreaticoduodenectomy for pancreatic ductal adenocarcinoma: a systematic review and meta-analysis. BMC Cancer. 2019;19:1–9.
6. Asbun HJ, Stauffer JA. Laparoscopic vs open pancreaticoduodenectomy: overall outcomes and severity of complications using the accordion severity grading system. J Am Coll Surg. 2012;215:810–9.
7. D'Cruz JR, Misra S, Shamsudeen S. Pancreaticoduodenectomy. StatPearls; 2023.
8. Tempero MA, Malafa MP, Al-Hawary M, et al. Pancreatic adenocarcinoma, version 2.2017: clinical practice guidelines in oncology. J Natl Compr Cancer Netw. 2017;15:1028–61.
9. Tan-Tam C, Segedi M, Chung SW. Whipple procedure: patient selection and special considerations. Open Access Surg. 2016;9:51–63.

Robotic Treatment of Duodenocephalopancreatic Tumors

35

Ugo Boggi and Cesare Gianfaldoni

35.1 Pancreatoduodenectomy and its Variants

A pancreatoduodenectomy (PD) involves the removal of the head of the pancreas, duodenum, bile duct, gallbladder, pylorus, and gastric antrum (PD according to Whipple), or with preservation of the pylorus and stomach (PD according to Longmire-Traverso). It is considered one of the most complex abdominal operations with a mortality rate of 3% and a morbidity rate of 40–50% at 90 days [1]. These high rates are justified only for pathologies characterized by high aggressiveness, symptoms, or lethality. The main indications for a PD are neoplasms or pathologies with a high risk of neoplastic degeneration of the head/uncinate process of the pancreas, the distal bile duct, the duodenum, or the periampullary region. In some cases, a PD can also be justified for highly symptomatic benign pathologies such as chronic pancreatitis of the head of the pancreas [2]. A PD can be performed in an open or laparoscopic modality, and current evidence shows that a robotic pancreaticoduodenectomy (RPD) is feasible with a safety profile equivalent to either an open or laparoscopic pancreaticoduodenectomy [3].

The pancreaticoduodenectomy is a complex surgical operation for several reasons:

1. It involves many steps on multiple visceral structures in a small region, requiring a lot of time and effort without losing concentration.
2. The consistency of the parenchyma and the anatomical location of the pancreas pose challenges, including the buttery texture and the close relationship with vessels such as the superior mesenteric vein and artery, the portal vein, and the hepatic artery.
3. An extensive lymphadenectomy is required in cases of neoplastic pathology [4].
4. The reconstructive phase is complex, as the continuity of the digestive tract must be re-established through three anastomoses (pancreaticojejunal/pancreatic-gastric anastomosis, hepaticojejunal anastomosis, and gastrojejunostomy/duodenojejunal anastomosis).
5. There is the possibility of having to perform vascular resections and reconstructions [5].
6. The treatment of possible complications, especially pancreatic fistula, adds further complexity to the procedure [6].

U. Boggi · C. Gianfaldoni (✉)
Division of General and Transplant Surgery,
University of Pisa, Pisa, Italy
e-mail: u.boggi@med.unipi.it;
cesaregianfaldoni@uslnordovest.toscana.it

© The Author(s), under exclusive license to Springer Nature Switzerland AG 2024
M. Milone et al. (eds.), *Scrub Nurse in Minimally Invasive and Robotic General Surgery*,
https://doi.org/10.1007/978-3-031-42257-7_35

35.2 Robotic Pancreaticoduodenectomy Surgical Steps

In accordance with the aim of this book, we will describe the robotic approach to the RPD procedure.

1. Induction of pneumoperitoneum through Veress needle or open technique. After positioning the camera's port at the level of the umbilicus, exploratory laparoscopy is performed using the robotic camera to confirm tumor resectability, absence of metastases, and the absence of any unexpected pathology. In the case of unexpected lesions, a biopsy is performed. Next, four additional ports are placed along a straight line above the umbilicus. The patient cart is then moved to the left of the patient, and docking is performed.

2. The liver is hung to the anterior abdominal wall by several sutures (Fig. 35.1).

3. Dissection of the hepatoduodenal ligament: The common bile duct, hepatic artery, and portal vein are identified and exposed, even by endoloop. The bile duct is marked with yellow, the arteries with red, and the veins with blue.

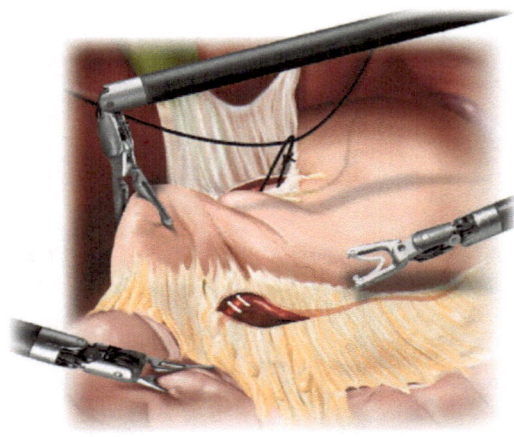

Fig. 35.2 Opening of the gastrocolic ligament from left to right until the right colonic flexure is mobilized. Identification, dissection, closure and division of the right gastroepiploic vessels. *Boggi, U., Perrone, V.G., Vistoli, F. (2018). Robotic Pancreatoduodenectomy. In: Boggi, U. (eds) Minimally Invasive Surgery of the Pancreas. Updates in Surgery. Springer, Milano.* https://doi.org/10.1007/978-88-470-3958-2_26

4. The gastroduodenal artery, which originates from the inferior surface of the hepatic artery, is identified, dissected, double-ligated, and divided.

5. The bile duct is divided between ligatures or a clip to prevent bile spillage during the procedure, and a swab is taken for culture. The frozen margin is sent for frozen-section histology.

6. The gastrocolic ligament is opened by proceeding from left to right until the right colonic flexure is mobilized. Then, the right gastroepiploic vessels are identified, dissected, clipped by Hem-o-lok, and divided (Fig. 35.2).

7. The first part of the duodenum is divided with a laparoscopic stapler loaded with a vascular cartridge.

8. The pancreatic neck is separated from the superior mesenteric/portal vein, and stay sutures are placed at the inferior and superior border of the gland. The gland is divided using a harmonic scalpel. The main pancreatic duct must be identified and cut sharply by robotic scissors, and the pancreatic margin is sent for frozen-section histology (Fig. 35.3).

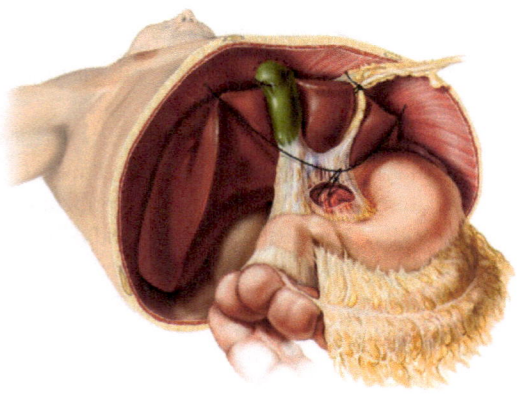

Fig. 35.1 The liver is hung to the anterior abdominal wall by several sutures. *Boggi, U., Perrone, V.G., Vistoli, F. (2018). Robotic Pancreatoduodenectomy. In: Boggi, U. (eds) Minimally Invasive Surgery of the Pancreas. Updates in Surgery. Springer, Milano.* https://doi.org/10.1007/978-88-470-3958-2_26

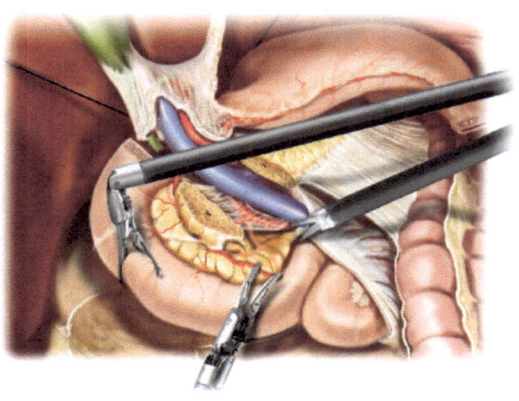

Fig. 35.3 Division of the gland by Harmonic Scalpel, division of the main pancreatic duct by robotic scissors. A frozen-section histology of the pancreatic margin is sent. *Boggi, U., Perrone, V.G., Vistoli, F. (2018). Robotic Pancreatoduodenectomy. In: Boggi, U. (eds) Minimally Invasive Surgery of the Pancreas. Updates in Surgery. Springer, Milano.* https://doi.org/10.1007/978-88-470-3958-2_26

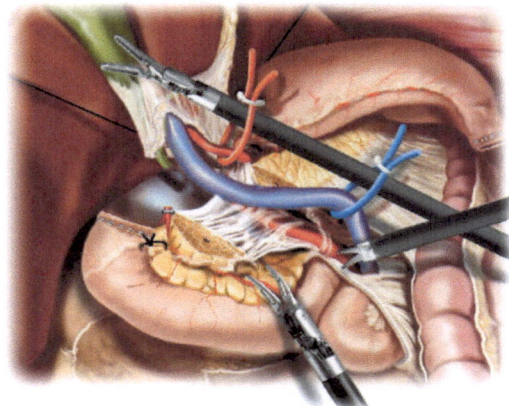

Fig. 35.4 Mesopancreas dissection. *Boggi, U., Perrone, V.G., Vistoli, F. (2018). Robotic Pancreatoduodenectomy. In: Boggi, U. (eds) Minimally Invasive Surgery of the Pancreas. Updates in Surgery. Springer, Milano.* https://doi.org/10.1007/978-88-470-3958-2_26

9. Duodenal kocherization: This involves the dissection of the duodenum-pancreas head block from the anterior surface of the inferior vena cava in a latero-medial direction until the left renal vein is visible.

10. The first jejunal loop is retracted to the right of the superior mesenteric vessels, and the jejunal mesentery is divided using a harmonic scalpel.

11. Mesopancreas dissection: The posterior margin of the pancreas is dissected along the periadventitial plane of the superior mesenteric artery with pancreaticoduodenal vessel ligation (Fig. 35.4).

12. The dissection phase is complete, and the specimen is free after cutting the first jejunal loop using a laparoscopic stapler loaded with a vascular cartridge (Fig. 35.5).

13. Three anastomoses are performed:

    (a) The pancreaticojejunal anastomosis can be performed in multiple ways. We typically do a duct-to-mucosa anastomosis using ePTFE 4/0 for the U-sutures and Polydioxanone 5/0 for the duct-to-mucosa a. In case the pancreatic parenchyma is too soft, a pancreatic-gastric anastomosis is done using Prolene 5/0.

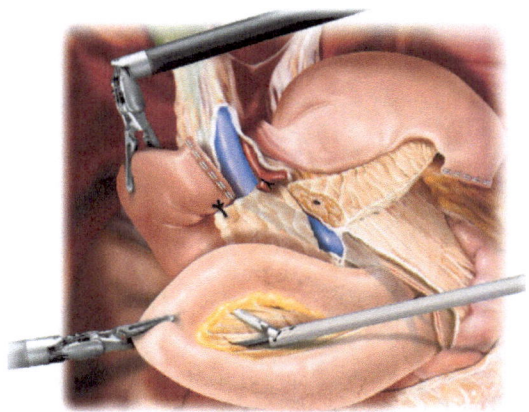

Fig. 35.5 Completion of the dissection phase after cutting the first jejunal loop. *Boggi, U., Perrone, V.G., Vistoli, F. (2018). Robotic Pancreatoduodenectomy. In: Boggi, U. (eds) Minimally Invasive Surgery of the Pancreas. Updates in Surgery. Springer, Milano.* https://doi.org/10.1007/978-88-470-3958-2_26

Sometimes, a stent is used in the Wirsung duct (Fig. 35.6).

    (b) The hepaticojejunal anastomosis is usually done in a single or double layer using half-running 5/0 polydioxanone.

    (c) The gastrojejunostomy/duodenojejunal anastomosis is done in two layers, with the outer layer typically using linen 3/0 and the inner layer using Vicryl 3/0.

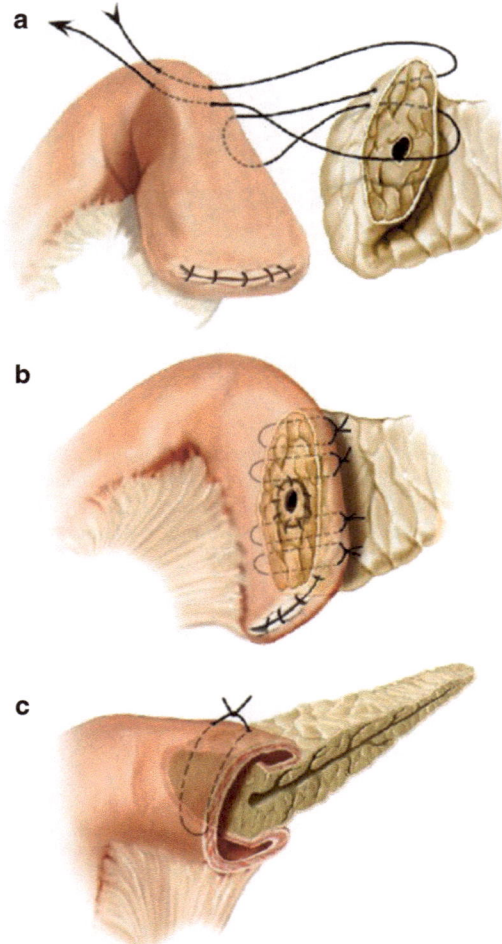

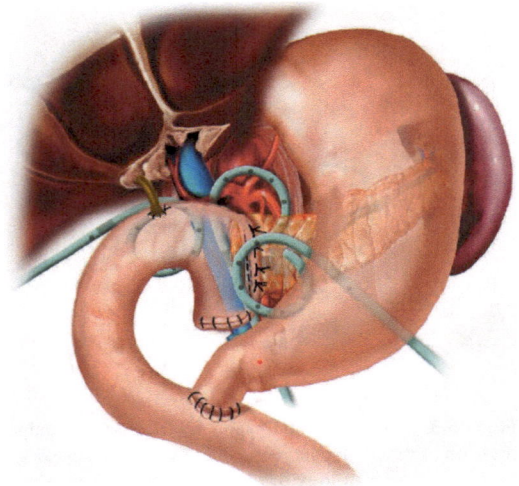

Fig. 35.7 Final view of the operating field. *Boggi, U., Perrone, V.G., Vistoli, F. (2018). Robotic Pancreatoduodenectomy. In: Boggi, U. (eds) Minimally Invasive Surgery of the Pancreas. Updates in Surgery. Springer, Milano.* https://doi. org/10.1007/978-88-470-3958-2_26

35.3 Patient Positioning and Preparation

To prepare for the procedure, the patient is positioned supine with legs apart, and the table is oriented at a 25° reverse Trendelenburg and tilted to the left. The arms are extended along the body (Fig. 35.8). To prevent the patient from slipping during the anti-Trendelenburg position, a vacuum silicone ball mattress is used, and a saddle is formed in the perineal area. The operative field includes the neck (usually the left lateral aspect to provide quick access to the external jugular vein in case of vascular reconstructions), thorax, abdomen, and roots of the thighs (access point to the saphenous veins, also in case of vascular reconstructions). Two sterile towels are used for the legs, one for each side of the patient, one for the caudal part of the sterile field, and one for the cranial one with the predisposition to use Rochard's retractor if conversion is necessary. The entire operating field is protected with a Steri-Drape.

Fig. 35.6 A modified Blumgart anastomosis. (**a**) first step of the mBlumgart anastomosis (**b**) When the anastomosis is completed, the jejunum moves to wrap over the pancreatic stump (**c**) The pancreatojejunostomy needs to be perfected at the upper and lower margins around the entire perimeter *Boggi, U., Perrone, V.G., Vistoli, F. (2018). Robotic Pancreatoduodenectomy. In: Boggi, U. (eds) Minimally Invasive Surgery of the Pancreas. Updates in Surgery. Springer, Milano.* https://doi. org/10.1007/978-88-470-3958-2_26

14. The specimen is removed through a Pfannenstiel incision, and hemostasis is achieved. Drain placement is performed, and we typically use two pigtail catheters (14 Ch). The wounds are then closed (Fig. 35.7) [7].

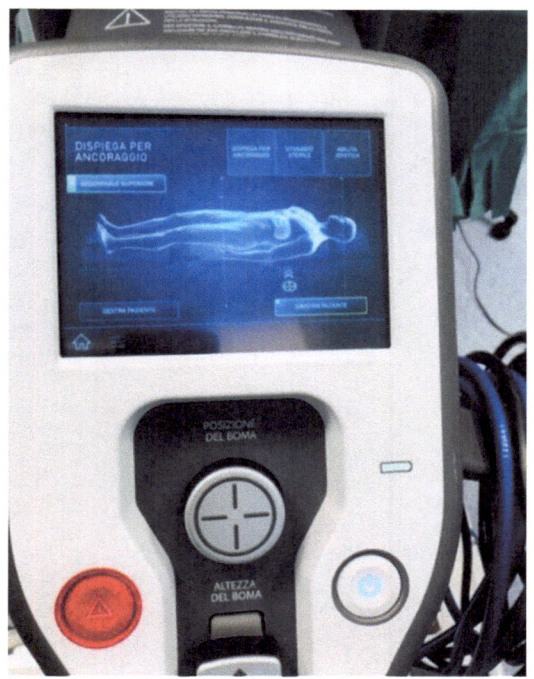

Fig. 35.8 Patient cart. *Our operatory room*

Prior to the procedure, 1–2 peripheral venous accesses are placed, and if necessary, even a central venous catheter (on the right side of the neck) is inserted. Finally, a nasogastric tube, bladder catheter, arterial access for invasive blood pressure measurement, and oximeter are also placed.

35.4 Operating Room Setup

The console is positioned at the foot of the patient, allowing the operating surgeon to maintain direct visual contact with the surgeons at the table. The assistant surgeon stands between the patient's legs, and one or two surgical assistants or residents assist with instrument exchange. The scrub nurse and instrument table are situated behind the patient to maintain a sterile environment.

When using the Xi system, the robotic tower is positioned to the left of the patient, while the vision cart, generators, and AirSeal System are located on the right side of the patient (Figs. 35.9, 35.10, 35.11).

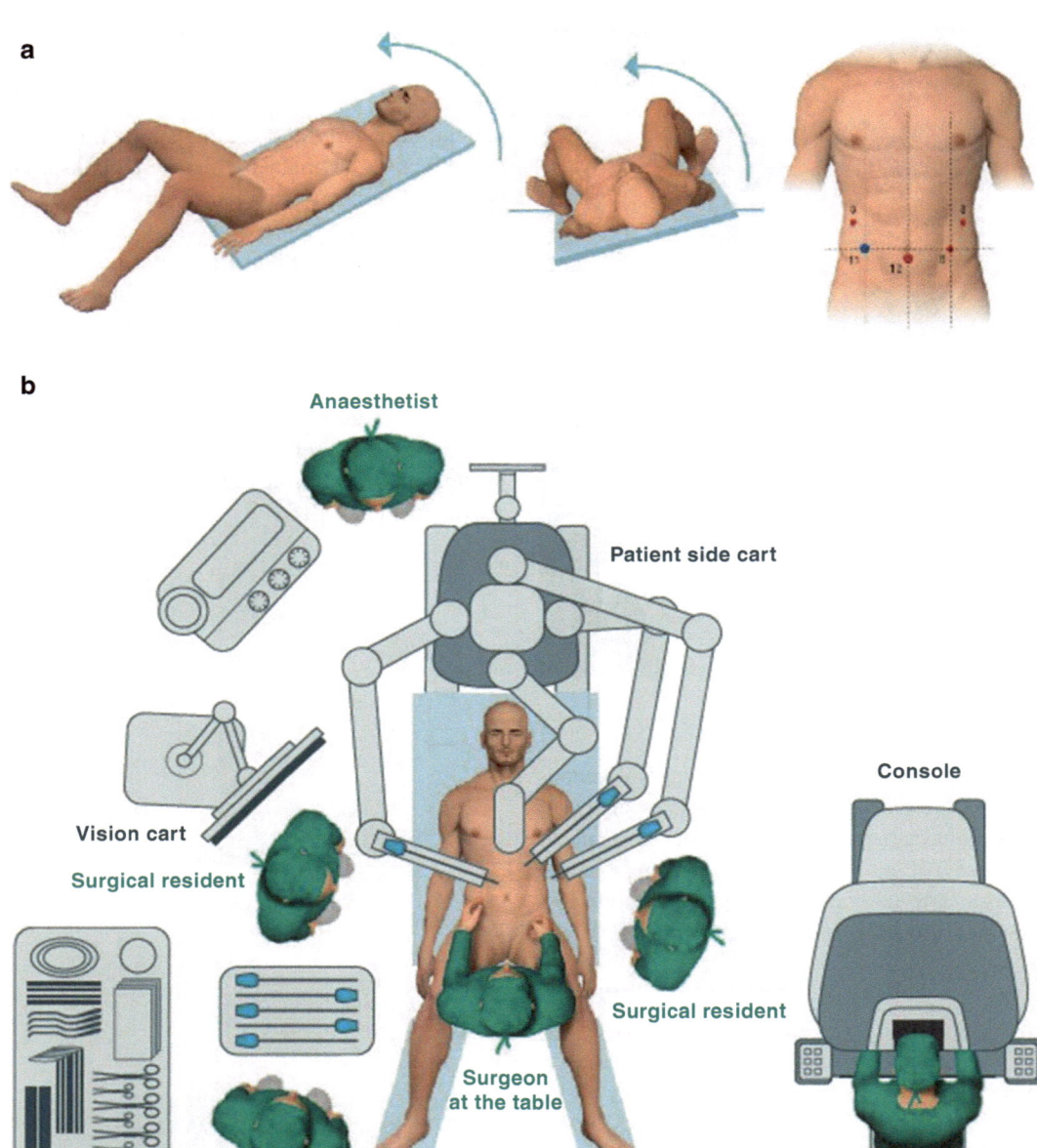

Fig. 35.9 Operating room setup. (**a**) patient position (**b**) operating room setup (with the Si system, the robotic tower is placed over the head of the patient, with the Xi system to the left of the patient) *Boggi, U., Perrone, V.G.,* *Vistoli, F. (2018). Robotic Pancreatoduodenectomy. In: Boggi, U. (eds) Minimally Invasive Surgery of the Pancreas. Updates in Surgery. Springer, Milano.* https://doi.org/10.1007/978-88-470-3958-2_26

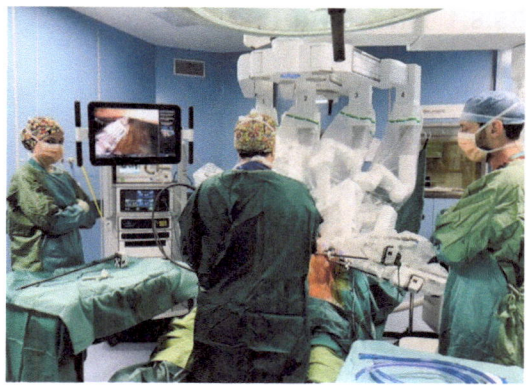

Fig. 35.10 Patient position. *Our operatory room*

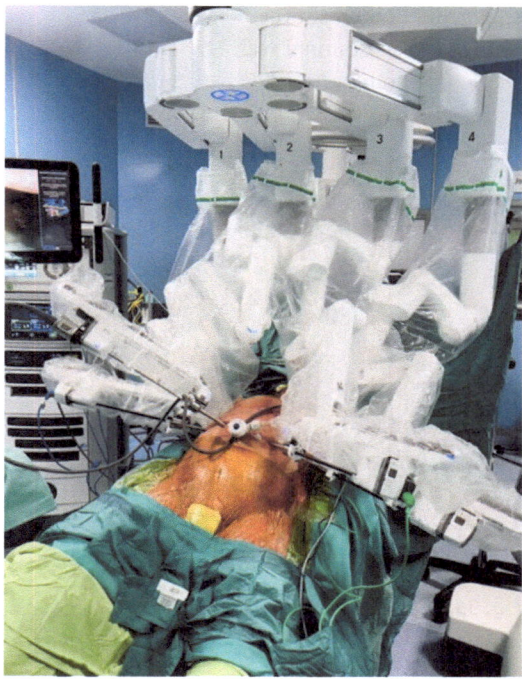

Fig. 35.11 Assistant surgeons position. *Our operatory room*

35.5 Instrument Table

- Tool pockets (3)
- Instrument arm drape and column drape (4)
- Cannula seal (4)
- Tip cover accessory (1)
- Electrosurgery (1)
- Thermos (1)
- AirSeal circuit
- Endoscopes (8 mm, 30°)

35.6 Robotic Instrument (Fig. 35.12)

- Monopolar curved scissors
- Maryland bipolar forceps
- ProGrasp forceps
- Cadiere forceps
- Large needle driver
- Medium-large clip applier
- Large clip applier
- Black diamond micro-forceps

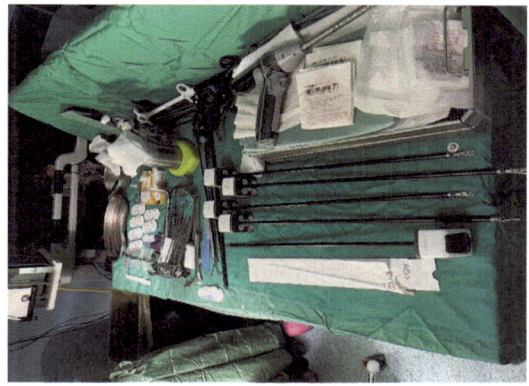

Fig. 35.12 Instrument table. *Our operatory room*

35.7 Laparoscopic Instrument Table

- Fenestrated grasper, long
- Babcock grasping forceps
- Clinch grasping forceps
- Metzenbaum curved scissor
- Maryland curved dissecting grasper
- Endoclip applier, small, medium, large
- Biopsy grasping forceps
- Right angle grasper
- Needle holder
- Endoscopic catcher
- Endo GIA stapler

35.8 Instrument Table for Conversion

- Gillies forceps (4)
- Monopolar coagulation forceps (3)
- Tissue forceps, no tooth, long (6)
- Tissue forceps, no tooth, medium (6)
- Debakey forceps, medium (2)
- Mikulicz abdominal wall retractor, long (2)
- Mikulicz abdominal wall retractor, short (2)
- Rochard abdominal retractor, long (2)
- Rochard abdominal retractor short (2)
- Abdominal spatula (1)
- Mathieu retractor (2)
- Richardson retractor (2)
- Farabeuf retractor (2)
- Yankauer suction catheter (2)
- Balfour abdominal retractor, two short blades, and two long blades (1)
- Scalpel handle, short no. 24 (2)
- Scalpel handle, long no. 24 (1)
- Scalpel handle no. 11 (2)
- Probe (1)
- Big kidney tray (1)
- Small kidney tray (1)
- Big sponge bowl (1)
- Medium sponge bowl (1)
- Small sponge bowl (1)

35.8.1 First Group (Fig. 35.13)

- Backhaus towel forceps (1)
- Mayo scissors, curved (4)
- Mayo scissors, straight (2)
- Mayo scissors, short (4)
- Metzenbaum scissors, long (1)
- Metzenbaum scissors, medium (1)

35.8.2 Second Group

- Backhaus towel forceps (1)
- Needle holder, long (4)
- Needle holder, medium (2)
- Needle holder, short (4)
- Needle "abdominal wall" holder (2)
- Needle holder, heavy (1)
- Needle holder, delicate and long (1)

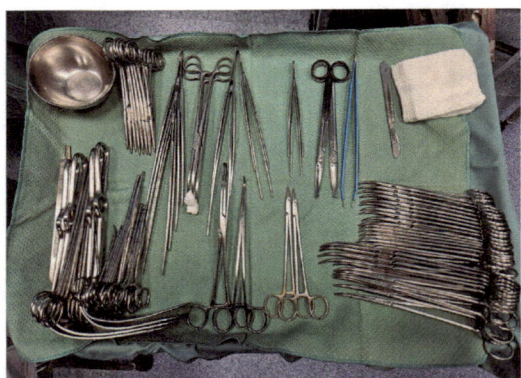

Fig. 35.13 Instrument table for conversion. *Our operatory room*

35.8.3 Third Group

- Backhaus towel forceps (1)
- Kocher forceps, long (4)
- Kocher forceps, medium (2)
- Allis tissue forceps, long (3)
- Allis tissue forceps, short (3)

35.8.4 Fourth Group

- Backhaus towel forceps (1)
- Mosquito forceps, curved (8)
- Mosquito forceps, straight (8)

35.8.5 Fifth Group

- Backhaus towel forceps (1)
- Crile forceps, straight (16)

35.8.6 Sixth Group

- Backhaus towel forceps (1)
- Crile forceps, curved (16)
- Delicate Crile forceps, curved (8)

35.8.7 Seventh Group

- Backhaus towel forceps (1)
- Foerster forceps (2)
- Kocher intestinal forceps (2)
- Crawford forceps (6)
- Long jaw ring forceps (2)
- Bengolea forceps (8)
- Mixter forceps (1)
- Big-tip Mixter forceps (1)

35.9 Instrument Table for Vascular Surgery

- Debakey forceps, long (2)
- Debakey forceps, medium (2)
- Robb spatula (1)
- Angiostat, angulated (2)

- Angiostat, straight (2)
- Angiostat, large and curved (1)
- Vascular needle holder (1)
- Potts scissors (3)
- Satinsky clamp, large (2)
- Satinsky clamp, small (1)
- Mixter forceps (1)
- Bulldog clamp, straight (3)
- Bulldog clamp, curved (2)
- Bulldog clamp, squared (2)
- Olive-tip catheter (1)

35.10 Tips and Tricks

Pancreatic surgery is a lengthy and exhausting procedure that requires a high level of concentration. It is crucial to ensure that the operation starts early in the morning and that all devices are in perfect working condition. Sterility must be maintained, and the patient's position must be secured, while instruments should be kept tidy.

To reduce the occurrence and amount of retroperitoneal fluid collections, all the retroperitoneal lymphatics must be constantly clipped. Therefore, clips of various sizes—small, medium, and large—should always be available, as well as vascular instruments.

The pancreatic gland is surrounded by large vessels, and metastatic cells can spread through lympho-neural tissue surrounding these vessels. Therefore, accurate lymphectomy may lead to unexpected vascular damage. In this regard, vascular instruments must always be available.

Given the duration of pancreatic surgery, shift changes are inevitable. To avoid errors or misunderstandings during handovers, a standardized, rapid, secure, and unambiguous procedure must be followed. The operating table must also be standardized so that every scrub nurse knows where everything is located.

Pancreatic surgery is particularly complex, and the surgeon must manage vital organs and vessels, making unexpected events possible. Therefore, it is crucial to be prepared for unexpected events and always ready to adjust the pace accordingly, as any unforeseen event in this type of surgery can endanger the patient's life (Fig. 35.14).

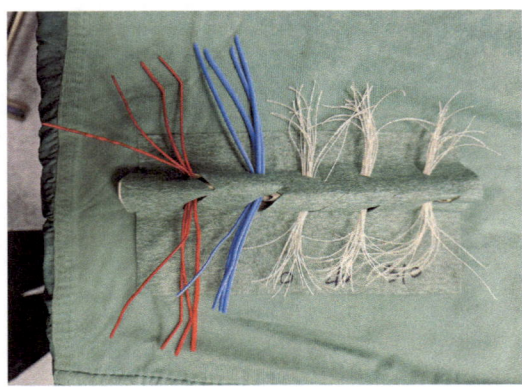

Fig. 35.14 Estote parati (be ready!). *Our operatory room*

35.11 End of the Operation

The scrub nurse must conduct a count of sponges and instruments with the circulating nurse and inform the surgeon of the results, clear away instruments and equipment, assist with dressing application, remove drapes, and prepare the patient for the recovery room. Finally, the scrub nurse must complete documentation and hand over the patient to the recovery room.

35.12 Conclusion

Being a scrub nurse requires anticipation, quick reaction, conscientious observation, as well as knowledge of anatomy and operative procedures. The scrub nurse works directly with the surgeon within the sterile field, passing instruments, sponges, and other necessary items during the procedure. As a member of the surgical team, the scrub nurse prepares and maintains a sterile field in which the operation can take place. Moreover, the scrub nurse is responsible for sponge counts, blade and needle checks, and instrument checks throughout the operation [8].

References

1. Hüttner FJ, Fitzmaurice C, Schwarzer G, Seiler CM, Antes G, Büchler MW, Diener MK. Pylorus-preserving pancreaticoduodenectomy (pp Whipple) versus pancreaticoduodenectomy (classic Whipple) for surgical treatment of periampullary and pancreatic carcinoma. Cochrane Database Syst Rev. 2016;2:CD006053.
2. Traverso LW, Kozarek RA. The Whipple procedure for severe complications of chronic pancreatitis. Arch Surg. 1993;128(9):1047–50 e 8368923, discussion 1051–3. https://doi.org/10.1007/978-3-642-77437-9_45.
3. Kauffmann E, Napoli N, Belluomini M, Miccoli M, Brozzetti S, Boggi U. Robot-assisted pancreaticoduodenectomy: safety and feasibility. Robot Surg. 2015;e 2:65–71.
4. Tol J A, Gouma DJ, Bassi C, Dervenis C, Montorsi M, Adham M, ... & Charnley RM. Definition of a standard lymphadenectomy in surgery for pancreatic ductal adenocarcinoma: a consensus statement by the International Study Group on Pancreatic Surgery (ISGPS). Surgery, 2014;156(3), 591–600
5. Kauffmann EF, Napoli N, Menonna F, Vistoli F, Amorese G, Campani D, Pollina LE, Funel N, Cappelli C, Caramella D, Boggi U. Robotic pancreatoduodenectomy with vascular resection. Langenbeck's Arch Surg. 2016;401(8):1111–22. https://doi.org/10.1007/s00423-016-149.
6. Bassi C, Marchegiani G, Dervenis C, Sarr M, Abu Hilal M, Adham M, Allen P, Andersson R, Asbun HJ, Besselink MG, Conlon K, Del Chiaro M, Falconi M, Fernandez-Cruz L, Fernandez-Del Castillo C, Fingerhut A, Friess H, Gouma DJ, Hackert T, Izbicki J, Lillemoe KD, Neoptolemos JP, Olah A, Schulick R, Shrikhande SV, Takada T, Takaori K, Traverso W, Vollmer CR, Wolfgang CL, Yeo CJ, Salvia R, Buchler M; International Study Group on Pancreatic Surgery (ISGPS). The 2016 update of the International Study Group (ISGPS) definition and grading of postoperative pancreatic fistula: 11 Years After. Surgery. 2017;161(3):584–91. https://doi.org/10.1016/j.surg.2016.11.014. Epub 2016 Dec 28. PMID: 28040257.
7. Boggi U, Signori S, De Lio N, Perrone VG, Vistoli F, Belluomini M, Cappelli C, Amorese G, Mosca F. Feasibility of robotic pancreaticoduodenectomy. Br J Surg. 2013;100(7):917–25. https://doi.org/10.1002/bjs.9135.
8. Mitchell L, Flin R. Non-technical skills of the operating theatre scrub nurse: literature review. J Adv Nurs. 2008;63:15–24. https://doi.org/10.1111/j.1365-2648.2008.04695.x.

Part X

Interventions Protocols in Abdominal Wall Surgery

Laparoscopic Preperitoneal Treatment of Inguinal Hernia

36

Enrico Lauro and Davide Lomanto

36.1 Introduction

The endo-laparoscopic approaches for inguinal hernias are:

- The Totally Extra-Peritoneal (TEP) repair
- The Trans-Abdominal Pre-Peritoneal (TAPP) repair
- The Intraperitoneal Onlay Mesh (IPOM) repair

The first two techniques are the most popular, while the technique with Intra-Peritoneal Onlay Mesh positioning (IPOM) is utilized today only in very selected and complex cases with a modified technique.

Both TEP and TAPP offer better results when compared to open techniques in terms of postoperative recovery, recurrences, and complication rates; they also have the advantage of reinforcing the entire myopectineal orifice through the posterior positioning of large prostheses [1–3].

E. Lauro (✉)
Department of General Surgery, St. Maria Del Carmine Hospital—Rovereto, APSS Trento, Trento, Italy
e-mail: enrico.lauro@apss.tn.it

D. Lomanto
Minimally Invasice Centre, National University Hospital, Yong Loo Lin School of Medicine, National University, Singapore
e-mail: davide_lomanto@nuhs.edu.sg

The main benefits of TEP over TAPP are the lower risk of injury to intraperitoneal organs (e.g., bowel, bladder) or vessels and the lower risk of postoperative peritoneal adhesions and seroma. On the other hand, TAPP offers the advantage of a diagnostic laparoscopy with immediate visualization of both inguino-crural districts (right and left) with direct control and management of the herniated content.

This can be extremely useful in emergency settings, in case of irreducible incarcerated hernias or suspicion of vascular bowel suffering.

36.2 Indications

- Primary, reducible hernias
- Recurrences of a previous anterior repair
- Fit for general anesthesia

36.3 Contraindications

- Non-fit for general anesthesia
- Acute abdomen with strangulated hernias or intestinal ischemia
- Respiratory distress
- Mesh repair in pediatric patients

36.4 Relative Contraindications

- Irreducible hernias
- Sliding hernias
- Inguinoscrotal hernias
- Previous prostatectomy or pelvic surgery
- Recurrence after posterior repair

A previous lower-pelvic abdominal surgery including prostatectomy is a relative contraindication since the risk of adhesion is unknown. Pelvic adhesions may result in more operative difficulties; for this reason, it is better to reserve the more complex cases for experienced surgeons. It should also be explained to the patient that there might be the possibility of conversion to transabdominal preperitoneal (TAPP) or, at least, to open technique.

A previous appendectomy does not usually represent a contraindication but needs further attention in the lateral dissection of the Bogros space.

A recurrence of TEP is a relative contraindication and can be addressed again in TEP or TAPP, especially by experienced surgeons.

Giant inguinoscrotal or sliding hernias are also a relative contraindication: The difficulty in managing the hernia content and the possibility of altered anatomy with a reduced operating space may increase the difficulties of the technique. Certainly, in these cases the posterior approach, either open (Stoppa) or endo-laparoscopic, produces the best long-term results.

36.5 Preoperative Preparation

A careful medical history and a careful physical examination are essential to correctly assess the patient, including the suitability to undergo general anesthesia.

In case of diagnostic doubts, it is advisable to proceed to further imaging studies by dynamic ultrasound (with Valsalva maneuver) of the inguino-femoral region or CT without contrast medium (unless in the presence of suspected vascular suffering). The combination of physical examination and dynamic US can produce a diagnostic accuracy of nearly 90%.

Concerning the informed consent, the risk of conversion to TAPP or open approach should be explained to the patient, depending on the difficulties of the procedure and the experience of the surgeon.

Likewise, the risks and complications should be clearly illustrated to the patient, such as the risks of vascular, nerve, or vas deferens lesions (male patients) and the possible formation of seromas especially in large and or direct hernias. Less common complications to be advised in endo-laparoscopic TEP are prosthetic infections (less frequent than the open approach) and the risk of developing chronic postoperative pain [4].

Antibiotic prophylaxis is recommended in the presence of risk factors for wound or prosthetic infections, based on the patient's condition (advanced age, use of steroids, immunosuppression, obesity, diabetes, neoplasms) or factors related to surgery (contamination, long operative time, use of drainages, presence of urinary catheter) [5–7].

Patients should also be advised to void their bladder before the procedure. In the case of complicated hernias (partially reducible, large defects) or urgent settings, it is advisable to use a urinary catheter, which can be removed at the end of the procedure.

36.6 Operating Theater Setup

36.6.1 Surgical Instrumentation (Fig. 36.1)

- 5-mm or 10-mm optics, 30°
- 1 Hasson trocar

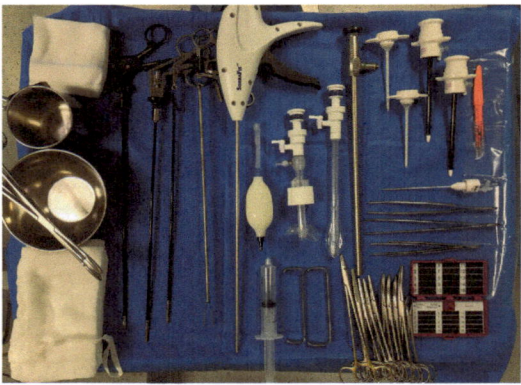

Fig. 36.1 Surgical instrumentation

- Two 5-mm trocars
- 1 balloon dissector (Spacemaker, Medtronic-USA, or similar)

According to the European Hernia Society (EHS) guidelines, the dissector balloon is recommended for surgeons in training, as it is useful for identifying the correct plane [5]. Blunt dissection with optics can be used safely by experienced operators, which is also cheaper.

- 2 atraumatic grasping forceps (Reddick)
- Maryland forceps
- Short or long bowel forceps
- Curved scissors
- Bipolar forceps bisect (optional) (Erbe, Gmbh, Germany)
- Prosthetics (10 cm × 15cm; 12 cm × 17 cm)

The use of prostheses of at least 10 × 15 cm is recommended. Smaller size meshes increase the risk of recurrence. Larger prostheses (12 × 17cm) are instead recommended in case of defects greater than 3–4 cm, sliding or inguinoscrotal hernias, following the EHS guidelines [5, 6].

Some prostheses are 3D anatomical shaped, allowing them to be safely placed in the preperitoneal inguino-femoral space without fixation; other meshes present a self-adhesive or self-gripping surface and do not require additional fixation.

- Fixation devices (tackers, fibrin glue, cyanoacrylate glue)

Following IEHS guidelines, the use of prosthesis fixation devices is recommended only for major defects (defects >3–4 cm) to avoid displacement of the prosthesis and reduce the risk of recurrence [6, 7].

Today, both absorbable and non-absorbable (to be preferred) tackers are available; they are used to secure the prosthesis to Cooper's ligament and rectus muscle medial to the inferior epigastric vessels and above the iliopectineal ligament. Fibrin or synthetic glues are available on the market, and many studies have now proven their effectiveness.

- Endoloops (pre-made tie loops) or plastic clips (Hem-o-lok)

All peritoneal breaches need to be repaired either with a simple endoloop, Hem-o-lok clips, or, in large defects, with absorbable sutures. All peritoneal defects must be obliterated to avoid the risk of internal hernias or intraperitoneal prosthesis exposition, dangerous visceral-prosthetic adhesions, and intraluminal erosion.

36.6.2 Position of the Patient and the Surgical Team

The patient lies in the supine position with both arms tucked along the body, and the operating table is placed in a slight Trendelenburg position (10°–15°).

The first operator places himself on the contralateral side of the hernia site. The assistant is on the same side in a more cranial position or on the opposite side of the operator. The monitor and the laparoscopic instrumentation (camera, insufflator, etc.) are placed at the patient's feet and in a slightly ipsilateral position to the treated hernia defect. The scrub nurse will be in a more caudal position than the first operator.

36.6.3 Surgical Technique

36.6.3.1 Access, Creation of the Preperitoneal Space, and Insertion of Trocars

Different techniques can be used to access and create the preperitoneal space, according to the experience and preference of the surgeon.

The most common is through a sub-umbilical incision, another is through the suprapubic insertion of a Veress needle in the preperitoneal space, and subsequent insufflation of CO_2.

The first access takes place through a sub-umbilical smiley incision of about 10–12 mm. The anterior fascia of the rectus muscle is exposed and incised, and the rectus muscle is retracted laterally (Fig. 36.2) exposing the retromuscular space.

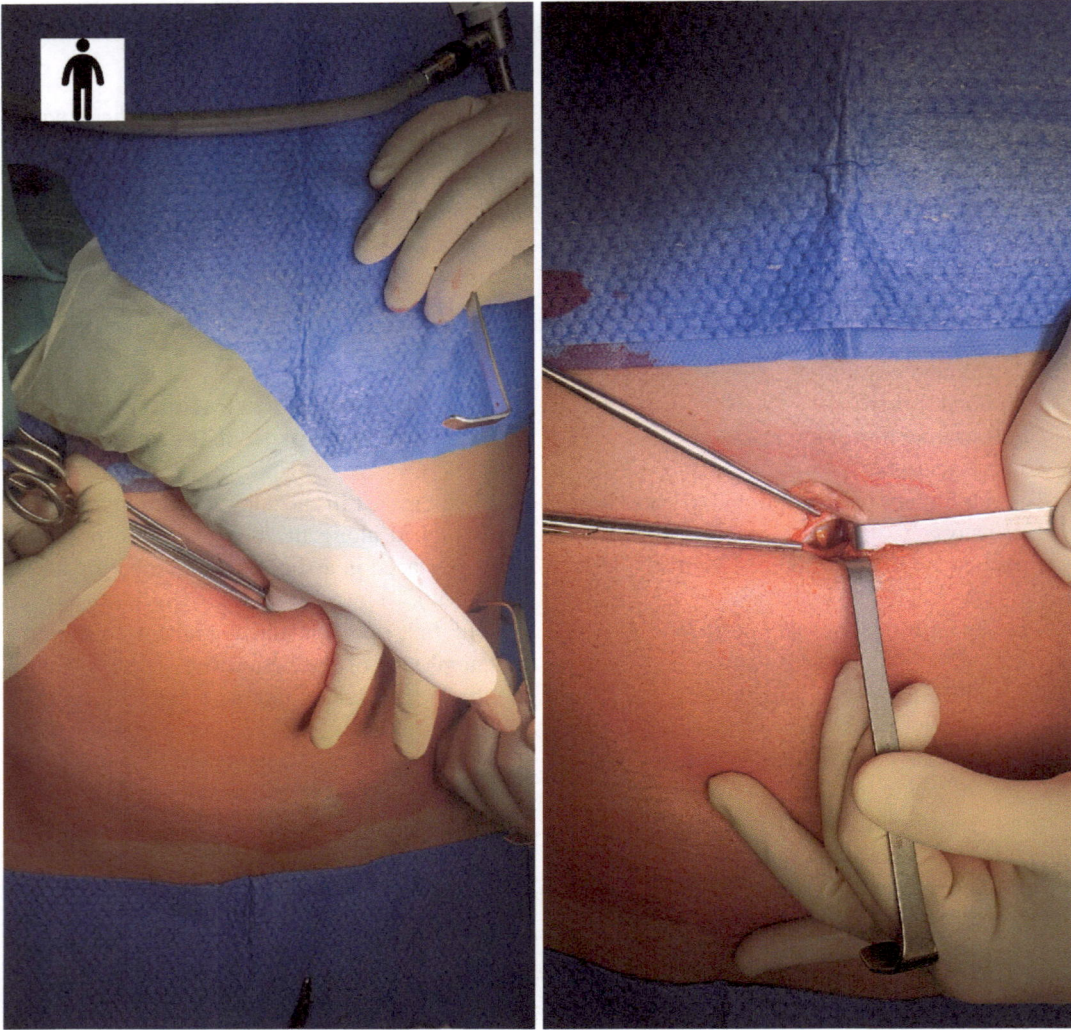

Fig. 36.2 Rectus muscle retracted laterally and finger dissection

At this point, there are two most common techniques to develop the retromuscular space:

- By blunt dissection
- Using a dissection balloon (Space-Maker, Medtronic-USA, or similar)

With the first method, the retromuscular space is created bluntly with the help of a gauze or finger. The operator can dissect the retromuscular space along the median line toward the pubis. Then a 10–12-mm Hasson trocar is inserted and using the camera the retromuscular tunnel can be developed. Once the pubic bone is reached, the other two 5-mm trocars can be placed safely under visual control along the midline tunnel.

The blunt dissection technique is recommended for experienced surgeons, and it significantly reduces costs.

With the dissection balloon technique, a special trocar with an inflatable balloon is used (Spacemaker, Medtronic, USA; PDB100 Medtronic, USA; etc.). There are two types of balloons in the market: one round-shaped balloon for unilateral hernias and another one kidney-shaped balloon for bilateral hernias. Using these

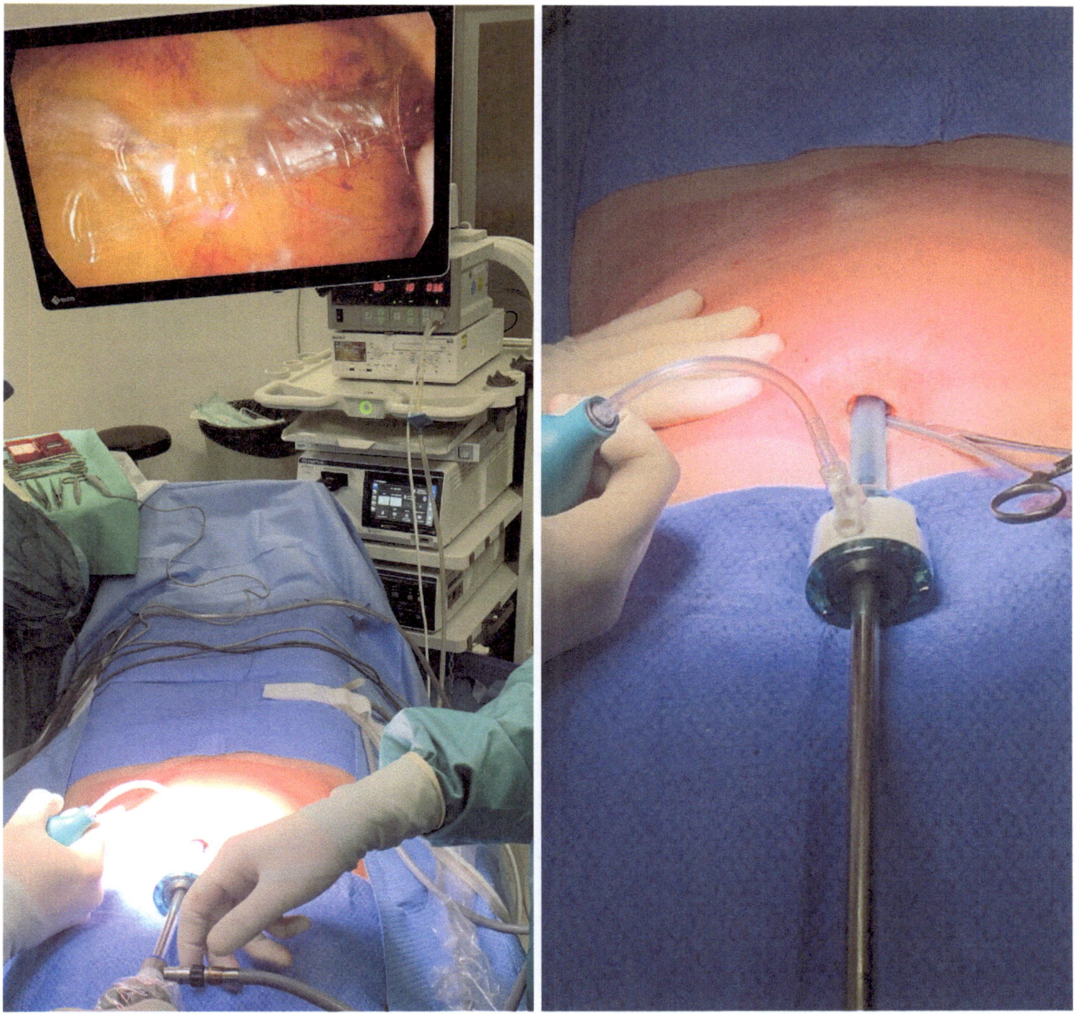

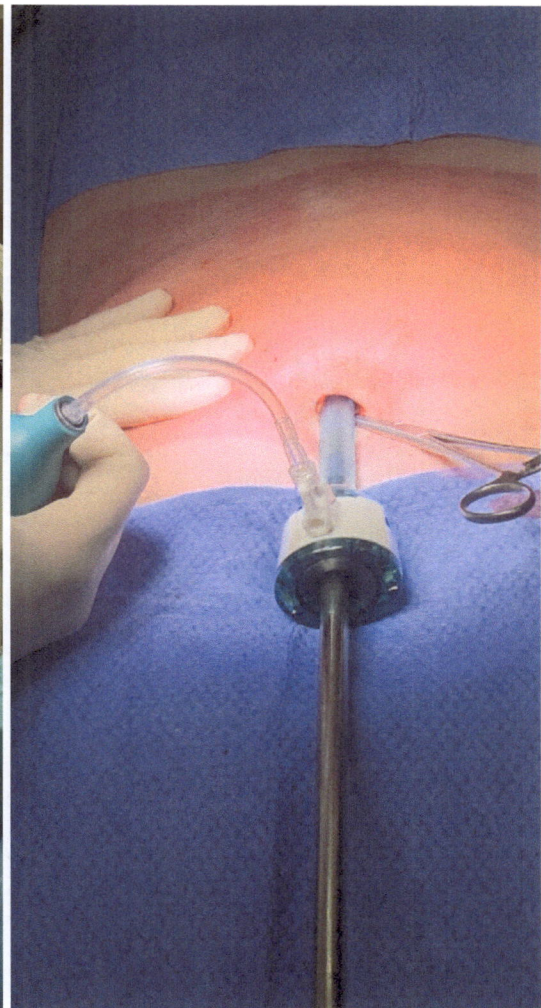

Fig. 36.3 Balloon dissector

types of balloon dissectors, the preperitoneal space is created by manually inflating air into the balloon connected to the tip of the trocar. The optic telescope is inserted inside the trocar dissector balloon ensuring a correct dissection of the preperitoneal plane (Fig. 36.3) under direct vision.

In this phase, it is important to verify that the epigastric vessels are detached from the peritoneal layer, remaining along the posterior aspect of the rectus muscles. It is also important to verify that no lacerations of vessels or the peritoneum occur, and this can be achieved through a slow, progressive insufflation.

At this point, the dissection balloon is deflated and extracted. Some of these trocars are now equipped with a system whereby it is possible to hold the trocar in place and extract only the balloon, while others require it to be removed before being replaced with a standard Hasson trocar.

Once the dissection is performed, regardless of the technique used, the remaining two 5-mm operative trocars can be placed along the midline under direct vision, to avoid damage to the underlying peritoneum, bladder, or intestine. The most distal 5-mm trocar is positioned about three fingers breadth above the pubis, and the other is in

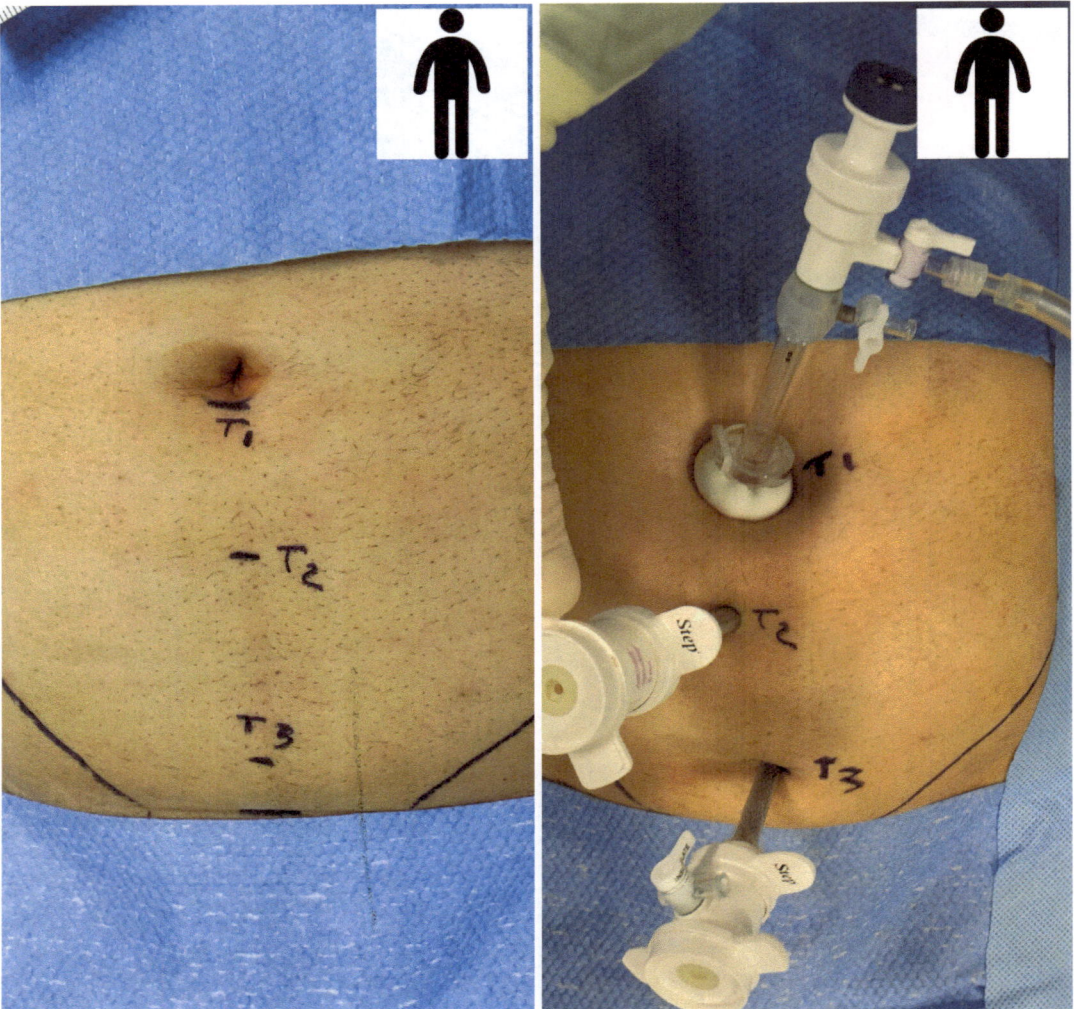

Fig. 36.4 Trocar placement

between this one and the umbilical access (Hasson trocar) (Fig. 36.4).

The working CO_2 pneumopreperitoneum pressure is approximately 12 mmHg.

36.6.3.2 Medial Dissection (Retzius Space)

The first dissection should be directed to the symphysis pubis. Using atraumatic forceps, the dissection should be along the linea alba, behind the rectus muscle toward the pubic symphysis and then below it for 1–2 cm. This allows to exclude

unrecognized obturator hernias and gain adequate space for the lower edge of the prosthesis.

In case of unilateral hernia, the limits of the medial dissection should be 1–2 cm beyond the midline.

36.6.3.3 Lateral Dissection (Bogros Space)

Proceeding laterally, toward the anterior-superior iliac spine (ASIS), the lateral space is created remaining below the epigastric vessels and above the peritoneal plane. This space is delimited by

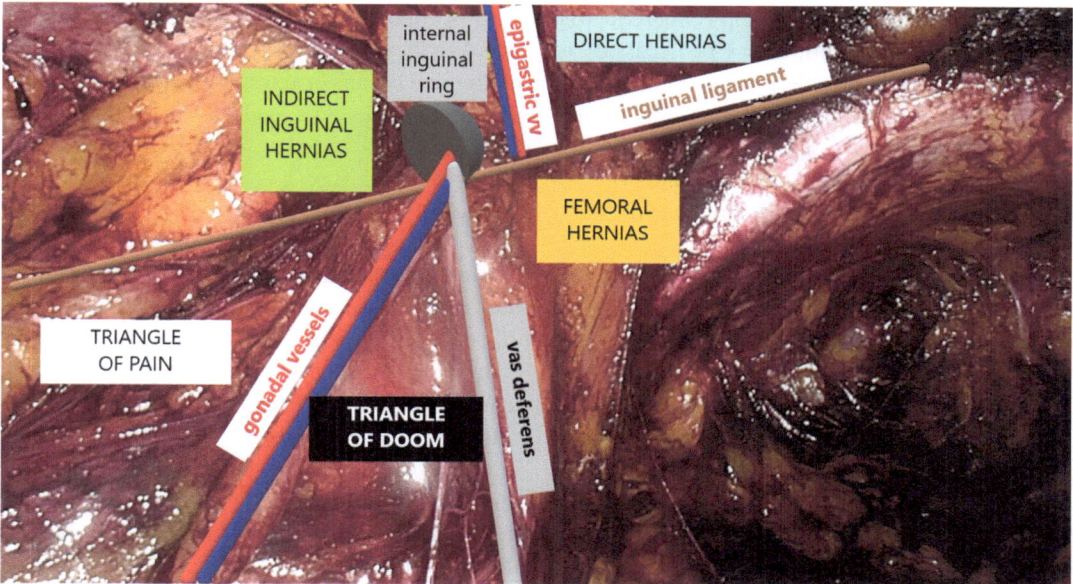

Fig. 36.5 Anatomic landmarks in endo-laparoscopic inguinal hernia repair

the two sheets of the transversalis fascia. The dissection is performed by dissecting the peritoneum toward the ASIS and downwards till the psoas muscle is visualized. Attention should be made to avoid dissecting further beyond the lumbar fascia, avoiding damage to the lateral cutaneous and the genito-femoral nerve. It is also advisable not to use direct electrocoagulation in this region due to the risk of indirect electric nerve damage. The limits of the lateral region are: inferiorly to the psoas muscle, superiorly to the ASIS, and cranially to the arcuate line.

36.6.3.4 Identification of the Hernial Sac and Its Reduction

Only once the dissection of both spaces (Retzius medially and Bogros laterally) has been completed, it will be possible to identify and repair all defects of the myopectineal orifice (MPO): direct, indirect, femoral, and obturator. This will allow the surgeon to visualize all the main anatomical structures, minimize any accidental damage, gain a wide space where to place the prosthesis and, in the event of accidental pneumoperitoneum due to an inadvertent lesion of the peritoneal sac, continue without impediments.

The exposure of the entire MPO should be complete at the end of the medial and lateral dissection and after the reduction of the sac (Fig. 36.5).

36.6.4 Hernia Reduction Technique

Direct Hernias: The internal oblique (or direct) hernias originate medially to the inferior epigastric vessels at the level of Hesselbach's triangle. The reduction can be easily achieved by separating the "pseudo sac" (transversalis) from the preperitoneal fat and the peritoneum, by pulling it gently forward. Attention must be paid to the posterior dissection adjacent to the pubic bone where there are the corona mortis anastomoses. This represents a vascular connection between the inferior epigastric vessels and the obturator-internal iliac vessels. Attention should be made medially to the bladder and inferior to the iliac vessels and the spermatic structures (vessels and vas deferens).

Femoral Hernias: The reduction of the hernia sac and its contents is achieved by gentle traction paying attention to the external iliac vessels, just lateral to the defect. If the content is not reducible due to a tight hernial port, it may be necessary to widen the defect using an electrified hook by performing the section of the hernia ring at the superomedial aspect. This will facilitate the reduction of the hernial sac and its contents.

Obturator Hernias: In the same canal where the obturator vessels lie it is sometimes possible to find herniation of preperitoneal fat or a real hernia sac. Like femoral hernias, gentle traction will allow its reduction.

External Oblique Hernias (Indirect): Lateral to the inferior epigastric vessels is the internal inguinal ring through which indirect hernias are formed. The standard approach to reduce an indirect hernial sac involves three simple steps: (1) the so-called slimming of the sac; (2) the separation of the peritoneal hernia sac from the spermatic structure; and (3) the division or reduction of the hernia sac.

Slimming of the sac can be achieved with gentle traction of the entire hernia content till the inferior edge is visualized, then the hernia sac is separated from the spermatic elements that stand along its lower margin; lastly, the reduction of the isolated sac by simple traction and peeling from the spermatic structure medially then laterally, and lastly medially along the space between iliac vessels and the bladder. Once isolated from the spermatic structure, a sac transection may be necessary in case of large, inguinoscrotal, or congenital hernias. The sac is not reduced *in toto* but transected to avoid damage to the testis from excessive traction maneuvers. In these cases, it is suggested to transect the sac with diathermy to avoid bleeding and to ligate its proximal part with a pre-made suture loop, or to divide the sac with diathermy after a proximal ligature is made to close the peritoneum.

Any lipoma of the cord, which is usually lateral to the indirect hernia sac, should be fully reduced either before or upon completion of the hernia sac reduction.

The reduced hernia sac should be further dissected up to the peritoneal reflection and medially from the attachment with the vas deferens at the level of a ligament that runs behind the vas and the spermatic vessels (*S-shaped ligament*).

It is important to close any peritoneal holes to avoid adhesions between the prosthesis and abdominal organs or internal herniations. For this purpose, plastic clips, endo-loops, or sutures can be used.

36.6.4.1 Mesh Repair

The last step is the repair of the defect and the reinforcement of the entire area corresponding to the myopectineal orifice with the use of a 10×15 cm synthetic mesh. The prosthesis is rolled and inserted through the Hasson trocar using a "*no-touch technique*" to minimize mesh infection. It is very important to reduce the risk of mesh infection that the mesh is placed into the preperitoneal space directly from its package and to avoid any contact with the skin. The mesh is then unrolled over the MPO making sure to cover all the hernia sites. Two centimeters of the mesh should be placed below the symphysis pubis while the upper margin should reach the inferior 5-mm trocar medially; laterally, the mesh should be lining over the psoas muscle (Fig. 36.6). It is important to ensure that the peritoneum is far behind the mesh and does not slip below the lower edge of the prosthesis to prevent a recurrence. In fact, the mesh should stand vertically and far from the peritoneal reflection to avoid a "clam-shell effect" upon desufflation.

In the case of bilateral hernias, the two prostheses should overlap medially by 1–2 cm.

According to the International Guidelines, the mesh should be fixed only in large hernias. In our opinion, it is adviced to fixed the meshes also in case of bilateral hernias, due to the large dissection

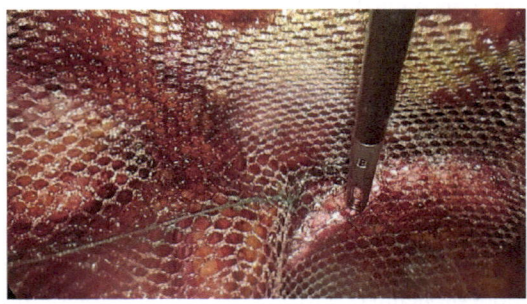

Fig. 36.6 Mesh reinforcement of the myopectineal orifice

of the preperitoneal space. The mesh is anchored with tackers or glue to avoid its dislocation. The points of fixation are the Cooper's ligament and the region medial to the epigastric vessels on the rectus muscle; if necessary, the prosthesis can also be fixed laterally to the epigastric vessels. A total of 5–6 tackers is usually enough.

It is advisable to avoid the use of tackers below the ilio-pubic ligament and to laterally consider 15–20% of abnormalities in the nerve path. This can avoid nerve damage and the risk of postoperative chronic pain.

3D shape or self-fixing/self-gripping meshes do not need additional fixation, minimizing the risk of iatrogenic nerve injury and chronic pain.

36.6.4.2 Hemostasis and Closure

At the end of the procedure, hemostasis is controlled, and the pneumoperitoneum is progressively desufflated by making sure that the lower edge of the mesh does not fold or the peritoneal reflection does not slip below the prosthesis. This is to prevent recurrences. It is useful to hold the lateral-lower edge of the prosthesis in position with atraumatic forceps during gas desufflation.

The endo-laparoscopic trocars are then removed, and the anterior rectus muscle fascia at the sub-umbilical port is closed with an absorbable suture.

36.7 Reduced and Single-Port Technique

Since the advent of laparoscopy, various surgical techniques with increasingly reduced access have been developed (mini laparoscopy, reduced and single-port technique, and needlescopic surgery) [8–10].

The "single-incision endo-laparoscopic surgery" (SPES) uses single-port access through which all the operative instruments, including optics, are inserted.

This minimally invasive approach has aroused much interest over the years, being used not only for hernia repair but also for cholecystectomies, colic resections, appendectomies, and adrenalectomies [11–14].

The advantages of these methods with reduced access are lower postoperative pain, less use of pain-relieving drugs, reduced hospital stay, and quick return to work.

However, these advantages are burdened by lower operative ergonomics, with a reduced operative field, difficulty in traction maneuvers, and conflict between the instruments due to a lack of adequate triangulation [15].

In addition, recent studies have shown comparable results as compared to the standard TEP approach in terms of operating time, postoperative pain control, and complication rate [16, 17].

36.8 e-TEP Technique

The enhanced view or extended TEP (e-TEP) technique was developed to solve the difficulties encountered during standard TEP (reduced operative and visual field, instrumental conflict).

The main novelty is to gain the retromuscular space also from different sites compared to the classic sub-umbilical access.

In the intention of the authors, this should allow easy creation of the extraperitoneal space, large surgical field, and flexible port setup.

e-TEP can be useful in difficult scenarios such as in obese or post-bariatric patients, short distance between the umbilicus and pubic tubercle, patients with previous pelvic surgeries, and large inguinoscrotal hernias [18, 19].

Regardless of the proposed variants, the main surgical steps remain the same as the standard TEP.

36.9 Postoperative Management

In the immediate postoperative period, it is recommended to proceed with:

- Postoperative resumption of oral intake as soon as possible and after 6 h.
- Adequate analgesia by limiting the use of opiates to avoid side effects (delayed recovery of bowel function, postoperative nausea, and vomiting). Heterocoxib and paracetamol are

recommended in the first 3 days and then ad hoc.

- The patient can be discharged on the same day or within 24 h once he is able to void and when all the discharge parameters are respected (e.g., stable vital signs, pain controlled by oral analgesics, nausea and emesis controlled).
- Follow-up is suggested at 1 week and 1 and 3 months.

36.10 Complications

Complications can be divided into intraoperative and postoperative complications.

Intraoperative complications can occur in 2–4% of cases and are mainly due to vascular, visceral, vas deferens, bladder, and lateral nerve lesions [20, 21].

Vascular lesions include lesions of the external iliac vessels, the lower epigastric vessels, the spermatic vessels, and the suprapubic arch including corona mortis.

The most frequent are accidental lesions of the epigastric vessels which can be minimized with the approach along the midline with positioning under direct vision of the operative trocars.

The lesion of the iliac vessels has catastrophic effects and must be avoided by paying attention to properly dissecting the sac along its lower edge, exerting gentle lateral traction on it and the elements of the funiculus, using a medial approach.

It is also mandatory to avoid the use of traumatic fixation in the region called the *triangle of doom*, between the vas deferens and spermatic vessels, due to the serious risk of injury to the iliac vessels.

Visceral lesions (bowel and bladder) can be avoided by careful dissection and by limiting the use of electrocoagulation as much as possible.

The use of bipolar forceps or short activations of the monopolar scalpel, at a power of use as low as possible, minimizes the risk of dispersion of electrical energy through the thin peritoneal layer.

Patients with previous pelvic surgery, presence of adhesions, inguinoscrotal or sliding hernias are more at risk of bladder damage. In these cases, bladder catheterization helps to minimize the risks of iatrogenic lesions which, eventually, can be treated endoscopically.

Nerve injuries can be avoided by careful lateral dissection, avoiding removing the thin layer of adipose tissue that covers the course of the nerves in the so-called *triangle of pain*, between the inguinal ligament and the gonadal vessels.

In this region, it is essential not to use clips or tackers to avoid damaging the nerves, preferring the use of glues or self-fixing/self-gripping meshes.

Injuries of the vas deferens and spermatic vessels can be minimized through proper anatomical dissection and avoiding excessive traction on these structures.

Any accidental peritoneal hole will be treated with clips, endoloops, or stitches to avoid exposure of the prosthesis or internal hernias.

Postoperative complications such as seromas can occur mainly in cases of very large hernias, typically in the 7–10th postoperative day, and do not usually require any treatment.

However, they can be mistaken for early recurrence. An ultrasound check is a fast and inexpensive way to make a differential diagnosis in case of doubt.

Usually, seromas undergo spontaneous resorption within 4–6 weeks. In the case of chronic (over 2 months), symptomatic seromas, needle aspiration in conditions of absolute sterility may be useful. After 4–5 months, persistent complex sero-hematomas may need surgical evacuation.

Early recurrences are usually due to imprecise patient selection, incorrect surgical technique, and inadequate mesh choice and fixation (especially in the case of large defects).

Incomplete dissection of the myopectineal orifice can lead to unrecognizing occult hernias [22].

36.11 Clinical Considerations and Conclusions

The totally extraperitoneal inguinal hernia repair (TEP) has been shown in various meta-analyses and clinical trials to reduce postoperative pain, decrease the consumption of painkillers, and allow an earlier return to work as compared to open techniques.

These benefits are most evident in the case of bilateral or recurrent hernias [1, 2, 7, 23].

As with any surgical technique, but especially in the field of hernia repair, careful patient selection coupled with adequate technical training is essential to obtain good results in terms of low recurrence and complication rates.

References

1. Feliu X, Clavería R, Besora P, Camps J, Fernández-Sallent E, Viñas X, Abad JM. Bilateral inguinal hernia repair: laparoscopic or open approach? Hernia. 2011;15:15–8.
2. Memon MA, Cooper NJ, Memon B, Memon MI, Abrams KR. Meta-analysis of randomized clinical trials comparing open and laparoscopic inguinal hernia repair. Br J Surg. 2003;90:1479–92.
3. Sartori A, de Luca M, Noaro G, Piatto G, Pignata G, di Leo A, Lauro E, Andreuccetti J. Rare intraoperative and postoperative complications after transabdominal laparoscopic hernia repair: results from the multicenter wall hernia group registry. J Laparoendosc Adv Surg Tech. 2021;31:290–5.
4. Lomanto D, Katara A. Managing intra-operative complications during totally extraperitoneal repair of inguinal hernia. J Minim Access Surg. 2006;2:165.
5. Simons MP, Aufenacker T, Bay-Nielsen M, et al. European hernia society guidelines on the treatment of inguinal hernia in adult patients. Hernia. 2009;13:343–403.
6. The Hernia Surge Group. International guidelines for groin hernia management. Hernia. 2018;22:1–165.
7. Bittner R, Bain K, Bansal VK, et al. Update of guidelines for laparoscopic treatment of ventral and incisional abdominal wall hernias (international Endohernia society (IEHS)): part B. Surg Endosc. 2019;33:3511–49.
8. Lau H, Lee F. A prospective comparative study of needlescopic and conventional endoscopic extraperitoneal inguinal hernioplasty. Surg Endosc. 2002;16:1737–40.
9. Carvalho GL, Loureiro MP, Bonin EA, Claus CP, Silva FW, Cury AM, Fernandes FAM. Minilaparoscopic technique for inguinal hernia repair combining trans-abdominal pre-peritoneal and totally extraperitoneal approaches. JSLS. 2012;16:569–75.
10. Goo TT, Lawenko M, Cheah WK, Tan C, Lomanto D. Endoscopic total extraperitoneal repair of recurrent inguinal hernia: a 5-year review. Hernia. 2010;14:477–80.
11. Trastulli S, Cirocchi R, Desiderio J, Guarino S, Santoro A, Parisi A, Noya G, Boselli C. Systematic review and meta-analysis of randomized clinical trials comparing single-incision *versus* conventional laparoscopic cholecystectomy. Br J Surg. 2012;100:191–208.
12. Fung AK-Y, Aly EH. Systematic review of single-incision laparoscopic colonic surgery. Br J Surg. 2012;99:1353–64.
13. Rehman H, Mathews T, Ahmed I. A review of minimally invasive single-port/incision laparoscopic appendectomy. J Laparoendosc Adv Surg Tech. 2012;22:641–6.
14. Goo TT, Agarwal A, Goel R, Tan CTK, Lomanto D, Cheah WK. Single-port access adrenalectomy: our initial experience. J Laparoendosc Adv Surg Tech. 2011;21:815–9.
15. Goel R, Lomanto D. Controversies in single-port laparoscopic surgery. Surg Laparosc Endosc Percutan Tech. 2012;22:380–2.
16. Fuentes MB, Goel R, Lee-Ong AC, Cabrera EB, Lawenko M, Lopez-Gutierrez J, Lomanto D. Single-port endo-laparoscopic surgery (SPES) for totally extraperitoneal inguinal hernia: a critical appraisal of the chopstick repair. Hernia. 2013;17:217–21.
17. Wijerathne S, Agarwal N, Ramzy A, Lomanto D. A prospective randomized controlled trial to compare single-port endo-laparoscopic surgery versus conventional TEP inguinal hernia repair. Surg Endosc. 2014;28:3053–8.
18. Andreuccetti J, Sartori A, Lauro E, Crepaz L, Sanna S, Pignata G, Bracale U, di Leo A. Extended totally extraperitoneal Rives–Stoppa (eTEP-RS) technique for ventral hernia: initial experience of The Wall Hernia Group and a surgical technique update. Updat Surg. 2021;73:1955–61.
19. Daes J. The enhanced view–totally extraperitoneal technique for repair of inguinal hernia. Surg Endosc. 2012;26:1187–9.
20. Tetik C, Arregui ME, Dulucq JL, Fitzgibbons RJ, Franklin ME, McKernan JB, Rosin RD, Schultz LS, Toy FK. Complications and recurrences associated with laparoscopic repair of groin hernias. Surg Endosc. 1994;8:1316. https://doi.org/10.1007/BF00188291.
21. Kraus MA. Nerve injury during laparoscopic inguinal hernia repair. Surg Laparosc Endosc. 1993;3:342–5.
22. Miguel PR, Reusch M, daRosa AL, Carlos JR. Laparoscopic hernia repair—complications. JSLS. 1998;2:35–40.
23. Cavazzola LT, Rosen MJ. Laparoscopic versus open inguinal hernia repair. Surg Clin N Am. 2013;93:1269–79.

Victor G. Radu

37.1 Introduction

Laparoscopic retromuscular repair of ventral hernias—the eTEP (Enhanced view Totally Extraperitoneal) approach represents the endoscopic alternative of the Rives-Stoppa (R-S) procedure. In larger defects, when the width of the defect closely approximates or exceeds two times the rectus width, it is necessary to add an additional muscular release, doing a TAR (Transversus Abdominis Release). In this case, the name of the procedure is eTEP-TAR.

The principles of this technique are [1]:

1. Closure of the defect.
2. Use uncoated mesh, placed outside of the abdominal cavity.
3. Minimizing mesh fixation.

To realize these principles, it is necessary to connect three spaces (Fig. 37.1) [2]:

1. The preperitoneal space, represented by the falciform ligament cranially and by the umbilical ligament caudally.
2. The retro-rectus spaces.
3. The pre-transversalis spaces, laterally to the linea semilunaris.

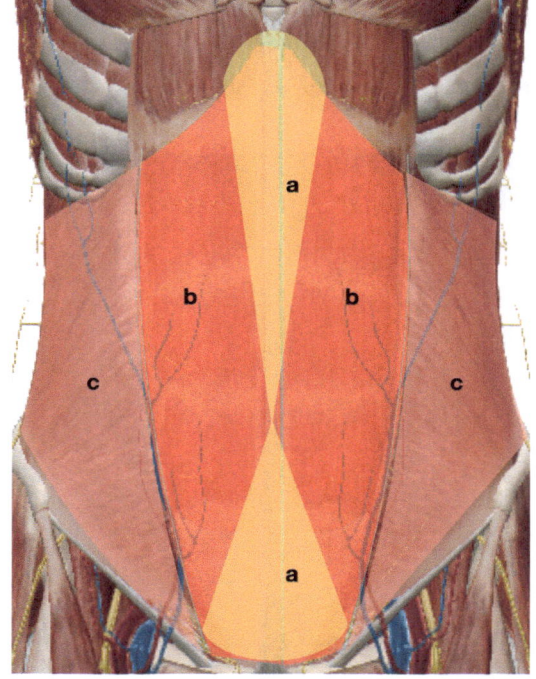

Fig. 37.1 Connection of the three spaces: preperitoneal (a), retro-rectus (b), and pre-transversalis (c)

The position of the patient on the table is very important [3].

- The bed is flexed up to 30°. In this way, the distance between the iliac crest and the costal margin is increased allowing an optimal ports placement and also avoiding the conflict

V. G. Radu (✉)
Life Memorial Hospital, Bucharest, Romania

between the surgeon's hand and the patient's thigh during the restoration of linea alba (Fig. 37.2).

- Supine position.
- Arms tucked to the trunk.

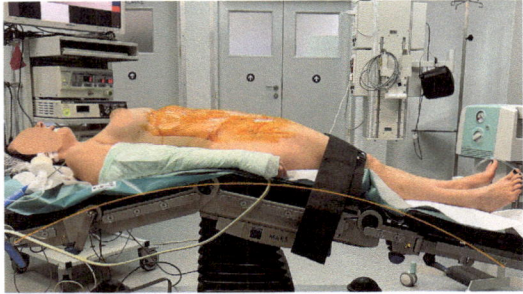

Fig. 37.2 Position of the patient

37.2 Ports Placement

The ports are placed medially to the semilunaris lines, in the opposite part of the abdomen to the hernia location (Fig. 37.3a, b) [4].

The surgical steps are as follows:

1. **Hernia Located on the Lower Part of the Abdomen**
   (a) Development of the left retro-rectus space.
   (b) Cross-over the midline anteriorly to the falciform ligament connecting both of the retro-rectus spaces.
   (c) Dissection of the retro-rectus compartment, cutting the medial aspect of the posterior rectus sheaths from cranial to

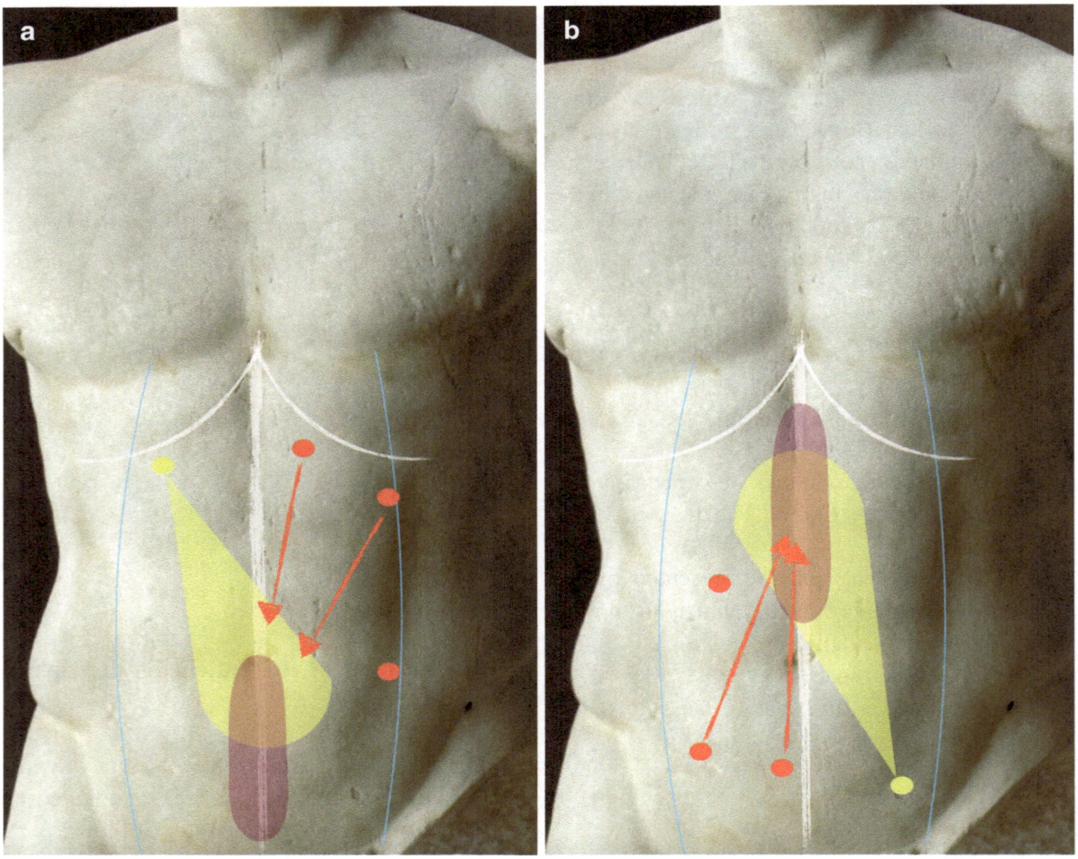

Fig. 37.3 Port placement in the opposite part of the abdomen to the hernia location: (**a**) hernia located in the lower part of the abdomen; (**b**) hernia located in the upper part of the abdomen

caudal (the medial aspects of the posterior rectus sheaths become the edges of
the defect).
(d) Reducing the hernia content.
(e) Measurement of the defect.
(f) TAR (if needed)
(g) Closure of the posterior layer.
(h) Restoration of linea alba, closing the
defect.
(i) Mesh placement.

37.2.1 Operating Theater Setting

The operating room (OR) setting in the eTEP
repair of the ventral hernias located caudal to the
umbilicus is performed as follows (Fig. 37.4):

- Operating table in the center of the theater.
- The laparoscopic tower positioned at the feet
  of the patient.
- The second monitor positioned to the right of
  the patient.

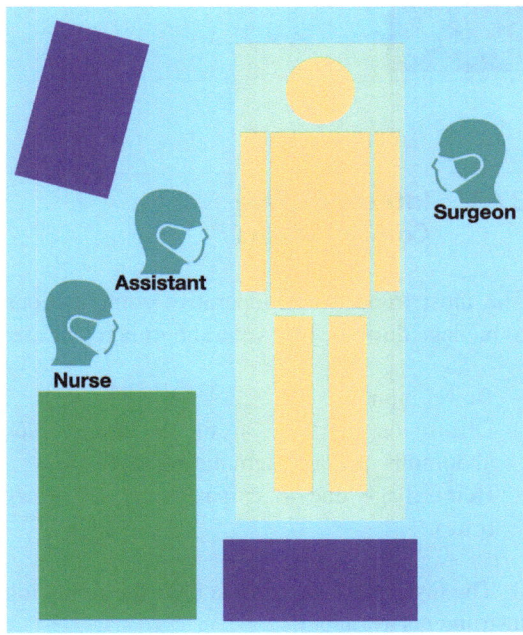

Fig. 37.4 OR setting in eTEP repair of ventral hernia
located caudal to the umbilicus

- Surgeon positioned at the left side of the
  patient.
- The assistant positioned at the right side of the
  patient.
- Instrument nurse to the right of the assistant.
- Serving cart to the right of instrument nurse.

2. **Hernia Located on the Upper Part of the
   Abdomen**
   (a) Development of the right retro-rectus
   space from cranial to caudal
   (b) Cross-over the midline anterior to the
   umbilical ligament, dissecting the Retzius
   space.
   (c) Dissection of the retro-rectus compartment from caudal to cranial, cutting the
   medial aspect of the posterior rectus
   sheaths which become the edges of the
   defect.
   (d) Reducing the hernia content.
   (e) Measurement of the defect.
   (f) TAR (if needed)
   (g) Closure of the posterior layer.
   (h) Restoration of linea alba, closing the
   defect.
   (i) Mesh placement.

37.2.2 Operating Theater Settings

The operating theater setting for the eTEP repair
of the ventral hernias located superior to the
umbilicus is performed as follows (Fig. 37.5):

- Operating table in the center of the theater.
- The laparoscopic tower positioned to left
  shoulder of the patient.
- The second monitor positioned at the feet of
  the patient.
- Surgeon positioned at the right side of the
  patient.
- The assistant positioned at the left side of the
  patient.
- Instrument nurse to the left of the assistant.
- Serving cart to the right of instrument nurse.

Fig. 37.5 OR setting in eTEP repair of ventral hernia located cranial to the umbilicus

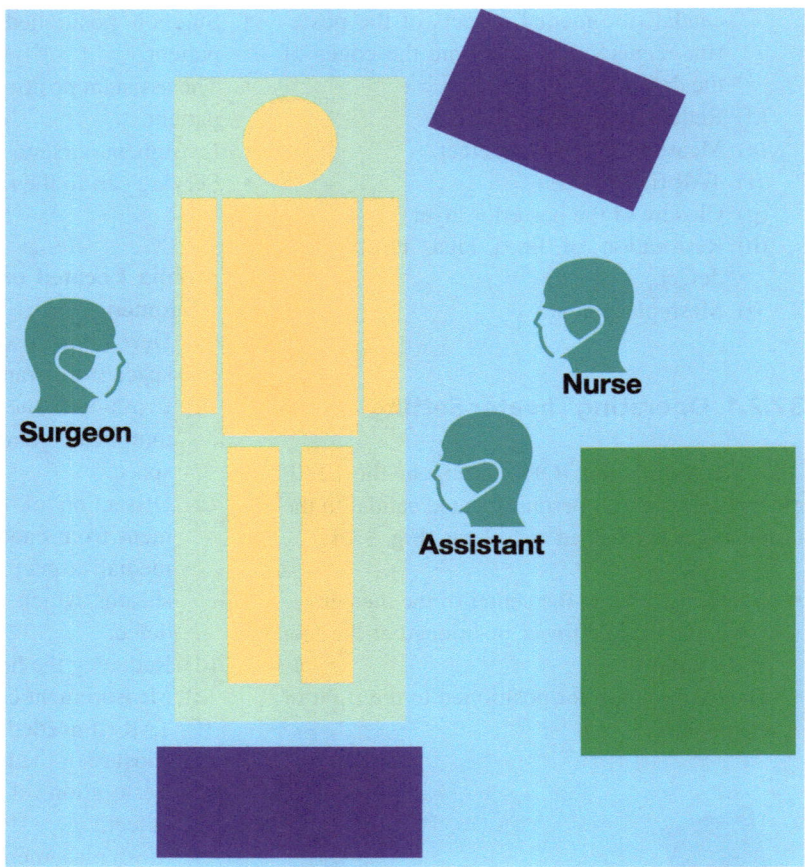

The Laparoscopic Instruments

- Optic port, or balloon trocar.
- Two 10-mm and two 5-mm trocars.
- Laparoscopic grasping forceps (Johann forceps; Park grasper).
- Hook monopolar cautery.
- Monopolar scissors Metzenbaum.
- Needle driver.
- Advanced energy 5-mm graspers (LigaSure, ultrasonic, etc.).
- Laparoscopic suction/irrigation system.
- Scope warmer or anti-fog solution.
- 10 mm 30° scope.

The Surgical Instruments

- Scalpel with stainless steel blade size of 11.
- Scissors.
- Needle driver.
- Surgical grasper 12 cm.

37.3 Intraoperative Complications

The most frequent intraoperative complications to manage during eTEP ventral hernia repair are:

- Bowel injury.
- Diffuse hemorrhage from the transversus abdominis or diaphragm during TAR.
- Hemorrhage due to epigastric vessel injury (rare).

The instrument nurse must have the following instruments available:

- Johann grasper.
- Needle driver.
- Scissors.

- Laparoscopic suction/irrigation system.
- 10 cm × 10 cm gauze to be passed to the assistant at the request of the surgeon
- Monofilament suture sutures resorbable: 4/0, 3/0, 2/0; barbed sutures resorbable: 3/0, 2/0; barbed sutures non-resorbable:0, 1.

References

1. Belyansky I, Daes J, Radu VG, Balasubramanian R, Reza Zahiri H, Weltz AS, et al. A novel approach using the enhanced-view totally extraperitoneal (eTEP) technique for laparoscopic retromuscular hernia repair. Surg Endosc [Internet]. 2017;32:1525–32. [cited 2017 Nov 30]; http://link.springer.com/10.1007/s00464-017-5840-2

2. Balasubramanian R. Signs and landmarks in eTEP Rives-Stoppa repair of ventral hernias. Hernia. 2021;25:545–50. https://doi.org/10.1007/s10029-020-02216-4.

3. Radu VG. Laparoscopic retromuscular repair of ventral hernias: eTEP and eTEP-TAR. Tech Innov Hernia Surg. 2020:1.

4. Radu VG, Lica M. The endoscopic retromuscular repair of ventral hernia: the eTEP technique and early results. Hernia. 2019;23:945.

Laparoscopic Extraperitoneal Treatment of Inguinal Hernia

38

Andrea Balla [ID] and Salvador Morales-Conde [ID]

38.1 Introduction

About 75% of all abdominal wall defect is represented by the inguinal hernia, and it is accounted that the lifetime risk to develop ranges between 3% and 27% [1–4]. Accordingly, inguinal hernia repair is one of the most commonly performed surgical procedures around the world [1, 2]. In 1887, Bassini first introduced the modern concept of surgical inguinal hernia repair, and since then, with the aim to improve postoperative outcomes, several surgical techniques and approaches have been proposed [1, 3, 5].

Several authors proposed different anatomical repairs (Shouldice, McVay) being undoubtedly the most important innovations in groin hernia repair, the tension-free hernioplasty concept using a prosthetic mesh proposed by Lichtenstein [1, 6]. This technique provided better postoperative results in comparison to the previous tension hernioplasty described in terms of pain, discomfort, and recurrence rate [1, 7]. Since the description of this technique, different anterior and posterior (Rives-Stoppa, Nyhus) open approaches have been described using a mesh [1, 6].

Although maintaining the tension-free hernioplasty concept, the introduction of the minimally invasive approach for inguinal hernia repair was another important innovation [8]. Minimally invasive inguinal hernia repair can be performed using two techniques: transabdominal preperitoneal (TAPP) and totally extraperitoneal (TEP) repair, both placing the mesh in the same surgical plane but through different approaches [9, 10]. Currently, these two techniques are equivalent in terms of postoperative outcomes such as pain, complications, hospital stay, return to daily activities, and recurrence rate [9, 10].

The aim of this chapter is to report the surgical instruments required and describe the surgical technique to perform the laparoscopic TAPP repair of inguinal hernia.

A. Balla (✉)
Unit of Innovation in Minimally Invasive Surgery, Department of General and Digestive Surgery, University Hospital "Virgen del Rocio," University of Sevilla, Sevilla, Spain

UOC of General and Minimally Invasive Surgery, Hospital "San Paolo", Civitavecchia, Rome, Italy

S. Morales-Conde
Unit of Innovation in Minimally Invasive Surgery, Department of General and Digestive Surgery, University Hospital "Virgen del Rocio," University of Sevilla, Sevilla, Spain

Unit of General and Digestive Surgery, Hospital Quironsalud Sagrado Corazón, Sevilla, Spain

38.2 Operating Theater Setting

The operating theater setting for laparoscopic TAPP repair is performed as follows (Fig. 38.1):

Fig. 38.1 Schematic operating theater setting in case of right inguinal hernia

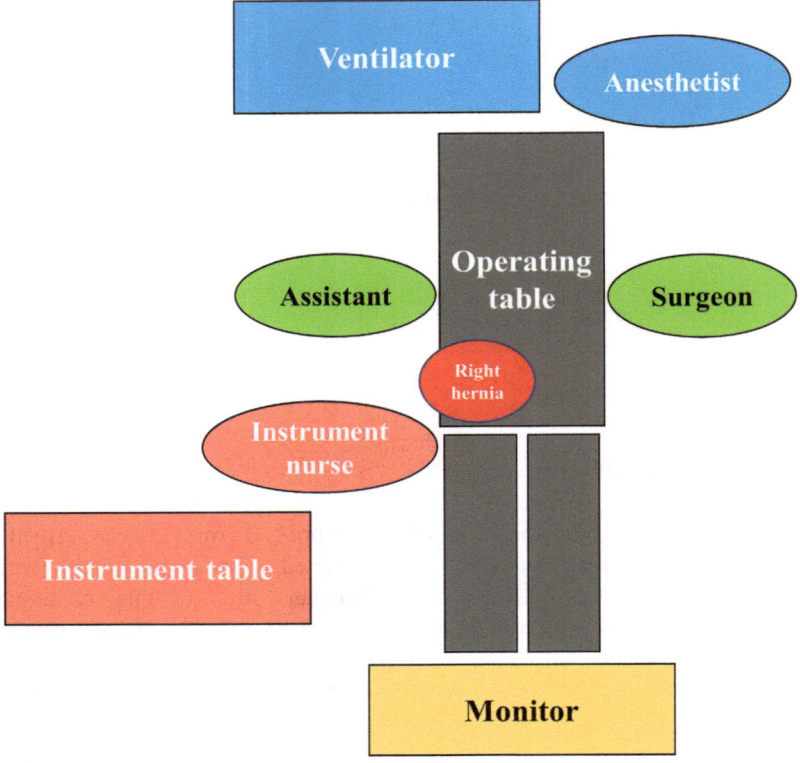

- The operating table is in the center of the theater.
- Surgeon is standing at patient's opposite side of the hernia to be repaired (although the access to the abdominal cavity is performed always from the left side of the patient).
- Assistant is standing on the other side of the patient, opposite the surgeon.
- Instrument nurse is to the patient's right side.
- Monitor is to the patient's feet.
- When performing the repair of bilateral hernias, the surgeon and the assistant will move from one side of the patient to the other, starting the repair of the right hernia, which means that the surgeon will start at patient's left side. The scrub nurse will stay in the same place independently of the side being repaired.

38.3 Patient Positioning

The patient is supine with adducted legs and both arms close to the body. Once the pneumoperitoneum is performed, the operative table is placed in the Trendelenburg position with an inclination of about 20°–30° and slightly to the side opposite of the hernia being repaired.

38.4 Surgical Instruments Required

Preparation of the Instrument Table

- Laparoscopic unit.
- 10 or 5 mm 30° optic.

- Conventional laparoscopic cable for monopolar cautery.
- One scalpel with stainless steel blade (size 11).
- Veress needle.
- Syringe for saline drop test.
- One 10-mm trocar.
- Two 5-mm trocars.
- Two laparoscopic grasping forceps.
- One laparoscopic scissor.
- One laparoscopic dissector.
- One laparoscopic needle holder.
- Small/large pore polypropylene mesh (3D Max, BD Bard, New Jersey, USA), depending on the case and the patient.
- Fixation device—options:
    - Fibrin sealant: Tissucol® (Baxter Healthcare, Deerfield, Illinois, USA).
    - Glues: cyanoacrylates.
    - Absorbable tackers (Medtronic, Minneapolis, Minnesota, USA).
- 3–0 absorbable barbed suture (V-Loc™, Medtronic, Minneapolis, Minnesota, USA) of 15 cm in length.
- Endoloop (Surgitie™, Medtronic, Minneapolis, Minnesota, USA).
- One open needle holder.
- One open tissue forceps.
- 0 absorbable multifilament suture (Polyglactin 910, Vicryl Rapide, Ethicon Endo Surgery, Cincinnati, Ohio, USA).
- One Mayo scissor.
- One skin stapler.

38.5   Surgical Steps and Related Instruments

1. **Pneumoperitoneum Creation and Trocars Placement**
    (a) Scalpel (blade 11).
    (b) Veress needle.
    (c) Syringe for saline drop test.
    (d) One 10-mm trocar.
    (e) Two 5-mm trocars.

The pneumoperitoneum is established with a Veress needle in the left hypochondrium

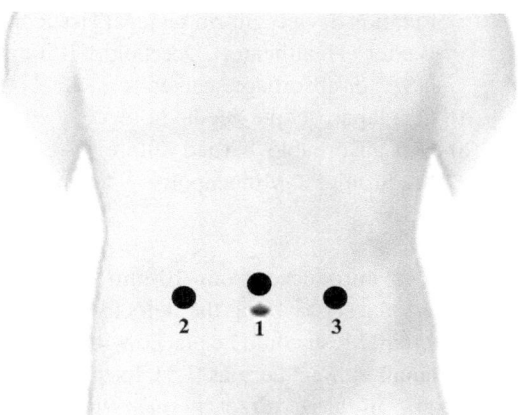

Fig. 38.2 Trocars placement to perform laparoscopic transabdominal preperitoneal (TAPP) inguinal hernia repair. (1) 10-mm trocar optic. (2 and 3) 5-mm operative trocars

(Palmer's point) and set at 14 mmHg. One 10-mm trocar is placed at the umbilicus for the 30° optic, and two 5-mm trocars are placed along the umbilical line at the right and left midclavicular lines (Fig. 38.2).

2. **Hernia Content Reduction and Peritoneum Opening**
    (a) Two laparoscopic grasping forceps.
    (b) One laparoscopic scissor with monopolar cautery.

After the exposition of the inguinal abdominal wall defect, if the hernia is incarcerated, the hernia content is reduced, combining gentle traction, and pushing from outside. Later, the peritoneum is opened, and the hernia sac is reduced. The cord is explored to detect a lipoma.

In case of direct hernia (M1–3), the fascia transversalis is plicated using an Endoloop (Surgitie™, Medtronic, Minneapolis, Minnesota, USA).

3. **Mesh Placement, Fixation, and Peritoneum Closure**
    (a) Two laparoscopic grasping forceps.
    (b) Small/large pore polypropylene mesh (3D Max, BD Bard, New Jersey, USA).

(c) Fixation devices: fibrin sealant (Tissucol®, Baxter Healthcare, Deerfield, Illinois, USA) or absorbable tackers.

(d) One laparoscopic needle holder.

(e) 3–0 absorbable barbed suture (V-Loc™, Medtronic, Minneapolis, Minnesota, USA).

Mesh is introduced from 10-mm umbilical trocar and placed covering the defect with sufficient overlap. Mesh could be placed without fixation, in small indirect hernias (L1), fixed by fibrin sealant, or in large direct hernias (M3) with absorbable tackers. The peritoneum is closed using a 3–0 absorbable barbed suture.

4. **Fascia and Skin Closure**

(a) One open needle holder.

(b) One open tissue forceps.

(c) 0 absorbable multifilament suture (Polyglactin 910, Vicryl rapid, Ethicon Endo Surgery, Cincinnati, Ohio, USA).

(d) One Mayo scissor.

(e) One skin stapler.

The fascia at umbilical incision site is closed by 0 absorbable multifilament suture. The three trocar skin sites are closed by a skin stapler.

References

1. Alarcón I, Balla A, Soler Frías JR, Barranco A, Bellido Luque J, Morales-Conde. Polytetrafluoroethylene versus polypropylene mesh during laparoscopic totally extraperitoneal (TEP) repair of inguinal hernia: short- and long-term results of a double-blind clinical randomized controlled trial. Hernia. 2020;24(5):1011–8. https://doi.org/10.1007/s10029-020-02200-y.

2. Jenkins JT, O'Dwyer PJ. Inguinal hernias. BMJ. 2008;336(7638):269–72. https://doi.org/10.1136/bmj.39450.428275.AD.

3. Lau WY. History of treatment of groin hernia. World J Surg. 2002;26(6):748–59.

4. Sartori A, Balla A, Botteri E, Scolari F, Podda M, Lepiane P, Guerrieri M, Morales-Conde S, Szold A, Ortenzi M. Laparoscopic approach in emergency for the treatment of acute incarcerated groin hernia: a systematic review and meta-analysis. Hernia. 2022;27:485. https://doi.org/10.1007/s10029-022-02631-9.

5. Zimmerman LM, Heller RE. Edoardo Bassini: his role in the development of hernial surgery. Surg Gynecol Obstet. 1937;64:971–3.

6. Lichtenstein IL, Shulman AG, Amid PK, Montllor MM. The tension-free hernioplasty. Am J Surg. 1989;157(2):188–93.

7. Scott NW, McCormack K, Graham P, Go PM, Ross SJ, Grant AM. Open mesh versus non-mesh for repair of femoral and inguinal hernia. Cochrane Database Syst Rev. (4):CD002197. 2002:CD002197.

8. Memon MA, Cooper NJ, Memon B, Memon MI, Abrams KR. Meta-analysis of randomized clinical trials comparing open and laparoscopic inguinal hernia repair. Br J Surg. 2003;90(12):1479–92.

9. Kler A, Sekhon N, Antoniou GA, Satyadas T. Totally extra-peritoneal repair versus trans-abdominal preperitoneal repair for the laparoscopic surgical management of sportsman's hernia: a systematic review and meta-analysis. Surg Endosc. 2021;35(10):5399–413. https://doi.org/10.1007/s00464-021-08554-3.

10. Aiolfi A, Cavalli M, Ferraro SD, Manfredini L, Bonitta G, Bruni PG, Bona D, Campanelli G. Treatment of inguinal hernia: systematic review and updated network meta-analysis of randomized controlled trials. Ann Surg. 2021;274(6):954–61. https://doi.org/10.1097/SLA.0000000000004735.

Robotic Transabdominal Preperitoneal Inguinal Hernia Repair (rTAPP)

Giampaolo Formisano, Adelona Salaj, Giulia Di Raimondo, and Paolo Pietro Bianchi

39.1 Introduction

Inguinal hernia repair is one of the most commonly performed general surgery procedures and accounts for almost 75% of all abdominal hernia procedures, with over 800,000 repairs in the USA per year [1]. Men are 10 times more likely to develop an inguinal hernia, with a lifetime incidence of 27% compared to 3% for women [2]. On the other hand, femoral hernias are detected twice as often in women. Definitive repair can be performed with different approaches, including conventional open anterior repair or transabdominal preperitoneal (TAPP)/ totally extraperitoneal (TEP) minimally invasive approaches. Recently, robotic abdominal wall reconstruction has gained popularity. Increasing trends in the number of inguinal hernia repairs being performed robotically have been noticed in the past year since it represents the ideal procedure for the training that is required before tackling most complex cases of ventral and incisional hernia.

Regardless of the approach, minimally invasive inguinal hernia repair should respect predefined principles to achieve complete exposure of the myopectineal orifice [3].

In this chapter, we will highlight patient position, operating room setup, instruments, docking, and the main surgical steps required for robotic TAPP (rTAPP) with the da Vinci Xi surgical system (Intuitive Surgical, Sunnyvale, CA, USA).

39.2 Indications

Indications to surgery is mostly based on symptoms, especially for male patients. Anyway, a long-term follow-up study revealed that crossover to surgery occurred in the majority of patients at 10-year follow-up; therefore, surgery should be considered in an elective fashion for surgically fit candidates [4, 5]. Indications to minimally invasive approach (both laparoscopic and robotic) are bilateral hernias, female patients and femoral hernias, and recurrent hernias after prior open anterior approach. Obese patients may benefit from TAPP repair. Unilateral hernias can be treated with TAPP according to patients' preference and surgeon's experience and background, especially in case of clinical suspicion of contralateral occult inguinal hernia.

39.3 Patient Position and OR Setup

The patient is placed supine on the operating table, with arms along the side and legs closed. All pressure points should be appropriately padded.

G. Formisano (✉) · A. Salaj · G. Di Raimondo
P. P. Bianchi
Department of General Surgery, ASST Santi Paolo e
Carlo, Dipartimento di Scienze della Salute,
University of Milan, Milan, Italy
e-mail: giampaolo.formisano@unimi.it

© The Author(s), under exclusive license to Springer Nature Switzerland AG 2024
M. Milone et al. (eds.), *Scrub Nurse in Minimally Invasive and Robotic General Surgery*,
https://doi.org/10.1007/978-3-031-42257-7_39

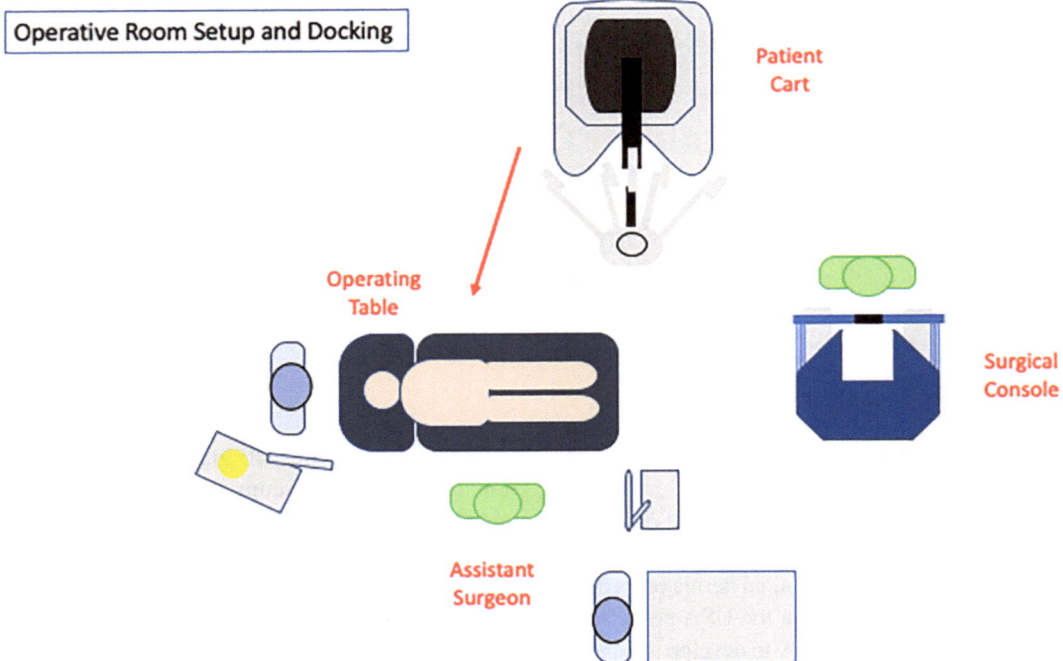

Operative Room Setup and Docking

Patient Cart

Operating Table

Surgical Console

Assistant Surgeon

Fig. 39.1 OR setup for robotic inguinal hernia repair

Surgeons and OR staff should consider a foam face pad as additional protection to the face from the elbows of robotic arms. Nasogastric tube (for pneumoperitoneum induction with a Veress needle) and urinary catheter are placed (they will be removed at the end of the procedure). A preoperative antibiotic was given less than 1 h before the beginning of the procedure. After pneumoperitoneum induction and trocar placement, the robot is docked from the left or right side of patient's table (da Vinci Xi system, with rotating boom, allows for extreme flexibility for OR setup for this specific procedure, that could be tailored according to specific OR features and available spaces). OR setup is independent from hernia's sidedness (Fig. 39.1).

39.4 Instruments and Docking

The following set of instruments is required to perform rTAPP:

- **Trocars:** Three 8-mm robotic trocars. We usually perform optical entry with a standard 12-mm AirSeal trocar (CONMED, USA) after

induction of the pneumoperitoneum with the Veress needle at Palmer's point (left subcostal area). Trocar-in-trocar technique is used for one 8-mm robotic trocar. Depending on surgeon's preference, optiview trocars with 0-degree laparoscopic camera or Hasson port can be required. 10- to 12-mm port should be considered if needed for larger/heavier weight mesh insertion.

- **Instruments**
  - Laparoscopic grasper
  - Laparoscopic needle driver
  - Laparoscopic scissors
  - Robotic 8-mm 30-degree camera
  - Robotic fenestrated bipolar forceps or force bipolar or Maryland bipolar forceps (all robotic instruments listed are from Intuitive Surgical, Sunnyvale, CA, USA), according to console surgeon's preference
  - Robotic monopolar curved scissors
  - Robotic needle driver or suture-cut needle driver
- **Sutures**
  - 3-0 absorbable sutures (12–15 cm length) for mesh fixation

- 3-0 barbed absorbable self-locking sutures (15 cm length) for peritoneal flap closure (materials, type, and length may vary according to operating surgeon's preference)
- Cyanoacrylate glue for mesh fixation
- 3-0/4-0 absorbable monofilament for trocar site closure
- If fascial closure is needed (10-mm trocar site)—0/2-0 absorbable braided suture
- **Mesh**
  - At least 10 × 15 cm flat sheet permanent mesh, according to the critical view of myopectineal orifice. 12 × 17 cm mesh can be used according to defect width and patient's anatomy. 3D meshes are also available in the market, according to surgeon's preference

39.5 Surgical Technique

The following key steps are performed:

1. Pneumoperitoneum induction with Veress-assisted or open technique and trocar placement.
2. Initial diagnostic evaluation (suture and mesh can be inserted during this initial phase according to surgeon's preference).
3. Robotic docking.
4. Peritoneal flap creation and sac/lipoma reduction.
5. Complete myopectineal orifice exposure (as per currently available guidelines).
6. Mesh placement and fixation.
7. Closure of the peritoneal flap.
8. Undocking of the patient cart.
9. Fascial (for 10-mm or larger trocar sites) and skin closure.
10. Removal of nasogastric tube and urinary catheter.

Pneumoperitoneum (PNP) is created using a Veress needle placed at Palmer's point (left subcostal area) using maximal pressure of 15 mmHg (then reduced at 6–8 mmHg). A 12-mm optical port is introduced in the right flank along the transverse umbilical line. Afterwards, two 8-mm robotic trocars are introduced under direct visualization at the level of the umbilical-supraumbilical area and in the left flank, along the transverse umbilical line, at 6–8 cm distance from each other, depending on patients' body habitus (Fig. 39.2). Before the trocar insertion, each port site was infiltrated with 10 mL bupivacaine. The patients are placed in a slight Trendelenburg position (5–10°), and the robotic cart is docked. Mesh and suture can be inserted prior to docking as a matter of time efficiency. Three robotic arms are used with the trocar-in-trocar technique in the 12-mm trocar. Alternatively, three 8-mm robotic ports can be used, with dedicated insufflation device for robotic surgery (AirSeal, CONMED, USA) if available. The 30°-up robotic camera is used. The two working arms are monopolar scissors and bipolar forceps. Large needle drivers or suture-cut needle drivers are used during reconstruction.

Peritoneal adhesions are divided, if present and needed, with particular attention to avoid bowel injury and damage to the peritoneum or fascia. Inguinal hernia repair is performed with creation of the peritoneal flap according to the standard transabdominal preperitoneal (TAPP) approach. Incision of the peritoneal flap is performed from the anterior superior iliac spine (ASIS) to the medial umbilical ligament. Medial umbilical ligament can be divided if necessary to gain more space for adequate dissection at the level of the pubic tubercle/Cooper's ligament. Inferior epigastric vessels should be identified during this initial step and preserved. Gentle traction allows for pneumoperitoneum to aid in the dissection along the relatively avascular plane and areolar tissue with minimal energy application. Dissection of the medial and lateral aspects of the myopectineal orifice should be performed before reduction of hernia sac and lipoma to identify proper anatomical landmarks. Early identification of the pubic tubercle and Cooper's ligament is helpful as constant landmarks to facilitate further dissection and clear complete exposure of the myopectineal orifice. Afterwards, the hernia sac and lipoma (if present) are identified, completely dissected, and

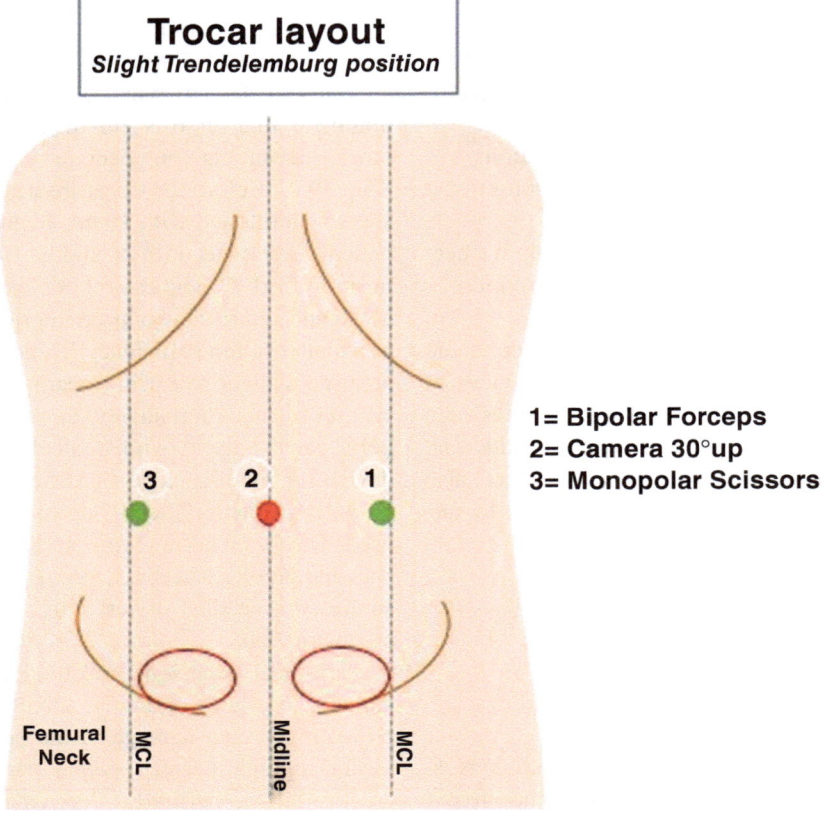

Fig. 39.2 Trocar layout for robotic inguinal hernia repair

reduced into the abdominal cavity. Vas deferens and gonadal vessels (round ligament in female patients) must be identified and preserved. Complete exposure of the femoral ring, just below and medial to the iliac vessels, must be obtained. Appropriate identification of the anatomical plane for dissection is of paramount importance to avoid nerve damage in the lateral area (triangle of pain) and major vascular injury (triangle of doom). Moreover, a correct plane of dissection in the medial aspect avoids undue bleeding and bladder injury.

In case of bilateral hernias, peritoneal flap and hernia reduction should be completed prior to proceeding. Two separate peritoneal incisions or one large flap can be performed for bilateral hernias, according to operating surgeon's preference. If creating two separate flaps, it must be ensured that the two separate dissection planes completely communicate in the preperitoneal

area at the level of the pubic tubercle to allow for medial mesh overlap.

Dissection of the myopectineal orifice is carried out according to the following steps [3]:

1. Identify and dissect the pubic tubercle across the midline.
2. Rule out a direct hernia and dissect the Hasselbach triangle.
3. Dissect at least 2 cm between Cooper's ligament and the bladder to avoid mesh displacement caused by bladder distension.
4. Rule out a femoral hernia.
5. Parietalyze the cord elements.
6. Identify and reduce cord lipomas.
7. Dissect peritoneum lateral to cord elements.
8. Perform the dissection, provide mesh coverage, and ensure that mesh and mechanical fixation are placed well above an imaginary inter-ASIS line.

9. Place the mesh (at least 10 × 15 cm, larger meshes may be required) only if the previous steps are completed, without any creases or folds.

Adequate dissection of the myopectineal orifice is of paramount importance. Appropriate surgical technique ensures that all present hernias or potential hernia sites are addressed and can be covered by a flat sheet mesh, thus potentially reducing the risk of recurrence (Figs. 39.3 and 39.4).

After dissection is completed, mesh placement is performed (Fig. 39.5). Macroporous permanent (light- or midweight) mesh are used. Several meshes are available for clinical use.

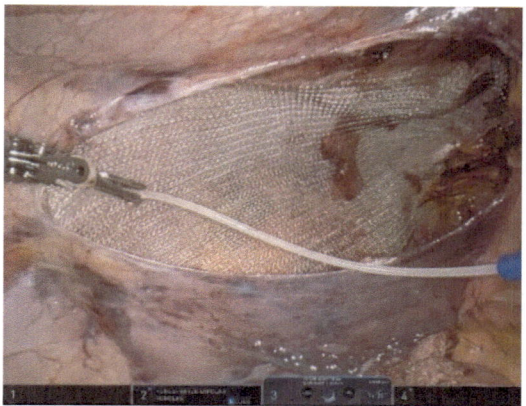

Fig. 39.5 Mesh placement (at least 10 × 15 cm), fixated with cyanoacrylate glue

Additional features such as 3D shape and self-gripping properties are used according to operating surgeon's preference. Of course, the mesh should be at least 10x15cm in diameter to allow for proper myopectineal orifice coverage in an adequately dissected space. Most of the available meshed can be introduced through a 8-mm robotic port in a folded configuration.

As far as fixation methods are concerned, data from the available literature show equivalent recurrence rates with different techniques of fixation (tacks, sutures, glue, or no fixation), even if lower rates of chronic pain may be associated with no fixation [6]. In our experience, we prefer glue fixation to avoid early mesh displacement or parachuting through larger defects. We avoid the use of tackers, especially if permanent. Suture fixation is usually performed in case of large direct defects, thanks to the capabilities of the robotic platform, at the level of Cooper's ligament or rectus muscle.

After mesh placement is completed, closure of the peritoneal flap is carried out with a 3-0 slowly reabsorbable running barbed suture. Any tears in the peritoneal flap must be repaired (Fig. 39.6).

Robotic cart is undocked, and trocars are removed under direct visualization to ensure for adequate hemostasis. Fascial defects of 10-mm or larger trocars are closed with absorbable sutures. The skin is closed with 3-0 or 4-0 interrupted absorbable sutures.

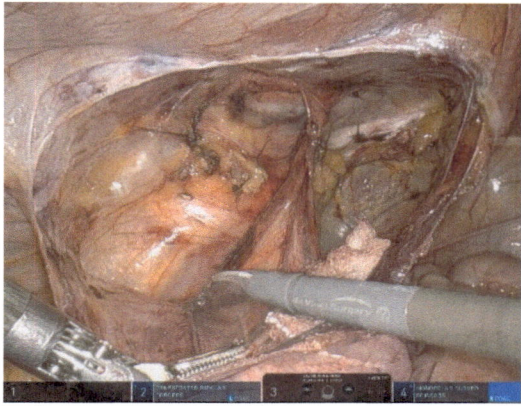

Fig. 39.3 Complete exposure of myopectineal orifice

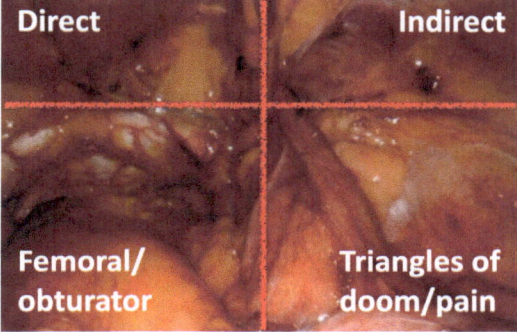

Fig. 39.4 Complete exposure of myopectineal orifice, all present hernias or potential hernia sites addressed

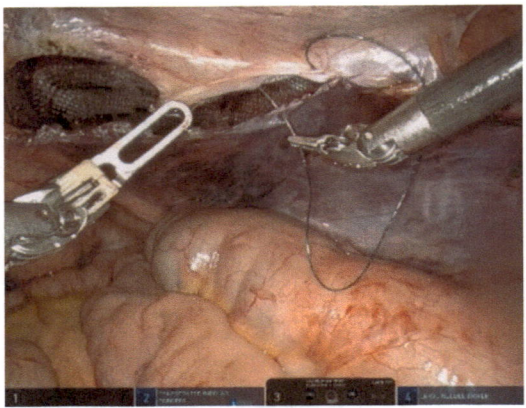

Fig. 39.6 Peritoneal closure with self-locking 3-0 barbed running suture

39.6 Discussion and Conclusions

Recently, the introduction of robotic surgical platforms has increased surgeons' enthusiasm by promising potential benefits not only for complex surgical procedures but also for robotic TAPP [7].

To date and to the best of our knowledge, few data are available in the literature regarding robotic inguinal hernia repair compared to conventional laparoscopic TAPP approach (mostly reporting single-center or single-surgeon experiences).

Ayuso et al. reported comparable outcomes of robotic vs laparoscopic inguinal hernia repair in a single-center case-matched study [8]. A recent multicenter study has shown comparable outcomes of robotic vs laparoscopic TAPP, except for a longer operative time in the robotic group [9]. However, longer operative time may still be attributable to the learning curve period of each center. Indeed, Muysoms et al. reported that rTAPP was related to a rapid reduction in operative time over the learning curve; once an adequate level of proficiency was achieved, the operative time to perform a rTAPP was comparable to laparoscopic procedures for both unilateral and bilateral inguinal hernia repairs [10].

On the other hand, Kudsi et al. demonstrated that robotic surgery may confer advantages over standard laparoscopy in terms of addressing more complex repairs by reducing conversion and recurrence rates [11]. Moreover, another potential advantage of robotic surgery has been reported in obese patients (comparable outcomes vs non-obese population) and recurrent inguinal hernias (lower postoperative pain and lower incidence of chronic groin pain) [12, 13].

In our experience, robotic inguinal hernia repair is a good procedure to start an institutional abdominal wall reconstruction program before tackling more complex ventral and incisional hernias (unpublished data), especially for specific residents' and fellows' surgical training.

To summarize, few data are available to date on robotic inguinal hernia repair. Robotic surgery may confer advantage in most complex cases (large hernias, recurrent hernias, obese patient population), even for experienced surgeons familiar with laparoscopic TAPP. Simpler cases may be the ideal procedure for the training pathway of residents and fellows in robotic surgery. Further large-scale prospective studies are needed to validate these findings and better understand whether the robotic platform offers substantial clinical benefit compared with conventional laparoscopy.

References

1. Rutkow IM. Demographic and socioeconomic aspects of hernia repair in the US in 2003. Surg Clin North Am. 2003;83:1045.
2. Haladu N'u, Alabi A, Brazzelli M, Imamura M, Ahmed I, Ramsay G, Scott NW. Open versus laparoscopic repair of inguinal hernia: an overview of systematic reviews of randomised controlled trials. Surg Endosc. 2022;36(7):4685–700.
3. Daes J, Felix E. Critical view of the Myopectineal orifice. Ann Surg. 2017;266(1):e1–2. https://doi.org/10.1097/SLA.0000000000002104.
4. Fitzgibbons R, Forse RA. Groin hernias in adults. N Engl J Med. 2015;372:756–63.
5. Fitzgibbons R, Giobbie-Hurder A, Gibbs R. Watchful waiting vs repair of inguinal hernia in minimally symptomatic men a randomized clinical trial. JAMA. 2006;3(295):285–92.
6. Andresen K, Fenger AQ, Burcharth J, Pommergaard HC, Rosenberg J. Mesh fixation methods and chronic pain after transabdominal preperitoneal (TAPP) inguinal hernia surgery a comparison between fibrin sealant and tacks. Surg Endosc. 2017;10(31):4077–84.

7. Waite KE, Herman MA, Doyle PJ. Comparison of robotic versus laparoscopic transabdominal preperitoneal (TAPP) inguinal hernia repair. J Robot Surg. 2016;10:239–44.

8. Ayuso SA, Marturano MN, Katzen MM, Aladegbami BG, Augenstein VA. Laparoscopic versus robotic inguinal hernia repair: a single-center case-matched study. Surg Endosc. 2022;37:631. https://doi.org/10.1007/s00464-022-09368-7.

9. Peltrini R, Corcione F, Pacella D, Castiglioni S, Lionetti R, Andreuccetti J, Pignata G, De Nisco C, Ferraro L, Salaj A, Formisano G, Bianchi PP, Bracale U. Robotic versus laparoscopic transabdominal preperitoneal (TAPP) approaches to bilateral hernia repair: a multicenter retrospective study using propensity score matching analysis. Surg Endosc. 2022;37:1188. https://doi.org/10.1007/s00464-022-09614-y.

10. Muysoms F, Van Cleven S, Kyle-Leinhase I, Ballecer C, Ramaswamy A. Robotic-assisted laparoscopic groin hernia repair: observational case-control study on the operative time during the learning curve. Surg Endosc. 2018;32:4850–9.

11. Kudsi OY, Bou-Ayash N, Kaoukabani G, Gokcal F. Comparison of perioperative and mid-term outcomes between laparoscopic and robotic inguinal hernia repair. Surg Endosc. 2022;37:1508. https://doi.org/10.1007/s00464-022-09433-1.

12. Kudsi OY, Bou-Ayash N, Gokcal F. Comparison of perioperative outcomes between non-obese and obese patients undergoing robotic inguinal hernia repair: a propensity score matching analysis. Hernia. 2022;26(4):1033–9. https://doi.org/10.1007/s10029-021-02433-5. Epub 2021 May 31.

13. Vitiello A, Abeid AA, Peltrini R, Ferraro L, Formisano G, et al. Minimally invasive repair of recurrent inguinal hernia: multi-institutional retrospective comparison of robotic versus laparoscopic surgery. J Laparoendosc Adv Surg Tech A. 2023;33:69–73. https://doi.org/10.1089/lap.2022.0209. Online ahead of print.

Laparoscopic Ventral Hernia Repair

40

Jacopo Andreuccetti, Ilaria Canfora, and Giusto Pignata

40.1 Introduction

Laparoscopic ventral hernia repair (LVHR) was developed as a minimally invasive approach to the abdominal wall.

Intraperitoneal Onlay Mesh (IPOM) technique was first described in 1993 by LeBlanc, and its application for incisional hernia repair is now widely spread [1].

The laparoscopic approach may be applied broadly to both initial and recurrent ventral and incisional hernias. Specifically, its benefits have been shown in the obese patient population among whom open repair is associated with a higher rate of wound complications and infection.

What we must always remember is that today there is no specific surgical technique for every single pathology. The concept of tailored surgery has been stressed in recent years in all fields of surgery, but it is in the abdominal wall surgery that it finds its maximum expression. The characteristics of the patient, the conformation of the abdomen, and the clinical history will direct us towards the most appropriate technical choice. Even if there is currently no upper limit of defect size that can be approached laparoscopically, we currently recommend laparoscopic intraperitoneal onlay mesh repair for defects ≤7 cm in greatest width [1].

J. Andreuccetti (✉) · I. Canfora · G. Pignata
General Surgery 2, ASST Spedali Civili of Brescia, Brescia, Italy

40.2 Surgical Steps

1. Adhesiolysis
2. Exposition of posterior rectal sheet
3. Hernia defect assessment
4. Mesh preparation
5. Pneumoperitoneum pressure reduction
6. Mesh fixation

40.2.1 Adhesiolysis

It is estimated that adhesions occur in 70–97% of patients who present incisional hernia after laparotomy. This is the lengthiest phase of ventral hernia repair. Advantages to a safe and effective adhesiolysis are provided by a magnified view of the abdominal wall and by a suspension of the adherent intestinal loops given by the pneumoperitoneum (Fig. 40.1). Operative bed movements are also considered fundamental to this step as well as a mild external pressure on the hernia sac.

Use of electrocauterization should be limited, and hemostasis should be provided with clips rather than ultrasonic dissector use. One must be aware of the proximity of the surrounding intestine, which may be hidden from view. At the end of adhesiolysis and the reduction of the hernia content, the omentum and the affected bowel must be inspected in order to identify any intestinal injury or bleeding [2, 3].

© The Author(s), under exclusive license to Springer Nature Switzerland AG 2024
M. Milone et al. (eds.), *Scrub Nurse in Minimally Invasive and Robotic General Surgery*,
https://doi.org/10.1007/978-3-031-42257-7_40

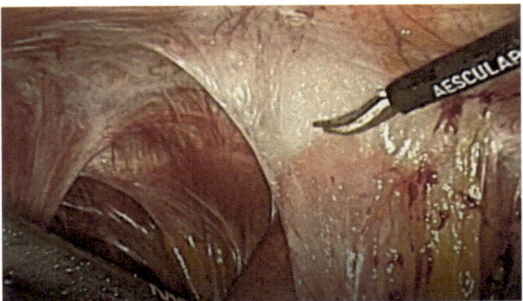

Fig. 40.1 Adhesiolysis with scissors in lateral incisional hernia defect

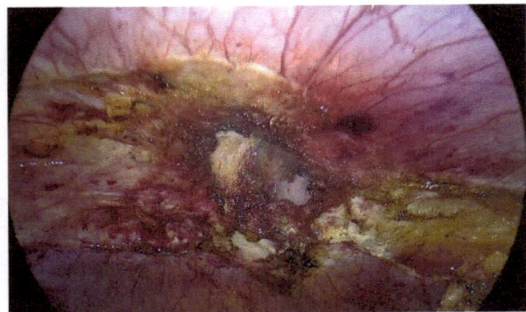

Fig. 40.3 Exposure of the posterior fascia

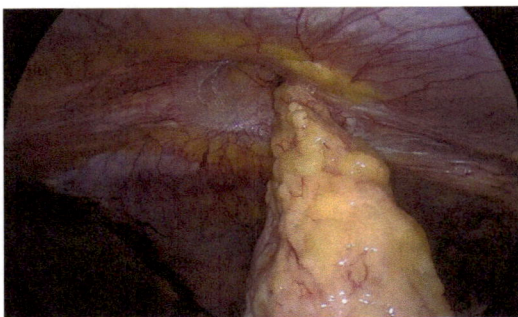

Fig. 40.2 Recurrent incisional hernia

40.2.2 Exposition of Posterior Rectal Sheet

In subxiphoid defects, the falciform ligament is divided to allow broad mesh overlap. It is fundamental to allow 5-cm mesh overlap which allows the uncoated side of the mesh to come in direct contact with the fascia in order to avoid mesh migration (Figs. 40.2 and 40.3). The falciform ligament is vascular and should be clipped or divided with energy dissection. Peritoneal fat that could hinder intraperitoneal onlay mesh (IPOM) placement should be removed.

Recurrent hernia with previous placement of intraperitoneal prosthesis can be a tough challenge. Obviously, an adequate removal of the prior mesh allows a better and safer placement of the new mesh, but often it is not possible. Sometimes mesh removal is too harmful to the abdominal wall, and it is therefore preferable to overlap the new mesh with transfascial sutures through healthy abdominal wall. If the bowel is

tenaciously adherent to prior mesh, it is preferable to cut off a part of the mesh and leave it adherent to the intestine rather than risking an accidental intestinal injury. The sac itself can be reduced or left in place.

40.2.3 Hernia Defect Assessment

Measuring the band defect is an essential step for a successful LVHR, as it allows an accurate estimate of the size of the mesh that should be placed [4].

A real advantage of laparoscopy over the open technique in the field of hernial repair is the possibility of providing direct visualization of the defect, which palpatorially is often inaccurate.

40.2.3.1 Defect Closure: IPOM vs IPOM Plus

The current practice of closure of the fascial defect during laparoscopic hernia repair, prior to mesh placement, is often dependent on the operating surgeon's routine preference.

In the IPOM plus technique, a muscle sheath is interposed between the skin incision and the mesh; this sheath plays an important role in preventing infection. In the case of IPOM, there is only subcutaneous tissue between the skin incision and the mesh [5–7].

Potential benefits of defect closure include reconstruction of a functional abdominal wall, closure of dead space that can lead to seroma formation, reduction in recurrence rate, and prevention of mesh eventration and bulging. However, more recent studies showed that there are no differences in the rate of seroma, surgical site infections, or hernia recurrence between a bridged repair (IPOM) or repair with fascial closure (IPOM plus).

40.2.4 Mesh Selection, Sizing, Introduction, and Placement

The main criterion of mesh choice is based on the concept that in the context of the IPOM the intestinal loops are in direct contact with the prosthesis.

Obviously, in order to avoid adhesions and intestinal fistulas, the presence of an adhesion barrier on its intraperitoneal side is essential; usually, this is a hydrophilic material that can be reabsorbed over time. At the same time, the parietal side should promote tissue ingrowth in order to facilitate repair of the defect and ensure a fixity of the prosthesis.

Most manufacturers of polypropylene or polyester meshes offer a product with an adhesion barrier on the visceral side. Typically, this is a hydrophilic component that resorbs over time. Alternatively, expanded polytetrafluoroethylene (ePTFE) is less adhesiogenic, and thus prosthetics composed of this do not have an additional adhesion barrier [8].

Whatever mesh is chosen, the size must provide adequate overlap of the defect. There is still a low level of evidence indicating the minimum overlap that should be for an LVHR, but nowadays most surgeons choose a 5-cm overlap of the defect, with acceptable recurrence rates.

The introduction of the mesh in the abdomen should provide:

- If adhesion barrier mesh is utilized, one must be able to recognize the coated visceral side and the peritoneal one.
- If transfascial sutures are chosen, those should be fixed to the prosthesis before its introduction into the abdomen.
- The rolled mesh must be introduced directly through a trocar to avoid any skin contact,

reducing prosthetic infections. This is why LVHR requires one 10-mm trocar [9, 10].

40.2.5 Pneumoperitoneum Pressure Reduction

Once the sutures are placed in the edges of the defect, the pneumoperitoneum pressure is lowered to 6–8 mmHg; this allows for easier closure of the defect with decreased tension.

40.2.6 Mesh Fixation

After the mesh has been placed with an adequate overlap, a method of fixation must be chosen:

- Tacks (helical or pronged, absorbable, or non-absorbable)
- Transfascial sutures
- Glue (Cyanoacrylate, fibrin glue)
- Some combination of these

The traditional technique involves placement of four transfascial sutures at equidistant points (Fig. 40.4).

Additional transfascial sutures can be placed, if necessary, to fix larger prostheses.

It is essential to fix the prosthesis on its perimeter to prevent the intestinal loops from coming into contact with the uncoated side. Tacks (Fig. 40.5) and glues can be helpful.

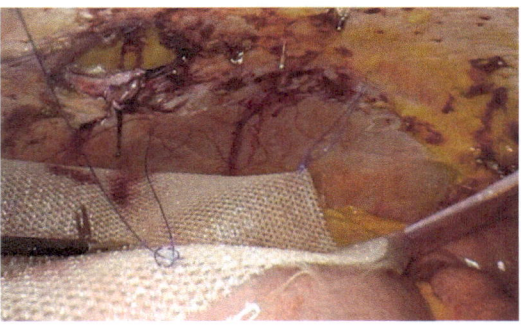

Fig. 40.4 Transfascial sutures

While suture is categorized as only absorbable or nonabsorbable, tacking options vary in design and material. Typically, tacks are helical or pronged, and available products vary in depth of penetration as well. There is no difference in literature, at least in short-term follow-up, in acute and chronic postoperative pain between the absorbable and nonabsorbable categories of tacks [11]. Tacks device can be utilized to secure the mesh around the perimeter between transfascial sutures in "single-crown" fashion or can be utilized without transfascial sutures, often in a "double-crown," with similar acute postoperative pain outcomes [12].

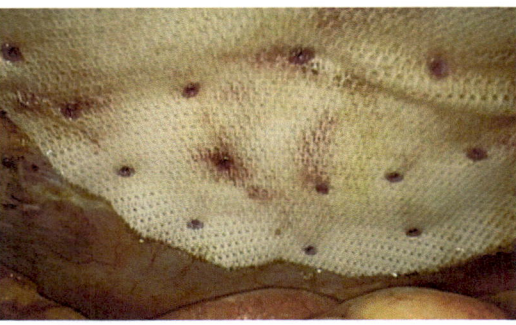

Fig. 40.5 Mesh fixation with tacks

40.3 Operating Theater Setting

The operating theater setting for an LVHR is performed as follows (Fig. 40.6):

- Operating table in the center of the theater.
- Laparoscopic column with vision cart positioned to the left of the patient.
- First operator on the right of the patient.
- First assistant at the operating table positioned on the right of the first operator.
- Instrument nurse to the right of the first assistant.
- Serving cart to the right of instrument nurse.

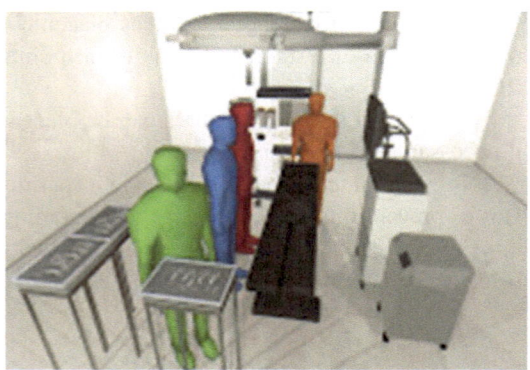
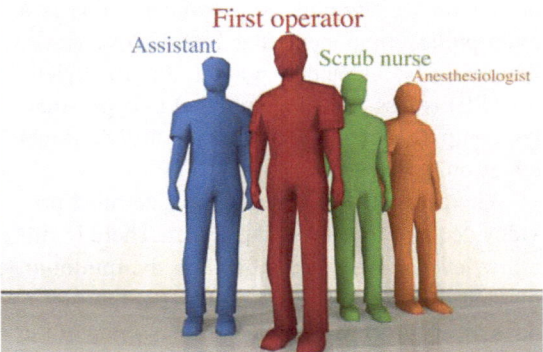

Fig. 40.6 Operating theater setting [13]

40.4   Patient Positioning

Patient positioning is performed as shown in Fig. 40.7:

The bed is placed in standard position. The patient lies supine with arms along the body. Laparoscopic rack is placed on the opposite side of trocar sites.

- Supine position.
- Legs together.
- Arms adducted along the body.
- Laparoscopic rank on the opposite side of trocar site.

Specific surgical drapes are used.

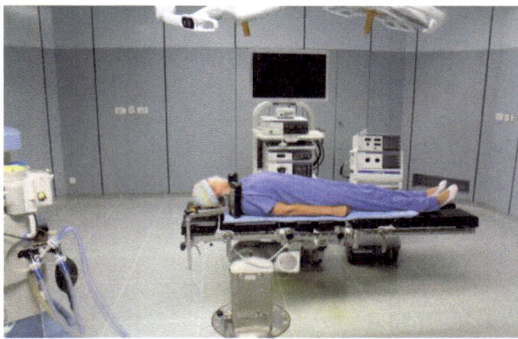

Fig. 40.7 Patient positioning [13]

40.5   Port Placement

A minimum of three trocars are placed. For the midline hernia defect, three lateral trocars along the anterior to the mid-axillary line are used including two 5-mm ports and one larger 10- to 12-mm port through which the mesh will be inserted. Additional port placement is often required for atypically located ventral hernias. Alternatively, you can place the largest trocar near the hernial defect so as to ensure the coverage of the defect with the mesh. This lateral trocar positioning allows a camera visualization and facilitates efficient adhesiolysis.

It can be useful for an additional 5-mm trocar on the contralateral side, providing a better positioning for tack fixation on the side of the initial ports. In cases of extensive adhesions, two 5-mm trocars (working port and camera port) on the contralateral side may be needed for a different vantage point to complete the adhesiolysis and hernia contents reduction.

Each of the ports should be placed under laparoscopic camera visualization in order to identify epigastric vessels and avoid bleeding [14].

40.6   Surgical Instruments Required

All the surgical instruments must be ready on the instrument table before the intervention begins (Fig. 40.8).

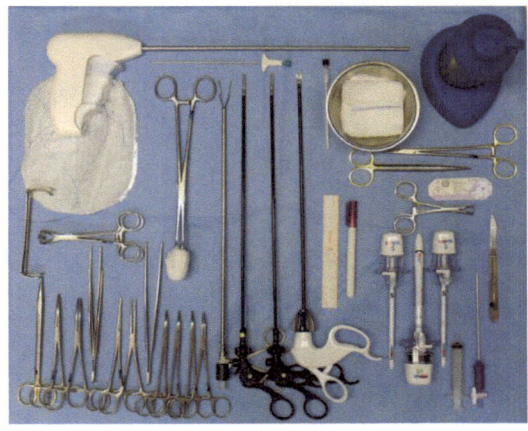

Fig. 40.8 Instrument table [13]

Instruments and Cables

- 30° and 5-mm laparoscope
- Cold light source cable
- CO_2 pipe and filter
- Monopolar electrocautery
- Patient return electrode (REM)
- Sterile instrument bag
- Monopolar and bipolar electrocautery cables

Laparoscopic Instrument Table (Fig. 40.8)

- Sutures: 2-0 not absorbable monofilament suture and skin wound closure sutures
- Surgical scalpel blade No. 23
- Gauzes
- Stainless surgical bowl
- Gross-Maier dressing forceps
- Two Bernhard towel forceps
- Veress needle and 10-mL syringe
- One 10-mm trocar
- Two 5-mm trocars
- Needle holder
- Two Backhaus forceps
- Two Farabeuf retractors
- Metzenbaum scissors
- Mayo scissors
- Two tissue forceps with teeth
- Two Kocher forceps
- Two Klemmer forceps
- Four mosquitoes forceps
- Bipolar laparoscopic forceps
- Laparoscopic scissors
- Two Johann forceps without ratchet handle
- Spinal anesthesia needles
- Demographic marker
- Sterile ruler
- Mesh fixation device
- Suture pass—Endo Close—Reverdin needle
- Thermos
- Intraperitoneal mesh

40.7   Surgical Steps and Related Instruments

Hasson Technique for Laparoscopic Access

- 1 scalpel (blade 11).
- 2 anatomical tissue forceps.
- 2 Mathieu retractors.

- 1 Nelson-Metzenbaum dissection scissors.
- 2 curved Kocher clamps to grasp fascia.
- 2 curved Klemmer clamps to grasp the parietal peritoneum.

Veress Technique for Laparoscopic Access

- Scalpel (blade 11).
- Veress needle.
- Syringe for saline drop test.

There is no substantial advantage of either closed Veress or Hasson open-access technique.

Vascular and intestinal injuries can occur with either method. First site of peritoneal access should be made in an area away from previous incisions. For the Veress technique, Palmer's point below the left costal margin is the safest area of placement.

40.7.1 Adhesiolysis

Indispensable tools are:

- 30°- and 5-mm laparoscope
- Monopolar electrocautery
- Bipolar laparoscopic forceps
- Laparoscopic scissors
- 1 Johann forceps without ratchet handle
- Laparoscopic gauzes

40.7.2 Exposition of Posterior Rectal Sheet

- 30°- and 5-mm laparoscope
- Monopolar electrocautery
- Bipolar laparoscopic forceps
- Laparoscopic scissors
- Two Johann forceps without ratchet handle

40.7.3 Hernia Defect Assessment

The required instruments for an accurate measurement of the defect are as follows:

- Spinal anesthesia needles

- Demographic marker
- Sterile ruler

Spinal needles can be used to mark the edges of the defect and to assist an accurate measurement, as well as a suture is inserted and held across the distance between the two spinal needles.

40.7.3.1 Defect Closure: IPOM Vs IPOM Plus

To perform an efficient defect closure, the laparoscopic instruments used are as follows:

- 30°- and 5-mm laparoscope
- 1 laparoscopic needle holder
- 1 Johann forceps without ratchet handle
- Laparoscopic scissors
- Barbed suture/monofilament

The choice of suture for plication of diastasis recti and defect closure may vary, but most authors choose slowly absorbable barbed suture (#0 V-Loc™ 180 Wound Closure Device, Medtronic Inc., Minneapolis, MN on a GS-21 needle measuring 30–45 cm).

Tips to facilitate adequate fascial approximation include decreasing the pneumoperitoneum to 8–10 mmHg, ensuring adequate visualization of the anterior rectus sheath with each stitch.

40.7.4 Mesh Selection, Sizing, Introduction, and Placement

- Intraperitoneal mesh
- Mayo scissors, necessary to shape the prosthesis according to the measurement
- 30°- and 5-mm laparoscope
- 2 Johann forceps without ratchet handle

40.7.5 Pneumoperitoneum Pressure Reduction

Operative room nurse in this phase should be ready to reduce pneumoperitoneum pressure to 6–8 mmHg when required by the surgeon.

40.7.6 Mesh Fixation

During mesh fixation should be on instrumental nurse cart:

- 30° laparoscopic endoscope
- Suture pass—Endo Close—Reverdin needle
- 1 laparoscopic needle holder
- 1 Johann forceps without ratchet handle
- Mesh fixation device (tacks, cyanoacrylate or fibrin glue, and monofilament suture) to perform mesh fixation, based on the surgeon's requests
- Laparoscopic scissors
- Intraperitoneal mesh

40.8 Intraoperative Complications

The most frequent intraoperative complications to manage during LVHR are basically two: hemorrhage and bowel injury.

40.8.1 Bowel Injuries

Bowel injuries can occur as thermal injury or traction injury, especially during adhesiolysis and hernia reduction. A meticulous adhesiolysis and close inspection for injury during laparoscopic are compulsory. Intestinal lesions should be immediately repaired either laparoscopically or laparotomically depending on the comfort of the surgeon.

Obviously, a bowel injury determines contamination of the operating field, compromising the ability to keep a prosthesis in place permanently.

40.8.2 Hemorrhage

Hemorrhage can occur basically in two technical steps of LVHR:

– Trocar positioning
– Fixation of the prosthesis

With any method of fixation, care should be taken to avoid injury to the epigastric vessels.

For the same reason, trocar positioning should be managed under laparoscopic vision.

An intraoperative bleeding can be managed with different surgical energy devices:

– Monopolar electrocautery
– Bipolar laparoscopic forceps

In these circumstances, the instrument nurse must have the following instruments available:

- Laparoscopic suction/irrigation system.
- 10 cm × 10 cm gauze.
- Endoscopic clip applier with titanium clips.
- Needle holder and monofilament suture with small gauge needle to attempt to repair the bleeding vessels.

References

1. LeBlanc KA, Booth WV. Laparoscopic repair of incisional hernias using expanded polytetrafluoroethylene: preliminary findings. Surg Laparosc Endosc. 1993;3:39–41.
2. Liakakos T, Thomakos N, Fine PM, Dervenis C, Young RL. Peritoneal adhesions: etiology, pathophysiology, and clinical significance. Recent advances in prevention and management. Dig Surg. 2001;18:260–73.
3. Sallinen V, Di Saverio S, Haukijärvi E, Juusela R, Wikström H, Koivukangas V, Catena F, Enholm B, Birindelli A, Leppäniemi A, Mentula P. Laparoscopic versus open adhesiolysis for adhesive small bowel obstruction (LASSO): an international, multicentre, randomised, open-label trial. Lancet Gastroenterol Hepatol. 2019;4(4):278–86. https://doi.org/10.1016/S2468-1253(19)30016-0. Epub 2019 Feb 12.
4. Birch DW. Characterizing laparoscopic incisional hernia repair. Can J Surg. 2007;50(3):195–201.
5. Suwa K, Okamoto T, Yanaga K. Closure versus nonclosure of fascial defects in laparoscopic ventral and incisional hernia repairs: a review of the literature. Surg Today. 2016;46:764–73.
6. Wennergen JE, Askenasy EP, Greenberg JA, et al. Laparoscopic ventral hernia repair with primary fascial closure versus bridged repair: a risk adjusted comparative study. Surg Endosc. 2016;30:3231–18.
7. Papageorge CM, Funk LM, Poulose BK, Philips S, Rosen MJ, Greenberg JA. Primary fascial closure during laparoscopic ventral hernia repair does not reduce 30-day wound complications. Surg Endosc. 2017;31(11):4551–7.
8. Bellón JM, Contreras LA, Buján J, Pascual G, Carrera-San MA. Effect of relaparotomy through previously integrated polypropylene and polytetrafluoroethylene experimental implants in the abdominal wall. J Am Coll Surg. 1999;188(5):466–72.
9. Bittner R, Bingener-Casey J, Dietz U, Fabian M, Ferzli G, Fortelny R, et al. Guidelines for laparoscopic treatment of ventral and incisional abdominal wall hernias (international Endohernia society (IEHS))—part 1. Surg Endosc. 2014;28(1):2–29.
10. Novitsky YW, Cobb WS, Kercher KW, Matthews BD, Sing RF, Heniford BT. Laparoscopic ventral hernia repair in obese patients: a new standard of care. Arch Surg. 2006;141(1):57–61.
11. Bansal V, Asuri K, Panaiyadiyan S, Kumar S, Subramaniam R, Ramachandran R, et al. Comparison of absorbable versus nonabsorbable tackers in terms of long-term outcomes, chronic pain, and quality of life after laparoscopic incisional hernia repair: a randomized study. Surg Laparosc Endosc Percutan Tech. 2016;26(6):476–83.
12. Wassenaar E, Schoenmaeckers E, Raymakers J, van der Palen J, Rakic S. Mesh-fixation method and pain and quality of life after laparoscopic ventral or incisional hernia repair: a randomized trial of three fixation techniques. Surg Endosc. 2010;24(6):1296–302.
13. Pignata G, Bracale U, Lazzara F. Laparoscopic surgery: key points, operating room setup and equipment. Springer International Publishing Switzerland; 2016.
14. Scott Davis S Jr, Dakin G, Bates A. The SAGES manual of hernia surgery. Springer International Publishing Switzerland; 2019.